Energy for Everything

Other titles in the
Women's Edge Health Enhancement Guide
series:

Busy Woman's Cookbook

Fight Fat

Food Smart

Foolproof Weight Loss

Get Well, Stay Well

Growing Younger

Herbs That Heal

Natural Remedies

The Inner Journey

Total Body Toning

Women's Edge
HEALTH ENHANCEMENT GUIDE™

Energy for Everything

Rejuvenation for the Mind, Body, and Soul

by Julia VanTine, Marie Elaina Suszynski, and the Editors of

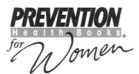

RODALE

© 2001 Rodale Inc.

All rights reserved. No part of this publication may be reproduced or transmitted in any form or by any means, electronic or mechanical, including photocopying, recording, or any other information storage and retrieval system, without the written permission of the publisher.

Prevention Health Books for Women and Women's Edge Health Enhancement Guide are trademarks of Rodale Inc.

Printed in the United States of America

Rodale makes every effort to use acid-free ⧜, recycled paper ♻

Cover design by Leanne Coppola

Illustrations by Shawn Banner, Judy Newhouse, and Tom Ward

Library of Congress Cataloging-in-Publication Data

VanTine, Julia.
    Energy for everything : rejuvenation for the mind, body, and soul / by Julia
VanTine, Marie Elaina Suszynski, and the editors of Prevention Health
Books for Women.
        p.   cm. — (Women's edge health enhancement guide)
    Includes index.
    ISBN 1–57954–349–9   hardcover
    1. Women—Health and hygiene.   2. Mental fatigure.   3. Fatigue.
    [DNLM: 1. Mental Fatigue—prevention & control—Popular Works
    2. Women's Health—Popular Works.   WM 174 V282e   2001]   I. Suszynski, Marie
Elaina.   II. Prevention Health Books for Women   III. Title.   IV. Series.
    RA778.V2848   2001
    613'.04244—dc21   00–012685

Distributed to the book trade by St. Martin's Press

2   4   6   8   10   9   7   5   3   1   hardcover

Visit us on the Web at www.rodalebooks.com, or call us toll-free at (800) 848-4735.

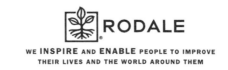

RODALE

WE **INSPIRE** AND **ENABLE** PEOPLE TO IMPROVE
THEIR LIVES AND THE WORLD AROUND THEM

About *Prevention* Health Books

The editors of *Prevention* Health Books are dedicated to providing you with authoritative, trustworthy, and innovative advice for a healthy, active lifestyle. In all of our books, our goal is to keep you thoroughly informed about the latest breakthroughs in natural healing, medical research, alternative health, herbs, nutrition, fitness, and weight loss. We cut through the confusion of today's conflicting health reports to deliver clear, concise, and definitive health information that you can trust. And we explain in practical terms what each new breakthrough means to you, so you can take immediate, practical steps to improve your health and well-being.

Every recommendation in *Prevention* Health Books is based upon reliable sources, including interviews with qualified health authorities. In addition, we retain top-level health practitioners who serve on the Rodale Books Board of Advisors to ensure that all of the health information is safe, practical, and up to-date. *Prevention* Health Books are thoroughly fact-checked for accuracy, and we make every effort to verify recommendations, dosages, and cautions.

The advice in this book will help keep you well-informed about your personal choices in health care—to help you lead a happier, healthier, and longer life.

Energy for Everything **Staff**

EDITOR: Debra L. Gordon

STAFF WRITERS: Deanna Portz, Alison Rice, Judith Springer Riddle, Elizabeth Shimer, Marie Elaina Suszynski, Mariska Van Aalst, Julia VanTine

CONTRIBUTING WRITERS: Marcia Cronin, Patricia Dooley, Diane Kozak, Jennifer Kushnier, Elizabeth B. Price, Bebe Raupe, Judy West, Ted Williams

COVER DESIGNER: Leanne Coppola

SERIES DESIGNER: Lynn N. Gano

PHOTO EDITOR: James A. Gallucci

ILLUSTRATORS: Shawn Banner, Judy Newhouse, Tom Ward

ASSISTANT RESEARCH MANAGER: Shea Zukowski

PRIMARY RESEARCH EDITOR: Anita C. Small

LEAD RESEARCHER: Elizabeth B. Price

EDITORIAL RESEARCHERS: Elaine Czach, Anne Dickson, Jennifer Goldsmith, Jennifer Bright, Jennifer Kushnier, Deanna Portz, Deborah Pedron, Staci Sander, Rebecca Theodore, Lucille Uhlman, Dorothy West, Teresa Yeykal

COPY EDITORS: Amy K. Kovalski, Kelly L. Schmidt

EDITORIAL PRODUCTION MANAGER: Marilyn Hauptly

LAYOUT DESIGNER: Donna G. Rossi

MANUFACTURING COORDINATORS: Brenda Miller, Jodi Schaffer, Patrick Smith

Rodale Women's Health Books

EXECUTIVE EDITOR: Tammerly Booth

VICE PRESIDENT AND MARKETING DIRECTOR: Karen Arbegast

PRODUCT MARKETING MANAGER: Guy Maake

BOOK MANUFACTURING DIRECTOR: Helen Clogston

MANUFACTURING MANAGER: Eileen Bauder

RESEARCH DIRECTOR: Ann Gossy Yermish

ART DIRECTOR: Darlene Schneck

PRODUCTION MANAGER: Robert V. Anderson Jr.

DIGITAL PROCESSING GROUP ASSOCIATE MANAGER: Thomas P. Aczel

OFFICE STAFF: Julie Kehs Minnix, Catherine E. Strouse

Prevention Health Books for Women Board of Advisors

Contents

Introduction. xiii

PART ONE
Where Did All the Energy Go?

Meet Carolyn: She's Everywoman, and She's Exhausted. 2

This Thing Called Energy. 11

Fxhaustion Only a Woman Could Know. 21

PART TWO
Energy Drainers

The New Workplace. 34

On the Home Front. 45

Relationships: Turning Sappers into Sustainers 65

Suffocating in the Sandwich Generation. 73

When Being Tired Means Something's Wrong 81

Energy and Emotions 92

PART THREE
Energy Chargers

Sleep: The Holy Grail 104

Food: The All-Day Energizer. 117

Vitamins and Other Supplements. 130

Moving Into Energy 140

Finding Energy the Alternative Way. 151

Play and Creativity. 166

Energy for Everything: A Year Later 176

Index 187

Introduction

Do you find yourself coveting sleep the way some women crave chocolate? Maybe you fantasize about checking into a hotel room alone and sleeping for 1 solid week. If so, you're not alone. "More energy" ranks right up there with "more time" and "more money" on many women's wish lists. Fatigue is one of the top 10 complaints—if not *the* top complaint—that send women to their doctors. Basically, we're exhausted. And it's no wonder.

Consider my typical day, which is probably not all that different from yours: I get up at 6:00 A.M., walk the dog, get the kids up and dressed, make various breakfasts and lunches, walk the dog (again), drive to work, cram 12 hours of work into 8 hours (if I'm lucky), drive home, get the kids, do the dinner rush, chauffeur the kids to soccer practice, clean the kitchen, fold the laundry, pay the bills, and try to remember to talk to that man in the corner who is my husband. I'm exhausted just writing it all down.

That's where this book comes in. From changing your work habits to discovering less labor-intensive methods to clean your house to finding ways to help yourself to the energy-enhancing benefits of exercise, this book will help you generate more get-up-and-go than a triple espresso.

This book will provide you with recipes for energy-enhancing foods and exercises to beat the afternoon doldrums that you can do either at your desk or at a stoplight. It will show you how to get your husband and kids to help with the housework, how to get rid of those mounds of energy-sapping clutter, and how to do something you thought only children did: play.

But this is more than a self-help book. In *Energy for Everything* you'll also learn about the experiences of a modern "everywoman" named Carolyn, who, like you and me, is exhausted. You'll follow Carolyn to work, to her son's soccer games, to the supermarket, even to the gym. Chapter after chapter, you'll watch as she integrates the ideas and tips given throughout the book into her life, eventually becoming more energetic, relaxed, and *alive*.

Like the other books in the Women's Edge series, this book is full of tips, illustrations, and new information that will reinvigorate you while improving your health, reducing your stress, and smoothing out the wrinkles in your life.

Debra L. Gordon

Debra L. Gordon
Women's Edge Editor

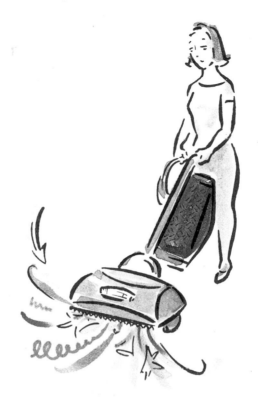

PART ONE

Where Did All the Energy Go?

Meet Carolyn: She's Everywoman, and She's Exhausted

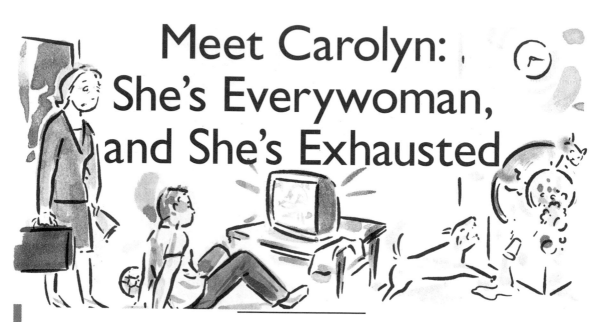

It's 6:15 P.M. Carolyn, a 49-year-old mother of two, walks in the door, throws her keys on the hallway table, and ponders one of Modern Woman's most perplexing dilemmas: Cook or Takeout?

It's a no-brainer. Her husband, Ben, an engineer who travels frequently, is in Ohio for the next few days. Anyway, her kids—Jocelyn, 13, in 7th grade, and Michael, 16, in 10th grade—would rather have pizza.

She wearily reaches for the phone. As usual, she's drained. Used up. Played out.

Exhausted.

Give Carolyn a choice among chocolate, sex, and a long, delicious nap, and she will invariably choose the latter. Her go-go-go schedule at work, equally demanding kids, and ailing mother keep her on the run from 6:00 A.M., when she rises, to 11:30 or midnight, when she puts away the vacuum cleaner.

The worst part: With her husband away much of the time, she's often forced to tackle the unremitting demands of modern life solo.

If you're shaking your head at Carolyn's plight, save some sympathy for yourself. Fatigue among women is, in fact, an epidemic. Women—especially those of us in our childbearing years—complain of fatigue more often than men. Let's call it female fatigue syndrome, or FFS.

Our tiredness isn't just physical, however. Research suggests that women's fatigue is a slippery condition with many intertwining causes, both biological (such as our menstrual cycles and menopause) and psychological (such as stress and depression). The sweeping social changes that have occurred in the workplace, our families, and our lifestyles in recent decades also contribute to FFS. But, we have to ask, why don't men seem so exhausted?

Let's play detective and take a closer look at Carolyn's life. Mission: to find out why she—and we—are so darn drained.

Round One: Carolyn Goes to Work

As an executive assistant to the president of a software company, Carolyn has a demanding full-time job, including long hours and high

THE DILEMMA OF THE SINGLE MOM

As demanding as our work and home lives can be, most of us don't have to go it alone. Yet there are nearly 10 million women in the United States who are raising children alone—more than a 200-fold increase since 1970. If you fall into this category, the worries and frustrations that come with the territory can drain your energy to the point where running on empty becomes the norm. "Many of our single mothers talk about feeling like prisoners—being shut into a child's world where nothing is more than 3 feet tall," says Mavis Hetherington, Ph.D., emeritus professor of psychology at the University of Virginia in Charlottesville. They're physically and mentally exhausted, she says.

"Sometimes they're exhausted because they can't sleep, worrying about how to keep food on the table and a roof over their kids' heads, about when their child-support payments will arrive, about the quality of day- or after-school care," notes Dr. Hetherington. And sometimes they're exhausted simply because of their reality. "Children are exhausting. Although you get the joys of being attached to a child, the mundane aspects of child rearing are not much fun," she says.

In fact, they take away precious rejuvenation time a single mom so desperately needs—the "Calgon take me away" moments as well as time with friends.

"Single mothers have sole responsibility for home, work, and children," notes Dr. Hetherington. "If there's an emergency—if there's a snow day or the babysitter doesn't show up—there are no other resources to draw on."

The following tips from Andrea Engber, founder of the National Organization of Single Mothers and author of *The Complete Single Mother*, can help stoke your energy.

Don't believe the hype. There are two kinds of fatigue, says Engber. There's the "earned" kind, like lack of sleep, and the kind caused by well-meaning marrieds who make you feel like single motherhood is simply too overwhelming to bear. "Dismiss their misconceptions," says Engber. "Tell yourself, 'It's as hard as I choose to make it.'"

Make time for you. You've heard this a million times. Now go do it. Ask friends for the names of their babysitters, drop your child off at your mother's house, or call in a favor. Then see a trashy movie, go for a long bicycle ride—do whatever floats your boat.

Make your own family rules. So your ex wouldn't abide a messy living room? Demanded dinner promptly at 6:00? Big deal. You make the rules now. And rule number one should be to abandon all hope of perfection. Do what works for you and your kids. When you're beat, ignore the living room clutter. Serve peanut butter sandwiches on whole-grain bread and milk for supper every other night, alternating with pancakes and fresh fruit.

Buy an egg timer. Set it for 20 minutes and tell your kids you're taking a timeout. Use the time to read, talk to a friend on the phone, surf the Net—whatever you know jump-starts your energy.

Nix the guilt. "Guilt is an exhausting emotion," says Engber. Repeat this mantra as often as necessary: I Can Only Do the Best I Can. Eventually, you'll come to believe it. For more information on the National Organization of Single Mothers, check out their Web site at www.singlemothers.org.

WOMAN TO WOMAN
She Has Energy to Spare

Diane Dobry brings new meaning to the word busy. This 44-year-old mother of two from Bethpage, New York, keeps a schedule that would bring many of us to the point of collapse. On a typical day, she is up by 5:30 A.M. By 7:24—the minute she has to dash around the corner to meet her 7:27 A.M. commuter train to New York City—Dobry has spent 30 minutes on the treadmill, gotten ready for work, and attended to motherly and housekeeping duties. After her 90-minute commute, she's at her desk at Teachers College at Columbia University, where she's the director of communications. More often than not, by 5:00 P.M., she still has energy to burn. Good thing. Because besides working full-time, she is working toward her master's degree in international education development. How does she do it? More important, why does she do it? Here's her answer.

There are so many things I want to do. And I could have done many of them 20 years ago, but I didn't. So I have to pedal twice as fast. I don't want to go to my deathbed saying, "Why didn't I do anything special?"

Of course, my life isn't perfect. My house has its share of dust balls under the bed. My sons grumble about my schedule. And yes, I do get tired. Some days, I'll put my head down on the desk and close my eyes. To catch up on sleep, I try to stay in bed late on weekends. But many times I have to get to a doctor's appointment before noon on the weekend, and then I go out to the gym or ride my bike. And on Sundays, I get up at 8:00 A.M. and ride 8 miles on my bike.

But unless I'm sick or have my period, I rarely feel wiped out. I have a lot of energy when I'm consumed by something.

Although it might sound as if I'm the multitasker from hell, living a balanced life is a priority. I even manage to squeeze meditation into my schedule. The more I learn about staying centered, the more energy I seem to have.

When I come home late, I spend time with my husband, Frank, and my kids before going off to bed. And I spend much of the weekends with my 16-year-old son, Kenny, and my oldest son, 18-year-old Jeff.

My advice is to make time for yourself. Sometimes I take a vacation day and go to a movie, take myself out to lunch, or just sit on the beach.

stress. She's wired—and not just emotionally. Armed with cell phone and pager, she practically beeps and chirps as she walks.

It's not unusual for her boss to call her at 10:00 P.M. Or for her to take work home. Which she dutifully does, unless she falls asleep on the sofa at 8:30 in front of her favorite sitcom.

Bet you can relate.

Women have *always* worked, whether on the farm or in the home. But whether for personal preference or financial reasons, an unprecedented number of us find ourselves locked in to the 40-hour-plus workweek.

Consider: In the years before World War II, "dual-career families"—that is, families in which both parents work—made up less than 10 percent of the American workforce. Now, 62 percent of families with kids under the age of 6 are dual career.

Not only are more of us working, we're working more. A 1998 national survey conducted by the Families and Work Institute in New York City found that women work an average of 44 hours a week—an increase of 5 hours a week since 1977. Another large study conducted by the same organization found that 68 percent of working parents with children under the age of 6 say their jobs require them to work very long and very hard—up from 55 percent in 1977.

One study looked at moms in 1965, who primarily stayed home, and moms in 1998, who primarily worked outside the home, and found that both sets spent about the same amount of time with their children. How could that be? The study found that moms in 1998 were taking time away from themselves. They slept 5 to 6 hours less per week—almost an hour per night—and they had 11 to 12 hours less free time for themselves per week—almost 2 hours per day.

Here's the irony: As our working hours have increased, so too has our sense that at work we sometimes feel more competent, more appreciated, and even more relaxed than we feel at home. Fact is, household and family obligations can make "home" work harder—and more frustrating—than paid work.

Eminent sociologist Arlie Russell Hochschild, D.Ph., Ph.D., of the University of California at Berkeley, spent three summers studying a company that offered "family-friendly policies," such as job sharing, part-time work, and telecommuting from home. What she found: Few men or women took advantage of them.

In the book based on her research, *The Time Bind: When Work Becomes Home and Home Becomes Work*, Hochschild found that one out of five workers preferred paid office work to handling frustrating family and household obligations. She writes, "Nowadays, men and women both may leave unwashed dishes, crying tots, testy teenagers, and unresponsive mates behind to arrive at work early and call out, 'Hi, fellas, I'm here!'"

Often, Carolyn calls out the same greeting.

DRIVING OURSELVES TO DISTRACTION?

If, between shuttling kids to soccer games and music lessons, cussing in traffic on your daily commute, and running never-ending errands, you feel like your mail should be delivered to your car, then Ford Motor Company has something for you.

Ford has teamed up with the Maytag Corporation to create the ultimate in a "personalized for your lifestyle" concept vehicle, named Windstar Solutions.

The minivan is designed to help women deal with the demands of their increasingly frantic lifestyles and achieve balance between their home and work lives, says Linda Lee, manager of the women's marketing and product office at Ford.

For women on the go, the minivan features a refrigerator, microwave, trash compactor, wet/dry vacuum, mini-washer/dryer, and voice activation technology called Home Connection, which ensures that important tasks are done without a glitch. From the driver's seat, we can use the Home Connection to turn down the thermostat, start or stop the dishwasher, or double-check if the kids *really* set the security alarm.

All this, plus an entertainment system that lets the kids watch a movie or play interactive electronic games while on the road (presumably to nip their are-we-there-yets in the bud).

"The media and consumer response has been amazing," Lee says.

But is a vehicle that can do it all really the answer to our prayers? Maybe not, says Joanne B. Ciulla, Ph.D., professor of ethics and leadership at the Jepson School of Leadership Studies at the University of Richmond in Virginia and author of *The Working Life: The Promise and Betrayal of Modern Work*. What it *will* do: Free up time that we'll spend . . . working.

"We live in a culture where the ideology is to pack in as much work as we possibly can," Dr. Ciulla says. "It's a kind of madness. The unanswered question here is, 'In what way does this vehicle improve a woman's quality of life?' I'm not sure it answers that question. It basically says, 'You can do your laundry in your car.'"

PAY YOUR DEBT!

Think losing out on a few nights—or weeks—of sleep is no big deal?

It's a huge deal for rats. Deprived of 70 to 80 percent of their normal sleep, laboratory rodents die in about 3 weeks.

And while no one's sure whether humans can die from lack of sleep, it definitely affects our bodies—and our quality of life.

We're talking about sleep debt—or, to sleep scientists, sleep deprivation—which is losing significant chunks of sack time for nights, weeks, or even months.

As many as 80 percent of Americans experience some degree of sleep debt in any given week. For women, one obvious reason is our frantic schedules.

"Women carry a disproportionate burden of home and family care, and many women with children work outside the home," says James Walsh, M.D., executive director of the Unity Sleep Medicine and Research Center at St. Luke's Hospital in Chesterfield, Missouri, and vice president of the National Sleep Foundation. With the exception of teenagers and shift workers, he says, working mothers may be most at risk for sleep deprivation.

The consequences of sleep debt go far beyond making us look like death warmed over.

In one study, men allotted 4 hours of sleep for 6 straight nights showed changes in thyroid function and metabolism. The researchers suggested that chronic sleep loss might also worsen certain age-related conditions such as diabetes and high blood pressure.

To find out how much debt you've racked up, turn to the Epworth Sleepiness Scale, a simple questionnaire sleep scientists use to measure sleep deprivation. (See "How Tired Are You?")

Or simply pay heed to the signs of sleep debt—becoming drowsy or falling asleep while watching TV, driving, or reading a book. (By the way, these activities don't make you drowsy because they're sedentary. They make you drowsy because you need sleep.)

Another sign of sleep debt: bitchiness. "Irritability is one of the hallmark symptoms of insufficient sleep," says Dr. Walsh.

It's fine to make payments on your sleep debt by sleeping later on weekends, as most of us do, according to Dr. Walsh. One caveat: If you sleep in a few days in a row, you may find yourself wanting to go to bed later and get up later, which will contribute to the groggy feeling on Monday morning. If you don't suffer any such ill effects, however, feel free to indulge yourself on the weekends.

Or simply nap, he suggests. "It won't interfere with your sleep unless you nap for more than an hour or two during the day, or close to your bedtime." (With respect to Dr. Walsh, however, most of us have as much chance of sneaking in a nap as we do of buying a winning lottery ticket.)

However you pay back your sleep debt, you'll know when that magic day comes, says Dr. Walsh. "You'll be able to sit down in front of the TV, or read a book, and be bored rather than sleepy."

Round Two: Carolyn Goes On "Second Shift"

When Ben is at home—which isn't often—he's glad to be there. It's his sanctuary from the cares of the modern world.

But not Carolyn's.

As soon as she steps through her front door, her "second shift" begins—cooking dinner, refereeing the kids' squabbles, doing laundry, the whole domestic goddess thing.

The "second shift" refers to the long hours of

family and household obligations we attend to before and after our "real" jobs. In her seminal book *The Second Shift: Working Parents and the Revolution at Home*, Dr. Hochschild calculated that women with full-time jobs who also did housework and child care worked about 15 hours a week more than men—an extra month of 24-hour days each year.

Sometimes, the shift starts before we get home. At Carolyn's house, both Michael and Jocelyn need to be ferried to and from piano and ballet lessons as well as Michael's baseball games and Jocelyn's soccer games, involving a crazy patchwork quilt arrangement of car pools, shortened workdays, and favors begged of the neighbors.

We didn't volunteer for the second shift. So why are we doing it?

In part, because of the feminist movement in the 1970s, when we made great inroads into the labor market. In the early days of feminism, "we accepted the career template that had been designed for men," says Phyllis Moen, Ph.D., a sociologist at Cornell University in Ithaca, New York, and director of the Cornell Employment and Family Careers Institute. So while we gained equal opportunity, "we were still playing by men's rules," she says. "Which means that we also had the 'right' to work 60 or 70 hours a week. And yet, on the domestic front, nothing was taken off the plate."

In one Canadian study of 153 women, fully 63 percent said that the combination of work (both inside and outside the home) was the main reason they were so exhausted. Commented one woman in the study, "I feel that I

HOW TIRED ARE YOU?

Sleep experts worldwide use the same assessment tool—the Epworth Sleepiness Scale—to measure folks' levels of daytime sleepiness. Now you can use it, too. Simply rate how likely you'd be to nod off in the following situations. Give yourself 0 points if you'd never doze off, 1 point for a slight chance, 2 for a moderate chance, and 3 for a high chance.

_____ Sitting and reading

_____ Watching television

_____ Sitting as a passenger in a car for an hour without a break

_____ Lying down to rest in the afternoon

_____ Sitting and talking to someone

_____ Sitting quietly after a lunch without alcohol

_____ Sitting in a car, stopped for a few minutes in traffic

_____ Total points:

 0–5 points: slight or no sleep debt
 6–10 points: moderate sleep debt
11–20 points: heavy sleep debt
21–25 points: extreme sleep debt

---

don't have time to breathe—with children, lunches, school assignments, housework, and a busy job, I feel overwhelmed. The only solution is to clone."

Or slack off on housework. In 1965, we spent 27 hours a week on housework; in 1995, 15.6 hours. "There are a lot more dust balls in the United States," says Ellen Galinsky, president of the Families and Work Institute.

But even being more relaxed about less-than-sparkling commodes can't make up for what we *really* need—a major rethinking of the traditional career path.

"Family-friendly work policies are merely window dressing around the old-style male ca-

JUMP START

Book It

Find your calendar. Pick a weekend you're free. (Pick one even if you're crazy busy.) Think of that beautiful but far-off bed-and-breakfast, craft show, or arts festival you've been dying to get to. Pick up the phone. Book yourself a room. Presto! Instant gratification—and "downtime" that's just for you.

reer model," says Dr. Moen. "We need to reinvent career paths that acknowledge that most workers—male or female—have family responsibilities."

Round Three: Carolyn Cares for Mom

Several times a week, Carolyn makes the 15-mile drive out to her mother's house. Since her mother's health began failing, Carolyn, ever the dutiful daughter, has been doing the older woman's laundry, buying her groceries, and visiting to keep her spirits up, often sipping tea and perusing old photographs for as long as 2 hours.

Carolyn's care of her mother is mirrored by an estimated 22 million caregiving households in America, triple the number in 1988. The most recent report of family caregiving in this country—conducted by the National Alliance for Caregiving and the American Association of Retired Persons—paints a vivid picture of the typical caregiver, 73 percent of whom are, not surprisingly, female.

The typical caregiver: a married woman in her mid-forties who works full-time. Moreover, 41 percent of all caregivers, male or female, have one or more children under 18 years old in the house.

Talk about a full plate.

Carolyn's lucky—she's not a "level 5" caregiver, defined as someone who provides constant care, or 40 or more hours of care per week. But even "part-time" caregivers such as Carolyn, who are at level 3 (providing 9 hours of care a week), can experience some stress and fatigue, says Gail Hunt, executive director of the National Alliance for Caregiving in Bethesda, Maryland. And the burden doesn't decrease even when an ailing parent moves into a care facility like a nursing home, says Hunt.

"Many women drive over to feed their parents," Hunt says. "And when we do focus groups, we hear all the time about women who get calls at 3:00 A.M. from the facility: 'We can't deal with her. She's all upset. You have to come over.'"

In the report, when caregivers were asked what kind of help or support they most wanted, the answer was, not surprisingly, "time for myself." That desire even beat out "help with housework" and extra money or financial support.

Round Four: Carolyn Takes a "Relaxing" Bath

It's 10:25 P.M. Carolyn has just finished unloading the dishwasher, folding the laundry, and paying bills. The kids are silent. The house is silent. Before her stretches a brief, shining gap of time before the grind begins again.

It's Carolyn Time.

She pads into the bathroom and fills the tub with warm water and lavender-scented bubble bath. (She's read that the scent of lavender helps reduce stress, and she needs all the help she can get.)

As she soaks, her mind relaxes . . . then suddenly recoils.

Will her mother eventually need to be moved to a nursing home? If so, how will they afford it?

Will she and Jocelyn bridge the ever-widening gap between them? As luck would have it, her daughter is entering puberty just as Carolyn is on the cusp of menopause, both intensely stressful transitions. While Carolyn knows that her daughter needs patience and support now, the constant bickering between them is wearing her down.

Will she and Ben ever have sex again? They've both been exhausted. She's contemplating a visit to Victoria's Secret.

Will she make the deadline for the report due next Wednesday?

And, heaven help us—Jocelyn has ballet at 3:00 P.M. tomorrow, the same time Michael has a soccer game, 20 miles out of town. She'll just have to call his friend Peter's mother—again—and plead for her to taxi Michael over to the game—again.

She drains the tub, feeling drained herself.

But not sleepy. Oh, no. She knows it will be hours before she falls asleep.

Stress and its kin, insomnia, are major causes of our fatigue. From 1985 to 1990—a mere 5 years—the proportion of people who reported "feeling highly stressed" more than doubled. And 1 million workers stay home on an average workday because of stress-related complaints.

Carolyn *wishes* she could stay home—to sleep. Whether because of worrying into the wee

> ### AMAZING ENERGY
> #### The Real Wonder Woman
>
> From humble beginnings in rural Mississippi, Oprah Winfrey, determined and charismatic, used her unflinching energy to become one of the most influential women in popular culture. Her accomplishments go beyond the world of television into such areas as publishing, music, film, philanthropy, education, health and fitness, and social awareness. She is one of only three women to own her own television and film production studios, Harpo, Inc. She received an Academy Award nomination for her film debut in *The Color Purple*. She started her own magazine, *O*, and she is a professor of management at Northwestern University. Additionally, she has established scholarships for hundreds of students and has donated millions of dollars to higher education institutions.
>
> It's no surprise Oprah was inducted into the National Women's Hall of Fame in 1994, and no wonder that President Clinton signed a bill in honor of her in 1993. She has made a difference to millions of people, has done the work of a thousand men, and still manages to look 15 years younger than her chronological age.

hours or a dawn-till-dusk schedule, she sleeps only about 6 hours a night.

It's hard to believe that in 1910, the era of ragtime and mutton-sleeved blouses, the typical American slept an average of 9 hours a night. These days, we get an average of 7 hours. And in a recent poll conducted by the National Sleep Foundation, 45 percent of respondents admitted that they sleep less to accomplish more.

Accomplish more—but give ourselves less.

In 1977, we working moms spent 96 minutes per workday on ourselves. By the turn of the century, that precious hour and a half has shrunk to just 54 minutes, according to the Families and Work Institute study.

What we couldn't do with those 42 long, luscious lost minutes!

Round Five: Carolyn Loses It— And Finds an Answer

It's 11:18 P.M. Carolyn is in front of the TV, waiting for the news to end so she can doze off to the soothing banter of Jay Leno. But she knows that tomorrow is going to be a killer, especially on 5½ hours of sleep.

A tear rolls down her cheek. Then another.

"I just can't face it. I just can't," she thinks.

She remembers how her life used to be—when she wasn't so tired, when she wasn't working 45 hours a week, when she and Ben and the kids would just pile into the minivan on a Saturday afternoon and take off for parts unknown for a picnic, a hike, or a day of cross-country skiing.

Then—and "then" wasn't so long ago—life seemed more of an adventure than a struggle. What happened?

She cries quietly, almost too exhausted for tears. Then she raises her head.

"That's it," she thinks. "Things have to change. There's more to life than dreaming of a nap."

In a burst of sleep-deprived inspiration, she draws up a list: Carolyn's Bill of Rights.

1. I have the right to 8 solid hours of sleep a night.
2. I have the right to turn off my cell phone and beeper at a reasonable hour.
3. I have the right to go "off-duty" to spend some time on *me*—to go out to dinner with a friend, to walk after work, to wax my legs and give myself a pedicure.
4. I have the right to ask my husband to help more with the kids and Mom.
5. I have the right to live a healthier life—in the foods I eat, the vitamins I take, and the exercises I do.
6. I have the right to play—with my husband, with my kids, on my own.

Carolyn, sick of being tired, has reached her breaking point.

How about you?

Come on. Tag along with Carolyn. Join her on a journey from energy bust to boom. By the end of this book, you, too, will know how to fight female fatigue syndrome. Learn real-world ways to jump-start your energy. Build an "energy tool kit" that will allow you to conquer the myriad causes of your fatigue, from the biological to the very, very personal.

If Carolyn can do it, so can you.

This Thing Called Energy

It's 6:00 A.M. and the sun is just peeking through the blinds in Carolyn's bedroom. She's still asleep, but her brain is already at work, signaling changes in critical chemicals and hormones throughout her body that serve as an internal alarm clock. By the time the buzzer blasts on the alarm beside the bed, her body temperature has begun to rise and tiny photoreceptors in her eyes have begun to signal a gland in her brain to slow its secretion of what some might call the sleep hormone, melatonin.

It's time to wake up.

But it takes a hot shower and three cups of coffee before her "sleep inertia," that grogginess that lingers like a bad dream, disappears. For the rest of the morning, Carolyn is on a roll—typing reports, tackling those toppling piles of paper, and planning her boss's business trip. Until 2:00 P.M. Suddenly, her eyes seem to have gained 10 pounds, and she has typed the same sentence over and over. She struggles through, though. Finally, she finds her second wind around 4:00 P.M., a blast that stays with her through the evening routine of dinner, car pooling, and dishes

until she conks out with just a brief kiss for Ben at 11:00 P.M.

Carolyn's energy peaks and valleys are endemic to us all. Some are our own doing, caused by late nights, caffeinated pick-me-ups, or heavy meals. But the conductor behind our energy levels resides deep in our brains. A complex clump of cells directs the symphony of daily hormone releases, body temperature changes, and blood pressure shifts called circadian rhythms. They developed in our early ancestors as an adaptation to the rhythms and cycles in nature—including variations in light, temperature, and food availability. But oddly enough, our circadian rhythms run on an average of a 25-hour cycle, which doesn't match the 24-hour time span it takes the Earth to spin once on its axis. So every day, we are forced to reset our natural 25-hour body clock to a 24-hour day, which is perhaps one more reason we're all so tired.

That's why it's so important that we understand the physical rhythms that guide our day. Only by becoming aware of them can we learn to modify our lives to maximize our peaks and plan for our valleys.

Living without Time

For 2 weeks, Lynne Lamberg, a medical writer from Baltimore, lived without time. "There were no clocks, no radios, no televisions, no windows, and no indications of time from the researchers with whom I interacted," says Lamberg, coauthor of *The Body Clock Guide to Better Health: How to Use Your Body's Natural Clock to Fight Illness and Achieve Maximum Health*. When she wanted to go to sleep, researchers shut down the lights; they turned them on again only when she told them she was ready to get up. Using volunteers like Lamberg, scientists hope to discover what happens to our body clocks when they're allowed to run on their own, natural schedule.

Lamberg spent her timeless days writing, reading, riding an exercise bike, listening to music, and taking tests to measure her alertness and mental abilities. She ate three meals a day. "One day they asked me to stay up as late as I could," she remembers. To stay awake, she lengthened the time between meals, trying to ignore her body's hunger clock (another player in our circadian rhythms) and suffering all the symptoms of jet lag. Without knowing why, she spent the time she normally would have slept now slumped over her desk, barely able to keep her eyes open, feeling physically ill. When what would have been her "sleep" time passed, she felt more alert. She went as long as she could before she crashed, having no idea how long she'd been awake. Later, she learned she managed to stay awake for nearly 23 hours, and slept for about 7.5 hours, stretching her day to about 30 hours.

ARE YOU A LARK OR AN OWL?

The science world refers to morning people as larks and evening people as owls. Owls tend to select later bedtimes and get up later than larks, and they tend to have a harder time adapting to social demands because much of the rest of the world rises and sets with the sun. "It's as if the clock just runs differently in different people," says Patricia Prinz, Ph.D., professor in the department of biobehavioral nursing and psychiatry at the University of Washington in Seattle.

Energy-wise, larks feel more vigilant in the earlier part of the day, while owls reach their peak in alertness later. In a study conducted at Leiden University in the Netherlands, morning and evening people rated their alertness six times a day for 2 weeks. The larks' alertness peaked between 9:00 A.M. and 4:00 P.M., and the owls' alertness gradually increased as the day progressed. The participants' energy levels rose and fell with their body temperature, further illustrating a link between body temperature and energy.

While scientists don't know for sure why we're a lark or an owl, or how we become that way, they do have some theories. One is that our early ancestors developed different sleep patterns so some of them could gather food during the day while others guarded the community at night.

Other scientists say that it may relate to the time of year we're born. A study at the University of Bologna in Italy showed that more morning people are born in autumn and winter, and more evening people are born in spring and summer. The proposed reasons behind this phenomena have to do with how much light we're exposed to as infants, which depends on the seasonal length of day. A related hypothesis is that circadian rhythms are established very early on by our first rhythms of light exposure, since fetuses in the womb are sensitive to light.

To assess whether you are a lark or an owl, take this short quiz.

1. If you had no obligations, what time would you choose to go to bed?
   a. Before 10:30 P.M.
   b. Between 10:30 and midnight
   c. After midnight

2. With no obligations, what time would you get up?
   a. Before 7:00 A.M.
   b. Between 7:00 and 9:00 A.M.
   c. After 9:00 A.M.

3. An hour before you go to bed during the workweek, how sleepy do you feel?
   a. Pretty okay
   b. Depends on the day
   c. Exhausted

4. A friend has asked you to exercise with her a few times a week. She suggests hitting the track from 7:00 to 8:00 A.M. How do you react?
   a. Ugh. There's no way.
   b. I think I'll be okay.
   c. No problem—morning's my favorite time to work out.

5. How alert do you feel in the first half-hour you're awake?
   a. Not alert—sleepy
   b. Depends on the day
   c. Alert and refreshed

6. In the morning, how much do you rely on caffeine to get you going?
   a. I'm a zombie without it; I drink it all morning.
   b. I drink it some days.
   c. I don't rely on caffeine at all.

SCORING:

1. a-0; b-2; c-4
2. a-0; b-2; c-4
3. a-4; b-2; c-0
4. a-4; b-2; c-0
5. a-4; b-2; c-0
6. a-4; b-2; c-0

0–5: You're a lark.
6–10: You have more lark than owl tendencies.
11–15: You aren't really either.
16–20: You have more owl tendencies.
21–24: You're an owl.

When she wasn't trying to break records for staying awake, Lamberg felt good in the lab. "I slept quite well, I was healthy, and I had as much, if not more, energy than usual. I just followed my biological clock." And her clock ran free on a 25-hour schedule.

On the last day of the study, Lamberg's researchers awakened her at a normal (according to the outside world) wake time, even though she had slept only 3 to 4 hours. "They then sat me in front of a bank of bright lights to help me readapt quickly to a normal schedule," she says. "I felt a little sleepy for the first couple of days, but I resumed my schedule quickly."

Once she reviewed the results of the study, Lamberg's attitude toward sleep changed. "In the lab, you sleep as long as you want, so I thought I was sleeping 9 to 10 hours instead of my usual 7," she says. "But I was surprised to learn that I slept only 7 to 7¾ hours each night, which is my internally determined amount of necessary sleep." Before the time lab, she woke every day to the alarm clock feeling groggy and tired. "Now, I don't pay attention to clocks," she says. "I just leave the blinds open and let light awaken me, and I always wake up at about the same time, even though my bedtime may vary an hour or so from night to night."

The Way It Works

There's a lesson to be learned in Lamberg's experience. Light drives energy. It works like this:

On various parts of our bodies—our eyes for sure, the backs of our knees, and other places possibly—are our body's version of solar panels: nerve endings called photoreceptors that absorb light. Once those photoreceptors pick up the light, they send a signal to the pineal gland, which is located in the brain, to stop producing melatonin, the so-called sleep hormone. One of melatonin's roles may have to do with body temperature. When it's dark, and melatonin is secreted, scientists suspect the hormone signals our body temperature to drop, which is ideal for rest. With light comes a cessation of melatonin and a gradually increasing body temperature, which is ideal for alertness.

The body temperature hits its low point at 4:00 A.M. Then, during the last hours of sleep, it starts to rise, helping us rise along with it. These aren't huge fluctuations—just 3 to 4 degrees—but they're enough.

That's why melatonin is often taken as a supplement to help with jet lag and sleep problems. The long-term effects of supplemental melatonin have not been thoroughly studied, however, so it should only be taken under the supervision of a doctor. Supplemental melatonin has many possible side effects, including drowsiness, headaches, nausea, morning dizziness, interactions with prescription medications, and adverse effects on people with some health conditions, such as diabetes and high blood pressure.

Body temperature continues to fluctuate throughout the day, even without any additional melatonin release. It rises during the mid- to late morning, which is one reason we often feel so energized during this time. Then, in early afternoon, it dips slightly—perhaps attributing to that postlunch slump. You know the one: You're in a meeting watching your boss's PowerPoint presentation and next thing you know, your cheek is

WOMAN TO WOMAN
She Learned to Reset Her Clock

Elizabeth Turner, 38, a flight attendant from Ontario, Canada, has been traveling overseas for 16 years. She's been to all the continents except Antarctica. She presently flies overseas four times a month. Elizabeth knows what it means to experience jet lag.

Jet lag definitely disturbs my life. My symptoms vary, but the disruption of my sleep cycle is the most obvious problem. When I have jet lag, my concentration decreases and I become "time disoriented." For the first 24 hours of a layover, I have to watch the clock to know whether I should be awake or asleep; relying on my internal sense of time is not an option. When I return home, I'm forgetful. When I don't rest after prolonged periods of jet lag, I have an increased incidence of viral infections—usually in the form of sties and cold sores.

I am affected by jet lag to some degree on each trip, but it's worse when I travel from west to east. It's also worse if I have an illness, such as a cold or the flu, or if it's the week prior to my period.

My family feels the effects of my jet lag as much as I do. Having kids forces me to deal with the situation in a proac-

resting on your coffee cup. Luckily, body temperature rises again, reaching its daily high, researchers suspect, in the mid- to late afternoon. That may account for the "second wind" we get around 4:00 P.M.—and explain why it's so hard to fall asleep at this time, says Margaret Moline, Ph.D., director of the Sleep-Wake Disorders Center at New York Presbyterian Hospital–Weill Cornell Medical Center in White Plains and New York City.

By 11:00 P.M., we've turned the lights out, melatonin production has already started, and our temperatures fall in preparation for sleep. Also, our heart and blood pressure rates drop in accordance with our body's natural rhythms.

tive rather than a reactive way. I can't make plans for the time right after I return from an eastern destination; I just know I'll be out of commission. I also let chores go undone when I am jet-lagged, so I'm left with a pile of them once my energy has returned. But it usually takes only a day or two until I'm feeling like myself again.

Despite the side effects of jet lag I've mentioned, I haven't been plagued by the bone-wearying fatigue that crippled me for the first 2 years of my career, which is probably because I learned to better manage it. I try to maintain a routine whenever I can. I go to bed at a regular time when I'm home. I also force myself to get some form of exercise daily, even when I travel. This can be as simple as a walk at my destination location, which I take as soon as I arrive, no matter how fatigued I am. On the subsequent days of my layover, I work out in hotel gyms or do laps in the pool, which helps increase my energy. I try to reset to local time when I arrive back in the West, which helps me adjust more quickly. I avoid taking naps, because the tease of sleep often leaves me feeling more exhausted. I maintain a healthy diet. I drink a lot of water and eat carbohydrates and vegetables like tomatoes and cucumbers. Finally, I stay away from sodium, since it dehydrates me.

The World around Us

Beyond our own biochemical brew, there are external cues that foul our circadian pacemakers. These cues, known in the science world as *zeitgebers*, German for "time givers," are what keep us on the 24-hour circadian schedule rather than the 25-hour timetable our bodies want to embrace.

Here are some cues that experts have identified, along with their suggestions to moderate them.

Travel between time zones. Remember when George Bush vomited and fainted at a banquet in Japan? The villain was jet lag. Travel disrupts our circadian rhythms, which leads to jet lag. It hits when we fly across several time zones, particularly west to east. For instance, if you fly from New York to London on a 6:00 P.M. flight, you arrive around 6:00 A.M. London time. But according to your body clock, it's still 1:00 A.M. New York time—and you should be in dream land. Try telling your body that. The sun is up, your photoreceptors have sent the message to your melatonin to shut down, and, according to some of your circadian rhythms, it's time to start a new day. Consequently, you've just lost a night's sleep. With jet lag come poor concentration, fatigue, insomnia, irritability, and, as President Bush demonstrated, an upset stomach.

To minimize jet lag's effects, follow these tips.

- Adjust your schedule slowly in anticipation of your trip. If you will be traveling to Europe, for example, go to bed a half-hour later on each successive night for several nights before you leave.
- Sleep as much as possible on overnight flights so you don't arrive with a sleep deficit.
- Guzzle fluids on the plane because dehydration can further confuse your sleep-wake cycle. But stay away from alcohol and caffeine, which can also play havoc with your rhythms.
- Reset your watch while you're on the plane to psychologically adjust to the new time.
- Stay in natural light as much as possible your first day in the new time zone. The more you stay indoors, the longer your jet lag symptoms last.

Erratic routines. "If your schedule is irregular, you can give yourself a kind of jet lag without

HOW IN THE WORLD DO THEY SLEEP?
Dreaming in Different Cultures

The significance of dreams varies across cultures. In some societies, dreams are thought to be unreal figments of the imagination, with no relevance to everyday life. In other cultures, however, dreams are considered valuable sources of information about the self and the future—as important as events in the waking world. Societies that place importance on dreams are called dream cultures. They include the Parintintin of South America, the Arapesh and Sambia of New Guinea, and the Azande of Central Africa.

While certain dreams pop up in most cultures—like being rooted to the ground when trying to run, falling, and flying—the symbolism of those dreams differs among societies. For instance, to the Parintintin of South America, an erotic dream means you desire the subject of the dream; in comparison, the Arapesh of New Guinea consider an erotic dream to be a form of actual intimate contact—it can even be considered adultery.

Then there are nightmares. The Azande of Central Africa see bad dreams as the process of being bewitched, while Parintintins view the anxiety a nightmare fosters as representative of a demon presence.

Some cultures go as far as to place social restrictions on dreams, creating rules about what kinds of dreams may be revealed and in what settings. The Sambia of New Guinea, for instance, hold the dreamer responsible for her actions in a dream, but only if she makes the dream public. So for a Sambian to publicly reveal a dream about killing someone would be similar to a Kamikaze mission.

lowest at night, when we are supposed to be sleeping," says Charmane Eastman, Ph.D., director of the Biological Rhythms Research Lab at Rush-Presbyterian-St. Luke's Medical Center in Chicago. Because they sleep when the rest of the world is awake, night-shift workers experience more interruptions to their sleep, such as noise, sunlight, and higher room temperature. So they are chronically sleep deprived. Since sleep helps rejuvenate our organ systems and our brains so that they function properly, this chronic lack of sleep jeopardizes health, on-the-job safety, memory, mood, and performance. Consequently, shift workers are at risk for concentration problems, weight gain, heart problems, and more colds and flu.

To beat the problems inherent in shift work, try the following measures.

- ➤ Reset slowly. Begin adjusting to a new work schedule several days before it starts. Maybe you changed jobs and now have to get up 2 hours earlier to commute to work. Then both go to bed and wake up 15 minutes earlier each day in the week prior to your actual first day, suggests Dr. Moline.

ever leaving where you are," says Dr. Moline. The 25 million Americans who work graveyard or split shifts know this very well.

"One reason it's difficult to perform well on the night shift is that performance parallels the circadian rhythm of body temperature, which is

- ➤ Adopt bedtime rituals. Wind down before bed by taking a warm bath, lowering the room temperature in your bedroom, and avoiding brain-activating activities, such as balancing your checkbook and watching a suspenseful movie.

- Darken your environment. On the way home from work, wear dark glasses to prevent your body from going into daytime mode. At home, darken your bedroom and bathroom with light-blocking curtains, and wear eyeshades while you sleep.
- Soundproof your surroundings. Unplug the phone, wear earplugs, and use a white noise machine, like a fan.

David Letterman. Our ancestors knew when to go to sleep and wake up. It got dark, they hit the hay. Sun came up, they followed. But with electric lights, alarm clocks, 24-hour Wal-Marts, late-night talk shows, and the Japanese stock exchange, the boundaries between night and day have not only blurred, they've disappeared. Sleep has become an afterthought, and that's the biggest detriment to balanced rhythms. Most of us need an average of 8 to 8½ hours of sleep a night, but we get only an average of 6 hours and 41 minutes.

"First and foremost, get enough sleep, and then all the rest follows," says Dr. Moline. "Adequate sleep is the amount you need to be alert and functioning during the day— without snoozing on the commuter rail to make up for what you physiologically need. But if you go to sleep late and wake up early, your brain may still want to be sleeping." That's why you feel groggy even after your third cup of coffee. Further, even 8 hours or more of sleep is no guarantee of energy. Just two 15-minute

WOMEN ASK WHY

Why am I so tired when we switch the clocks to Daylight Saving Time in the spring?

When that dreaded April weekend arrives, we're asked to go to bed and wake up an hour earlier than usual. This can be difficult, especially for night owls. For example, if you set the alarm for 7:00 A.M. in the new time, it will actually ring at 6:00 A.M. in the old time—thus forcing you to get up an hour earlier. Similarly, if you plan to go to bed at 11:00 P.M. in the new time, it will really be 10:00 P.M. according to your body clock, so you won't be able to fall asleep.

Within a few days, however, your body clock should reset itself to match your watch. If not, you could be sleep-deprived or have a sleep disorder, so check with your doctor. To help your internal hands adjust, the National Sleep Foundation recommends the following steps.

- On the Saturday night before the time change, get at least 8 hours of sleep.
- In the fall, delay bedtime by a half-hour on Saturday night, and go to bed at your regular time on Sunday. In the spring, go to bed at your regular time on Saturday, but get up a half-hour earlier on Sunday morning. Most important, make sure you see the sunlight when you wake up.
- Take a nap before 4:00 P.M. on the Sunday of the change.
- Get 8 hours of sleep that Sunday night.

Experts consulted
Margaret Moline, Ph.D.
Director of the Sleep-Wake Disorders Center
New York Presbyterian Hospital-Weill Cornell
*   Medical Center*
White Plains and New York City

Charmane Eastman, Ph.D.
Director of the Biological Rhythms Research Lab
Rush-Presbyterian-St. Luke's Medical Center
Chicago

JUMP START
Breathe

Daily stress makes us take short, sluggish, shallow breaths, which cuts the intake of energy-providing oxygen. One way to remedy this is to put one hand on your belly; quickly breathe in and out through your nose, pushing your belly against your hand with each breath. Keep the breaths short and fast, like panting during labor, except this time you're using your nose instead of your mouth. Deep breathing exercises are also effective for providing your body with more oxygen.

disruptions in an 8-hour night, either by your child or your partner's snoring, can affect your energy level the next day, she says.

To get a good night's sleep, experts suggest the following tips.

- Relieve some stress before bed. Do something that relaxes you before you retire. Talk to a trusted friend on the phone, or meditate.
- Designate worry time. A troubling thought at 3:00 A.M. can be a major sleep interruption. So set aside time in the day to think about situations that are bothering you and how to remedy them.
- Skip the nightcap. Alcohol at bedtime may help induce sleep at first, but it will disrupt your rest later in the night by awakening you, giving you nightmares, or leaving you with a headache in the morning.

Seasons. Lack of sunlight in the winter may lead to seasonal affective disorder (SAD), a form of depression in which you feel sad only during certain months of the year.

Scientists aren't sure why some of us feel down when the weather turns cold, but they suspect it has to do with a disruption of our circadian rhythms. Long winter nights may cause us to secrete more melatonin. The hormone's sedating effects may render us depressed. If you have had less energy and felt anxious and depressed for two consecutive winter months, you may be suffering from SAD and should talk to your doctor. A common treatment is light therapy, which involves exposure to special lamps that are 10 to 20 times brighter than normal indoor lights.

Weekends. We can't treat ourselves to a noon wake-up on the weekends and then expect to joyfully leap out of bed at 6:30 A.M. come Monday morning. The price we pay is Sunday insomnia—when we lie in bed wide awake at our normal 11:00 P.M. bedtime. "What's going on is that the brain is not in the 'go to sleep' zone yet," says Dr. Moline. If this happens to you when you sleep late, wake up at the same time every day, even on the weekends, to keep your rhythms balanced.

When Your Rhythms Are Out of Whack

Like a tiny mountain spring that eventually turns into a raging river, fatigue is the catalyst for a host of repercussions that arise from haywire circadian rhythms. They include problems in the following areas.

Safety. Each year, about 100,000 automobile crashes are caused by driver drowsiness, killing more than 1,550 people. Half of us admit we drive while drowsy. And nearly 17 percent of us have actually fallen asleep at the wheel.

To avoid becoming one of these statistics, experts recommend the following preventive measures.

- Take a 15- to 20-minute nap before driving if you are too sleepy to drive safely. Even a small dose of sleep will make you more refreshed and capable of driving.
- Bring a talkative passenger. Conversation is a great eye-opener.
- Be extra careful when driving between 2:00 A.M. and 6:00 A.M., when your circadian rhythms are in sleep mode, or avoid driving at these times altogether.
- Recognize the warning signs of driving fatigue: eyes closing or going out of focus, thoughts wandering, or your car drifting off the road. If you experience drowsiness, you should not be behind the wheel.

Productivity. "Fatigue can impair our ability to work and do what we care about in life," says Patricia Prinz, Ph.D., professor in the department of biobehavioral nursing and psychiatry at the University of Washington in Seattle. Disturbed circadian rhythms put us into slow motion, and everything requires more effort. We hit the snooze button three times, spend an extra 10 minutes in the shower searching for alertness, and down half a pot of coffee before we hit the road—already an hour late.

Once at work, the exhaustion in our bodies affects our minds, making it harder to concentrate. We also feel stressed and out of control when we're tired, so we're less likely to deal with a computer glitch or a troublesome employee with the calm and finesse required.

Relationships. We may exhibit the same irritability toward our families as toward our computers when we're tired. "Fatigue can make you short with your loved ones because you're con-

Amazing Energy
Taking Wing

Phoebe Snetsinger of Webster Groves, Missouri, began bird-watching as a hobby in the mid-1960s, building her skills, enthusiasm, and life list. Throughout her lifetime, she spotted 8,040 of the 9,700 known bird species. She personally saw 85 percent of the world's species, including every bird "family" on the official list. Snetsinger's passion for birding really took wing upon her doctor's proclamation in 1981 that she had incurable cancer and less than a year to live. She survived her cancer but died years later in a van accident, in 1999.

serving your energy," says Dr. Prinz. Our emotional reserves have shrunk and we're less adaptable. We feel as if we barely have enough energy to take care of ourselves, much less worry about others.

Adjusting to Your Own Clock

You don't have to be a victim to your rhythms. There are ways you can control them, instead of allowing them to control you.

Keep an energy diary. "Be aware of your own patterns and when you function best," recommends Cheryl Dellasega, Ph.D., associate director of research in general internal medicine at Pennsylvania State University's Hershey Medical Center. For one day, set the alarm on your watch or pager to go off every hour; then write in your "energy diary" how you feel at that particular time.

Measure your rhythms. Although you can't measure everything yourself (you'd need a doctor, for instance, to figure out hormone fluctuations), you can measure your temperature, says Dr. Moline. Take your oral temperature every hour from the time you wake up in the morning to the time you go to bed. (Don't exercise on the day that you're taking readings, and avoid eating or drinking before taking an oral temperature because both activities raise your body temperature.) Then map the temperatures on graph paper or a spreadsheet, recording each hour's reading. Plot your temperature on the vertical axis and the time of day on the horizontal axis. You may see peaks during the high-energy times you noted in your diary, and valleys during your low-energy times.

So you've mapped your cycles and you know that you have downtimes in the afternoon. Now what do you do? Well, you aren't going to change those downtimes. Just as people's per-

sonalities typically don't change—you have to change how *you* react to them—so it is with our circadian rhythms. You can shift your entire rhythm forward or backward, as when you adjust to a new time zone, but you'll still see the same peaks and valleys throughout the day. What you *can* change is the way you react to those rhythms. If you know you dip after lunch, for instance, don't schedule intense work during that time, or build a 15-minute nap into your daily calendar.

Another tip: Read the rest of this book. It's filled with practical information on maximizing your peaks and preparing for your valleys as well as eliminating the energy-depleting effects of stress and day-to-day life.

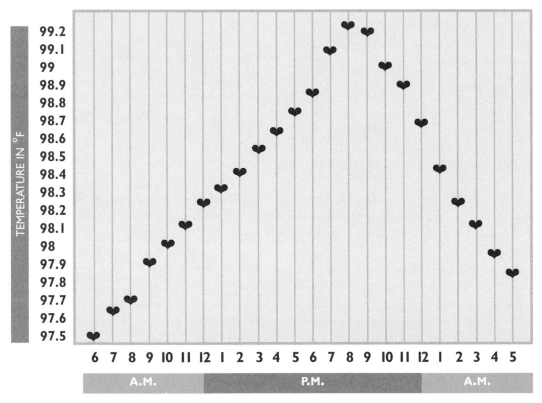

This is an example of what your temperature plot will look like. These are Carolyn's temperature readings over the course of 24 hours.

Exhaustion Only a Woman Could Know

She races along the deserted shoreline, the sand massaging her toes with every step, the rhythmic crash of the waves and squawk of the seagulls a mesmerizing symphony of sound. Off in the distance she spots the silhouette of a young man. She squints, her eyes gradually widening in shock as she draws closer. Can it be . . . is it really . . . Paul McCartney?

Suddenly Carolyn bolts awake, her sheets soaked with sweat. She peeks at the alarm clock, only to find its red numbers glaring 3:12 A.M. with the irritation of a blinking neon sign. Not again! She scrambles out of bed and staggers down the stairs for a glass of ice water. As she rounds the corner, she's startled to see the kitchen light already on. There sits Jocelyn at the table, her head propped on her hand.

"What's the matter?" Carolyn asks, as she holds an ice cube against her steaming skin.

"Can't sleep, Mom." Then the girl glances at her mother. "Why are you all sweaty?"

"Hot flashes. You'll know in 30 years or so. Why can't *you* sleep?"

"I dunno. I usually sleep like a rock. Come to think of it, I've had trouble sleeping a couple times these past few months, and you know, it's always been when I'm on the rag."

"Really? I wonder what that's all about," says Carolyn, as she warms some milk for her daughter on the stove. "Hey, I was having this really cool dream before I woke up. . . ."

Jocelyn sips the warm milk while she and her mother talk about their dreams. They connect. And something good comes of a sleepless night.

Hormones: A Culprit behind Female Fatigue

As Carolyn and Jocelyn have discovered, some of our exhaustion—and disturbed sleep—comes from the very things that make us women. Our hormones.

Hormones do more than prime us for pregnancy and strengthen our bones. They mold us into who we are. They give us our feminine curves, our supple skin, and our high-pitched giggles. In fact, estrogen and progesterone are about the only things that keep us from sitting around in smelly sweats, noshing beef jerky and

WOMEN ASK WHY

Why do we menstruate?

The intended biological function of the female reproductive system is to reproduce. Every month, your uterine lining thickens in response to a rise in estrogen levels. After you ovulate and the egg is released, your body makes progesterone, which helps the lining of the uterus become more receptive to the embryo. If pregnancy occurs, there's no shedding of the lining; if no pregnancy occurs, your hormone levels decrease, the lining of the uterus sheds, and the whole cycle starts all over again. So basically, menstruation's true function is to tell you you're not pregnant.

Women used to get their first period later, have more babies, breastfeed longer, and die earlier—all of which meant they ovulated (and menstruated) less. In fact, up until this century, a woman ovulated only 160 times in her life; today, a woman may ovulate up to 450 times. And many women suffer debilitating premenstrual symptoms like fatigue, irritability, bloating, nervous tension, breast tenderness, mood changes, depression, and increased appetite.

I have some patients with terribly difficult menstrual periods. When they're not bleeding, they feel great. When they have their periods, they may be confined to bed or unable to function at their jobs. For these women, I sometimes prescribe a daily steady-dose birth control pill. They schedule their periods for three or four times a year and decide for themselves when they'd like to menstruate. That way, it doesn't happen when they're on vacation or when they have to give a big presentation at work.

I'm not ready to suggest that every woman stop menstruating for convenience's sake. But as far as we know now, there's no medical reason why she couldn't. I wouldn't recommend this for life, but I think it's okay for a couple of years, after which a woman should reevaluate the situation.

Expert consulted
Samantha Pfeifer, M.D.
Assistant professor in the department of
*   obstetrics and gynecology*
University of Pennsylvania Medical Center
Philadelphia

belching as we watch men in skates fight over a puck about the size of a mayonnaise jar lid.

The challenge is keeping our hormones in check. When they're balanced, we feel as energized as that annoying pink bunny. But they naturally have more peaks and valleys than the Swiss Alps, which can leave us feeling like we just *climbed* the Alps. Fortunately, there are ways to recognize those high and low points, and steps you can take to minimize the energy-sapping valleys.

That Time of the Month

You know it's coming. It has been about 20 days since your last period and you're so sluggish you feel like you're moving in slow motion.

"Most women complain about fatigue the day or so before their periods and the first day or two of their periods," says Ricki Pollycove, M.D., an obstetrician/gynecologist and director of patient education at the California Pacific Medical Center Breast Health Center in San Francisco. We're tired then because of dropping levels of estrogen and progesterone, which affect various other hormones and body systems and processes, including:

- Serotonin. This brain chemical/hormone is involved in sleep, mood, pain, and appetite. Higher levels of serotonin increase the amount of deep sleep we get each night and improve our overall well-being. And higher levels of estrogen support higher levels of serotonin. So when estrogen levels drop, so, too, does the amount of serotonin in our brains. One way to boost serotonin levels is with vigorous physical exercise, says Dr. Pollycove.

- Metabolism. Some women require higher levels of estrogen to keep their metabolisms working at peak efficiency. Since metabolism is what turns food into fuel, if it's running at half speed, so are we. So during our periods, when estrogen levels drop, we're dragging. To find out if you have low estrogen levels, ask your doctor about a saliva test that can be used to measure your hormone levels, Dr. Pollycove suggests.

- Stress hormones. There's a synergistic effect between estrogen and stress hormones, such as cortisol and adrenaline. The more stress we're under, the more stress hormones we release, which seems to plunge our estrogen levels even lower. All the more reason to pencil in a massage just before your period starts.

- Sleep. Progesterone's role in a woman's cycle is to prepare her uterus for pregnancy. But if she's not pregnant, levels drop just before her period, sending a signal to slough off the blood-rich lining of her uterus. In the years before menopause, when our ovaries slow down their progesterone production, sleep

WOMEN ASK WHY

Why is it so hard to fall back to sleep when I wake up in the middle of the night?

If you are waking up at 3:00 or 4:00 A.M. and can't get back to sleep, it's often an indication of depression. Usually, this isn't the "woe-is-me-life-is-terrible" depression, but the "I-have-so-much-to-do-and-can't-get-it-all-done" depression we all occasionally experience. The problem grows when this mental stewing meets with age-related decline in deep sleep. By our forties and fifties, most of us have outgrown the deeper stage 4 sleep and begun to experience a higher percentage of lighter-stage sleep. Add in perimenopausal hot flashes, and you've established a pattern of early morning awakening and insomnia.

Another factor in early awakening is the rapid eye movement (REM) phase, a stage of sleep that gets proportionately longer toward the morning hours. During other phases of sleep, body temperature is controlled the way it would be during the day: When we're cold, we shiver; when we're hot, we sweat. During this stage, however, we lose the ability to control body temperature. So if you've had an especially bad bout of night sweats and you're not awake already, the chill of the wet sheets will almost certainly wake you.

Physical activity between 3:00 and 6:00 P.M. should help prevent you from waking up in the middle of the night. Exerting yourself alerts your brain that your body needs to rebuild its tissues and muscle. When you go to sleep, your brain responds by going into the deeper stage 3 or 4 sleep, where restoration occurs. Without exercise, your brain stops generating stage 3 or 4 sleep as you age. If you have trouble waking up, get your exercise in the early morning hours.

Expert consulted
Donna Arand, Ph.D.
Clinical director
Sleep Disorders Center of Kettering Medical
  Center
Kettering, Ohio

CAN HRT IMPROVE SLEEP?

Imagine going to sleep in Siberia and waking up in Tahiti, and you'll have some understanding of what 4 in 10 peri-menopausal and menopausal women experience each night. These women suffer from sleep interruptions caused by night sweats and sleep apnea. This pattern of repeated waking—up to six times per night, 5 nights a month—can lead to insomnia, fatigue, depression, and other problems.

You don't even have to be in full-fledged menopause to experience night sweats, because sleep is one of the most sensitive indicators of hormonal changes, says Marla Ahlgrimm, a registered pharmacist and president of Women's Health America, a Madison, Wisconsin, pharmacy devoted to women's health issues. "I've seen sleep disturbances start up to 10 years before menopause," she says.

According to studies, hormone-replacement therapy (HRT) can help prevent night sweats and ease sleep apnea. "Your brain is very sensitive to hormonal changes, so that's why we use HRT—it restores the balance, and with it your sleep," says Ahlgrimm, author of *The HRT Solution: Optimizing Your Hormone Potential.* In one study, for instance, the sleeping brain waves of 11 postmenopausal German women were tested with and without estrogen patches. Estrogen improved their rapid eye movement (REM) sleep, reduced sleep interruptions, and improved their slow-wave, deep sleep—the most restorative sleep we get.

After menopause, our sleep is more likely to be disturbed by sleep apnea, which affects one in four women age 65 and older. Some women even develop it by age 50. Again, HRT can help. One study found that when menopausal women who had sleep apnea took estrogen replacement for 3 weeks, they increased their total REM sleep and were better able to get oxygen while sleeping. One theory suggested by study authors is that estrogen may directly influence how the brain regulates breathing during sleep.

There is no age determinant for HRT, Ahlgrimm says. She has seen women as young as 40 benefit from HRT for insomnia. If you think HRT might help you, discuss it with your doctor.

disturbances plague us even more. For some women, using progesterone just before their periods may help, says Dr. Pollycove. It may, however, result in increased water retention.

You might try applying a progesterone cream, available at health food stores, before hitting the sack, suggests Dr. Pollycove. For best results, apply the cream on your abdomen or the inner parts of your arms or thighs. Use the cream every night for the last 10 days of your cycle. (Day 1 of your approximately 28-day cycle is your first day of bleeding.) Or, ask your doctor about a progesterone pill such as Prometrium. This prescription drug works much the same as the cream. However, your doctor may want to measure your progesterone levels first before prescribing progesterone supplements, says Dr. Pollycove.

Moving Into Menopause

Noticed that your sleeping attire has become, ahem, significantly *less* with each passing year? Maybe, it's your love life, but it's just as likely to be your hormones.

The hot flashes so prevalent as we approach menopause result from dropping estrogen levels. During a hot flash, blood rushes to the surface of your skin until you feel like you're standing in a furnace. Not only do you sweat, but your breathing and heart rate also speed up. Experts

WOMAN TO WOMAN

She Has More Energy after Her Hysterectomy

Upon seeking a second opinion for help with her troublesome periods, Linda Mehl, 50, of Alburtis, Pennsylvania, was told she needed a hysterectomy. Today, the pain and fatigue that plagued her for years is gone. This is her story.

When I was 46, my periods started getting painful, heavier, and more frequent. One time my period lasted 14 days. Some days I was so drained that I couldn't even think. The veins in my legs swelled up and I got moody, but I told myself it was a normal part of aging. My first gynecologist thought hormone-replacement therapy would regulate my cycle. Well, it helped with my mood swings, but it really didn't change my periods. I scheduled an appointment with a new doctor at the hospital where I worked. An MRI showed I had cysts in my ovaries and a tumor on my cervix; later, my new doctor found I had endometriosis as well. He ordered a hysterectomy.

I was scared and had to do a lot of praying. But by that time, my uterus was so enlarged, it pushed up everything into my chest area. Believe me, my hysterectomy was a godsend.

After the surgery, I was in the hospital for 3 days. When I came home, my husband and kids had moved our sleeper sofa to the living room so I wouldn't have to climb the stairs. That was so nice. I don't know how people cope without a loving support group. All the sisters from the Catholic hospital visited and brought food. My daughter came home to cook dinner at night. I think my friends' prayers were a big part of my healing.

The doctors said I should take 6 weeks off from work. At that time, I had been working as a secretary in a large hospital, and it wasn't a "sit-behind-the-desk" kind of job. I went back after 4 weeks but stayed in the office and didn't walk around much. For about 6 months after the surgery, day-to-day life was tiring, but strenuous activity really knocked me out. I had trouble walking my mile every day and couldn't swim as many laps as before. My next-door neighbor, who'd also had a hysterectomy, would say, "It's okay, your body's just shutting down to heal. Give it time." She helped me realize that when I sat down and relaxed, my energy would build back up again.

I'm a firm believer in "you are what you eat." I fixed less red meat and more broiled fish and chicken, and really watched my fat intake. I ate smaller meals more often, and that seemed to help my energy level. My doctor also had me on special vitamins, similar to prenatal vitamins, for 6 weeks to build up the iron in my blood.

Two months after the surgery, my doctor told me the tumor on my cervix was nonmalignant. It sounds crazy, but I hadn't even considered cancer—I'd just felt so much better. Now that it's a year later, I have much more energy than I did before the surgery, probably because I don't have those heavy periods.

speculate we get hot flashes because the climate control center in the brain reads the perimenopausal drop in estrogen as a drop in body temperature and tries to warm things up to compensate.

Flashes (or "Baby Boomer Power Surges," as some women call them) are especially prevalent at night because the part of the body that "turns on" a hot flash is sensitive to levels of estrogen, sugar, and alcohol, all of which drop while we sleep, Dr. Pollycove explains.

One solution (other than not drinking before bed) may be low-dose birth control pills, which contain about ¹⁄₅ to ¹⁄₃ the amount of estrogen found in traditional birth control pills, says Dr. Pollycove. They've been found to help with hot flashes, sleep disturbances, fatigue, and PMS symptoms.

Another reason for sleep disturbances as we enter menopause has to do with that traditionally male hormone, testosterone. Just as men's bodies produce the hormone estrogen, our bodies produce small amounts of testosterone. Because our bodies make such a tiny amount of the hormone—1/15th of that found in men—we're very sensitive to any fluctuations. Just a slight drop in testosterone can disrupt our normal rate of metabolism and leave us feeling drained, not to mention less than interested in sex, or, as some women with low testosterone describe it, having a "dead" sex drive.

Our ovaries make about one-third of our testosterone, so if a woman has a hysterectomy and also has her ovaries removed, there will be a sudden drop not only in estrogen but also in testosterone. Many doctors don't know this, and so they fail to warn their patients. If you've had this operation and noticed a corresponding decline in sex drive and energy, ask to have your testosterone levels tested.

Natural menopause, however, may eventually have much the same effect. That's what happened to Susan Rako, M.D., a Boston psychiatrist who, in 1996, brought the often

WHAT DOES "TIRED" MEAN?

Beat. Bushed. Burned out. Used up. Spit out. Spent. We have so many different words to describe fatigue, but what do they *really* mean? To some women, being tired means that they can't lift a finger to wash another dish. To others, it means that they're so cranky they want to sit in their cars and scream at the top of their lungs. Still others define it as not being able to even get out of bed in the morning.

But when we finally go to the doctor, chances are all we say is, "I've been really tired lately."

Fatigue is such a broad term that it's almost useless in diagnosing a condition, says Dianne Delva, M.D., associate professor of family medicine at Queen's University in Kingston, Canada.

Lab tests aren't much better: One study showed that less than 10 percent of laboratory tests for fatigue helped determine a diagnosis. Instead of ordering a bunch of costly tests that don't yield any information, Dr. Delva and her colleagues at Queen's University devised a new way to get to the root of fatigue.

Their revolutionary method? Talking.

Asking specific questions about how fatigue affects your life is the most effective way to help your doctor uncover the problem, says Dr. Delva. "You can run a race and feel fatigued. You can be up all night and feel fatigued. But the cause and the way you feel are quite different in those two situations," she points out.

Many times the problem can be resolved without any further medical treatment, just with minor adjustments in sleeping, eating, exercising, or working habits. In fact, almost half of all women who tell their doctors they're fatigued are actually depressed.

One objective indicator of fatigue is its relation to time.

overlooked problem of testosterone deficiency to the forefront with her book *The Hormone of Desire: The Truth about Testosterone, Sexuality, and Menopause*. She discovered that she had low levels of not only estrogen but also testos-

It's either acute, prolonged, or chronic. Acute fatigue, lasting less than 1 month, is often easier to diagnose, because chances are you know the cause. If you have the flu, for example, you probably wouldn't even mention fatigue to your doctor because you'd already know why you're so tired. Another reason might be pregnancy; some of the more intense fatigue we experience occurs within the first trimester.

Prolonged fatigue typically lasts between 1 and 6 months. Often, women who are depressed will have prolonged fatigue—it doesn't develop overnight, but over a couple of months of worry, sadness, stress, or sleepless nights. The same with hypothyroidism, in which the thyroid doesn't produce enough of its hormone, resulting in low energy levels. If you don't seek help for these conditions, you may stray into chronic fatigue territory—more than 6 months of exhaustion.

Chronic fatigue is definitely not something you should try to cope with on your own, cautions Dr. Delva, since it could reflect a serious health concern. For instance, chronic fatigue could be a sign of type 2 diabetes. Left untreated, it could lead to kidney or heart disease, blindness, strokes, and other health problems.

The message in all this: Be specific, says Dr. Delva. If you're not sure what's making you tired, become a cub reporter and ask questions: *Whom* do you feel most tired around? *What* are you doing when you are tired? *When* during the day or month are you most tired (and how long has it been like this)? *Why* do you think you feel this way? *How* exactly does being "tired" feel?

This information is like gold to your doctor, but if she's not used to asking, she may feel more comfortable with tests. Don't let that stop you—use your gift of gab to get better. And best of all—no needles!

No wonder. Tests showed she had almost no testosterone in her system.

Dr. Rako was 47 at the time and going through perimenopause, the several years of irregular periods that most women experience before periods totally cease. During these transition years, our ovaries not only begin producing less and less estrogen, they make less testosterone as well. What's more, the other significant source of testosterone, the adrenal glands, also produce less as we age.

Further, if we choose estrogen- or hormone-replacement therapy for menopausal symptoms, the treatment actually *decreases* the level of usable testosterone in our bodies even more. That's because estrogen boosts levels of globulin—a substance that binds and inactivates some of the testosterone—thereby keeping a pool of testosterone in our bodies that we can't use. Thus, the more estrogen, the less usable testosterone.

A study at Baylor College of Medicine in Houston found that giving estrogen-replacement therapy to 28 postmenopausal women for 12 weeks caused their testosterone levels to drop 42 percent. On the other hand, several other studies show that women treated with supplemental estrogen and testosterone have greater energy and a better sense of well-being than those treated with estrogen alone. In the past, doctors were reluctant to give women supplemental testosterone because too much could make them feel irritable and anxious, develop facial hair and acne, and increase their risk of developing diabetes and high cholesterol.

terone. Her symptoms appeared gradually over a period of 3 to 4 months. As for her energy level, she says that she felt "flat." "It affected everything," she remembers. "My zip. My zest. My libido."

HORMONE TESTING: TO SPIT OR NOT TO SPIT

There are two ways to measure your hormone levels: blood and saliva.

The major difference between the two tests is that the saliva test measures only "free" hormones, while the blood test checks only for the "bound" form. The hormones that are "free" are the ones ready to latch onto receptors in your cells and make things happen. The "bound" hormones are attached to a substance that removes them from your system, thus rendering the hormones useless.

Since the blood test measures only bound hormones, it may misinterpret your hormone levels as being "normal" despite low levels of free hormones, says Mark Stengler, N.D., director of natural medicine at Personal Physicians clinic in La Jolla, California, associate clinical professor at the National College of Naturopathic Medicine in Portland, Oregon, and author of *The Natural Physician*. So on this front, the saliva test wins.

The saliva test is the new kid on the block, notes Ricki Pollycove, M.D., an obstetrician/gynecologist and director of patient education at the California Pacific Medical Center Breast Health Center in San Francisco. "It got a bad reputation a few years ago because it wasn't very reliable, but they've since fixed that," she says. Still, many doctors would rather use the more tried-and-true blood test.

This is too bad, because a blood test costs about $300, while the saliva test is closer to $110—not to mention that many of us would rather spit into a tube than be pricked with a needle.

"With all of these pluses, I can guarantee you the saliva test is the way of the future," says Dr. Stengler.

Today, more doctors test and treat women for testosterone deficiency, says Barbara Sherwin, Ph.D., professor of psychology, obstetrics, and gynecology at McGill University in Montreal, Quebec. If you suspect a testosterone deficiency is to blame for your fatigue and low libido, find a doctor who's willing to test your hormone levels and, if necessary, treat you with supplemental testosterone.

The Butterfly in Your Throat

Just below your Adam's apple (or Eve's apple) sits a butterfly-shaped gland called the thyroid. Call it the energy gland. It produces hormones that, like bosses who love to micromanage, have a hand in nearly every body system, from your heart rate and body temperature to how fast you metabolize food.

A thyroid that doesn't pump out enough hormones is a common (and often overlooked) cause of fatigue—so common, in fact, that as many as 10 percent of all women may have some degree of thyroid deficiency. In fact, we make up the vast majority of the 11 million Americans with underactive thyroids.

Because of the gland's far-reaching effects throughout the body, an underactive thyroid can cause a slew of symptoms, ranging from fatigue, depression, and constipation to dry skin, hair loss, hoarse voice, sensitivity to cold, muscle or joint aches, and increased menstrual flow.

One of the critical areas affected by a decrease in thyroid hormones is metabolism. So while that extra scoop of ice cream and couch potato habits may indeed be the cause of the extra 20 pounds you're carrying, so, too, could an underactive thyroid. Typically, the hormone "turns on" adrenaline-like parts of cells that speed up the rate at which we turn food into energy. Too little output means it's that much harder for your cells to burn the fuel they need for energy. Ergo, fatigue and weight gain.

The most common cause of an underactive thyroid is autoimmune hypothyroidism, sometimes called Hashimoto's thyroiditis, or Hashimoto's disease, after the Japanese doctor who first described the disorder. The immune systems of women with this condition attack and damage their own thyroid glands, leaving them unable to pump out enough hormones. Autoimmune hypothyroidism tends to run in families, so it's best to know your family history.

An underactive thyroid is also common in women who've had radioactive iodine to treat an *over*active thyroid and those who've had radiation to treat head or neck cancers.

Yet another reason we're more susceptible to underactive thyroids is, you guessed it, another imbalance in female hormones. If your estrogen levels are high compared to your progesterone levels, it can throw off your thyroid hormone levels, says Mark Stengler, N.D., director of natural medicine at Personal Physicians clinic in La Jolla, California, and associate clinical professor at the National College of Naturopathic Medicine in Portland, Oregon, and author of *The Natural Physician*. Called estrogen dominance, it occurs when there is not enough progesterone to balance the effects of estrogen. High estrogen levels sup-

> **JUMP START**
> *Talk*
>
> Call a friend, and then walk around your house or office while you have a cozy, 10-minute conversation.

press thyroid-stimulating hormone (TSH), a messenger hormone sent from the brain to tell the thyroid to make thyroid hormone. If the message can't get through, the thyroid hormone doesn't get produced.

We're also more at risk for hypothyroidism simply because we tend to live longer than men. As with many body systems, the older we get, the less effectively our thyroids work.

Usually, all it takes to diagnose hypothyroidism is a simple $25 blood test called a thyroid-stimulating hormone test. But don't put it off. Hypothyroidism that goes undiagnosed for too long can lead to high cholesterol and increase your risk of heart disease. That's one reason the American Thyroid Association recommends that all women 35 and older have a routine thyroid test every 5 years.

Treatment is also simple: taking synthetic thyroid hormones, perhaps for the rest of your life. Once your doctor determines the right dose, you'll have to get your thyroid hormone levels rechecked about once a year.

Some naturopaths and herbalists recommend kelp supplements to boost thyroid hormone production. Kelp is high in iodine, which can stimulate thyroid hormone production if you have an iodine deficiency, says Adrian Dobs, M.D., associate professor of endocrinology and vice chair of the department of medical clinical research at Johns Hopkins University School of Medicine in Baltimore. But since we get plenty of iodine in our diets (thanks to iodized salt), raising iodine levels won't improve our thyroid function, she says. In fact, studies show *hyper*thyroidism, or an overactive thyroid gland, is much more common in regions where people have diets that are high in iodine.

The Hormone before the Hormone

Erase wrinkles! Live longer! Boost your sex drive! Fight disease!

That's the promise for the "miracle" hormone, the fountain of youth, DHEA. Short for dehydroepiandrosterone, DHEA is a precursor to testosterone and estrogen. Preliminary research is now being conducted to determine what role, if any, DHEA levels play in predicting fatigue, low sex drive, and bad moods. "DHEA and testosterone levels go hand in hand," says Arthur Schwartz, Ph.D., researcher and microbiologist at Temple University Medical School in Philadelphia, who has been studying DHEA for 25 years. You can, in fact, have a decline in testosterone levels and still have normal DHEA levels. So even though your ovaries could be producing less testosterone because you are on birth control pills, are undergoing menopause, or have just had a hysterectomy, your level of DHEA—produced predominately by the adrenal gland—would remain unchanged.

Our DHEA levels are highest when we're in

WOMEN ASK WHY

Why do older women seem to need less sleep?

First of all, the belief that older women need less sleep is a fallacy: You may seem to need less sleep than you used to, but you need the same amount of sleep at any age—about 8½ hours.

In fact, our average total sleep time increases slightly after age 65, but instead of sleeping all our hours in one nighttime block, we break up our sleep in daytime naps and don't sleep as long at night. Daytime drowsiness is not an inevitable result of aging, however. Falling asleep frequently during the day can interfere with your ability to sleep at night. When you feel sleepy, try going for a walk, gardening, or doing other outdoor activities that will help you maintain alertness.

As we age, many things interfere with our ability to get all our sleep at one time. Our sleep/wake rhythms become less distinct. We suffer from bladder problems. We may experience arthritis, osteoporosis, heart disease, heartburn, or any number of medical maladies, all of which affect the quality of our sleep. And if you've ever looked at the instructions that come with your prescription drugs, you know that many medicines can cause drowsiness or sleeplessness, both of which may affect nighttime sleeping. If you think your sleeping problem may be associated with your medication, discuss it with your doctor, who may be able to find a substitute that doesn't affect you so dramatically.

our twenties; as we age, our adrenal glands produce less DHEA. By the time we hit our seventies and eighties, they're producing only 30 percent of what they made when we were younger.

The key to curbing this DHEA decline is to keep your adrenal glands healthy, says Ray Sahelian, M.D., a physician in Marina del Rey, California, and author of *Mind Boosters: A Guide*

Another problem may be advanced sleep phase syndrome. That's when your head starts bobbing in front of the 6:00 P.M. news, but you're getting up before the sun. While there's a tendency for advanced sleep phase syndrome to develop as we age, it doesn't mean you're doomed to this fate. Your best course of action is to spend time in the daylight between 4:00 and 6:00 P.M., keep bright lights on once it gets dark, and try to stay up a little later than normal. Then go to sleep in a pitch-black bedroom. This marked difference in light and darkness will send a signal through your optic nerve to a little pacemaker in your brain—called the suprachiasmatic nucleus—that it's time to produce the sleep hormone, melatonin. This "pacemaker" may develop lesions as we age, affecting our circadian rhythms and sleep/wake cycles. Providing extra clues through lighting helps it do its job more efficiently.

Another reason you may experience sleep problems as you age is lack of activity. If you're sitting in front of the TV all day, you're keeping your body in low gear, so it doesn't know whether it's supposed to be awake or asleep. And, of course, getting exercise during the day will improve anyone's sleep at night—no matter what age.

Expert consulted
Donna Arand, Ph.D.
Clinical director
Sleep Disorders Center of
    Kettering Medical Center
Kettering, Ohio

doctor to check your DHEA levels. If they're low, talk to her about DHEA supplements. In one German study, 24 women whose adrenal glands didn't produce normal amounts of DHEA reported feeling more energetic and less depressed after taking 50 milligrams of DHEA for 4 months.

But don't self-supplement with DHEA. "It's a double-edged sword," Dr. Sahelian says. "DHEA and other hormones available over the counter have benefits, but they can do harm if misused." They could cause irritability, acne, thinning hair, and menstrual cycle changes. "These are all signs you're taking too much or don't need to be taking it at all," he says.

And because we convert DHEA into other hormones, Dr. Sahelian adds, supplementing with DHEA may increase the risk of breast cancer and other reproductive cancers.

to Natural Supplements That Enhance Your Mind, Memory, and Mood. That means adopting a healthy, active lifestyle. No surprises here: Exercise regularly; eat a balanced, low-fat diet with adequate omega-3 fatty acids (found in coldwater fish like tuna, salmon, and mackerel); get enough sleep; and learn ways to reduce stress.

If you do have unexplained fatigue, are depressed, and have a low sex drive, ask your

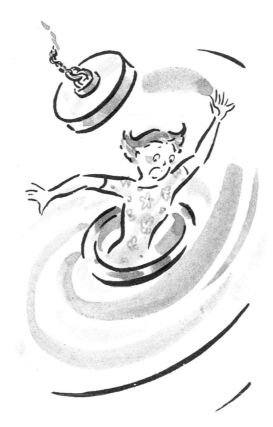

PART TWO

Energy
Drainers

The New Workplace

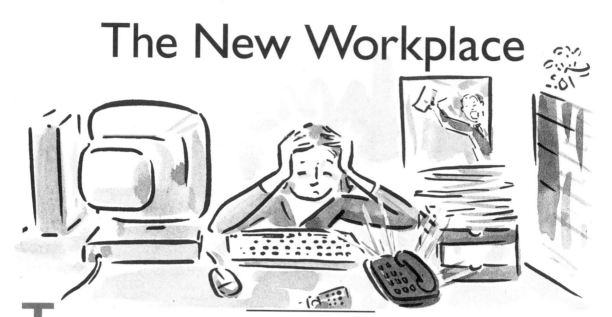

This is the school nurse. Jocelyn is ill. Can you pick her up?"

Carolyn freezes on the other end of the phone. She glances at the pile of work teetering on her desk. "Not today," she moans inside. But, ever the competent mother, she calmly says, "I'll be right there," and hangs up.

She nearly tiptoes into her boss's office, praying he'll be in a good mood. And although she gets the go-ahead to leave, it's accompanied by that suspicious one-raised-eyebrow look she hates. She ignores it. She has no other choice; Ben's away on business again.

On the way home from the middle school, with Jocelyn moaning in the back seat from painful menstrual cramps, Carolyn's beeper chirps. It's her boss, of course, and the terse message on the display tells her to check her e-mail from home and hurry back to the office—he needs the monthly budget compilations immediately. Once home, Carolyn quickly checks her e-mail and gives Jocelyn an ibuprofen fix. Then she's back on the road. She grips the steering wheel with white-knuckled hands as she drives—partially because she's in a hurry, but also because of the mounting pressures of work and home pushing down on her shoulders.

It's a common scenario for millions of working mothers—a never-ending workplace where the traditional boundaries between home and job have blurred to the point of indistinctness. Forget 8-hour days; these days, we're working 24/7.

To escape burnout and maintain excellence on all fronts, we have to take care of ourselves, says Filomena Warihay, Ph.D., president of Take Charge Consultants, an international management training and organizational development firm in Downingtown, Pennsylvania. "The key to success in this rapidly changing business world is knowing what to stop—as well as what to start."

The Workplace of Today

In 1960, a panel of government authorities predicted big changes in the workplace because of budding technological advances. Number one: more free time. Boy, were they ever wrong. Granted, technology has simplified some aspects of our lives—we can talk on our cell phones in the office bathroom and make plane reservations on our computers. But these "conveniences" aren't shaving any hours off our workdays. In fact, they're adding them—we're working 3 hours longer each week than in 1980, we're taking 20 percent less vacation time, and the phrase "leisure time" has been tossed in the backs of our closets like the suits bearing the same name.

"Expectations have changed along with the tools and technology," says Kathleen Conroy, vice president of client relations at xylo.com, a work/life solution provider in Bellevue, Washington. "We're expected to be on call virtually around the clock."

Organizational changes have occurred along with technological advances. Companies are downsizing, temporary employees are replacing full-time ones, and we get raises based on our contributions to company profits rather than our tenure. "The old psychological contract between employer and worker, where the worker gives her loyalty and the employer guarantees long-term employment, is dead," says Dr. Warihay. Today, the employee brings a skill, and the employer provides employment as long as that skill is needed.

"Changes in the workplace are both positive and negative," says Sharon Keys Seal, certified professional business coach and president of Coaching Concepts in Baltimore. "They're positive in that many companies are looking at the 'whole em-

HOW IN THE WORLD DO THEY SLEEP?
The Siesta

For centuries, people in Spanish-speaking countries have embraced the siesta, the nap portion of a 2- to 3-hour midday break designed to refresh and reenergize. It doesn't mean they work less, just that the typical workday begins earlier and ends later, with dinner served around 9 o'clock at night. But this ancient tradition is giving way to the demands of modern life.

In 1999, Mexican officials formally ended siestas for all government employees, forcing them to work regular 8-hour days to synchronize their schedules with North American trading partners. The pressures of a global market and foreign interests have endangered the tradition in Spain as well. The change is known as *semana inglesa* (English week), and it means that the 24-hour-7-day-a-week American influence is taking over.

Although the idea of a siesta for an entire society has probably seen its day, don't count it out completely, says Margaret Moline, Ph.D., director of the Sleep-Wake Disorders Center at New York Presbyterian Hospital-Weill Cornell Medical Center in White Plains and New York City. "Regardless of the culture, we're still talking about sleep need," she says. "Each individual generally needs 7½ to 9 hours each day to be fully functional. How we account for those hours is the variable, especially in these times, when sleep deprivation is more and more common."

Employees who do not get a 3-hour midday break may still get a half-hour rest period. In Barcelona, for instance, a massage and a half-hour nap costs $7 through a chain of siesta parlors called Massages for 1,000.

Even in America, several companies have developed nap rooms and encourage their employees to take catnaps of 15 to 30 minutes in hopes of improving productivity. There have been several studies into the effectiveness of such naps, but Dr. Moline sees an overriding issue. "If you have chronic sleep deprivation, a 20-minute nap won't help you. The goal should be to get the optimal amount of sleep every day. In today's world, that's a challenge."

ployee' and trying to accommodate needs like security, safety, and flextime. They're negative in that employees are expected to work longer and harder."

Workplace changes have hit working women, who now make up about 60 percent of the workforce, particularly hard. Although some women's magazines glorify the woman who made her first million before age 30, jogs and swims daily, has three kids, and works more than 60 hours a week, the reality is that she provides an unrealistic ideal for the rest of us, contributing to our own burnout.

In addition, our values are changing. We're rewarded much less for an afternoon at the zoo with the kids than for a productive day at the office, so it's no surprise many of us choose to devote our time to the latter. The result: less time spent with our families and friends. We're geared away from feeling all right about making other things like our families, friends, health, volunteer work, and vacations a priority, areas of life that are crucial for personal and societal well-being, says Barbara J. Distler, Psy.D., a licensed clinical psychologist in Chicago.

Regardless of our salaries or status, the factors contributing to burnout in working women are remarkably similar.

The I've-got-to-be-perfect factor. Males supposedly feel more stress than females before age 12, but we make up for it from then on. A survey from Northwestern National Life Insurance Company showed that female employees suffer more from burnout and stress-related illnesses than men, and they're more likely to quit their jobs. "Part of the reason for this is that many women grew up in an era when they had to be better than men in the same position to

HOW IN THE WORLD DO THEY SLEEP?
The History of the Bed

According to an Egyptian proverb, one of the worst experiences in life, ranked up there with falling in love with someone who doesn't love you back, is, "To be in bed and sleep not." Hence a comfortable bed is a crucial part of a healthy, happy life. The significance of a good night's sleep has remained constant throughout history, but like so many trends, the bed itself has gone through some major cosmetic changes over the years.

The first documented bed existed in the Neolithic period 10,000 years ago. Not much is known about this bed, except that it was a very primitive model. Almost 7,000 years later, in 3400 B.C., Egyptian pharaohs decided to raise the bed off the ground; King Tut's "mattress" sat atop an ebony and gold bed.

The Romans followed with a luxury bed decorated with gold, silver, or bronze, and a mattress they stuffed with feathers, reeds, hay, or wool. The Romans were also the first to adopt the concept of a water bed; the sleeper lounged in warm water until she was drowsy, and then was lifted onto a mattress and rocked to sleep. Must have been nice.

survive," says Dr. Warihay. "So they confuse perfection with performance."

The dual role factor. At a time when the number of working women is at an all-time high, no equivalent household revolution has emerged to counteract this increase. Nearly one-third of us earn more than our partners, yet still do the bulk of housework and child rearing. Then, too, more working women than ever are single or taking care of elderly parents. "Many women feel conflicted—there are greater opportunities in the work world—and at the same time, there are more family and personal demands on them," says Dr. Warihay. Luckily,

During the Renaissance, mattresses were covered with velvets, brocades, and silks on the outside, and the inside was constructed from pea pods, straw, or feathers stuffed into coarse ticks.

The rope bed was born during the 16th and 17th centuries; the mattress was stuffed with straw or down and placed on a bed frame strung with a latticework of rope. In the late 18th century, it was replaced with the cast iron bed and cotton mattress, which proved less attractive to bugs than previous models. The first coil mattress was patented in 1865, and innerspring mattresses entered the picture in the 1930s.

The Western version of a futon celebrated its 60th birthday in 2000, and we can thank the innovative 1950s for foam rubber mattresses and pillows, and the 1980s for the creative portable air bed.

Despite its brief appearance during the Roman era, the modern water bed didn't emerge in its full glory until the 1960s. At the same time, it was joined by its competitor, the adjustable bed.

Consistent with the "more is better" philosophy of today, space to sleep has replaced the once valued ebony, gold, and silver. King- and queen-size beds are the preferred sleeping item of the 21st century.

adds Conroy, a new generation of young men and dads is sharing more of the housework, but we probably won't see the results of this trend for a while.

The blurry line factor. When we got the laptop on the first day of our new jobs we thought, "What a perk!" But with that perk came a hidden message: "Use me at home." The Internet further expands our workdays—we can connect with e-mail, electronic files, and coworkers around the world at all hours of the day or night. Work follows us home and perches on our shoulders like a pet parrot, its beeping beeper, ringing cell phone, and never-ending e-mail a constant reminder of its presence. "Because it has become so much harder to protect our time away from work, we are at a much greater risk of burning out," says Dr. Distler.

The I-hate-my-job factor. The amount of joy we get from our jobs has a bearing on whether or not we burn out, says Dr. Warihay. Numerous things help or hinder our workplace happiness. Good relationships with subordinates, colleagues, and superiors are important, and even taking a coworker out for lunch to celebrate her promotion can give you a burst. A feeling of control over your job—in which you have a clear picture of what is expected of you, how to do it, and where it fits into the company as a whole—is also important. Stimulating work is an obvious, yet necessary, plus; if you love what you do, you'll be more likely to do it well.

On the flip side, numerous things can jeopardize our job satisfaction. A difficult boss who behaves unpredictably, places you in frustrating situations, and damages your self-confidence drains your job satisfaction faster than a corporate takeover. Shaky job security—not knowing whether your job will be there tomorrow after a merger or acquisition—has a similar effect.

The I-have-a-life-too factor. Women who don't have children are experiencing work burnout too, in part because they are sometimes expected to pick up some of the slack of the working mothers, says Carlla Smith, Ph.D., professor of industrial and organizational psychology at Bowling Green State University in Ohio. For example, the working woman without children has to change meeting times to accommodate the working mother. Hence, she has less

ARE YOU A WORKAHOLIC?

Workaholic tendencies can lead to a vicious circle. "The workaholic refuses to delegate, she wears herself thin, and her productivity suffers," says Sharon Keys Seal, a certified professional business coach and president of Coaching Concepts in Baltimore. Because of this, the workaholic is at a high risk for burnout.

To find out if you are on the road to becoming a workaholic, or if you're already there, check off the statements that apply to you fairly regularly.

_____ I take work home with me.

_____ I put family obligations after work responsibilities.

_____ I feel like the company will go under without me.

_____ I think I can handle any workload, no matter how large.

_____ I would rather do the work myself than delegate it to others.

_____ I feel I can do my job better than others in my department.

_____ I check my e-mail at least every hour when I am at work, even if I'm not expecting an important message.

_____ I work more than 40 hours in a week.

_____ I call the office when I'm on vacation.

_____ I think about work when I'm at home.

If you checked off at least two items on this list, you may be on the way to wearing a workaholic badge. If four or more items apply to you, you're already there. Read over the tips in this chapter on how to tackle work burnout.

time to spend with her friends or family. "There's no longer just the 'dual role' work/family balance—the new area is work/life balance," says Dr. Smith.

The Resulting Burnout

"It's essential to recognize the difference between a 'slump' and burnout," says Dr. Warihay. True burnout is a form of depression, the kind of stress that isn't fixed by a relaxing weekend on the beach.

Burnout also has implications beyond our own lives. "The more we suffer from burnout, the more health and emotional difficulties we'll be faced with as a society," says Dr. Distler.

The signs of burnout include:

Behavioral red flags. Changes in behavior are the earliest signs of occupational stress. In the first stages of burnout, you may begin to avoid coworkers, ignore work responsibilities, pay less attention to your appearance, and make more frequent mistakes. "You may also find yourself becoming irritable, defensive, arrogant, and insubordinate," notes Dr. Warihay. Eventually, dramatic behavioral changes may occur. "You may be a neat person and then suddenly become really sloppy, for example," she says. Or you may find yourself indulging in a nightly cocktail and cigarette after years of not drinking or smoking.

Emotional warning signs. If you can't remember the last moment you had to yourself, you may be on the cusp of burnout. Feelings of being overworked, unappreciated, and out of control at work are additional signals. Difficulties with your spouse or children are another sign. "When you're burned out, you're likely to become anxious, insecure, sad, and preoccupied, and you may no longer get pleasure out of activities you once enjoyed," says Dr. Warihay.

Physical symptoms. Emotional stress affects us physically. For example, stress is a bigger culprit in elevated cholesterol levels than diets high in cheese and eggs. In fact, some tax accountants' cholesterol levels rise sharply just before April 15, then fall back to normal shortly after the tax filing deadline. In addition, if you're burned out, you're more likely to experience frequent illnesses, fatigue, sleep disturbances, changes in appetite, indigestion, headaches, and sexual dysfunction, says Dr. Warihay.

Preventing and Tackling Work Burnout

The remedy for burnout is not as obvious as the problem itself. "Some women decide to quit altogether and stay home," says Dr. Smith. But many of us can't afford that option. And there's always the fear that if we drop out of the workforce, our only option for reentry will be in a lower position.

If you're feeling burned-out and quitting isn't an option, you need to look for other options. "If you wait to the point of illness or depression, you'll limit your alternatives," says Dr. Smith. Here are a few suggestions.

Declutter your workload. Take an objective look at your tasks,

WOMAN TO WOMAN
A Bad Boss Forced Beth to Quit

Beth, 53, an executive secretary from Emmaus, Pennsylvania, left her job after spending almost 10 years working for a boss who made her life miserable. Finally, she could take it no longer, and she got out. Here is her story.

An administrative assistant to the CEO at a large health care retirement community, I didn't feel overworked—workload has never been an issue for me. But my boss was very difficult. She micromanaged everyone, changed her mind all the time, was sometimes hours late to meetings with coworkers and customers, and was dishonest. When I went into work, I never knew what kind of day I was going to have. It was a terrible way to work.

The stress I felt at work affected my personal life. I was often down, and I lost a lot of weight. But I felt like I had to stay. I was a single mom, and my youngest son had cerebral palsy. My work was two blocks from my house, so I knew I could get home quickly if he needed me. I also had a lot of vacation days, so I could take time off to take him to radiation treatments when he got sicker with Hodgkin's disease.

When my son's health deteriorated and I had to take some time off, I didn't hear from my boss once. She showed no support. Then he died. She came to my house and told me to take as much time as I needed. But then when I took her up on her offer and requested 2 weeks off after the funeral, she gave me a terrible time. When I returned to work, she had demoted me in title but not in workload.

Then came my epiphany. I was in charge of planning a trip to New York City for 25 fellow employees. We had a wonderful day—except my boss, that is, whose behavior was awful. Sitting on the quiet bus on the way home, suddenly I thought, "Why am I doing this?" So I wrote my letter of resignation and quit 30 days later without having another job lined up.

Luckily, after a much-needed 3-week vacation to Scotland, I found another job fairly quickly. Today, I feel much better. My new boss is fair and honest. I have no regrets about leaving that job.

JUMP START

Blink

We blink one-third less often when working at a computer, resulting in dry eyes, eye strain, and energy drain. To jump-start your energy, close your eyes and blink several times. If that doesn't help, try eyedrops (but stay away from ones that get rid of the red; your eyes may become dependent on them). And to prevent the problem, make sure that the middle of your computer screen is 4 to 8 inches lower than your eyes (when you look down, your eyelids should be partly closed, which helps keep your eyes lubricated).

and clean out the unnecessary. "Every month, try to stop doing at least two things—no one is likely to even notice," says Dr. Warihay. For example, erase all forwarded e-mail jokes and chain letters before opening them, or transcribe only those portions of the budget meeting that really matter instead of unnecessarily documenting every word spoken. And finish your projects both at work and at home. "Having a lot of incomplete projects is like cosmic constipation," says Dr. Warihay.

List your to-dos. "We feel more energized when we actually get things done," notes Conroy. Start your workday by listing your tasks and how long you have to do them. For example, "I have to make five phone calls and type three reports between 2:00 and 5:00." Then reward yourself with an energizing activity each time you cross something off. When you finish a report, call your spouse or partner to give your brain a change of pace, or grab a quick snack with a coworker.

Exercise for work. "If you ride a bike 5 miles on Sunday, filing on Monday will seem like a piece of cake," says Janet O'Mahony, M.D., a physician in internal medicine at Mercy Medical Center in Baltimore. "But if your most strenuous daily activity is walking to the vending machine, you'll feel exhausted just answering the phones." Exercisers miss fewer days of work, are in better moods, and are mentally and physically healthier overall than their sedentary coworkers. "It's simply being 'in shape'—the more activity you do, the more activity you are able to do comfortably," Dr. O'Mahony says.

Eat for energy. "Your body uses food for fuel, so it will stall on an empty tank," says Dr. O'Mahony. For maximum energy at work, eat something in the morning (even if it's only a piece of fruit or a granola bar). For lunch, a meal brought from home, such as a tuna fish sandwich or stir-fry leftovers from last night's dinner, is usually more nutritious than fast food eaten on the go. And since most of us don't eat dinner until after 6:00, an American version of what the English call afternoon tea is a good idea. "Bring in some fruit or yogurt to eat in the afternoon so you won't be tempted by those leftover stale breakfast doughnuts sitting in the lunchroom," Dr. O'Mahony suggests.

Laugh it off. "Bad days aren't so bad if you can laugh at adversity," says Dr. O'Mahony. This doesn't mean you shouldn't take your job seriously, but it's the woman who can see the hidden humor in a printer paper jam or an unreasonably grouchy coworker who tends to view potentially stressful situations more objectively.

Make friends at the coffee machine. Social support is a major stress reducer at work, and studies show that women with work comrades are absent less often. "Make it a point to rub shoulders with the people at work who energize you," recommends Conroy. Grab lunch with them, or spend a few minutes at the end of the day catching up with one another.

Synthesize your life. "Efficiency means getting more done by doing less work," says Dr. O'Mahony. Have a routine you follow every day. For example, pack lunches and iron clothes the night before, and use that time in the morning to relax and energize yourself with a cup of herbal tea and an engrossing magazine before you leave for work. At work, keep things neat and orderly. Maintain an alphabetized filing cabinet, put your scattered desk papers into piles so your disorganization doesn't stare you in the face, and periodically dust off your work space so you work on a clean slate. "When you're organized, you don't have to waste time looking for things, and you generally do a better job," says Dr. O'Mahony.

Listen to the serenity prayer. "A sense of confidence and competence comes from recognizing the elements over which you have some control and focusing your energy in that direction," says Dr. Warihay. For example, you *can* control how much time and effort you put into preparing a report, but you have no control over whether or not your boss chooses to feature it in her upcoming presentation.

Leave without a trace. Periodic rest and relaxation is very important for a healthy body and work attitude. If you can't afford a vacation to Fiji, try a camping trip or head to the beach—someplace

WOMEN ASK WHY

Why am I tired at the end of the workday even though all I did was sit at my desk?

You're probably not being stimulated enough physically, and, depending on your job, you may not be getting adequate mental stimulation either. Physically, you're sitting in one position for 8 hours, which is fatiguing. You miss out on the periodic increases in circulation you get from moving around. Sitting all day can also lead to pressure on your joints and muscles. And if you're parked in front of a computer for 8 hours, you're straining your eyes, which can make you even more tired.

If your daily tasks are somewhat mundane, you may not have enough mental action to keep you energized. Some managers actually encourage their employees to play computer games like solitaire for 10 minutes or so when they feel psychologically bored. The games help you shift gears mentally, so you can be more productive when you return to the task at hand.

To keep from going home feeling like you've physically moved the furniture in your cubicle (even though you've just sat on it), move around throughout the day. Get away from your desk at lunch and walk around the building. You don't have to walk for an hour every day—just 10 minutes here and there when you get a chance.

If it's not a convenient time to leave your work area, swivel your chair away from your computer and do some stretches and deep breathing. If you have an office mate or two, have one of you lead stretching exercises every hour or so—it will build camaraderie as it energizes you. Or, if your office approves, listen to some uplifting music on headphones while you type.

Expert consulted
Cheryl Dellasega, Ph.D.
Associate director of research in general
*   internal medicine*
Pennsylvania State University's Hershey
*   Medical Center*

where you're not wired to your cell phone or the Internet. Although it's often hard to fit vacations into our busy schedules, "you need to draw the line in the sand at some point, just say no, and go," Conroy says.

The Energizing Work Environment

If our lives sometimes feel like a Dilbert cartoon, it's no coincidence. Studies show that we're in our cubicles for one-third of our waking hours. So make the atmosphere in there as pleasant as possible. Here are some suggestions for sprucing up your cube.

Make it cozy. Put some throw pillows on your chairs. Bring in a small desktop fountain—the gurgling will soothe you as you work. Plants also make a nice addition, and they give off energizing oxygen. "Fresh cut flowers are visually pleasing, and they smell good," says Conroy. So splurge on a bunch, or ask for a weekly flower delivery as a birthday or anniversary present.

Invigorate with color. Warm colors, like reds, oranges, and yellows, provide energy. Red makes our hearts beat faster, and yellow is thought to make us more creative and communicative. In addition, green helps us concentrate. On the other hand, whites, blues, and blacks can have a depressing effect. You probably don't have the freedom to repaint your work space, but you can probably hang an energizing red and yellow poster or painting.

THE FENG SHUI CUBICLE

Feng shui is the Chinese art of placement. Its tenet is that the placement of objects in an environment has a profound effect on the inhabitants. Feng shui has been around for 3,000 to 5,000 years in China, and it's becoming more popular here in the West. We can apply feng shui to our work cubicles to maximize our energy, productivity, and prosperity at work.

Feng shui is based on the same theory as acupuncture: a balance of the five elements—water, earth, fire, wood, and metal. "It involves the flow of energy, called chi, in and outside the environment," says Michelle Sayres, a feng shui and real estate consultant in Greenbrae, California.

In an office or cubicle, the ideal place for a desk is facing the door, catty-corner to a corner of the room. "You want to be able see everyone who enters the doorway, giving you maximum control, authority, and concentration," says Sayres. If you can't face the entrance, place a mirror in such a way that you can see the door. "This restores your power," she explains.

In addition, you want to represent water in your working space in some way because water is the element for career. "You can have a little desktop fountain in your office space," says Sayres. "The sound of the fountain is soothing, too; just make sure the pump isn't too loud and the water isn't making a gushing sound, which can be distracting."

"An aquarium is also a great addition to your work space because the fish symbolize prosperity," says Sayres. But it's critical to keep your fish tank clean and your fish healthy. If a tank has algae, it has a negative effect.

"Water can also be represented figuratively in a free-form shape," says Sayres. Any free-form object will work to symbolize water. You can use a shiny black rock to represent water, because black is the color for water. "You can also use something silver, or a mirror, which has the reflective quality of water," Sayres says.

There's an ideal place for the water symbol in your office or cubicle. "In feng shui, we use a map called a *bagua*," says Sayres. You take the space you're working with and divide it into 9 smaller squares, 3 by 3. As you're looking into the space, look at the 3 squares that are closest to you. The one on the left is knowledge, the one on the right is helpful people and travel, and the one in the center is career. "Ide-ally, you want to have the fountain in the career third—the center imaginary square on the wall with a door or en-trance," says Sayres.

The water symbol will also provide a constant reminder of your career goals. "Feng shui is the unique combination of psy-chology, design, and intention," says Sayres. So if you put some-thing on your desk to represent water and, therefore, career, every time you see the item, whether you realize it or not, it will enhance your career. "It's one more way to condition your subconscious to what you want to achieve," she explains.

Wood is the element for wealth, and plants represent wood, so a plant is also an excellent addition to your work space, says Sayres. Any type or size plant will do, although rounded leaves are preferable. If your back is to the door, a standing plant at the entrance to your office or cubicle can provide protection, so you feel enclosed. "I like to use or-chids," Sayres says. But as with the fish tank, if the plant is not clean and alive, its effect is negative. "A clean, good-quality silk plant is far superior to a semi-dead, live plant," she notes. "While some of this may seem like common sense, it's so often overlooked. Remember, feng shui is a process: Don't expect immediate results, but be happy if you receive them."

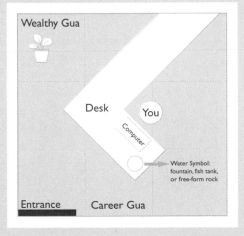

Put motivation in view. Decorate your work space with items that stimulate and energize you, such as paintings, inspirational sayings, and pictures of your family trip to Disney World. Collect meaningful quotes and feature a new one on your bulletin board each morning. "Even using a handmade, interesting pottery coffee mug versus the company-issued Styrofoam cups can make a big difference," notes Seal.

Energize with effervescence. Pleasant fragrances stimulate nerves in our bodies that promote wakefulness. Peppermint and citrus have specifically been shown to increase energy and concentration, for example. So put a little bowl of dried peppermint or lemon rind on your desk, or use some citrus or peppermint essential oils. The diffusers that plug into electrical outlets also provide a nice scent.

Create ideal illumination. "Lighting is a very important piece of a well-designed work space," says Conroy. If possible, you want your light to be on your desk and your task, because lights from above or behind force you to work in a shadow. Ask if the overhead lights can be turned off, and bring in a desk lamp from home, if that suits you better. Lightbulbs that are red-yellow in color are best at boosting mood.

Mold your mood with music. Listening to music while you work can both relax and energize you, says Cheryl Dellasega, Ph.D., associate director of research in general internal medicine at Penn State University's Hershey Medical Center. If you need a boost, plug in some energizing tunes; if

SHOULD YOU QUIT?

You're tired, you're bored, and you think you may be burning out. Should you stick it out or find another job?

The decision to stay or go definitely depends on the situation at hand, says Kathleen Conroy, vice president of client relations at xylo.com, a work/life solution provider in Bellevue, Washington. Some scenarios are toxic and necessitate an immediate change. But if you're considering switching jobs because your company is going through a rough period, or simply out of boredom, you may want to think twice before you jump ship.

Although frequent job changers are usually viewed favorably in smaller start-up and technology companies, larger, more mature organizations look at them with an eye of suspicion.

"The ability to see through challenging situations, overcome obstacles, and creatively problem-solve are all demonstrated by someone's long-term career track within a given company, particularly if in that company you're progressing and being promoted," says Conroy.

Instead of immediately reaching for the Help Wanted ads when you start to feel a little burned-out, first conduct a self-analysis. Think about whether it's your job that's making you unhappy or the way you're perceiving it. "Make sure you've done everything in your control to exhaust the possibilities for improving the surroundings you're presently in, because the grass usually isn't greener on the other side," says Conroy. Both people and the companies they work for go through rough periods. "And organizations are going to trade off problems," Conroy says. So you may leave because you dislike the lower pay in your present job, only to find that a slightly higher salary somewhere else means a whole lot more hours.

How Companies Are Combating Employee Burnout

If you're reading this on the couch in your pajamas, with your pesky work parrot hanging out on your shoulder, try not to get too discouraged—changes are in the works. "Employers are becoming more understanding because they themselves are experiencing the strain of balancing work and home," says Dr. Smith. Some employers offer support services such as life-improvement seminars, on-site child care, and flex-time, and they welcome their employees to come to them with problems. "Although workplace reorganizations may not be happening fast enough for someone in the middle of all this, things certainly are changing. It's the wave of the future," Dr. Smith says.

In the meantime, you can take advantage of what is available to you. For example, if you're having trouble with a supervisor or co-worker, talk to someone in human resources, or ask your boss how you can do a better job, says Dr. O'Mahony. The other thing to keep in mind is that your job is *just* your job. "There are clearly other things that are more important in life," she points out. "If your job was great all the time, you wouldn't be paid to go there."

you're feeling frazzled, soothing music can calm your nerves. Just be courteous of your neighbors and wear headphones if they find your auditory escape distracting.

On the Home Front

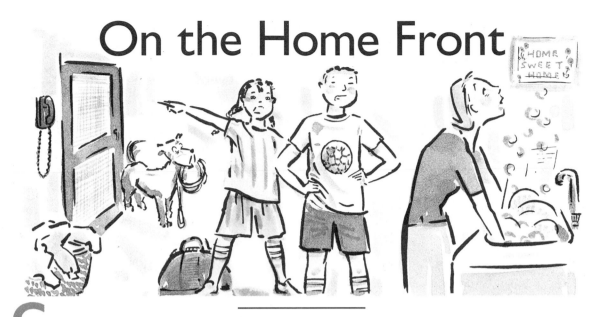

Carolyn glances at her watch, realizing with a start that it's already 5:30. She needs to leave work immediately to get Michael to soccer practice.

As soon as she puts her key in the door at home, however, her stomach begins churning. The blast of rap music that meets her in the living room, coupled with the sight of unwashed breakfast dishes in the sink, is enough to start her head pounding. She yells up the stairs for Michael to turn down the music and get ready for soccer. Then she throws the mail on the ever-growing stack on the hall table and heads for the kitchen, picturing the inside of her freezer and wondering if there is anything in it for dinner. She sets a package of frozen hamburger aside and yells again for Michael to hurry up.

And thus begins her evening.

During the next 4 hours, Carolyn drives to and from the soccer field twice, fixes dinner for the family, cleans up the kitchen, does two loads of laundry, calls her mother to say hello, searches frantically for the permission slip Michael needs for school, and checks Jocelyn's homework, resulting in a tense discussion about why leaving reports until the last minute is a generally bad idea.

By 9:00 P.M., Carolyn is exhausted but still working; she irons Ben's shirts while watching her favorite TV program. She keeps thinking that she should straighten the house, or at least tackle that pile of mail and newspapers, but she just doesn't have the energy.

It should come as no surprise that life on the home front can be even more draining than life in the workplace. If we're lucky, we feel some degree of control at work. The schedule is predictable, our duties and responsibilities are spelled out, the chain of command is clear. And at least we know *someone* is going to empty the trash and vacuum the floor.

At home, it's a different story. The schedule changes daily, no one wants responsibility, and on some days it seems no one—or everyone—is in charge. Plus, our to-do list is endless and repetitive. After all, you never finish washing dishes or doing laundry the same way you finish a report. So for many of us, home life spins out of control, draining us of energy.

"Comfort and engagement at home have diminished to the point that even simple cleanliness and decent meals—let alone any deeper

THE FENG SHUI WAY

Sometimes a room just doesn't feel right. Even if we've moved the furniture around, something about the room still may not suit us. It may be that the room is out of balance and it's time for some feng shui.

This ancient Oriental art is a popular way to harmonize manmade environments, especially your home, says Sophia Tang Shaul, a traditional feng shui practitioner and instructor and co-owner of 168 Feng Shui Advisers of Burbank, California. "When the energy of a house is balanced, it can create better health, better finances, and better relations," she says.

Here are a few general ways to put feng shui to work for you.

Take a minimalist approach. "Nature abhors a vacuum," says Bonnie Primm, a trained feng shui practitioner and adjunct faculty member at Old Dominion University in Norfolk, Virginia. "So we fill it up with things we love, things we don't love, things we've outgrown, things that are outmoded, other people's things, broken things, all kinds of things."

That spells trouble in any home, but in feng shui terms it blocks not only the doorway to your house but also the energy in your life. "Energy can't move beyond the clutter," Primm notes. "But it's more than just the clutter, it's what the clutter takes away from us. It steals our energy because we're worried about it."

Remain in your element. Each of us has a primary element tied to a number based on our birth year. Those numbers also relate to a *bagua*, the blueprint-type chart that is used in feng shui to tell you what areas of your house relate to what aspects of your life. Find your element by adding the last two digits of your birth year and, if the number is less than 10, subtracting it from 10 to get your number. If it's greater than 10, you add the two digits of that number and then subtract from 10. For example, if you were born in 1949, add 4 and 9 and get 13. Then add 1 and 3 and get 4, which, subtracted from 10, equals 6, which makes you a "metal" person.

Number 1 relates to the element water; 2, earth; 3, wood; 4, wood; 5, earth; 6, metal; 7, metal; 8, earth; and 9, fire. Certain colors, shapes, and traits are associated with each of those elements, and each person has a primary number and two secondary numbers.

Knowing your element is a beginning toward balancing your home. For instance, an earth person who lives in a very square house, with square rooms and furnishings, may need to soften things up with some round or arched shapes.

Here are some feng shui remedies to try.

Use mirrors, the aspirin of feng shui. Mirrors represent water. They balance its lack in many rooms. They also can bring in something a room

satisfaction—are no longer taken for granted in many middle-class homes," writes author Cheryl Mendelson in *Home Comforts: The Art and Science of Keeping House.* "Homes today often seem to operate on an ad hoc basis."

Our home life has contracted, Mendelson says. As we clean less, cook less, and entertain at home less, we risk losing the knack. Increasingly we become strangers in our own homes and lose that sense of solace that a home provides.

But you can bring your home life out of chaos and clutter. In the next few pages, we'll show you how to establish a peaceful home, a home where you and your family go to regroup, relax, and refresh.

lacks, through reflection, or can reflect out something you want to exclude. For instance, if you have an unfriendly neighbor, hang a mirror so that it reflects back toward his house.

Hang some crystals, mobiles, or chimes. When these items are hung in places where there isn't enough light or air, they provide movement and stir up good energy.

Use colors that support you. Neutrals will generally calm, while certain colors, like red, empower us and lift our energy. Too much red, however, can take energy away. In fact, anything taken to excess is not good.

Pay attention to shapes. If you have a very square room with very square furniture, consider angling your furniture to break the lines and maybe using an oval rug and a round table covered with a soft, flowing cloth. Or, if a room has too much wood, consider adding some metal to cut it, such as a brass planter.

Add an aquarium. The glass and water represent the water element; the square shape is earth; the stone pebbles represent metal; the plants are wood elements; and the fish are fire. Ah, perfect balance.

Dispose of certain symbols. Unless your life needs a little stirring up, you'll probably want to get rid of tempestuous symbols, such as pictures of fighting or storms or fiery scenes. Instead, use symbols that take you to a peaceful place, such as seashells gathered on a restful trip to the beach or a picture of a couple of beach chairs or a mountain stream.

Light the way. If there are rooms where you want more energy, use more light—natural, artificial, or reflected. If a room is too energized, lessen the light.

Position for power. In the bedroom, the bed should face the door yet be as far away from the door as possible.

Keep work and rest separate. Don't set up a modern office in the bedroom, because the more you plug in, the more energy is circulating, and the more tired you'll feel.

Pick up some plant power. Plants such as pothos, philodendron, and snake plant are particularly good for absorbing electromagnetic energy, while pointy plants that come down break up energy and may not be desirable in a creative, energized environment.

Create some kitchen cures. We need the fire of the kitchen stove to nourish us, so the stove should not be next to the refrigerator or sink, which represent water and could extinguish our fire energy. If they are adjacent, put a piece of red tape between them for separation.

Exorcising the Expectation Demon

There are actually researchers out there who get paid to study housework. (Bet they don't have any dust bunnies under *their* beds.) Thanks to them, we have actual studies to back up what we've known in our guts since we got married: We do more around the house than he does. About 60 percent more, according to one Ohio State University study. In fact, women list housework as one of the leading causes of fatigue. Overall, we're doing two-thirds of the household work, ranging from cleaning the house to scheduling the kids' dentist appointments.

Why, then, do our standards still include such things as a sparkling refrigerator and weekly dusting? Who actually sees the inside of our refrigerators? Are we bad mothers if there are fuzzy things in the back and spilled juice on the shelves? Of course not. So listen up, ladies: It's time to jettison the June Cleaver image and the guilt that accompanies it.

"You have to get rid of the idea of perfect and best and adopt the idea of 'this works,'" says Margaret Sanik, Ph.D., a time allocation expert and associate professor of consumer sciences at Ohio State University in Columbus. "The first thing you have to realize is that the world doesn't fall apart if all those expectations are not met."

Focus on what really matters to your family. When Dr. Sanik first married, for instance, she folded her husband's socks and underwear. "Why'd you do that?" he asked her. Now she concentrates on the things that are appreciated, like home-cooked meals.

If your children would be just as happy with slice-and-bake chocolate chip cookies as with made-from-scratch ones, don't knock yourself out making the from-scratch ones. If you're the only one who ever sees the upstairs bathroom and you don't mind showering in a gritty bathtub, leave the cleaning for next week. Dr. Sanik also has never made it a habit to check her children's homework, and she still has two straight-A students. But, she cautions, one size won't fit all; know what works for your family.

Other expectations to jettison:

- Polishing silver. Keep it under wraps so it doesn't tarnish.

- Drying dishes. That's what air is for.
- Balanced meals. Every meal doesn't have to have a vegetable and a starch. It doesn't matter when you get your five fruits and veggies a day, just so long as you get them.

WOMAN TO WOMAN
She Left Her Family to Find Herself

Norma Graham, 51, of Lincoln, Massachusetts, married her college sweetheart at age 21. After 13 years, they had their first child, Lauren. Norma took a couple of years off, then returned to work as a Spanish teacher, had several devastating miscarriages, and, 7 years later, had another daughter, Jillian. About that time, Jack started his own company, and soon after, Norma's parents died. Her secure world crumbled. Her loss of identity and depression became so great that, at age 47, she temporarily left her family to find herself. Here is her story.

When Jack began his business, we had some rough times. After the birth of Jillian, I went back to work sooner than I wanted to, because we needed the health insurance and there was so much anxiety and risk involved.

A year into all of this, my mother became ill with a series of debilitating strokes. My parents lived in Florida, and my father cared for her for 3 years in their small condominium. It took a lot out of all of us. After she died, he was determined to live on his own. He did for 2 years, but it was with a giant hole in his heart that I tried to fill but couldn't.

In the meantime, my oldest daughter turned 13. We are Jewish, so it was time for her bat mitzvah. My daughter chose to dedicate her speech to her Opa, her grandpa. On the day he was to come here, he had a heart attack and wasn't able to travel. We limped through the whole thing. The next day, I flew down, but he had another heart attack. I stayed for 8 weeks caring for him until he died.

For 2 years, I was in a fog. It was like my stability had been ripped out from under me. I had a fear that I was going to die before I could do some things I wanted to do. I asked my husband if I could do two things—study at Harvard and go on an archaeological dig. He agreed.

I attended Harvard to study Spanish, linguistics, and archaeology for a year, after which I found an archaeological dig taking place on the island of Mallorca off the coast of Spain, in the Mediterranean. I left home a scared, nervous, depressed heap of middle-age anxiety, trying to get some sense of myself and where my life was going. I was filled with self-pity and fear and pressure and worry.

Finding Roman artifacts was thrilling beyond belief. Some were 2,000 years old, and we found pottery that traced back to the Bronze Age. It was a lot of hard work. We had to walk a mile or so through an olive grove filled with goats, and up and down steep cliffs. We dug all day in the hot sun. What a total departure from my suburban mommy life.

I discovered a lot about myself. It gave me time to look at what I had. Missing my father would never go away, but the depression eased. I realized that I was a lucky person, and I really had a wonderful life.

Before that trip, I had never cultivated *me*. I was always helping my husband or being a teacher or being a mother or being a perfect daughter. I learned that I could go to school and be successful, and that I could learn something just because I wanted to. The dig proved that I could pick an adventure and make it work. It gave me a sense of strength and self-worth and independence that I had never taken the time to discover. Part of me wanted the adventure to go on, but by the end of the experience, I couldn't wait to get home.

Now I look at my beautiful photographs and think of the peace of sitting on the veranda overlooking the Mediterranean and the long walk down to the water and the steep climb back up. How primitive it was and how glorious!

- Fund-raising. Forget selling candy and gift wrap for the PTA. Write a check instead.
- Ironing. You have four choices: Don't buy clothes that need ironing; get everything dry-cleaned; pull clothes out of the dryer when they're still slightly damp; accept the wrinkled look.
- And the golden rule of lowered expectations: If it isn't dirty or can't be seen, don't clean it.

Escaping from Housework Hell

Unfortunately, there's only so far you can go with your new, lowered expectations before you hit rock bottom and a dirty, messy house becomes more of an energy drainer than cleaning it would be.

You have two choices: Hire a housekeeper or enlist the family. If you choose the first, you can skip down to the next section in this chapter (and write the Great American Novel in your free time). Otherwise, join the rest of us in learning how to delegate. Start with the fruit of your loins.

"Mothers who feel like they have to do everything for their kids are really burdening themselves," says Catherine A. Chambliss, Ph.D., psychology professor and department chair at Ursinus College in Collegeville, Pennsylvania. And they're not doing their kids any favors. By the time our children are teenagers, they should know how to cook, clean, do laundry, and, in general, have control over and responsibility for most aspects of their lives, she says. "We should view the development of independence as one of the prime goals of mothering," Dr. Chambliss says.

And don't go light on the boys. A Swarthmore College study shows that the chore gender gap—the difference between the time girls and boys spend on housework—doubles from 2 hours to 4 between the freshman and senior years in high school. That leaves more time for the boys to spend on extracurricular and leisure activities. And we already told you about the disparity between the housework you do and what your husband does.

To get the kids and your husband to do their fair share, you first have to get their attention. You can try the civilized way of setting up a meeting and calmly explaining the facts of 32 loads of laundry a week, two bathrooms to clean, and a dog that hasn't been bathed since your high schooler was in diapers. Request a second meeting if necessary. If, by the third meeting, your family still doesn't catch on, a more dramatic approach may be required: You could go on strike, or picket the house. Somehow, says Susan Schenkel, Ph.D., a clinical psychologist in Cambridge, Massachusetts, you need to let them know the ways they're making it needlessly hard for you and how they can help you. "You won't always have immediate success, since you're dealing with human behavior, and change can take time, but it pays to be persistent."

Now that you have their attention, where do you start?

Share the responsibility. When it comes to household chores, the more consistent you are as a parent, the quicker your kids will comply, says Deniece Schofield, a home-management consultant and author of *Confessions of a Happily Organized Family.* Routine household chores teach a child about responsibility, family, participation in groups, and many other valuable life skills.

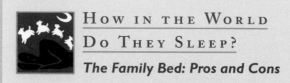

HOW IN THE WORLD DO THEY SLEEP?

The Family Bed: Pros and Cons

Since we're already getting as few as 6 hours of sleep a night, why would any woman invite her kids into bed with her?

Some mothers say that having their babies sleep with them and their partners actually results in more sleep. Instead of getting up to feed their babies, especially when nursing, they can just let the baby feed while they doze. And with the parents only an arm's length away, the baby doesn't have to scream and fully awaken to get their attention, so she's easier to get back to sleep, says Aletha Solter, Ph.D., developmental psychologist, founder of the Aware Parenting Institute in Goleta, California, and author of *The Aware Baby.*

Some families go beyond the baby stage in cosleeping, however, using a family bed until their kids are age 3 or older, says Dr. Solter. That's fine, she says, as long as it feels right. Proponents of the family bed say it's a safe way to bond with a child. Most children are comfortable moving to their own beds sometime between ages 3 and 8, but they should still be given closeness at bedtime if they request it.

Others disagree. In 1999, the U.S. Consumer Product Safety Commission warned parents not to sleep with their babies. Between 1990 and 1997, they reported 515 infant deaths linked to sleeping in adult beds, 121 of which resulted from an adult rolling on top of the baby. Other deaths resulted from suffocation between a mattress or other object, from lying face down on a water bed, or from strangulation in headboard rails.

Even a 2-year-old can pick up her toys. Starting with young children, have them spend 5 minutes a day straightening their rooms. Then they won't have those whiny hours on Saturday trying to find that one particular action figure or doll they absolutely must have. If you start your 3-year-old sorting laundry, by the time he's 11 or

Other critics charge that inviting kids into your bedroom is immoral, but Dr. Solter says that's nonsense. "If you want to be intimate, there are other rooms in the house," she notes. "And there is no evidence that child sexual abuse is more common in families that cosleep. In fact, I suspect that it might even be less common."

To ensure a safe family bed, Dr. Solter recommends the following rules to anyone who shares a bed with an infant.

- Avoid drinking alcohol or taking tranquilizers or anti-depressants before bed.
- Never smoke in the room where your infant sleeps.
- Use a firm mattress, not a water bed, feather bed, beanbag chair, or couch.
- Keep a tight fit between the mattress, headboard, and wall, and use a bumper pad around the edge of the bed.
- Never put your infant on a pillow.
- Always lay your baby on her back to sleep.
- Do not sleep with your infant if you are extremely obese because you are at risk for inadvertently smothering her.
- Keep pets and stuffed animals out of the bed.
- Tie back long hair so your infant will not become entangled in it.
- Do not let your infant share a bed with another child unless an adult is between them.
- Do not place your infant near curtains with dangling strings.
- Never leave a baby alone in an adult bed.

12, he should be measuring out the Downy and spraying stain remover.

By the time your child is 8 or 9, you have an official extra set of hands at your disposal. Children can vacuum, dust, set and clear the table, help with preparing a meal, unload the dishwasher or wash the dishes, and clean a bathroom.

Once they hit their teen years, they can do almost anything (involving housework, at least) you can do.

Schedule it. Recognize that housework is an infinite task. If you don't make a schedule and stick to it, you'll never get free. For example, do laundry 1 or 2 days a week and don't worry about it the rest of the time. Let everyone in the family know the schedule to eliminate constant interruptions from someone looking for clean socks, Schofield recommends.

Appoint an assistant. In large families, name young assistants for a week to help with chores such as laundry, kitchen duties, and yard work. This person can also be the designated go-fer. Rotate the duties and post a schedule.

Create a card file. To enlist her children, organizing guru Barbara Hemphill of Raleigh, North Carolina, wrote each household chore on an index card and assigned it points, based on difficulty and desirability. For example, vacuuming the family room might be 5 points; feeding the pets all week, 10 points, and cleaning the bathrooms, 15 points. Each child had an envelope with his or her name on it and points assigned based on age and ability. The children chose which tasks they wanted to do each week to reach their assigned points and put those cards in their envelopes. If the tasks weren't completed by noon Saturday, the child lost TV privileges for a week. "One of the reasons it worked was it gave the kids so much control over what they did and when they did it—and the kids monitored each other," says Hemphill, author of the *Taming the Paper Tiger* books.

Create a chore chart. This can be as simple as a handwritten, color-coded chart that divides chores among family members and lists daily, weekly, and monthly responsibilities, or it can be a fancy spreadsheet. Rotate chores weekly or monthly so no one tires of them. Check out the Internet site www.shiftschedules.com to download a free weekly family chore spread-sheet.

Be absolutely, unequivocally clear. This is obviously necessary with young children, but no less so with teenagers, who are better than Bill Clinton at skating along the edge of the truth. Tell a 13-year-old to wash the dishes, and he'll likely wash *only* those dishes in the sink, not the ones on the counter or table. Nor will he wipe the counters or clean out the sink. Write it out, if necessary, but don't leave it open to interpretation.

Make it a family affair. Some chores are more tolerable if tackled together. Host a clothes-folding session where everyone folds clothes while watching a favorite video or TV show. Designate a time of the day or week, such as 5 minutes before dinner, when everyone puts away anything left out of place that day. Or establish a Sunday night pickup-party, when everyone goes around the house putting away the weekend detritus and finishes up with a bowl of ice cream. You can use TV commercials for a little cleaning or straightening competition—who can pick up all their things first, clean a mirror quickest, or empty all the trash cans on one floor before the program resumes?

Create a ransom box. Kids won't clean up?

At the end of the day (or week), collect every wayward object in sight and stash the items in a box or bag. On Saturday, the owners may regain possession by doing a chore or paying a ransom for each item they reclaim.

On the husband front:

Put it in writing. The more you nag him, the less likely it is that he'll do what you want. So make a list on Friday night of every chore you both need to accomplish on the weekend, sign up for the ones you can handle, and get him to sign off on the ones he can do. He may not take on as much as you'd hoped, but at least he has

SEX: THE SUPER ENERGIZER

For many of us, sex is just one more thing to squeeze into a busy day. But it's worth the effort, says Linda De Villers, Ph.D., a certified sex therapist and psychologist based in El Segundo, California.

"Although it will take a little time and energy to be sexual, bothering to work it into your busy schedule can have its benefits by helping you maintain a sense of sanity and balance in your hectic life," Dr. De Villers says.

When a couple has been married awhile, continuing to make sex a priority vitalizes the marriage as well as the body. "It's an excellent alternative to the energy-zapping possibility of a straying partner," she notes.

On the physiological side, when we have an orgasm, there is a definite release of tension, Dr. De Villers says. Our bodies produce endorphins, the so-called feel-good hormones that are the body's natural painkiller, leaving us a little euphoric.

Our bodies also release the hormone oxytocin during sexual orgasm. A preliminary study at the University of California, San Francisco, suggests oxytocin is associated with maintaining healthy relationships and healthy psychological boundaries, both of which could have energizing effects. Social situations, as well as sexual, may induce oxytocin release, and the presence of the hormone may make good relationships more rewarding. Women in the study who were in committed relationships released more oxytocin in response to positive emotions than did single women.

And, let's not forget an added bonus: Sex is exercise—good for the heart and the muscles. Research indicates that from both a biological and a psychological standpoint, the principle of "use it or lose it" gains in importance as we get older, Dr. De Villers says. The uterine wall thins if postmenopausal women stop having sex, and the effects may begin in their forties, during perimenopause.

On an emotional level, sex improves our self-esteem and increases our intimacy and communication with our partners, says Barbara Bartlik, M.D., clinical assistant professor of psychiatry at Weill Medical College of Cornell University in New York City.

The question is when to find the time. Dr. De Villers recommends setting aside time to make it a nourishing experience. A warm shower or bath can help a busy woman make the transition, and a nap can be the perfect finish.

Or try oral sex. You don't have to do much if you are on the receiving end; just lie there and enjoy it. "You can let go of tension, if you focus on it, and it's likely to be a stress buster," notes Dr. De Villers.

signed on to the team. An added plus: You'll get better response from the kids if you present a united front.

Play to their strengths. If you're married to your own personal version of Tim the Toolman, who's a klutz when it comes to hammer and nails, but who earns a good living, is willing to run errands and chauffeur the kids, and gives you foot massages every night, count your blessings and stop feeling like a martyr for doing things you're good at. You may be surprised at how much more cooperation you get once you quit nagging.

Housework Hints

Now that you have your workforce organized, there are ways to get the job done faster and better, leaving you with more energy for the other 20 things on your to-do list (like sleep).

Assemble supplies. Keep a tote of cleaning supplies in a central location on each floor of your home, near where they'll be needed. For instance, every bathroom sink should be stocked with bathroom cleaner, glass cleaner, paper towels, and a sponge, and the hall closet should have dusting spray and rags. You can pick up a cheap vacuum cleaner at a garage sale for the upstairs.

Stop dirt at the door. Encourage family and friends to leave their shoes at the door, and keep a handy basket nearby. Put a couple of mats on both sides of doors leading to the outside to trap dirt.

Simplify bedding. A comforter instead of a bedspread saves valuable seconds on bed making each morning. After you wash sheets, fold a matched set and store it inside a matching pillowcase. That way, there's only one thing to grab when it's time to change the sheets.

Separate laundry once. Once a week, put three laundry baskets in the hall and have all family members sort their laundry by colored, whites, and delicates. When the laundry is clean, pile each person's into an individual basket, leave it in that person's room, and forget the agony of putting away laundry (until you need the baskets for next week's loads).

Line wastebaskets with grocery bags. If you're using plastic bags, keep a few extras stuffed in the bottom of each wastebasket to make for quick changes.

COLOR YOUR WORLD

Certain colors are associated with certain moods, and a fresh coat of paint can work wonders. Is the kitchen always the most chaotic room of the house? Try blue for a more tranquil, leisurely atmosphere. Family room dark and sunless? Make the most of existing light and warm the atmosphere with white, off-white, or yellow. Cozy up a large, cold room with rich, warm colors like burgundy.

Consider the language of colors:

Pink: Soothes and promotes affability and affection

Yellow: Cheers and energizes

White: Energizes, unifies, and, in combination, enlivens other colors

Black: Strengthens and encourages discipline (maybe try this in your teenager's room?)

Orange: Cheers and stimulates appetite and conversation

Red: Stimulates and dramatizes

Green: Balances, refreshes, and encourages emotional growth

Purple: Comforts, spiritualizes, and encourages intuition

Blue: Relaxes, refreshes, and promotes peaceful moods

Make a sock drawer. Designate one drawer for all the white socks in the house. Then just throw them in, unmatched, and let people pull them out as needed.

Clutter Control

You can have the cleanest house in the world, but if there are piles of clutter everywhere, you're never going to reclaim your lost energy. The problem is moving beyond that there's-so-much-to-do-I-feel-so-overwhelmed-so-I-just-won't-do-anything feeling. When you're feeling like that, the piles grow larger, the clutter grows thicker, and the confusion looms larger. Yet if you spent just a few minutes up front taking care of the little things, like sorting the mail, filing the bills, and cleaning the closet, you could recover an extra 6 days a year that researchers estimate are spent looking for misplaced items.

"Physical clutter is not an irrelevant detail," Dr. Schenkel notes. "People vary in their tolerance of clutter, but if you have limited time and a lot to do in it, you want to have a house that's streamlined."

Clutter is a sign of postponed decisions, says Schofield. In some homes, it's a flashing neon sign, constantly reminding us that our lives are out of control. But you don't need to be a neat-freak to want some element of order in your home. The more organized you are, the more time you'll free up for spontaneity and stress-reducing fun, our ultimate goal. To that end, we've created the *Prevention* Decluttering Plan. With a little upfront time invested—one weekend ought to do it—and some new habits, you can reclaim those lost 6 days and do something really important with them—like lie on a beach.

Streamline your stuff. Like a good weight loss plan, decluttering your life takes preparation. Organizing guru Hemphill sums it up in her mantra: "Have nothing in your home that you do not know to be useful, think to be beautiful, or love." Yet much of what we hang on to are things we think might be useful or valuable *someday*, such as clothing you'll wear when you lose 20 pounds, memorabilia from trips you would rather forget, flower vases for fresh flowers you never have. In the meantime, these things get in the way of real life and suck up pre-

cious time. Hemphill remembers severe floods in North Carolina in
1999, and how easy it was for people
to look in their closets and cabinets
and share things with people who
needed them. Do that on a continual basis, and life gets simpler.

You certainly don't need to wait
for a flood to declutter your house.
Start with one room, three boxes,
and a trash can. Put things you must
keep in one box, things you want to
give away, sell, or donate in the
second, and things you aren't sure
about in the third. You know what
to use the trash can for. Move
quickly. If you aren't sure about
something, put it in box three.
When it's full, seal it and store it.
After a year, if you haven't needed
anything in it, get rid of it (but don't
open it or you risk becoming reat-
tached).

Here are some questions to ask
yourself as you sort.

- Is it a duplicate? After all, how
  many whisks, spatulas, coffee
  makers, and plastic containers
  do you really need? Must you
  have bags and bags full of other
  bags?
- Can I easily find the item or information somewhere else if I
  get rid of it?
- Am I keeping this because I
  think it will become valuable? If
  so, find a collector now and get
  rid of it. It probably won't be very valuable
  in your lifetime anyway.
- Is this a family heirloom? If so, see if there's
  a family member you can pass it along to. If
  you plan to will it to someone, consider

doing it early to avoid battles after you're
gone.

- Is this souvenir really worth saving? Sometimes a picture and a few words in an album
  will suffice.

- Am I keeping this because I don't want to offend the giver? If the giver must know, be honest and say that it doesn't fit your lifestyle and you passed it along to someone who could really use it.
- What's the worst possible thing that could happen if I don't save this item? This works with everything from clothes and kitchenware to books and papers.

Look forward, not backward. Don't try to catch up on years' worth of filing and sorting. "Today's mail is tomorrow's pile," Hemphill says. If you start by trying to deal with the backlog, you'll never catch up. Move it out of the way and set up a system to start from where you are today.

Now you're ready to move on to maintenance.

Toss as you go. Keep a box in every closet of every room. When something doesn't fit or breaks, or you think you could live without it, drop it in. When the box is full, decide what you'll donate and what you'll throw away.

Fill a treasure chest. Put another box in each closet marked "treasures" to hold all those keepsakes that can quickly take over a dresser or desk.

Recycle. We're not talking about putting out the cans and bottles for the trash man. We're talking about those piles of magazines you just can't bear to throw away because they seem so much more substantial than newspapers. Donate them to a hospital, nursing home, or day care center, or just bring them into work and put them in the coffee room for the taking.

Free your refrigerator. Get a three-ring binder for each child and some plastic sheet protectors. Put each child's name on the outside,

---

TAMING THE PAPER TIGER

Use the following tips from organizing guru Barbara Hemphill of Raleigh, North Carolina, author of the *Taming the Paper Tiger* books, to help gain control of those mounds of paper accumulating in your house.

- Always open mail by the trash.
- Pay regular bills, utilities, and loans with automatic transfers.
- Slow the tide of junk mail coming into your home. Use the Direct Marketing Association's Mail Preference Service. The trade organization will notify its 4,600 members that your name should be removed from its mailing lists. Be sure to include the names of all members of your household. But keep in mind that this won't stop local junk mail or the ever-burgeoning number of new companies sending out bulk mail. Write to: DMA Mail Preference Service, PO Box 9008, Farmingdale, NY 11735-9008. They also provide a similar service for telemarketing at DMA Telephone Preference Service, PO Box 9014, Farmingdale, NY 11735-9014. You can also check out the ideas at www.stopjunk.com or www.privatecitizen.com.
- To curb offers from credit cards and other financial companies, contact the Opt-Out Service, run by major

---

then let them fill it with their special artwork and stories, class pictures, awards, report cards, and other memorabilia that typically clutters up your refrigerator, bulletin board, and walls. For bulky art projects, take a Polaroid picture and include it in the book. Arrange the photos by grade in the binder.

Set up a center. Quick! Where's your birth certificate? This month's electricity bill? Your dog's shot records? Not sure? Then you need a paper management system, which is really just a fancy way of saying you need to put all your important papers in one place. It could be a desk in the kitchen, or an actual study, but you should keep it convenient to the heart of the house,

credit agencies, at (888) 567-8688. The service allows you to remove your name from the list of names pre-screened for credit offers by the four major credit reporting agencies. You can opt to have your name removed for 2 years or permanently. This may not stop all the offers you'll receive, but it should reduce the influx.

- Never file a permanent change of address form with the post office, because the postal service sells its lists, and your junk mail will follow you. It's better to send your own change-of-address post cards.

- Don't enter sweepstakes or respond to surveys or contests, because those, too, will get your name on more lists.

- Don't send back warranty cards; your warranty begins when you buy the product. The only reason to return a card is to find out about product recalls. If you do return it, fill out only your name, address, and product's serial number. If you check that you're interested in other products or services, you'll be sure to hear from other marketers.

- Look for boxes to check on magazine subscriptions, credit card applications, bills, and other forms that allow you to opt off of mailing lists.

which is typically the kitchen/family room. Gather a file cabinet and folders, telephone, office supplies, calendar (paper or electronic), clock, stamps, wastebasket, and recycling box. Set up three trays for sorting: "in box," "out box," and "to-file box."

Get the picture. Photographs seem innocent enough, but they quickly morph into a pack rat's worst enemy. Somewhere along the way we got this idea that we have to organize pictures perfectly—labeled and in scrapbooks (if you still feel this way, go back and reread "Exorcising the Expectation Demon" on page 47). Maybe you could keep up the first year of your first kid's life—before she walked—but by the time she's old enough to wear a bra, you're probably drowning in thick packets of photos. Try this: Scrawl a few notes on each envelope of pictures when you pick them up. Then put them in a shoe box with no lid. At the end of the year, put the appropriate pages from a calendar in the box with the photos, providing notes to refer to.

File it where you need it. If you can't remember the last time you saw your kitchen table or counter, get a portable plastic file box for the kitchen. It holds about 15 hanging files and can organize things like takeout menus, tickets and invitations to upcoming events, coupons, papers you need to sign, and correspondence to answer. Used in combination with a calendar, it can clear a lot of clutter and save a lot of time.

Keep a calendar. The refrigerator remains the central posting place for many families because, sooner or later, we all go there. A family calendar, an erasable memo board, and a magnetic refrigerator caddy for papers that need signing or immediate attention can all be posted on family central. If the kids have something that requires parental involvement—such as a sports practice or baking for school—make a rule that if it's not on the calendar, you're not obligated to drop everything and take care of it. Calendar codes, such as P for Pending, can remind you to check the hanging file box for more information.

Create and use a personal planner. "It's absolutely my brains on paper," says Schofield. "It really takes the pressure off if you put everything in one place." Start with a planner or custom design one using a small, loose-leaf notebook. Include yearly and daily calendar

---

JUMP START

Run

Hit the stairs and run up and down them until you feel your blood flowing.

---

pages, birthdays and other significant dates, important phone numbers from business contacts to contractors, family clothing sizes, project ideas and notes, and a pouch for short-term papers, such as directions, coupons, or tickets. The notebook will evolve over time depending on your own personal needs, but don't hesitate to add things such as wallpaper, fabric, and paint samples; committee notes and phone lists; reading lists; and memorable thoughts and quotes.

Carry a waiting bag. Fill a bag with things you never seem to have time for and carry it with you, so you can tackle them in bits and bites while stuck in traffic, watching baseball practice, or waiting in a doctor's office. You can include such things as bills to pay; bank statements to balance; reading material for work, school, church, or pleasure; invitations and announcements; thank-you notes; stationery; greeting cards; and craft projects.

Conquering Kid Chaos

Ever feel like your mail ought to come to you in care of your minivan? That you spend more time shepherding your kids to activities than you do sleeping? No surprise. A 1997 study by researchers at the University of Michigan's Institute for Social Research shows that children today have 75 percent of their weekday programmed, an increase from 40 percent in 1981. That means only 6 hours of free time now, com-

pared to 9.5 hours 20 years ago. Of the children studied, more than half of their time was spent playing organized sports.

This dramatic change in family life is largely related to mothers working outside the home, says Sandra Hofferth, who coauthored a study on how children spend their time. And while she is careful not to make judgments about the changing pace of life for kids, her study supports the impression that kids (and moms) are leading more hectic lives, with time carefully parceled out among school, afterschool care, sports, ballet, karate, piano, horseback riding, and "play dates," with less time for pure play and family meals and conversation.

In this era of unprecedented wealth and fast-paced culture, it's harder for parents to slow down and set appropriate limits on the family's expenditures of time and money, says Dr. Chambliss. Families with two working parents sometimes feel like they have to buy the latest of everything and sign their kids up for every available activity to make up for the lack of time together, she explains. Sometimes, she says, it's easier to buy another new computer or let them play another sport than to expend the emotional energy explaining why it's not necessary—or not going to improve their lives. In families where there's a single breadwinner, parents may feel apologetic about their lack of wealth and make unreasonable personal sacrifices in order to keep up with their neighbors. Bottom line: No one puts the brakes on, and home life becomes a frenetic race between activities and taking care of *things*.

Slow down and make sure your priorities are in the right order. Ask yourself:

Are we doing what's important to us? Many female clients who come to Ruth Klein, a clinical psychologist and owner of The Marketing Time Source, say their families are important, but their schedules tell another story. They are rarely home, and when they are home, everyone is so busy running in different directions that there is no family time.

"What you role-model is what others perceive is important to you," Klein says. Her three children always knew their activities were important to her by the amount of time she spent attending their soccer, tennis, and volleyball games and theater performances. Similarly, her family's nutrition and health are important, so she spends time shopping for and preparing healthy foods. Conversely, Klein preserves time for her family and herself by paying $10 for a courier service to deliver packages across town, or $16 to hire a college student to assist with the family dinner on Friday evenings. The student arrives near the end of dinner, makes coffee, serves dessert, and cleans the dishes and kitchen floor—while mom enjoys her family.

Are we doing too much? You need to periodically appraise your family's extracurricular activities. If your son is crazy about a particular sport, group, or lesson, and you like socializing at the events and watching him develop, it may be worth the time. But if he's ambivalent and you resent the effort or expense, it may be time to drop it. Even if he likes the activities, if you're stressed by overcommitments, you need to establish priorities.

Why are we doing this activity? Don't assume that just because the neighbor's child is participating in three activities, those three things will be good for your child. An introverted child may need more time to herself to explore the world in her own way.

Further, don't take on the responsibility for exploring these questions alone, says Dr. Sanik. "It's everybody's job to be a happy, well-adjusted family," she says. "Kids learn about family life at home, and you don't want your kids to learn that it's mom's responsibility to do all this stuff."

Even if you set a rule, as many parents do, of one extracurricular activity at a time per child, if you have three children, things are still going to be pretty hectic—especially when you add chores, schoolwork, and birthday parties. To help with the chaos, try using planning sheets just for the kids. These include each child's weekly household chores, sports and other lessons, social activities, and any recurring or big school projects. File them in your hanging file or a family organizer notebook. Then, when a child asks to add something to her schedule, tell her to check her planning sheets. It breeds an atmosphere of family cooperation and mutual responsibility, Schofield says.

Transitioning between the First and Second Shifts

If you think evening rush hour describes the drive home, you haven't entered a house with kids just before dinnertime.

But before we get to the food part, we need to focus on the relaxation part. And it should start before we ever step foot in the house.

Use your drive time. On the drive home from work in the evening, instead of fretting about traffic or what went wrong with your day, think ahead to how you can organize your evening and carve out a niche for yourself. Decide what you can accomplish that evening, and when it's done, promise yourself you'll take some true downtime.

Delay dinner. We rarely take the time for cocktails anymore, but there's something to be said for that pre-dinner relaxation. "Most moms have this fantasy that as soon as they get home from work, they need to produce great meals for their families," says Alice D. Domar, R.N., Ph.D., a Harvard Medical School psychologist and director of the Mind/Body Center for

Women's Health, Mind/Body Medical Institute; and author of *Self-Nurture: Learning to Care for Yourself As Effectively As You Care for Everyone Else.* "The last thing you need to do is walk in and start cooking." Take a breather. It may be 5 minutes in a quiet place; a 30-minute walk alone or with your dog, spouse, or kids; a glass of wine or a quick nap in a hammock. It should be something to get you out of your work mode and ready to relax and reconnect with your family. With a quick, healthy snack, the children can wait a few minutes for dinner.

Focus on what's good. Seventy percent of what happens to us each day is neutral, 15 percent is positive, and 15 percent is negative, but we tend to focus on the bad, says Dr. Domar, who looks for ways in her own life to counteract this tendency. For example, when she walks through the door in the evening, Dr. Domar asks everyone who is there to tell her what happened new or good in their day. The "New or Good" game forces everyone to look at their day in a different way by focusing on the positive.

Create a sacred space. We need a place to sit and calm ourselves, a place to shift out of the stress of ordinary activities and get back to ourselves, says Judith Orloff, M.D., a Los Angeles psychiatrist and author of *Dr. Judith Orloff's Guide to Intuitive Healing: Five Steps to Physical, Emotional, and Sexual Wellness*, who lectures on the interrelationship of medicine, intuition, and spirituality. It may be a table with a candle, incense holder, flowers, a bowl of fruit, or other favorite objects, or it may be as elaborate as an altar. It should be a place

TECHNOLOGY: ENERGIZER OR ENERGY ZAPPER?

It's a rare purse or minivan these days that doesn't sport a cell phone. Even our kids are carrying beepers. And half of all Americans use computers, up from 36 percent in 1993, according to a 1999 U.S. Census Bureau survey.

While technology has simplified some tasks for us, it has also blurred the boundaries between home and office and made our home lives a maze of multitasking, says Helen Seltzer, president and chief operating officer of MessageClick, a high-tech unified messaging service.

Technology can become tyrannical, placing more demands on our already limited time and energy, cautions Susan Brace, Ph.D., a medical psychologist in private practice in Los Angeles. Some psychologists argue that we live so fast in this technological era that we don't live at all. We stand on the sidelines talking business on our cell phones, rather than reveling in our children's achievements. We retreat to our home offices to eke out a little more work, rather than spend time with our families.

Used with restraint, however, technology can be a godsend to the energy- and time-starved woman. "The key is to have and use technology at our demand, not to let technology gone crazy make you 'on demand,'" Seltzer says.

Women want technology to help them gain control of their lives, Seltzer believes, which primarily means the ability to be in contact with family members at any time. Knowing where our children are and being able to reach them whenever we need to gives us a sense of control over our lives, and thereby energizes us.

that's all our own, away from the hustle and bustle of the household. Spend at least 5 minutes there when you get home from work, just sitting and breathing.

Managing Mealtime

Most experts agree that eating dinner together strengthens the family. Early on, it's important to

There are three keys to successfully integrating technology into your life, Seltzer says: It must be simple, provide information on demand, and be mobile. Mobility is particularly important to working mothers. On any given day, less than 30 percent of executives are mobile during the workday, while 70 percent of working moms are, she notes.

Here are a few ways today's wired world can make our lives easier.

- Bank online, including having your paycheck directly deposited and bills automatically paid.
- Shop online, having gifts wrapped and mailed directly to the recipient, saving you hours in long post office lines.
- Stay connected. Studies show that women use e-mail more than men to communicate with friends and family. To a large extent, it has replaced letter writing and phoning, because it's quicker than letter writing and not as intrusive as phoning, Seltzer says.
- Cut down on clutter. Spend a weekend entering addresses, telephone numbers, birthdays, anniversaries, and other annual events into your computer, in addition to time-saving lists such as instructions for house sitters and what to pack for holidays. Draw up a sample grocery list you can print out each week and keep on the refrigerator, circling each item that's needed. Or register dates. You'll never miss another birthday or anniversary if you take advantage of free Internet reminder sites, such as www.rememberit.com, which e-mail you with reminders.

teach young children table manners and to instill family values and rituals, but the lessons and benefits don't end there. Communication is one of the main ingredients of the family meal, and it's also a key to raising emotionally healthy children, according to the National Safety Council. Ticklish topics—such as peer pressure and schoolwork—are more easily approached across the dinner table.

One study found that teenagers categorized as well-adjusted ate with their families an average of 5 days a week, while poorly adjusted teens ate with their families only 3 days a week.

The study didn't discover just what it is about family meals that helps teens deal with the pressures of adolescence—just that they do. If your family rarely has meals together, think about clearing some time.

Coordinate schedules to keep several nights a week clear, and if you can't clear enough nights, try breakfast some days. But it doesn't count if you keep your nose in the newspaper or eyes on the television.

Having family meals does require planning. And at 4:00 P.M. every day, 60 percent of us still have no idea what we're fixing for dinner.

The key is planning ahead.

Make a list. Once a month, list your family's 15 favorite (and easiest) meals, shop for the ingredients, and put them in a designated place where they won't be gobbled up before you need them. Then post a list of menus on the inside of a cupboard door and, each morning, decide what to make that day, depending on what's going on with the family. Set out the recipe, and whoever gets home first starts dinner.

Delegate, delegate, delegate. Assign each member of the family (depending on age and ability) a particular night to cook. No complaining, however, if they don't have a green vegetable or if they serve the same thing every week.

Retire the short-order cook. Too many of us fall into the trap of cooking different meals for everyone in the family. We'll spend all night preparing, serving, and cleaning up food to accommodate various tastes and schedules. If someone must miss a meal or refuses to eat what's served, let that person fend for herself—that's why microwaves were invented.

Have the basics. In addition to such staples as cooking oils, vinegars, sugar, flours, canned milk, herbs, and spices, your pantry might include such things as pastas, sun-dried tomatoes, canned tomatoes, tuna, anchovies, olives, chickpeas and other beans, salsa, refried beans, taco kits, rice, soy sauce, hoisin sauce, plum sauce, bean sprouts, and water chestnuts. Freezer standbys include frozen vegetables such as green beans, corn, peas, and spinach; pita bread; butter; frozen waffles; ginger (simply slice off a frozen piece); bags of chopped onions and peppers; packaged, deboned chicken breasts and other meats; sausages and bacon; and extra cheeses.

Prepare as you put away. Just back from the grocery store? Before you stash that ground meat in the freezer, toss it into a frying pan and brown it, then freeze it for quick additions to spaghetti sauce or casseroles. Wash salad greens and store them in a plastic bag in the refrigerator; grate cheese and freeze in bulk; chop some onions and green peppers and freeze in plastic bags; and clean and cut up veggies and fruit for snacks and lunches.

Think double. It takes about 6 minutes to throw together one meat loaf; it takes 7 minutes to make three. With just an extra minute, you have two meals in the freezer. Dovetail processes as well as dishes, such as using the food processor to shred cheese for tonight's tacos,

QUICK DINNERS

Here are a week's worth of quick dinners (complete with shopping list) that can be prepared in about 20 minutes using canned, frozen, or otherwise partially prepared products.

Shopping/Pantry List

Meat/Poultry/Fish:
Pork loin chops
Boneless chicken breasts
Frozen, peeled shrimp
Salmon steaks

Produce:
Asparagus
Bagged salad greens
Broccoli florets
Fresh vegetables for pizza topping
Seasonal fruit

Other:
Spice rub or marinade for pork

Couscous
Sun-dried tomatoes
Vinaigrette dressing
Pasta
Pine nuts
Canned chicken broth
Frozen vegetables for stir-fry
Bottled stir-fry sauce
Rice
Prepared pizza crust
Sesame seeds
Udon noodles

Dairy:
Parmesan cheese
Eggs
Milk

cabbage for tomorrow's coleslaw, and carrots for vegetable meatballs.

Cook for leftovers. Consider a week in the life of a roasted chicken. Cook two or three at one time, and after the first night, you can use leftovers in chicken curry; tossed with pasta and broccoli; on an open-faced chicken, avocado, and tomato sandwich; in quesadillas or burritos; mixed with veggies for a quick frittata or omelette; and, finally, cut up and made into soup, using the carcass for stock. Similarly, a large batch of meat loaf does yeoman's duty as the makings for manicotti, meatball stroganoff, stuffed grape leaves, and, of course, meat loaf

Meal Plan

Sunday: Grilled pork loin chops with prepackaged spice rub or marinade (cook enough for leftovers), quick-cooking couscous, and grilled asparagus, marinated with salt, pepper, olive oil, and lemon

Monday: Leftover pork thinly sliced atop a salad made from prewashed, bagged greens, sun-dried tomatoes, and a vinaigrette dressing

Tuesday: Pasta with deboned chicken breasts (chopped), prepackaged broccoli florets, and pine nuts in a sauce made from a canned chicken-stock base, topped with grated Parmesan cheese

Wednesday: Use the leftover pasta (chicken, broccoli, and all) to create a frittata, mixing it with eggs, milk, and more Parmesan and cooking in a frying pan until firm

Thursday: Frozen shrimp, Oriental vegetables, a bottled sauce, and rice make a delicious stir-fry

Friday: Take a night off and let the kids throw some toppings on a prepared pizza crust

Saturday: Make a quick meal fit for company with pan-seared, sesame-encrusted salmon, Japanese udon noodles, and a fruit salad, using a couple of seasonal fruits, with some of the salad greens and vinaigrette left over from Monday

sandwiches. Even extra mashed potatoes can be recycled into potato puffs, potato pancakes, or shepherd's pie, or used as a thickener for soups and sauces.

Make it snappy. Don't hesitate to use some prepared or partially prepared foods to make life easier. There are more and more high-quality convenience products out there, including bags of vegetables that need only the addition of some ground turkey to make a nutritious stir-fry.

Never run out. Always have a running shopping list, accessible to the whole family. It's even more efficient to have one set up by cate-

gories. Schofield suggests: breads and cereals, canned goods, convenience foods, dairy and eggs, frozen foods, health and beauty aids, household and miscellaneous, meat, produce, and staples and condiments. To take it a step further, organize your list according to your grocery store's layout; many stores will give you a guide.

Shop smart. For must-have, non-perishable items such as toothpaste, shampoo, and detergent, always buy two. When one runs out, add it to the shopping list; it saves emergency runs to the store.

When It's Time to Pay

So you've evaluated your priorities, delegated the heck out of everything, and decluttered and organized until your house echoes, but you're still dragging.

Maybe it's time to hire help. "If you're working 60 hours a week and you don't want to be seen as a nag, you follow the organizational lead and outsource—get someone else to clean," says Dr. Chambliss. "It's the way to go in two regards. First, you're getting assistance in liberating time for more important activities. And it can help you detach a little from the whole emotional issue. If you get outside help, it's no longer your thing."

Decide what chores you'd most like to dump—and do so. Hire a housekeeper, a gardener, a cook, a courier service, a chef, a caregiver, or a college student. Even if you can't afford a weekly housekeeper, it'll give you a big energy boost to hire a couple of college students to help with the annual spring cleaning.

There are many professional organizations geared toward personal needs, such as the National Association of Professional Organizers. For an hourly fee, a pro will help you sort through the clutter that has become your life and get you started on a new, less time-consuming track. (Call 512-206-0151 or visit their Web site at www.napo.net.)

Similarly, the United States Personal Chef Association provides resources on another fast-growing profession—catering to the time- (and energy-) starved. With a click of a mouse or a phone call, you can hire a personal chef to buy groceries and come to your home once a week or so and fix meals to your liking, to be frozen and thawed when you need them. They'll even freeze individual portions for families in which everyone eats on a different schedule. Call (800) 995-2138 or visit their Web sites at www.uspca.com or www.hireachef.com.

Low on cash? Swap meals with a neighbor, organize car pools, even grab a friend and clean each other's house together—the work will go faster and be more fun.

And fun, after all, should be part of life on the home front. "If you're not having any fun, find some."

Relationships: Turning Sappers into Sustainers

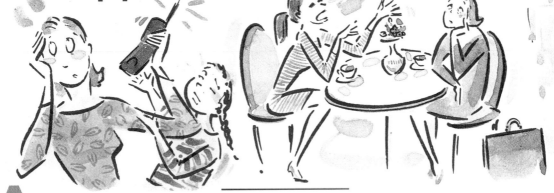

As Ben climbs into bed, Carolyn rolls her back to him. "Not tonight," she thinks. It's a familiar feeling; sex is the furthest thing from her mind most nights. She feels guilty over her lack of desire and sad for the loss of passion in their relationship. Although she still loves Ben, these days, sex seems like just one more item on her increasingly long to-do list.

Plus, she ended up hosting the book club tonight for the 3rd month in a row. Somehow, the group seems to know that she'll offer to play hostess when no one else will. She doesn't mind too much because it's one of the few times she's able to enjoy her women friends. But it also means rushing home from work to clean up the house and make dinner for eight people.

And today, of course, her boss decided at 4:45 P.M. that he wanted her to stay late to get some contracts in the mail. With her annual review just a month away, she just didn't feel in a position to argue, especially since she's hoping for a promotion and a raise. Ever the good employee, she pasted a smile on her face and said, "Sure, no problem."

There's no question that the care and feeding of the people in our lives require a tremendous amount of time and energy. Too often, we focus only on meeting everyone else's expectations and ignore our own needs, which leaves us spent. Yet if we could learn how to balance what we give with what we get from our relationships, the people in our lives could actually turn into energy sustainers instead of energy sappers.

"Relationships can be extremely energizing if there is mutuality, if we *allow* them to be two-way rather than trying to be the source of all giving," says Maria M. Mancusi, Ph.D., a clinical psychologist in Springfield, Virginia.

Sapper or Sustainer?

While men are usually defined by their achievements, women seem to be defined by their relationships. Helping others and being available to listen and provide support is a central role in our lives.

Think you're immune? Take a pencil and paper and jot down all of the roles you fill during an average week—wife, mother, daughter, friend, employee, chauffeur, tutor, housewife, boss, neighbor, church volunteer, social coordinator—the list goes on.

"There's a big debate about how all these relationships affect our energy levels," says Simone Ravicz, Ph.D., a psychologist in Pacific Palisades, California, and author of *High on Stress: A Woman's Guide to Optimizing the Stress in Her Life*. Some experts believe that we have a limited amount of energy and that the more roles we perform in life, the less energy we have—like a pie that gets cut into smaller and smaller slices. It's a concept that psychologists call the scarcity theory.

Dr. Ravicz, however, has another view. Tackling multiple roles boosts our self-esteem, while a strong social-support network actually increases our energy levels. This theory is called the enhancement hypothesis. "The mere fact that you have several roles doesn't mean in and of itself that you'll have less energy," she says.

It's a hard concept to grasp, especially since so many of us end up feeling like a limp dishcloth by the end of the day. The difference, says Dr. Ravicz, is how many energy drainers we've integrated into our roles and relationships.

Stress. Studies show that while men stress out over infrequent events like loss of income, we stress out over everyday events that involve those close to us. We worry about our best friend's divorce. We stew over an unreasonable request from the boss. We wonder how long an ailing parent will be able to manage independently. All of this mental caretaking drives up our stress levels, wearing us out physically and mentally.

WOMAN TO WOMAN
She Learned to Say No

Therese Hadley was everybody's yes-woman. Chronically overcommitted, the 45-year-old working mother of three grown kids from Los Angeles said yes to everyone until she burned herself out and finally learned how to say no. Here's her story.

I have a tendency to want to help people. In my job as an inventory control specialist, I'm known for my willingness to help out. Coworkers would frequently show up at my desk with questions about new procedures. And instead of turning them away, I usually walked them through each step of the process. The problem was, I often helped so much that I ended up doing the other person's job in addition to my own.

Then, people at work started coming to me for help with personal problems—financial problems, marital problems, kid problems. I became the office sounding board. But taking on everyone else's problems soon began taking its toll on me. I started to feel very tired. Even simple activities like doing the dishes seemed to wear me out. I'd do something and then I would need to rest. Instead of going out to play bingo with my friends, I sat at home on the couch.

Too much give, too little take. We become drained when those around us make constant demands but give nothing in return. "Women are socialized to give, give, give," says Dr. Ravicz. "Our socialization has trained us to feel obligated to be responsive to the needs of others, even at the cost of our own. We're not socialized to draw boundaries, so we end up giving too much." The irony is that by spreading ourselves so thin, we often end up disappointing the very people we're trying to please. And because of social conditioning, we feel guilty when we reach out for support. The answer, says Dr. Ravicz, is

One day, a coworker confided that his wife was dying of cancer, and asked if I'd help him find a facility to care for her. I made several calls and found information about several nearby nursing homes. Later, he asked if I would go to the facility to help him sign the papers. Unable to say no, I did. A month later, he came to me with another request. He had brought his dying wife home and needed help caring for her. Would I help by coming over and changing her clothes?

I realized then that I just didn't know how to say no. I said to myself, "What's wrong with this picture?" I had tried to be all things to all people and in the end, nobody, especially me, was satisfied. Ultimately, I became emotionally and physically exhausted. When people came to me for help I said, "I'm having a bad time; I've taken on everyone's problems, and I don't have the energy anymore."

I also realized it was time to get professional help for my yes-woman syndrome. After spending some time in counseling, I've learned that the art of managing my relationships with others actually starts with managing myself. For instance, I've learned how to draw boundaries. Before I say yes to any request, I ask myself, "How is this going to affect me as a person?" These days, when coworkers ask for help doing a job, I simply give them the information and tools they need and stay focused on my own job.

the superficial relationships in our lives, we spend too much time with our masks on; there's no time to be authentic," says Dr. Haber.

Biting our proverbial tongue. The minute we start denying, repressing, or suppressing our feelings to those we're involved with, our energy is drained. It's like driving a car with one foot on the accelerator and the other on the brakes. "If you don't express how you feel, then you wind up covering up the feeling, and that takes energy," says Dr. Haber.

Your husband asks if you would mind having a colleague over for dinner tomorrow night. You think to yourself, "No way! I have such a long day tomorrow; I don't want to do it." But instead of saying that, you say, "Oh, sure."

As women, we're socialized to be agreeable and "nice," so we usually go along with a request even if it makes us angry, uncomfortable, or resentful. By not voicing how we feel, we limit our options, explains Dr. Haber. If you said to your husband, "Tomorrow is a busy day for me, I don't know if I can do this," then the two of you can work out a compromise. Maybe you can go out for dinner instead, or schedule it on another night.

Not spending enough time alone. The most important relationship is the one you have with yourself. An hour or even a half-hour of by-yourself leisure time each day is a necessity for refueling your energy, not a reward for completing all of your tasks. That means spending quality time taking a walk, meditating, reading, or even soaking in a hot bath. As long as you enjoy it, the activity will energize you, says Dr.

to remember that healthy, life-sustaining relationships are a two-way deal.

Lack of intimacy. Ironically, a lack of close relationships with our spouses and partners as well as our friends can be just as draining as a plethora of them, says Sandra Haber, Ph.D., a New York City psychologist who specializes in women's issues. Intimate relationships help balance our emotional bank accounts by giving us time to just be ourselves. They are the few special relationships in our lives in which we feel comfortable seeking out as much support as we give. "When we spend all of our time tending to

Haber. The key is to plan for it, not to just wait for free time to appear. Usually, the only way to create time for you is to take it away from some other activity.

Learning to Give and Take

There is nothing that drains your energy more than trying to change another person's behavior. In fact, it's draining for both of you. The path to energizing your relationships is more a matter of shifting your own perceptions, reevaluating your own expectations, or redefining the way you communicate, rather than expecting others to change.

"It's an American myth that you should always tell someone when you're upset with them to try to get them to change," notes Karen Fingerman, Ph.D., assistant professor of human development at Pennsylvania State University in University Park. "That may be good advice for some married couples, for example, but not for every relationship." Instead, you need to focus on changing how you perceive or react to the other person. By making one positive change in each of these relationships, you can get what you want: more energy.

Agree to Disagree with Your Mother

Accepting Mom for who she is seems to be the key to easing mother-daughter tensions, according to Dr. Fingerman's research. She's found

WOMAN TO WOMAN
The Death of a Marriage

The happily-ever-after part of the marriage ceremony is something that Linda Oberdorfer, 42, of Allentown, Pennsylvania, believed in with all her heart, right through 10 years of a failing marriage. But when the sleepless nights and exhaustingly frustrating days became too much, she gave up and filed for divorce in 1997. Here's her story.

I got married forever, I thought, like my parents did. So when there were problems, we went through marriage counseling. I think women tend to want to fix things, so it took a long time for me to see that there are things that just can't be fixed. Being in a failing marriage is like rowing a boat upstream; you never get anywhere, no matter how hard you work at it. All of my energy was going into a relationship that was not going to work. No matter how "perfect" I tried to be, no matter how clean the house was, or how fabulous dinner was, it was never enough.

The mental and physical drain of trying to keep everything together and "just right" is exhausting. So is the face you wear in public. I smiled when I felt like crying, and that was exhausting work. Finally, I knew I had to emotionally separate.

My then-3-year-old son and I moved 1,100 miles away from Florida back to my hometown. But it was very difficult for me to readjust to single life. I worried whether I had done the right thing by leaving my husband and if I could face the future without him. It took 9 months before I felt strong enough to get a full-time job.

I kept it together for my son; I didn't want my child to see me turn into an emotional wreck. But it was very tough, and my friends and family couldn't help. It wasn't until I found a good divorce counselor, someone with no emotional attachment to my situation, that I realized every woman has

that in the most positive mother-daughter relationships, the daughter is able to view Mom's annoying traits as simply that: annoying traits, not deliberate acts designed to drive her crazy.

to deal with divorce in her own way. It was very difficult for me to admit failure. My marriage had failed. And when I moved back to Allentown, I left everything behind except for our clothes. I was starting over completely. I had left my home, my husband, and my stuff, and I really felt adrift. I was very afraid that I couldn't support my son and myself. I've always been an independent sort, and to be so dependent on others was upsetting. I also felt overwhelmed at the prospect of raising my son alone and taking care of all of the day-to-day things like laundry, shopping, and child care. I just didn't know if I could manage it all. I was really lacking self-esteem. The last few years of my marriage seemed to have taken all the fight out of me.

The experience allowed me to come to terms with the course my life had taken and to grieve for the death of my marriage. Professional counseling allowed me to see that I didn't have to do it all; I could take one day at a time. Being the perfect mother, daughter, employee, or friend just wasn't in the equation. My counselor also helped me realize that I didn't have to make all of these life decisions at once, but rather, I could take the time to think things through, acting on them when I felt strong enough. For instance, I didn't have to accept the first job I was offered.

Eventually, I was hired as a marketing manager at a publishing company and found that there is nothing more energizing than working and making my own way. I began working out, devoting 1 hour each day to exercise. This was my time for physical and mental release. As a bonus, I became really fit, which was great for my self-esteem.

It took 2 years for me to develop the courage to try another romantic relationship, but I'm thankful to have found a wonderful person. I even think I might like to get married again, something I never thought I'd say. For now, though, I'm just enjoying life. It's great to feel this good.

"Daughters who are able to say, 'That's how Mom is,' or 'That's just her way,' fare best," Dr. Fingerman says. On the other hand, when daughters perceive their mother's attention as an intrusion, or as critical in some way, the relationship suffers.

Acceptance is a matter of shifting your perception of the situation, she says. For example, maybe your mother has lousy taste in clothes. When you open the baby clothes she bought for your children, you can either laugh about it and chalk it up to a simple flaw in your mother, or you can view her gift as an intrusion, your mother foisting her taste on your kids when she knows full well that's not what you want them to wear. Which one do you think is more energy draining?

It helps to understand that part of the reason you see things differently from your mother is because you're each at different points in your lives, Dr. Fingerman says. The good news, however, is that research shows that your relationship with Mom actually improves with age.

Lean on Your Friends

Research shows that friends, not spouses or partners, are often the best sources of emotional support. While men are more likely to name their spouses or girlfriends as their main source of support, women are more likely to name other women, usually friends, sisters, or their mothers, explains Susan Lynch, Ph.D., director of the bachelor of social work program at the University of Arkansas at Little Rock.

The problem is that even with our friends, we tend to be more comfortable giving support than getting support. For us, reciprocity is a big

FALLING IN LOVE AGAIN

He sits there in his recliner watching TV, and you wonder if you still love him. Can you fall in love with him again?

"You can fall out of love just as easily as you fall in love," says Marilyn Fithian, Ph.D., codirector for the Marital and Sexual Studies Work and a licensed marriage and family counselor in Long Beach, California. "The most important thing is to decide what love is to you."

Look beyond passion to find the answer. "Friendship is the crucial element," Dr. Fithian says. "Without a genuine enjoyment of spending time together, there's not much point to any relationship." Even the best relationships can get stale, however. Here are some things she recommends to stave off boredom.

Separate. Just temporarily! Take a vacation away from him. "Sometimes you don't know how much a relationship means until you miss your partner for a while," she says.

Surprise each other. Arrange a surprise trip for just the two of you. Have the bags packed and the kids camped elsewhere when he gets home from work. Sometimes, all you need to do is go to a motel across town. The key is to do something off-kilter.

Touch. Counselors often use caress exercises with couples in crisis. "This usually goes on for 2 to 3 hours—touching, kissing, hugging, and patting." They learn to appreciate the closeness and sensuousness of touch without the pressure of sex having to be the ultimate end result.

Share. Maybe you're not really into fishing, but he is. Once in a while, ask to tag along. Your partner will appreciate the effort and be more inclined to get involved in something you really enjoy.

Relax. Take a walk around the neighborhood or go out for ice cream. Do some of the simple things you did together before you got married. And take your time with the things that have always naturally spawned communication.

issue. When we get something from a friend, our comfort levels go way down, Dr. Lynch says, and we want to pay it back quickly. So when we're stressed and overburdened, we avoid unloading on our friends because we're not sure we can reciprocate. We're afraid that they'll see us coming and say, "Oh no, there's Susan; all she does is complain."

"Give yourself permission to need support," says Dr. Lynch. "Cultivate your friendships with women. They tend to be the least demanding and the most supportive of relationships, yet they are the first thing we cut from our busy lives." Your best bet is to seek out friends with whom you can laugh. The most energizing friendships are fun friendships.

Rekindle the Flame with Your Spouse or Partner

Nearly one in three women ages 30 to 60 aren't interested in sex, according to the National Health and Social Life Survey, a study of sexual behavior in American adults. It's a sure bet that our chronic lack of energy is part of the problem. So is the fact that when two people have been together for a long time, sex can get dull and stop feeling personal.

"Touching does a lot in terms of adding energy to a relationship," says Marilyn Fithian, Ph.D., codirector for the Marital and Sexual

Studies Work and a licensed marriage and family counselor in Long Beach, California. "It adds spark back into a marriage." By taking time to caress, hug, and kiss more often, she says, you can restore the passion and energy in your relationship. To help her clients reconnect emotionally, physically, and spiritually with their partners, Dr. Fithian prescribes a touch exercise she calls caress therapy. Couples begin by spending 30 minutes to 1 hour simply touching and caressing each other's hands, faces, and feet. You can use a massage oil, but make sure you pick it out together.

Couples gradually work up to a 3-hour duration. "We've had couples holed up in a room for an entire weekend doing caress exercises but never having intercourse," Dr. Fithian says. "It meant so much more in terms of being in love. The goal here isn't sexual. It's a great way to discover each other again on a very personal level."

Keep It Positive with People at Work

Negative people drain energy. Listening to a coworker whine about her workload, her manager, or her working conditions is a real downer, says Filomena Warihay, Ph.D., president of Take Charge Consultants, an international management training and organizational development firm specializing in

WOMEN ASK WHY

Why is parenting a teenager just as exhausting (if not more) than parenting a newborn?

Just as you're never prepared for the enormous time and physical energy required to deal with a baby's needs, neither are you prepared for the intense emotional energy required to cope with a questioning, rebellious teenager who is seeking independence. But there are ways to survive the teen years without taking to your bed.

Choose your battles. How many moms get into hideous battles with their daughters over music? Take a stand on the important issues. You'll have a much better chance of success.

Be consistent. Develop a set of family values (curfew, study time, relationships with siblings) and stick to them. When these values are challenged, be consistent in how you deal with each situation. You are the best person to instill these values within your child. Truthfully, that's all you can do—and then hope they'll take effect when your child encounters influences you can't control.

Reinforce the positive. Just as you did when your child was little, emphasize your teen's triumphs, whether they're big or small. Some parents show emotion only when their adolescents misbehave. It's important to spontaneously comment on something your teenager does that you appreciate.

Minimize the negative. Don't overreact; limit your response when you're angry. Don't say things that you'll regret.

Keep score. Start a diary in which you record each problem and argument, including what set off the episode, how long it lasted, and what helped. Instead of worrying about how the situation makes you feel, concentrate on what is actually happening.

Expert consulted
Maria M. Mancusi, Ph.D.
Clinical psychologist
Springfield, Virginia

AMAZING ENERGY
The Tightly Tied Knot

Paul and Mary Onesi celebrated their 80th anniversary in 1998, becoming the longest-married couple in the United States. Their marriage has endured the Great Depression, two world wars, the Cold War, and 80 years of uncelebrated Valentine's Days. No flowers on Valentine's Day? Not for this couple. The Onesis seem more inclined to sensibility than sentiment. When reporters asked for the secret behind their matrimonial record, Mrs. Onesi chalked up their success to a simple strategy. "If you have trouble, you go talk about it, argue, and get over it," she said. Mr. Onesi waved off their accomplishment, giving more attention to the fact that too many marriages don't work. "In our family, no one ever wanted to get divorced because no one wanted to tell Grandma and Grandpa," added Laura Cerrillo, one of the couple's 28 grandchildren.

positive change in the workplace in Downingtown, Pennsylvania. You may try to help by offering a solution such as, "You can talk to your manager about the problem." But the whiner responds with, "Yeah, but she won't listen." You offer another suggestion, and the whiner retorts with another, "Yeah, but . . ."

"The downward spiral continues until you are exhausted, and the whiner starts whining about you and your inability to understand or be helpful," says Dr. Warihay. A surefire way to avoid the whiner and keep your workday energized is to ask a couple of questions. "What would you like to have happen instead?" or "What are you going to do to get what you need?"

Overall, says Dr. Ravicz, "Relationships can wear us out, but they are also what get us through our day-to-day crises. Self-management and balance are the name of the game."

And balance starts by learning to set boundaries. To establish a comfort zone, you need to know what you are willing to do and what you're not willing to do. The most important thing we can learn, she says, is how to say no when we're stretched too thin.

Learn to say no nicely. Now that you know how many times you're willing to host a meeting or help a friend out, or how many minutes you're willing to spend on the phone, you have to learn how to tell people in a firm, yet gentle, way when you've reached your limit.

Keep it simple and polite. Resist the urge to overexplain. "Sorry, I can't this time" or "I have plans that day" are the most effective. The other person may try to change your mind if you offer up too many details. ("You would rather clean your house than spend time with me?")

Buy some time. Tell the other person that you'll think about it, and then consider the best way to say no.

Make it a policy. Your "no" has less sting when it sounds like a rule. "I'm sorry, but it's my policy to never lend money to friends."

Suffocating in the Sandwich Generation

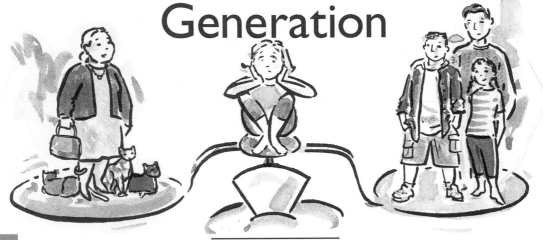

The sun warms Carolyn's face as she steps outside. "It's going to be a beautiful Saturday," she says to herself. "Too bad I'll be cleaning Mother's house all day."

As she drives to her mother's house, Carolyn thinks about the challenges of the past year, and how her 79-year-old mother's arthritis has become so severe that the older woman can no longer cook or clean. Even getting dressed has become a chore, especially if there are buttons to be fastened.

Enter Superdaughter.

Giving up what little free time she has, Carolyn has been cleaning her mother's house, paying the bills, and bringing her dinner most days. But lately, it doesn't seem to be enough. Sometimes when she stops by after work, her mother is still wearing a bathrobe. Even worse, her mother's health problems are multiplying. The arthritis is getting worse, and her doctor just diagnosed her with hypertension, prescribing even more drugs.

Lately, Carolyn has been thinking about an assisted-living facility for her mother, where someone can help with everyday activities like dressing and bathing. But every time she's about to bring it up, an overwhelming sense of sadness and guilt silences her. This woman, who never completed college, managed to raise three children on a secretary's salary after her husband died at age 34. To see her unable to even tie her own shoes breaks Carolyn's heart. If she sends her mother to a nursing home, she'll feel like she's turning her back on her mother. So Carolyn has simply added the job of Caregiver to her already crowded résumé.

Carolyn's situation is far from unique, and it's going to become even more common. The number of people age 65 and older is expected to grow from 13 percent of the population in the year 2000, to 20 percent in the year 2030. Our parents (often our mothers because women live longer than men) are also living longer (the 85-plus crowd is the fastest-growing demographic in the United States) and remaining at home instead of moving into nursing homes. Today, 23 percent of households in this country contain at least one person who is caring for an older relative or friend. And the kicker is that 73 percent of those caregivers are women.

Just when we think our lives can't possibly get any busier, we're given another role to play. So how do we maintain our energy (and sanity), manage our time, admit we can't do it alone, and find the resources to help?

Why We Do It All

Who wrote the rule that said we are the ones who should care for Mom and Dad (or our mothers- and fathers-in-law)? Where are our brothers and our husbands?

"There's an expectation that women will do it, and that they're more comfortable and experienced doing the job," says Ramsey McGowen, Ph.D., associate professor in the department of psychiatry and behavioral sciences at East Tennessee State University in Johnson City. But before you start blaming the men, consider our own complicity in this. After all, if we didn't still buy into the old stereotype about "women's work," would we still be the ones doing most of the housework and child care?

Gender isn't the only factor. If it were, why are your sisters at the mall on Saturday afternoons while you're running Mom's errands? "Almost invariably, there's a caregiver in families," says Barbara Ensor, Ph.D., a psychologist at the geriatric facility at Stella Maris in Baltzimore. "You can pick them out when they're children." They're the babysitters, the ones making dinner every night, or those supervising bath time.

HOW IN THE WORLD DO THEY SLEEP?
Sleeping on the Space Shuttle

Imagine spending the night attached by Velcro to the bedroom wall. Well, just how did you think the astronauts slept onboard the space shuttle?

It may not sound too comfortable, but NASA goes the distance to make sure shuttle crews sleep soundly, says Marianne Rudisill, Ph.D., an aerospace technologist in manned systems at NASA Langley Research Center in Hampton, Virginia. Finding ways to help the astronauts sleep can be a problem, she says. There's no gravity in space, so crew members can't simply lie down on their beds.

What's more, in low orbit above the earth, there isn't even a clear distinction between day and night. The shuttle goes around the earth every 90 minutes, so the astronauts see 45 minutes of light and then 45 minutes of darkness throughout their missions.

On missions with a single-crew shift (those with four or five astronauts), everyone sleeps at the same time. To stay connected to NASA and to hear shuttle alarms, at least one crew member, usually the commander, wears a headset while he sleeps. Unlike the other astronauts on board, the commander and pilot must sleep at their szztations on the flight deck, strapped into their seats in a small area about the size of an airplane cockpit. All crew members have the option of wearing eye covers to keep those frequent "sunrises" from waking them. Specially designed, lint-free cotton

Then there's the big G: Guilt. Our parents did so much for us for so long and made so many sacrifices; now it's our turn. We should put them before anything else the way they put us before anything else. It's a role reversal, only we also have to cope with long-buried resentments and fears of their deaths. Once they die, we realize that we're no longer anyone's child.

shades (similar to the cushions on lawn chairs) are attached by Velcro to the windows to further block the sun. They must be lint-free because the lack of atmosphere on board means no air circulates. Fans help move the air, and any lint from the shades could get trapped in the shuttle's filters. But the fans cause another problem when crew members want to sleep: noise. Soft, squishy ear plugs, just like the ones we use here, help the astronauts get their 8 hours of sleep.

The crew members who don't spend the night on the flight deck usually sleep below, on the shuttle's windowless mid deck. When it's time to call it a night, they simply float into lint-free sleeping bags with armholes (kind of like sleeping-bag pajamas) and zip themselves in. The bags keep their legs and feet in place despite the lack of gravity. Some astronauts keep their arms inside their sleeping bags so they don't bump into equipment or other objects as they sleep.

Velcro patches and attachment pins on the sleeping bags let the astronauts nuzzle up to a wall and lock in for the night. On missions using more astronauts, crew members sleep in shifts in rigid sleep stations that allow them to close the door, strap in, lay on their sides, curl up, or roll over.

The astronauts, incidentally, follow Central Standard Time, says Dr. Rudisill. On missions with a single shift, the astronauts in low Earth orbit "sleep when the people in Houston sleep."

The Job Itself

There's an old saying, "Who cares for the caregiver?" Usually, the answer is no one. Caring for a parent is like adding a full-time job to your life. Many caregivers spend 20 or more hours each week in the role, doing everything from dusting to driving to opening mail and paying bills.

That can lead to major health problems, aside from the obvious exhaustion. A National Family Caregivers Association survey found that caregivers experienced more headaches, stomach problems, back pain, sleeplessness, and depression than they did before they began the role. The problems weren't limited to physical health, either. Episodes of frustration, anxiety, and sadness also increased.

And this is for the long haul. "It's not a sprint, it's a marathon," says Mary Pipher, Ph.D., a psychologist and the author of *Another Country: Navigating the Emotional Terrain of our Elders*. We might be able to care for Mom around the clock when she has 6 weeks left to live, but we'll never be able to keep up that frenzied pace for 5, 10, or even 20 years. "Some people get burned out at the very point when their parents are in desperate need," she says.

Not only do our extra responsibilities cut into our family and free time, they often disrupt the hours we spend at work. Half of all caregivers who are employed have to change their work schedules—going in late, leaving early, or taking time off in the middle of the day. While some companies provide time off, many caregivers must use their own vacation time or cut their hours at work. And since nearly 25 percent of caregivers still have children at home, they're not only getting the 3:00 P.M. call saying that Susie got home safely, they're also getting the 10:00 A.M., noon, and 2:00 P.M. call from Mom complaining of dizziness.

Also, little chores for our parents tend to turn into big projects. When we want to make a fast trip to the store, Mom wants to stop for coffee

WOMAN TO WOMAN
She's Caring for Mom Long Distance

Rona Buchbinder's 90-year-old mother has one request: that she live in her own home. The problem is that Rona lives in Silver Spring, Maryland, and her mother lives in Venice, Florida. Her mother also has osteoporosis, high blood pressure, and ulcers, and takes numerous medications, many of which have side effects. So caring for the older woman from four states away is a challenge. Here's how Rona manages.

Independent hardly begins to describe my mother. She's lived in Florida for 25 years and she wants to stay there, even though my sisters and I are a day's drive away. In the past year, she's broken her hip and a bone in her upper arm when she fainted because of the medication she was taking.

Neither my sisters nor I consider ourselves her primary caregivers. My mother is her own primary caregiver, and she wouldn't have it any other way. Her body may be failing, but her mind is still sharp, so we let her make her own decisions. After she broke her hip, she lived with my sister in New Jersey for 4 months. Then we had a big family meeting in which we asked her to move north with us. Her response? "I'm going back to Florida." We flew back with her a week later. Her smile when we arrived was worth the entire trip.

We arranged for a 24-hour home health aide to do her cooking, shopping, and laundry. Mom can still shower, dress herself, and make her own bed.

My sisters and I continually keep in touch with her. One of us calls her every day, and we all visit periodically. I'm lucky because my job gives me family leave, and I have plenty of days off to visit. What worries me most is that if and when something happens, I can't get there very quickly.

Dealing with Mom may be frustrating at times, but the fact that she's always lovable counterbalances those frustrating interactions. The best part of this experience is being able to spend more time with her. She has a positive outlook on life, and we have a good time together. We laugh, and she sings, plays the piano, and tells jokes. My friends all love her, too. It's wonderful to give her back some of the love and attention that she gave me for so many years.

and a bite to eat, which she nibbles at for an hour. We want to drop off some dinner and sprint to our son's soccer game, but Dad has a list of chores he needs to complete *now*.

Then there are the age-old parent-child issues. If Mom didn't work outside the home, she might have no idea how stressful it is to commute, what it's like to report to a boss every day, and how hard it is to be a supermom. And if you're a caregiver to your father, who never washed a plate or cooked a meal in his life, he's not going to have a clue about your "second shift" of home and family obligations.

So you need to do some educating. Talk about your frustrations at work, laugh about the difficulties of raising kids, and be open about your day-to-day activities, Dr. Ensor suggests. This will help your parents understand you better and make your job as caregiver easier. But remember the Golden Rule of the adult child: "You can't tell your parents what to do," Dr. Ensor says. "That just doesn't work. They are still the parents."

Avoiding Burnout

Start by giving your parents as much control of their lives as possible. Even if someone else has to handle your mother's finances, let her decide who does it, if she can. If Dad is going into an assisted-living facility, take him on the tours with you so he can ask questions.

Let him make choices, such as whether he'd like a room by the kitchen or by the garden. If you're hiring a home health aide, let your mother interview the best two and choose one.

Still, like parenting, this is a job that only gets tougher, so you have to keep an eye peeled for burnout. Experts say you're doing too much if:

- You haven't talked to a friend in 2 weeks.
- You haven't gone out socially in at least a week.
- You're getting fewer than 7 hours of sleep a night.
- You're getting sick more often than usual.
- You're smoking or drinking more often than usual.
- You don't have the energy to talk about your stress.
- You can't concentrate, whether you're reading a book, balancing your checkbook, or following a recipe.
- You're more forgetful than usual.
- You're missing out on things you really want to do, such as going to your kids' baseball games.
- You're more irritable than usual.
- You start to think that Mom is faking her symptoms.

If you recognize yourself in any of these symptoms, you desperately need the one thing caregivers lust after most: time for yourself. You need the caregiver-in-control plan. Here's how it works.

Step 1. Lay out your own life. Take a daily calendar and fill in the days and hours with everything you do outside of caring for your parents: work, cooking, chauffeuring, laundry, cleaning, shopping, paying the bills. And don't forget to schedule yourself in.

> ### JUMP START
> #### *Tongue Tickle*
>
> Feeling sleepy? Take the tip of your tongue and tickle the roof of your mouth. It's one way some astronauts stay awake when in orbit.

Whether it's an hour every day, or an entire evening every week to take a bubble bath, read a book, or watch your favorite television shows, you deserve it.

Step 2. Lay out your parent's life. List everything that needs to be done for your parent and see what you can reasonably fit into your schedule, such as having your parent over for dinner three times a week and doing her laundry on Wednesdays.

Step 3. Show your parent your schedule. When your parent sees your schedule on paper, she'll realize just how frantic your life really is. Not only will it provide a blast of reality, but also it may help assuage some of your own guilt, says Dr. McGowen. Even if she's too sick to understand, seeing all of this on paper will make it clearer to you that you can't make dinner, clean the house, do three loads of laundry, *and* check on your parent in the 1 hour between work and dinner.

Step 4. Call a meeting. Gather your parent, husband, kids, relatives, and any neighbors and friends willing to help. Make sure they understand the seriousness of the situation and where it's going in the future. Bring pamphlets and medical records (with your parent's permission) to update them on her health. Then show them your schedule so they also understand just what the term Superdaughter really means. Yes, you're pawning some of the guilt

WHERE TO GET HELP

There's an entire world of people out there willing to help with caregiving, sometimes on a volunteer basis. Services include home-delivered meals, household repairs, cleaning, yard work, bathing, dressing, cooking, laundry, running errands, health care, and companionship.

- The National Association of Area Agencies on Aging (www.n4a.org) provides the Eldercare Locator, which helps identify nationwide information and referral services to help with care for the aged; (800) 677-1116
- National Institute on Aging; www.nih.gov/nia
- American Association of Retired Persons (AARP); www.aarp.org
- National Association for Home Care (NAHC); www.nahc.org
- American Association of Homes and Services for the Aging; www.aahsa.org
- Alzheimer's Association; www.alz.org
- National Family Caregivers Association; www.nfcacares.org
- National Alliance for Caregiving; www.caregiving.org
- Other local charities and organizations you can contact include United Way, Family Services of America, Jewish Family Services, Catholic Charities, Protestant welfare agencies, the American Red Cross, the Visiting Nurses Association, social service agencies, and local churches. For organizations in your area, check your phone book.

- Use a transportation service specifically for older adults.
- Hire a teenager to mow your parent's lawn or do her grocery shopping, kind of like a mother's helper in reverse.
- Sign up for a Meals on Wheels program to deliver hot meals.
- Ask out-of-town relatives to visit for a week to give you a break. Or, set up a time for your parent to visit them. If they don't have the time but want to help out, suggest that they chip in for laundry or maid service.
- Suggest jobs that match your relatives' strengths and weaknesses. If your sister can't be in the same room with your parent without fighting, assign Sis the bill-paying job so that the two don't have to talk.
- Keep your parents active, and help them find their own circle of support. Look for activities at your local senior citizen's center, and volunteer opportunities at libraries, hospitals, and schools. The busier they are, the more in control and happier they'll be.

off on them, but if it makes it harder for them to turn down your plea for help next time, it's worth it.

Step 5. Brainstorm solutions. Some ideas:
- Hire a maid (for you or for your parent).
- Assign duties to the kids. They can cut the grass, read to Grandma, or, if one of them drives, take her to some of her doctor's appointments.

Step 6. Maintain. Don't stop after one meeting. The core group of people who have agreed to care for your parent should meet at least every 2 weeks in the beginning to keep lines of communication open. You may want to rotate responsibilities after a few weeks.

Step 7. Seek support. Sign yourself up for a support group. "People don't understand that one of the reasons we're so busy is because we're

WHEN ENOUGH IS ENOUGH

A day may come when your parent requires more than you, your relatives, or friends can handle. Admitting you can't do it all doesn't mean turning her over to strangers. These days, there are a variety of options available for the elderly.

Adult day care. These centers offer services for older adults who have paralysis or early dementia, or who are in wheelchairs. Fees are around $70 a day and are often charged on a sliding scale basis. The staff provides a variety of services and scheduled activities, including crafts, exercises, minimal medical care, and bathing. Trained nurses are available to give medications.

Home health care. A skilled nurse capable of providing medical treatment can visit your parent's home daily for about $70 a day. If your parent's needs are a result of hospitalization, Medicare may cover the costs. A home health aide, who provides personal assistance with dressing, bathing, and feeding, may cost $10 to $18 an hour.

Assisted-living facility. This is the newest entrant on the long-term-care continuum, providing 24-hour service but with far more independence than a nursing home. Mom gets help with personal care, from bathing to receiving hot meals, but in an apartment-like setting. Monthly costs range from $1,000 to $4,000 and are rarely covered by insurance.

Board and care. These facilities typically offer many of the amenities of an assisted-living facility, but in a smaller, more homelike atmosphere—often in a private home. Costs range from $350 to $3,000 a month and are rarely covered by insurance. You can find out about board-and-care homes in your area by contacting your local office on aging, which is usually listed in the blue pages of the phone book. Another option is to contact the Eldercare Locator at (800) 677-1116 for information.

Nursing home. This is the last step on the long-term care continuum. Only adults who require significant medical and personal care are admitted to nursing homes, which cost $4,200 to $4,700 per month. Medicare covers the first 100 days in a nursing home only after a hospital stay. Once your parent's condition improves, her stay is no longer covered. Half of all nursing home residents wind up on Medicaid.

Continuing-care retirement communities. These facilities offer different levels of care (often on one site) ranging from apartments for independent living to nursing homes. The advantage is that your parent doesn't have to adjust to a new environment as her health needs change. Most require a hefty entrance fee, as much as $50,000 or more, as well as monthly fees of $1,000 to $4,000.

For information on state guidelines, patient rights, and recent government inspections of local nursing homes, call your state's long-term care ombudsman. You can find your ombudsman on the National Citizens' Coalition for Nursing Home Reform Web site at www.nccnhr.org.

For help with a parent who doesn't live near you, try a geriatric care manager. You can find one through the Eldercare Locator or visit the Web site of the National Association of Geriatric Care Managers at www.caremanager.org. Fees range from $50 to $100 for the initial consultation. Be a smart consumer when looking for a care manager by pricing several managers and making sure they have either a background in nursing with experience in geriatrics or a master's degree in social work.

trying to do everything ourselves," Dr. Pipher says. But building a community of people who support us saves time and energy. You'll find resources through other members, and you may find companions for your parent. Most important, however, you'll be able to talk to a group of people who know exactly what you're going through. To find one near you, check with the National Alliance for Caregiving and the National Family Caregivers Association (see "Where to Get Help" on page 78), or look for information at community centers or your local church.

Moving Forward

Once Carolyn joined a support group, her life was transformed. She met a friend whose mother lives in an assisted-living facility that she adores. Carolyn was able to introduce her mother to the older woman and suggest that her mother think about moving into the same facility. Her mother agreed. Now that the facility does Mom's laundry and cooks her meals, Carolyn has more time to just *be* with her mother, going to movies, for walks, or simply sitting and talking.

When Being Tired Means Something's Wrong

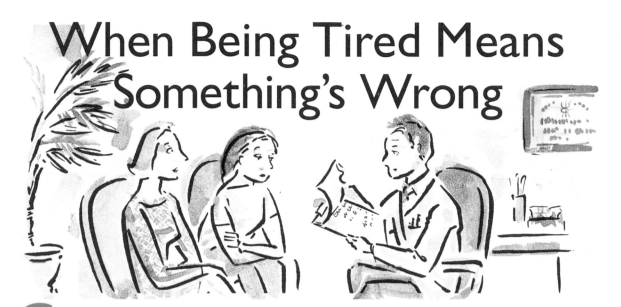

Good to talk to you, too—hope you feel better tomorrow!" Carolyn sighs as she hangs up the phone. Her friend Marcia, a collegiate partner-in-crime and fellow soccer mom, has chronic fatigue syndrome (CFS). She'd had a really bad day today after spending the weekend at a soccer tournament. The games were over, but Marcia's day-after pain had just started, and it was worse than any New Year's Day hangover.

"Why do I always do this to myself?" Marcia had asked in a voice so weak Carolyn had to strain to hear. "Why can't I just take it easy like my doctor recommends?"

"Because you've never taken it easy," Carolyn had answered honestly, thinking of Marcia's nonstop energy in college. Her friend would stay up all night preparing a presentation or writing a paper, only to spend the next night dancing until dawn. After college, Marcia worked full-time and went to business school, simultaneously earning promotions and her M.B.A. in record time. Was it any wonder that the word *relaxing* wasn't in her vocabulary?

Then Marcia's doctor told her she had CFS, which was once known as the yuppie flu. Carolyn remembers her reaction when Marcia broke the news to her. "Chronic fatigue syndrome?" Carolyn had scoffed aloud. "What woman with a husband, kids, job, house, and family *doesn't* have chronic fatigue syndrome?"

Years later, she still cringes when she recalls that flippant remark. CFS has proven to be a tough competitor even for an all-star like Marcia to beat. While she has improved, she still isn't 100 percent and doesn't know if she ever will be again. "Thankfully, there's nothing wrong with me that a good night's rest won't help," Carolyn thinks to herself as she goes upstairs to fold the laundry before bed.

Chronic Fatigue Syndrome

When we're juggling work, family, and home, chronic fatigue seems like a way of life. But CFS represents a serious health problem that's difficult to diagnose and challenging to treat.

Yet CFS is relatively benign compared to other health issues. "The good news is that it won't shorten your life. It won't put you in a wheelchair. It won't lead to other problems," says Mary B. Duke, M.D., associate professor of internal medicine and pediatrics at the University of Kentucky in Lexington. And although there's no known cure for CFS, it's not an incurable disease. About half of CFS patients recover from the disorder, most of them within 5 years.

As many as 800,000 people nationwide have the condition, three times as many women as men.

For many women, CFS starts like "the flu from hell," says Dr. Duke. Only this flu never seems to go away, leaving you tired and weak, with your energy spent after seemingly minor exertion. You may think you're just extraordinarily exhausted from finishing last month's big project at work, but sleep doesn't help. Many people who have CFS turn to exercise, telling themselves, "If I just work out, I'll get my energy back." But their efforts backfire, leaving them barely able to get out of bed the next day. Other symptoms include:

- Memory and concentration problems
- Sore throat
- Unrefreshing sleep
- Tenderness in the lymph nodes (Located in the neck, armpits, abdomen, and groin, these glands fight infection.)
- Muscle pain
- Joint pain without redness or swelling

OTHER COMMON CULPRITS OF FATIGUE

Not every woman's fatigue can be chalked up to a busy schedule and too little sleep. But neither is a bad case of exhaustion always something as serious as CFS. "Most of the time, there are other explanations," says Mary B. Duke, M.D., associate professor of internal medicine and pediatrics at the University of Kentucky in Lexington.

Springtime allergies can make us both restless and woozy, especially with decongestants and antihistamines. The flu can leave us prostrate on the couch. Sometimes, the culprit is even less obvious. "Sinus infections can be low-grade infections with vague symptoms," says Elizabeth Burns, M.D., professor of family medicine at the University of Illinois at Chicago.

These concerns may sound minor, but their impact on our energy levels isn't. Fighting an infection is a major task for our bodies. When bacteria or a virus appears in our bloodstreams, cells known as lymphocytes start making antibodies, disease-fighting molecules that recognize and match the unique proteins of the bacteria or virus. Those antibodies go into our bloodstreams and attack the invader. Our temperature rises in response to inflammatory chemicals that reset our internal thermostat. We're hot to the touch, yet we get the chills as our muscles try to warm up to our new, higher body temperatures. We feel exhausted because our energy is being diverted to battle the virus.

If it's an invader you haven't seen before, prepare for bodily combat. "When your body is being challenged by a virus your system has never seen, the virus builds up in numbers before your immune system has the antibodies to fight it off—and you are one sick puppy," says Dr. Burns.

Allergies may not be as dramatic, but they're just as unpleasant. Between the congestion, the postnasal drip, the snoring from stuffed-up noses, and the sometimes stimulating, sometimes sedating side effects of the medications we're taking, sleep is darn hard to come by. So it's no wonder we sleepwalk through the day when pollen counts are high.

But there are multiple ways to beat energy busters like colds, allergies, and the flu.

Pick simple medications. If allergy or cold medicines leave you hyped up at night, take a simple antihistamine such as Benadryl before sleeping; it tends to be more sedating. If daytime drowsiness is your problem, choose a decongestant, which is generally more stimulating, though it can cause sleepiness. Follow package instructions for the dosage. Talk to your doctor if over-the-counter drugs don't work for you; newer prescription medications such as Allegra and Claritin-D may have less dramatic side effects, says Dr. Burns.

Take long, hot showers. When your nasal passages are blocked as a result of colds, allergies, or sinus infections, the steam and moisture of showering can help drain them.

Buy a humidifier. Running a humidifier adds moisture to the air, which is helpful if you have a cough. Keep the humidifier clean, however; if you don't, the mold spores that result will aggravate your symptoms even more.

Rest. Go to bed early. Sleep in. Nap. Call in sick. Return to the office too soon, and you may have a relapse.

Drink. You need lots of fluids when your body's fighting off a virus. Colds are often accompanied by fever, which increases your breathing rate and makes you sweat more. And your body is trying to get rid of the waste products created in the battle between your immune system and the infection. All of this can lead to dehydration, says Dr. Burns. To stay hydrated, drink enough water, hot tea, and juices that you go to the bathroom about every 2 hours.

Choose C. When you have an infection, take 500 to 1,000 milligrams of immune-boosting vitamin C hourly up to six times daily. If you start experiencing diarrhea, slowly cut back to an amount that you can tolerate, says Liz Sutherland, N.D., a naturopathic physician with the National College of Naturopathic Medicine's Natural Health Sciences Research Clinic in Lake Oswego, Oregon. Vitamin C has been shown by many studies to reduce the duration of cold and flu symptoms.

Try echinacea. Take this immune-enhancing herb in tincture form (more effective than the pill form) hourly at the first sign of a cold or flu, suggests Dr. Sutherland.

See a doctor. If you're bringing up green or yellow mucus, you may have a sinus infection, which often requires antibiotics.

> Headaches that vary in their severity or pattern compared to previous headaches

If you're experiencing any four of the above symptoms and you've felt severely fatigued for 6 months or more, talk to your doctor about CFS. Be prepared for lots of tests: blood work, urinalysis, a thyroid test, even cognitive exams that ask about your concentration or memory. Before your doctor can diagnose you with CFS, she needs to rule out everything else that can cause fatigue, such as depression, sleep problems, and autoimmune diseases.

What's Happening?

No one really knows what causes CFS, but some researchers speculate that extreme stress or a viral infection such as a cold or flu may somehow send your immune system into overdrive, leaving your body fighting as though you had a perpetual case of the flu. Other theories suggest that the central nervous system is responsible, as physical or emotional stress activates various glands, leading to the increased release of stress hormones.

Researchers are also looking at the role low blood pressure plays, since both CFS patients and those with a condition known as neurally mediated hypotension, or NMH, seem to experience dizziness, light-headedness, or fatigue after standing for a long time or in warm places. Researchers think medications for NMH may help CFS patients as well.

CFS may have connections to both our minds and our bodies—not just one or the other. According to one study, those with CFS reported more negative life events and infections before the syndrome's onset than those without CFS. "This mind-body link makes sense intuitively," says Susan K. Johnson, Ph.D., assistant professor of psychology at the University of North Carolina at Charlotte. "But it's very hard for people to grasp that model." Doctors need to acknowledge that CFS is a real disease, she says, but patients also need to accept the fact that their lifestyles or thought patterns may contribute, too. "The connection of CFS with stress is a tricky one," she says. Learning to reduce both physical and emotional stress is an important component in recovery.

Finding Help

One of the single most important steps in recovery from CFS is finding a doctor who believes you even have the disease. This sounds simple, but it's often not. Validation may be more important in CFS than other chronic illnesses precisely because it's less socially legitimate, says Barbara Saltzstein, a lecturer in psychiatry at Harvard Medical School. She found that women with CFS who were diagnosed early and found a CFS-friendly physician who was optimistic about their future health reported more improvement than those whose physicians were not CFS-friendly.

If your doctor is skeptical about CFS, call a nearby medical school and ask if they have a CFS clinic. Rheumatologists, immunologists, and primary care physicians also treat CFS. Although there's no cure for CFS yet, there are several approaches to treatment.

Antidepressants. Prescribed in small doses, antidepressants (generally, selective serotonin reuptake inhibitors such as Prozac or the older tricyclic drugs) help you sleep better. They may also ease the muscle and joint pains that trouble some people with CFS.

NADH. Shorthand for nicotinamide adenine dinucleotide, NADH is a substance that helps the cells in your body produce energy—a process that is disrupted in CFS patients. In one study, 31 percent of those who took the dietary supplement for 1 month felt better compared to the 8 percent who took a placebo. Be aware that some people have reported nervousness, loss of appetite, and stomach upset in the first few days of taking the supplement. NADH is available at health food stores; follow label instructions regarding dosages.

Emotional therapy. A specific psychotherapy approach known as cognitive behavioral therapy may be helpful in coping with the emotional frustration of CFS. "CFS can be devastating to successful women who are used to performing and achieving; this lifestyle has become part of their identity," says Dr. Duke. "But when all they can do is walk to the mailbox and wash their hair in a day, that doesn't feel like success. Cognitive behavioral therapy helps them redefine what success is."

Exercise. As unappealing as it sounds when you feel perpetually exhausted, you need to move your muscles. Otherwise, both your cardiovascular system and your muscles will get weaker and weaker, making everyday tasks such as climbing stairs, carrying laundry, and even just taking a shower that much harder. Dr. Duke suggests working in up to 30 minutes of aerobic, low-impact exercise such as walking or bicycling daily.

Relaxation. "Women with CFS tend to overdo it," says Billy Brennan, a mental health practitioner at Harborview Medical Center's Chronic Fatigue Clinic in Seattle. "When they're having a good day, they try to get as much done as possible." To guard against overexertion, keep a notebook in which you jot down your activities and look for connections. Were you spent on Thursday after 6 hours of shopping on Wednesday, but okay on Monday after only 3 hours of Sunday gardening? Maybe 3 hours is your physical limit.

Multivitamins. "Taking a multivitamin is not a cure," cautions Dr. Duke. "It's nutritional insurance for those who don't eat right." Some researchers have suggested that people with CFS are deficient in magnesium or B vitamins, but Dr. Duke says that hasn't been proven.

Support. A chronic health problem such as CFS can be socially isolating. Check your local newspaper for support groups that can offer companionship and understanding.

Fibromyalgia

After a Saturday spent raking leaves, hauling mulch, and hiking up and down a football field, only a superwoman with arms of steel wouldn't be tired and sore, right?

Don't be so quick to explain your pains away.

For some, muscle soreness and fatigue may signify something more serious than weekend overexertion. It could be fibromyalgia, a chronic disorder that results in muscle pain, sleep problems, and fatigue.

"Fibromyalgia feels like the worst case of flu ever imaginable," says Carole Kenner, D.N.S. (Doctor of Nursing Science), professor and director of the Center for International Affairs at the University of Cincinnati, who has fibromyalgia herself. Other symptoms include morning stiffness, regular headaches, bowel problems, jaw pain, and chemical sensitivities to smells such as perfume or cigarette smoke.

What's Happening

One result (or symptom) of fibromyalgia is an insufficient amount of serotonin, a neurotransmitter that regulates sleep and perception of pain. Women with fibromyalgia also may have low levels of cortisol, a hormone that gives us the energy we need in intense situations. But there is plenty of a chemical known as Substance P, which may intensify pain perception.

Complex and still not fully understood, fibromyalgia is easy for doctors and patients to miss. "The sleep problems and fatigue makes it easier to dismiss the pain as everyday aches and pains," says Dr. Kenner. "We think, 'I must have picked up my grandchild wrong,' or 'I must have carried something too heavy.'"

We sometimes blame our fatigue on a bad night's sleep—a common complaint among fibromyalgia patients, who often have trouble either falling or staying asleep.

In many ways, fibromyalgia resembles CFS, leaving some to speculate that the two conditions are simply different points on a continuum. Like CFS, fibromyalgia primarily affects women and its symptoms include pain, fatigue, sleep problems, and cognitive difficulties. And like CFS, fibromyalgia has an unidentified cause and is a diagnosis of exclusion, meaning that your doctor must rule out all other causes for your fatigue and pain. She'll also do a "tender point" exam, checking the sensitivity of 18 specific areas on your body. If you've been in chronic pain for at least 3 months and have tenderness in 11 or more areas located near your knees, elbows, butt, and the base of your skull, you probably have fibromyalgia.

Some doctors suspect fibromyalgia is triggered by an infection, injury, or stress that somehow affects the central nervous system. Others blame an immune system that is in perpetual overdrive.

Finding Help

Many women with fibromyalgia live with symptoms for 5 to 7 years before they're diagnosed. If you don't want to spend the next decade feeling inexplicably exhausted, start looking for a doctor who's knowledgeable about fibromyalgia. You can call the Fibromyalgia Network at (800) 853-2929 or visit their Web site at www.fmnetnews.com for a list of fibromyalgia-friendly health care providers. You might also want to try the rheumatology department at a nearby medical school.

Once you find a doctor, talk with her about therapies—both conventional and alternative—as well as lifestyle modifications. Commonly used medications include antidepressants, which may reduce your pain and help you sleep as well as boost your mood, since depression often accompanies fibromyalgia. Although nonsteroidal anti-inflammatory drugs (NSAIDS) are often prescribed to ease the muscle pain of fibromyalgia, there's no proof that they work, and they may lead to intestinal problems resulting in food allergies, an overactive immune system, or even irritable bowel syndrome.

But don't rule out alternative therapies. In one study, researchers found that nondrug therapies provided more energy and pain relief in fibromyalgia patients than antidepressants, muscle relaxants, or NSAIDs. They include:

SAM-e (S-adenosyl-L-methionine). More commonly used for treating osteoarthritis, SAM-e (found in health food stores) can also act as an antidepressant and pain reliever for people with fibromyalgia. Doses up to 1,200 milligrams daily are considered safe. This supplement may increase your blood levels of homocysteine, a significant risk factor for cardiovascular disease. To keep homocysteine levels down, SAM-e should be taken with folic acid and vitamins B_6 and B_{12}.

5-HTP (5-Hydroxytryptophan). Besides reducing the number of painful "tender points," 5-HTP may help with the pain, stiffness, and fatigue of fibromyalgia by providing the precursor for the serotonin you lack, says Liz Sutherland, N.D., a naturopathic physician with the National College of Naturopathic Medicine's Natural Health Sciences Research Clinic in Lake Oswego, Oregon. A typical dosage is 300 to 900 milligrams per day, usually divided into 2 or 3 doses throughout the day. Some research suggests that taking 100 milligrams of 5-HTP three times a day combined with St. John's wort extract (300 milligrams standardized to 0.3 percent hypericin three times a day) and magnesium (200 to 250 milligrams three times a day) produces very good results, Dr. Sutherland says. The form of magnesium is very important, she adds. "I specifically recommend magnesium citrate, malate, succinate, or fumarate."

When buying 5-HTP, be certain to purchase a reputable brand. In the past, some brands of this supplement were found to contain trace amounts of a contaminant that caused serious symptoms that are associated with eosinophilic myalgia syndrome (EMS), which is characterized in the acute stage by flulike symptoms, intense muscle pain, and an increase in blood eosinophil counts. The following brands were confirmed to be free of the contaminant: Natrol,

FOOD SENSITIVITIES: A HIDDEN ENERGY SAPPER

Many naturopathic doctors think that food allergies (more accurately known as food sensitivities or intolerances) sap our energy just as much as ragweed season. "When you have a sensitivity to a food, your body doesn't break it down fully," says Liz Sutherland, N.D., a naturopathic physician with the National College of Naturopathic Medicine's Natural Health Sciences Research Clinic in Lake Oswego, Oregon. As a result, these incompletely digested food molecules sneak into the bloodstream through openings in your stomach and intestinal linings. Because these molecules are larger than the body expects, your immune system sees them not as food but as foreign invaders, and fires up your body's defenses just as if it had encountered a cold virus.

"This constant low-grade immune response is very irritating to the body," Dr. Sutherland says. You feel tired and foggy because all of your energy goes toward fighting off that ice cream cone you ate.

If you suspect a food sensitivity, confirm it by cutting the questionable food out of your diet for 4 to 6 weeks. (Common offenders are dairy, soy, corn, and gluten, which is found in wheat, oats, rye, barley, couscous, and other grains.) Then slowly reintroduce the food and see how you feel. If you eliminate more than one item, allow 3 days between adding each food back into your diet.

You can also ask your doctor to test you for food sensitivities, but if you tend to have a delayed allergic reaction to certain foods, you may be out of luck—some food allergy blood tests pick up only on immediate immune responses.

Nature's Way, TriMedica, Country Life, and Solaray.

Chiropractic. In one small study, 15 to 30 sessions of chiropractic manipulation eased the pain, reduced fatigue, and improved sleep in a group of women with fibromyalgia.

Acupuncture. The ancient Chinese practice of inserting needles at specific points in the body to relieve pain may temporarily relieve the pain and morning stiffness of fibromyalgia. The National Institutes of Health, after reviewing numerous studies, concluded that acupuncture may be useful as an "adjunct treatment" for fibromyalgia.

As with CFS, there are several other things you can do that may improve your condition, including exercise, relaxation techniques, and cognitive behavioral therapy.

Lupus

No two women are alike. Especially when it comes to an autoimmune disease like lupus (shorthand for systemic lupus erythematosus). "Three women with lupus can talk and discover that they have no symptoms in common," says Tammy Olsen Utset, M.D., M.P.H., assistant professor of clinical medicine at the University of Chicago.

The disease sends your immune system out of control, attacking your own tissues and cells, causing swelling and pain. In some women, it's constant. Others have cycles of remissions, when they feel healthy and well, and relapses, when the disease flares up. Some experience severe fatigue; others may start losing their hair. Additional symptoms of lupus include:

WOMAN TO WOMAN

After Breast Cancer, She Races for the Cure

Jan Shaw, 36, always considered herself an athletic woman. In high school, she'd played several sports. As an adult, she could walk for miles without stopping. Then she was diagnosed with breast cancer. Four months of chemotherapy left the once-energetic Gilbert, Arizona, resident weak and tired—feelings she'd rarely encountered before. But neither cancer nor chemo could turn Shaw into a couch potato. In the spring of 2000, she began training for Race for the Cure, a 5-K running race that raises awareness and money for breast health education, screening, and treatment as well as breast cancer research. Here is her story.

I learned about the lump in my breast when I was 33, during a get-to-know-you-visit with a new physician. My husband, baby daughter, and I had just moved, and this was just a routine doctor's visit. Until he found the lump.

After a biopsy determined that it was cancerous, my doctors removed the lump right away, along with four lymph nodes. But then they found cancer in one of the lymph nodes. So I went back for a second operation to have the rest of my lymph nodes removed. Three weeks later, I started chemotherapy.

Looking back, the chemo wasn't as bad as I thought it would be. I had heard stories that it would make me sick, but my treatments included antinausea drugs, so I was okay.

- Joint and muscle pain
- Unexplained fever
- Skin rash on the face
- Chest pain when breathing deeply
- Fingers and toes that turn colors in the cold or when stressed
- Unusual sensitivity to the sun, with 15 minutes of exposure resulting in sunburn, fatigue, or joint pain
- Swelling in the eyes or legs
- Swollen glands

But it definitely affected my energy levels, and I noticed the difference after my first treatment. I used to be able to stroll around the mall with my daughter all day. I could walk until I dropped. With the chemo, though, I tired much more easily. I'd have to lie down and rest. Near the end, I'd take a day off work after each treatment. And I'd go to bed at 9:00 P.M., roughly 2 hours earlier than before I got sick.

Today, I'm in remission and in training for my first 5-K: Race for the Cure in Phoenix. I learned about the race from a friend. Unbeknownst to me, she had run the race "in honor" of me, wearing my name on her runner's tag just as others were running in memory of their mothers, grandmothers, and wives. Her gesture meant so much to me, and running Race for the Cure became something I wanted to do for myself.

I started training slowly. The first time I went out, I walked about 1 mile, which was definitely not as far as I wanted to go. But my stamina came back quickly. Once I could walk 4 miles, I began walking and jogging. In only 2 months, I found that I had more energy, especially in the morning.

I have another reason for running this race: my father. He went through such a tough time when my mother died of ovarian cancer. I know it must have shaken him when he found out I had cancer, yet he was such a pillar of support. I want to run for him, too, to show him that I'm going to be just fine.

♦ Recurrent and frequently multiple canker sores

"If you have three or more of these symptoms, it's probably worth seeing a doctor," says Rosalind Ramsey-Goldman, M.D., associate professor of medicine at Northwestern University Medical School in Chicago.

Whatever your symptoms, you usually feel worn out from your body's fight against itself. The inflammation may be one reason for the fatigue, but it could also be the sleep problems or the anemia that often goes along with a chronic disease like lupus.

What's Happening

The prevalence of lupus among women, and especially women between the ages of 15 and 45, has many experts suspecting that hormones may play a role, particularly estrogen. Other theories blame stress, sunlight, certain medications, and viruses for the disease. Lupus also seems to have a slight genetic link, so if you have a family history of lupus, let your doctor know.

As hard as lupus is for researchers to understand, it's often just as tough for family members, who may be unwilling to pick up the slack for a mom who doesn't look or sound sick to them. "You don't get any sympathy the way someone with crutches and a cast might," Dr. Utset says.

Finding Help

You may have to see more than one doctor to get the help you need. While rheumatologists specialize in diseases such as lupus, you may need a nephrologist for kidney problems or a dermatologist for rashes. There are several prescription treatment options.

Steroids. Fast and effective, steroids are usually the first line of therapy for serious flare-ups. But they may increase your risk of osteoporosis, diabetes, high blood pressure, and other conditions, so many doctors look for other options.

Immunosuppressive drugs. Medications such as methotrexate sodium (Rheumatrex) or azathioprine (Imuran) may be easier on your body than steroids alone, says Dr. Ramsey-Goldman. "Sometimes, two drugs at lower doses give you better control with fewer side effects." But if you choose this route, you should discuss vaccinations against tetanus, hepatitis B, and the flu with your doctor because these "steroid-sparing drugs" treat lupus by suppressing your overactive immune system. Your lupus will be under control, but you'll be at greater risk for colds, flu, and anything else that comes around.

Antimalarials. Used for treating malaria, drugs such as hydroxychloroquine sulfate (Plaquenil) also help the skin and joint problems associated with lupus by reducing inflammation and ratcheting down your hyperactive immune system.

NSAIDs. Nonsteroidal anti-inflammatory drugs such as ibuprofen (Advil, Motrin) and naproxen sodium (Aleve) can ease the pain, swelling, and fever of lupus, but talk to your doctor before buying a bottle of over-the-counter ibuprofen: You may need a higher dosage than the one listed on the label.

There are some other strategies you can try as well.

Stay in the shade. Sunshine can trigger a flare-up. To protect yourself, stay inside from 10:00 A.M. to 2:00 P.M., when the sun's rays are at their strongest. Other times, wear a hat, long sleeves, and an SPF-30 sunblock.

Take notes. Problems with memory or concentration are a common challenge for women with lupus. Keep your edge by carrying a small notebook and pen to jot down everything from your grocery list to phone numbers.

Exercise. "You need to get regular rest, but that doesn't mean that you should be a lump the

WOMEN ASK WHY

Why am I so tired during the first trimester of pregnancy?

Nobody knows precisely why we feel so fatigued in the early months of pregnancy, but hormones probably play a role. These symptoms aren't psychological; before women discover that they're pregnant and start changing how they eat, drink, or exercise, they often report feeling fatigued or nauseated. That's how many women first realize they're pregnant.

During the first 3 months, there's a major increase in two hormones: human chorionic gonadotropin, or hCG, and progesterone. When women use products that contain progesterone, such as hormone-replacement therapy, birth control pills, and even hormones for early pregnancy support, they often say they feel drowsy.

But not every woman reports fatigue or nausea—some get lucky with a symptom-free first trimester. Others may just be more sensitive to their hormones. Then there are women who describe a fatigue that seems to be out of proportion to how pregnant they are—to the point where they can't get out of bed. When they see ultrasound images of

rest of the time," says Joan Merrill, M.D., chief of rheumatology at St. Luke's–Roosevelt Hospital Center in New York City. She urges women to pursue moderate exercise, such as walking, swimming, and bicycling. "When people have a chronic illness and let themselves waste away, they only get sicker."

Be heart smart. Lupus patients may have an increased risk of heart disease, which makes it especially important for them to eat a heart-healthy diet low in saturated fat, control their blood pressures, and watch their cholesterol levels.

Find good fatty acids. Research has shown that omega-3 fatty acids, found in such fish as

their pregnancy, they say, "That's how little the baby is? How can I feel the way I feel?" But usually the women who suffer the most also describe the most dramatic improvement when the first trimester ends. They just wake up one day and feel better.

Many women survive those 3 months by being good to themselves. They stay in bed an hour later and go to bed an hour earlier. They do low-impact exercise. They modify their work environments. It can be tough, however, because many women are superstitious about telling people they're pregnant or don't want their employer or coworkers to know just yet. Taking a nap can seem like the ultimate tip-off when they're already forgoing caffeine and alcohol.

So early pregnancy can be stressful, especially for women in the workforce, but that stress often subsides around the time they start feeling better physically and decide it's okay to share the news of their pregnancy.

Expert consulted
Shari Brasner, M.D.
Obstetrician-gynecologist
Manhattan
Author of Advice from a Pregnant
    Obstetrician

sardines and salmon, and gamma-linolenic acid (GLA), which is present in black currant oil and evening primrose oil, can reduce the painful inflammation in autoimmune diseases such as lupus. Researchers don't know exactly how they work, but one theory about evening primrose oil is that it blocks the effects of prostaglandins, body chemicals that cause inflammation.

Mark Stengler, N.D., director of natural medicine at Personal Physicians clinic in La Jolla, California, associate clinical professor at the National College of Naturopathic Medicine in Portland, Oregon, and author of *The Natural Physician*, recommends at least 3 grams of omega-3 fatty acids and 150 to 400 milligrams of GLA daily for those with inflammatory conditions like lupus or arthritis. Check how much GLA the evening primrose oil contains to determine the exact dosage. He also suggests taking both of these fatty acids at the same time, particularly if you plan to keep taking them for more than a few months. Naturopaths believe that long-term solo use may create an essential fatty acid imbalance in the body, which could worsen existing conditions.

Drink your milk. Both the steroids used to treat lupus and the physical inactivity too commonly associated with it can increase your chances of osteoporosis. Take 1,200 to 1,500 milligrams of calcium a day split into two doses, says Dr. Ramsey-Goldman, because your body can absorb only so much calcium at one time. She also suggests increasing your intake of dairy products such as low-fat cheese and yogurt.

Energy and Emotions

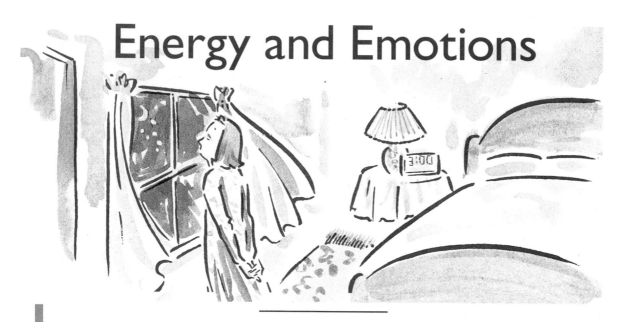

It's Monday morning, and Carolyn drags herself out of bed feeling oddly numb (in addition to exhausted). She goes through the motions of getting the kids off to school and herself to work, but the feeling remains. It scares her because it reminds her of that bad spell she had 2 years ago, when a blanket of despair seemed to suffocate her.

It started right around the time her mother began demanding more time and energy. Her daily routine, which was already insane, grew worse with regular calls and visits to ensure that her mother's needs were met. Added to the pressures of work and of raising two children, the extra duties sent her over the edge.

As the months passed, she found it harder and harder to get out of bed. She no longer looked forward to going to work, and there were days when she would just sit in her car and cry. When she got home in the evening, she felt like she had nothing left for her husband or children. All she wanted to do was sleep; yet most nights, she would lie awake for hours, or if she did fall asleep, her eyes would snap open at 4:00 A.M.

and that would be the end of her rest for the night. Eventually, her husband convinced her to see a doctor.

After 6 months of medication and talk therapy, Carolyn felt better and stopped treatment. Now, 2 years later, she's wondering if depression, her old nemesis, is back.

Carolyn is right in viewing her sleep problems and fatigue as a possible warning sign of depression, says Laura J. Miller, M.D., chief of the women's services division at the University of Illinois at Chicago. Nearly everyone who is depressed, and many who experience other mental disorders, will have disturbed sleep patterns of some sort, she says. It may be difficulty falling asleep, sleeping too much, nightmares, middle-of-the-night wakefulness, or other irregular sleep patterns.

"It's an individual thing, so everybody needs to do a personal appraisal," says Catherine A. Chambliss, Ph.D., psychology professor and department chair at Ursinus College in Collegeville, Pennsylvania. "But I urge people to take disrupted sleep somewhat seriously, to recognize that a good night's sleep will have an effect not only on your energy the next day but also on your cognitive and emotional functioning."

Fatigue or Depression?

When is what you're feeling simply fatigue? And when is it depression or anxiety? If you're merely worn out from juggling responsibilities and running all over the place, you're probably going to sleep well and wake up feeling refreshed and energized after a good night's sleep, says Dr. Chambliss. Like many overscheduled women, you might have a little difficulty going to sleep, but your body will do its best to restore itself.

"Women who aren't depressed and who are busy with their careers and their families realize that their lives have tremendous meaning," says Dr. Chambliss. "They recognize the value of what they're doing and, if they're lucky, are appreciated by others for what they're doing."

On the other hand, "the hallmarks of depression are hopelessness and helplessness," she says. "It's chronic despair and the inability to do anything about it. If you find yourself feeling that there's nothing you can do but give up, it's usually time to see a physician or therapist." These are the symptoms of clinical depression, according to the National Mental Health Association.

- A persistent sad, anxious, or "empty" mood
- Sleeping too little or sleeping too much
- Reduced appetite and weight loss, or increased appetite and weight gain
- Loss of interest or pleasure in activities you once enjoyed
- Restlessness or irritability

AMAZING ENERGY
Oh, My Aching Lips

Think Louis Armstrong had a tough kisser? Mark and Roberta Griswold of Allen Park, Michigan, locked lips continuously for a record 29 hours. Throughout their attempt, they and eight other couples had to follow rigid rules: They had to remain standing without rest breaks, and they had to keep their lips constantly touching. Asked how they were able to withstand kissing for more than one day, Mark said the secret was comfortable underwear, while Roberta attributed it to 16 years of practice. While fatigue was speculated to be the reason for stopping, the winners claimed it was the need to go to the bathroom. Their world-record kiss won them a weeklong trip to (where else?) Paris, the City of Love.

- Persistent physical symptoms that don't respond to treatment, such as headaches, chronic pain, and constipation and other digestive disorders
- Difficulty concentrating, remembering, or making decisions
- Fatigue or loss of energy
- Feeling guilty, hopeless, or worthless
- Thoughts of death or suicide

If five or more of these symptoms last longer than 2 weeks, or if the symptoms are severe enough to interfere with your daily routine, you should see a doctor.

Depression: A Woman's Nemesis

When we're depressed, neural circuits in our brains that are responsible for sleep, moods, thinking, appetite, and behavior fail to function properly, and critical neurotransmitters (the chemical messengers that enable brain cells to communicate with one another) are out of balance.

The effects of depression on sleep can be measured on an electroencephalograph (EEG), which consistently shows a delayed rapid eye movement (REM) cycle among depressed patients. When we're deprived of REM sleep—the dream state—we become far more emotional, reactive, and unstable.

Patients with other mental disorders also don't function as well when they're not sleeping well, says Dr. Chambliss. "One of the functions of sleep is to stabilize emotional reactivity, and if sleep is being disrupted by mental disorders, there can be real, measurable consequences," she says.

Another reason for sleep problems is that when we're depressed, we spend more time sitting and fretting, and so we don't tire our bodies out for a good night's sleep. We may respond to our fatigue in a passive way, such as consuming more alcohol or caffeine, or smoking a lot. We work against our body's rhythms. On the other hand, sleep frequently becomes a means of escape for depressed patients, adds Dr. Chambliss.

All in the Hormones?

"There's an epidemic of stress and depression right now," says Alice D. Domar, Ph.D., a Harvard Medical School psychologist, director of the Mind/Body Center for Women's Health, Mind/Body Medical Institute,

WOMAN TO WOMAN

She Battled Depression and Won

Ann Barry Burrows, 42, of Norfolk, Virginia, knows that she has to keep a close check on her mental health because too much stress or fatigue can cause a flare-up of her multiple sclerosis (MS). Since her diagnosis 16 years ago, Burrows has scaled back her full-time career as a journalist and learned to say no to people and jobs that demand too much. She also has gained spiritual strength and forged friendships with people who share her joy for life. Still, once in a while, things can creep up on her; around the time she turned 40, she sank into a deep depression. Here is her story.

Things were piling up on me: My only child, Morgan, had entered second grade and was becoming more independent by the day. I had left a job editing a parenting magazine because the hours had expanded and the uncertainties and pressures were too great. I was trying to figure out what would come next. My husband had recently been promoted, and we had less and less time together. Communication was limited at best.

I realize now that much of my depression was about missing my father and searching for fatherly guidance, but at the time I didn't see that. My father died when I was a year old, and my mom remarried when I was 9. My relationship with my stepfather has been difficult at times, but I've always been close to my parents and my five younger siblings.

That's why it hurt so much when one of the sisters I'd helped raise made an issue over my husband's previous divorce. She said she didn't believe the Roman Catholic church recognized our marriage. She didn't want us to stay at her house with her children. That really hurt.

I'd buried that hurt and was trying to ignore it until I received a phone call from my mother one day. She was accommodating my sister in saying that we couldn't stay at her home during the upcoming holiday gatherings while my sister's family was there.

Suddenly, I felt like an emotional orphan. I've since learned that depression can be set off by both real and imagined grief, and I was grieving for my lost family.

I went into a very bad emotional cycle. I was drained from worry, and my outlook was bleak. Everything seemed overwhelming. I didn't want to get out of bed in the morning. I thought my body was just telling me that I needed more rest.

This time, rest didn't bring relief; it led me into a vicious circle. I was tired all the time, so I would sleep too much, which would make me tired. And I would eat for comfort, then berate myself. For the first time in my life, I couldn't work. Writing is usually easy for me and a source of satisfaction, but I had to force myself to go through the motions. The avoidance of burdens added the bigger burden of guilt. It all led to a feeling of hopelessness.

Providence led me to a Christian counseling service. The counselor worked with my husband and me on our communication skills and helped me come to grips with other family issues. Through prayer, my gratitude grew for my family and what I did have.

I tried talking with my mother several times, and we made some progress, but mostly I gained understanding, acceptance, and forgiveness. It's easy to love people who love you in return, but that's not all there is to loving.

My depression lasted from September to January, and in the midst of it I had an MS attack. I started taking prednisone for it; a side effect of the medication was that it lifted my spirits.

I also had a therapeutic night in the hot tub, sharing wine and stories with some girlfriends, which helped me regain my sense of community and know I wasn't alone with my problems. Everyone empathized and supported me.

I found a therapist who specializes in guided meditation and imagery. He helped me find a quiet place within myself. I realized through meditation that I could take all my problems and let the crucial one bubble up and crystallize. That's how I focused on the relationship with my two fathers, and through that, I gained a stronger relationship with my spiritual father.

I'm in good health now and have a quiet spirit. Whenever I need to, I can take 20 to 30 minutes to get into this relaxed state. I'm not just coping but conquering. There are times when there is so much joy in my life that I can hardly stay in my skin.

and author of *Self-Nurture: Learning to Care for Yourself As Effectively As You Care for Everyone Else.* Over the course of a lifetime, about 1 in 5 women will be diagnosed with depression, compared to only 1 in 10 men.

One reason may be our hormones. A study by the National Institute of Mental Health showed that the depressive mood swings of premenstrual syndrome (PMS) result from an abnormal response to normal hormone changes during the menstrual cycle. Women with a history of PMS experienced relief from their depressed moods when their sex hormones estrogen and progesterone were temporarily "turned off" by a drug that suppressed the function of the ovaries. The symptoms returned within a week or two after the hormones were reintroduced. Women with no history of PMS had no effects from the hormonal manipulation, indicating that sex hormones don't *cause* PMS but *trigger* PMS symptoms in women with a vulnerability to the disorder. Researchers are still trying to determine why some women get PMS and not others.

Additionally, many women who are depressed have an overactive hormonal system that regulates their bodies' response to stress. Normally, when we're threatened physically or psychologically, the hypothalamus, the region of the brain that manages hormone release from our glands, increases production of corticotropin releasing factor (CRF). That stimulates the pituitary and adrenal glands to release more of their hormones, thus

ANXIETY DISORDERS

Depression isn't the only mental disorder that can sap your energy. Anxiety disorders, the most common group of mental disorders, can disrupt sleep. If you feel anxious because you're about to undergo surgery or because your marriage is falling apart, that's normal anxiety. But if you constantly anticipate disaster and worry about every part of your life, from what to fix for dinner to what to give as a gift, you have generalized anxiety disorder. It usually isn't diagnosed unless you've spent at least 6 months worrying excessively.

Generalized anxiety disorder makes it hard to relax. Though sleep problems may be less common than with depression, the worrying can make it difficult to fall asleep or stay asleep. "People with anxiety disorders tend to have energy, but the energy is channeled in ways that aren't helpful, such as worry, obsession, constantly imagining worst-case scenarios, overreacting to stress, and exaggerating negative things in the environment," says Catherine A. Chambliss, Ph.D., psychology professor and department chair at Ursinus College in Collegeville, Pennsylvania. "They're energized, but it's not a pleasant state."

Panic, another form of anxiety disorder, is a feeling of terror that can strike suddenly and repeatedly with no warning. Symptoms include a pounding heart, chest pains, light-headedness, nausea, flushes or chills, sweating, shortness of breath, tingling, shaking or trembling, feelings of unreality or being out of control, and even a fear of dying. Attacks can occur anytime, even during sleep. Panic disorder is twice as common in women as in men and can become disabling if not treated. The exhausting physical symptoms and loss of sleep from nighttime attacks can leave you feeling drained during the day.

There are many other anxiety disorders, including obsessive-compulsive disorder (OCD), post-traumatic stress disorder, and phobias. All involve irrational fears, and some affect sleeping habits. For example, people with post-traumatic stress disorder often are awakened by nightmares of the trauma they experienced, says Laura J. Miller, M.D., chief of the women's services division at the University of Illinois at Chicago.

preparing our bodies for the fight-or-flight reaction. Our bodies respond with reduced appetite, decreased sex drive, and heightened alertness. This is a good reaction in the face of real danger, but research suggests that persistent overactivation of this hormonal system may leave us exhausted and lay the groundwork for depression. For instance, when depressed patients with elevated CRF levels are treated with antidepressant drugs, the reduction in their CRF levels corresponds to improvements in their depressive symptoms.

Low levels of serotonin and norepinephrine also seem to play an important role in mental disorders. Women naturally have lower serotonin levels than men, which may be one reason we're more prone to depression. That may also explain part of the reason for the sleep disorders of depression. Higher levels of serotonin increase the amount of deep sleep we get every night and improve our overall well-being. When levels drop, as they do when we're depressed, our sleep is disrupted.

Types of Depression

Depressive disorders can take many forms, but there are three common types.

Major depression. A combination of symptoms interferes with work, study, sleep, eating, and the ability to enjoy once-pleasurable activities. If depressive symptoms last for 2 weeks or if you have recurring thoughts about suicide or death, see your doctor, because major depression is likely. Episodes of major depression may occur only once, but they often reoccur periodically.

Dysthymia. A milder but longer-lasting depression, dysthymia can go untreated for years, draining happiness and energy from your life and the lives of those around you. Symptoms may be the same as for major depression but are often long-term, and they may make others think you're just grouchy or gloomy. You may be constantly pessimistic, guilt-ridden, irritable, withdrawn, or easily hurt by others for no apparent reason. You may have trouble getting along with others at home, work, or school. Dysthymia usually isn't diagnosed until you've been depressed for most of the day, more days than not, for at least 2 years.

Bipolar disorder. Also called manic-depressive illness, this disorder is characterized by mood swings. Sometimes the mood switches are dramatic and rapid, but most often they are gradual. In the depressed part of the cycle, you can have any or all of the symptoms of major depression.

In the manic part of the cycle, you may be overactive or overtalkative and have a great deal of energy, which is often misguided. An inability to sleep (sometimes for days) or a decreased need for sleep is another symptom in the manic phase. Others include inappropriate displays or excitement, high energy levels, the need to talk constantly and loudly, wild racing thoughts, distraction, sudden increase in sexual desire, impaired judgment, embarrassing behavior, and dangerous risk taking.

Know Thyself

If you've had one kind of mental disorder at some time in your life, you're more likely to ex-perience another, either of the same kind or of a different type. So it's important to keep a finger on the pulse of your mental health. In fact, after one episode of depression, there's a 50-percent chance of a recurrence; after two episodes, that risk increases to 75 percent.

It's equally important not to let sleep disturbances and fatigue go unnoticed, or to try to drown out your problems with alcohol or other drugs.

"When they hit problems in life, a lot of people will use alcohol to help them relax and fall asleep," Dr. Chambliss says. It may help you fall asleep, but it also can wake you up in the middle of the night and make it difficult to fall back to sleep. Thus, alcohol deprives you of your full sleep cycle, which can result in emotional problems.

Drinking alcohol can become a vicious circle: You drink because you're stressed; then you don't sleep well and you're tired the next day, so you drink more to relax and get to sleep. This leads to a stream of nights with poor sleep and increases the risk or severity of depression or anxiety disorder.

Similarly, you may consume more caffeine because you're tired and that, too, can disrupt your sleep patterns, Dr. Chambliss says. You should also be aware that as you age, you might not handle caffeine or alcohol in the same way you did when you were younger.

Seeking Solutions

Start with a visit to your doctor to rule out any medical conditions or medications that may cause symptoms similar to depression. Some, including anemia, thyroid disease, and calcium imbalance (your parathyroid gland doesn't process calcium properly or you're getting too much or too little) are common among middle-age women. Even women who have adjusted their diets to eat more iron can suffer from anemia during perimenopause because the blood loss during prolonged, heavy periods is greater than they are accustomed to, says Dr. Miller.

If your physical health is fine, the next step is a psychological evaluation from a psychiatrist or psychologist. Research shows that most of the 19 million Americans who experience a depressive illness each year can be helped if they receive appropriate treatment, often including a mix of medication and talk therapy. You can go the alternative route or the traditional route, or combine the two. Traditional therapies include:

Short-term therapy. Typically involving 10 to 20 weekly sessions, short-term therapy is best used when your symptoms are mild but have been around for a while and are causing consistent unhappiness. Also used with anxiety disorders, it teaches you to change specific actions and to understand and change your thinking patterns. There are two major types of short-term therapy.

- Cognitive behavioral therapy focuses on changing negative styles of thinking and behaving. Instead of thinking that everything is going to go wrong on a given day, you begin to look for the good in your life and to think of yourself as worthy.
- Interpersonal therapy focuses on problems in your personal and social relationships. The therapist helps you see how you interact with other people and helps you work on changing that behavior to improve relationships. For example, if you feel like your husband and children walk all over you, you'll learn how to express your needs and get them met.

Long-term psychodynamic therapies. Best used with severe depression, long-term psychodynamic therapies attempt to resolve internal conflicts. Because you look inside yourself to un-cover and understand emotional conflicts, your therapy may involve looking back at unresolved problems from childhood, such as abuse and neglect, and working through them to a resolution. It may last for months or years, as long as you and your therapist think you are improving and growing as a result of the therapy.

Antidepressants. Prozac is the brand name for fluoxetine, the first in a new generation of antidepressants. It's one of a class of drugs called selective serotonin reuptake inhibitors (SSRIs), which also includes Paxil, Luvox, and Zoloft. These and newer medications that affect neurotransmitters in our brains, such as dopamine, serotonin, and norepinephrine, generally have fewer side effects than tricyclics, the older class of drugs used to treat depression. To find the right drug for you, your doctor may have to try several medications or dosages, and you may have to take the medication for as long as 8 weeks before you feel the full therapeutic effect.

Lithium. For years, lithium was the drug of choice for treating bipolar disorder. It was scary stuff because the range between an effective dose and a toxic one was small. Now, however, several other drugs have been found to control mood swings, and anticonvulsants such as divalproex sodium (Depakote) and carbamazepine (Tegretol) are generally considered the first choice for treating acute mania. Both of these anticonvulsants can have serious side effects, such as lowered white blood cell counts, skin rashes, gastrointestinal disturbances, and liver dysfunction, so careful monitoring is necessary.

Benzodiazepines. Although antidepressants are also used to treat some anxiety disorders, such as panic attacks and phobias, more commonly used are benzodiazepines, which include alprazolam (Xanax), diazepam (Valium), and chlordiazepoxide (Librium, Librax, Libritabs). These antianxiety medications help calm and relax you while clearing away troubling symptoms. Benzodiazepines are generally prescribed for brief periods of days or weeks or intermittently because you can become dependent on them and have withdrawal reactions when you stop taking them.

Other medications. Prescribed for general anxiety, buspirone (BuSpar) must be taken daily for 2 to 3 weeks before its effects are felt. Other medications occasionally prescribed for anxiety disorders include antihistamines, barbiturates such as phenobarbital, and beta-blockers such as propranolol (Inderal, Inderide).

Nondrug Options

You're not limited to just therapy and medication when working through emotional problems; here are some alternative strategies that you can try.

Exercise. Any kind of exercise is good, but getting outside is best because nature and sunlight have a way of lifting your spirits. Exercise can complement traditional treatments in those who are clinically depressed and prevent depression in those who don't have the illness. One study of hospitalized depressed patients found significant reductions in depression among those who participated in an aerobic exercise program, but not in a control group who did just occupational therapy. Another study found improvement in a group of patients assigned to 8 weeks of walking and jogging, but

MEDICATIONS THAT AFFECT YOUR SLEEP

Psychotropic medications, which affect your mental state, usually have one of three effects on sleep.

- They make it easier to sleep by treating an underlying condition.
- They are sedating.
- They make it more difficult to sleep.

The most commonly used psychotropics are antidepressants, which are also prescribed for anxiety disorders and eating disorders.

Tricyclics are the oldest antidepressants still in use, and they tend to have a sedating effect on most people. When you take tricyclics and they are effective, the first thing you'll notice is that your sleep patterns improve, even before you begin to feel better, says Laura J. Miller, M.D., chief of the women's services division at the University of Illinois at Chicago.

If they make you groggy during the day, however, your doctor may need to change your dosage. They also may not be a good choice if you are already exhausted from pregnancy or parenting small children, or if you are already sleeping too much because of depression.

The most widely prescribed class of antidepressants is selective serotonin reuptake inhibitors (SSRIs) like Prozac. Eventually, they help you reclaim normal sleep patterns, but they can make you nervous and jittery for 2 to 3 weeks. Some women have to take a sleeping pill to get them through that adjustment period, says Dr. Miller.

Drugs belonging to a newer class of antidepressants, such as Effexor, affect more neurotransmitters in the brain, which means that their effects on sleep are more unpredictable. They can be sedating, activating, or have no effect on your sleep patterns.

The key, Dr. Miller says, is to communicate with your doctor about any problems you're having with medications, including troublesome sleep changes. Be as detailed as possible. Keep a sleep journal or ask your doctor for a mood chart on which you track your mood, sleep patterns, and medications so that your doctor can see the connections.

no improvement in those assigned to recreational therapy or a waiting list.

Any form of exercise may work, though most studies have been conducted with running, walking, or other aerobic exercise. One study found similar improvements between groups who ran or lifted weights for 8 weeks. That study also concluded that mood improvement did not depend on achieving physical fitness.

How exercise eases depression remains unclear. Psychologically, exercise may give us a greater sense of mastery, which is important when we feel a loss of control over our lives, says Dr. Miller. Analysis of 51 studies linked exercise to a small but significant increase in self-esteem. It also gets our minds off what's bothering us. And it may improve our health, physiques, flexibility, and weight, all of which put us in a better mood, she adds. Just being able to eat without worrying about gaining weight can increase our pleasure and sense of self-control.

Intense exercise has been shown in some studies to increase brain serotonin. And beta-endorphins, chemicals that reduce pain and can make us euphoric, have been linked to the runner's high that comes after intense exercise.

One thing that is clear is that exercise completed 4 to 6 hours before bedtime makes us sleep better. This is important because disturbed sleep is both a symptom and an aggravating factor in depression. A controlled clinical trial of 32 depressed adults found that a program of weight-training exercise done three times a week for 10 weeks improved the quality of their sleep and lessened their depression.

Socialize. Walking with a friend or a group is doubly beneficial because you get exercise and the bonus of conversation and company. People

WOMEN ASK WHY

Why do I get so tired in winter?

It may be your body's way of making sure you recover from the winter holidays, it may be a seasonal depression, or it may be the human version of hibernation.

The holidays can wipe you out completely. There's so much to do from mid-November continuing through New Year's. You eat more, drink more, and socialize more, which makes you more tired.

And you tend to exercise less in the winter because of jam-packed holiday schedules and cold weather. Like animals that hibernate, you burn energy faster when it's cold, so your body wants to slow down and conserve that energy.

Sometimes, just the feeling of being trapped inside makes you depressed, especially if you live in an area with harsh winters. You may want to stay in bed and pull the blanket over your head until spring arrives. In the Northeast and Midwest, social activities are curbed. People don't plan things because the weather is so unpredictable. Weddings, graduations, and other celebrations are geared toward spring and summer.

Or the problem may be seasonal affective disorder, commonly known as SAD, in which a lack of sunlight causes depression. Although summer depression can occur, SAD most

who aren't willing or likely to depend on others and people who are hostile or aggressive (thereby having fewer friends and social support systems) are more likely to relapse into major depression, according to a University of Washington study.

"Social support is a tremendous buffer against depression," Dr. Domar says. "And for today's working moms, time with friends is the first thing to go." We also tend to isolate ourselves when we're depressed. So reach out. Attend classes, concerts, lectures, church or synagogue,

often begins in late fall or early winter and goes away by summer. It occurs more often in northern climates, and it's four times more common in women than in men.

Symptoms of SAD may be similar to those seen in other forms of general depression: increased appetite, especially a craving for sweet or starchy foods; weight gain; heavy feeling in the arms or legs; a drop in energy level; fatigue; a tendency to oversleep; difficulty concentrating; irritability; increased sensitivity to social rejection; and avoidance of social situations.

If the winter blahs seem to be affecting your daily life, it's time to see a doctor. She may suggest light therapy, in which you sit under or near a specially made light box or a light visor for 30 minutes each morning. She may also recommend medication or behavior therapy, either alone or together with light therapy.

One initial treatment of SAD is to get sun on your face by going for a midday walk outside. Whether you have depression or just the blahs, it's important that you continue to exercise. Exercise makes you feel better, reduces depression, and keeps you healthier.

Expert consulted
Alice D. Domar, Ph.D.
Director of the Mind/Body Center for Women's
   Health, Mind/Body Medical Institute
Beth Israel Deaconess Medical Center
Harvard Medical School

a book club, or anything else that suits your personality.

Get religion. A study conducted by Patricia Murphy, Ph.D., assistant professor in the department of religion, health, and human values at Rush-Presbyterian-St. Luke's Medical Center in Chicago, shows that religious beliefs lower levels of depression and have an even greater impact on lowering levels of hopelessness.

Relax. Numerous studies have shown that meditation, guided imagery, and muscle relaxation alleviate symptoms of anxiety and depression. Dr. Miller suggests that one way to relax is with a quick abdominal exhalation of breath—one or two exhalations every second. Relax on the inhale. Breathing with your abdomen and diaphragm calms the sympathetic nervous system that regulates your blood pressure and pulse, making you feel more relaxed and energized, Dr. Miller says. A therapist trained in these areas can tailor a regimen of exercise and relaxation to suit your particular disorders and symptoms, she adds.

Try an herbal therapy. In Germany, hypericum, the concentrated extract from St. John's wort (*Hypericum perforatum*), is used more than any other medication to treat depression. German researchers say that it is safer and just as effective for treating moderate depression as the antidepressant drug imipramine, with fewer side effects.

Although it is sold as a dietary supplement at health food stores in the United States, the Food and Drug Administration does not allow any antidepressant claims for St. John's wort. The National Institutes of Health, however, is conducting a 3-year study in the United States on the effectiveness and proper dosages of hypericum.

Unblock your energy. Chinese medicine, which combines the use of herbs and acupuncture, may help with depression and anxiety. "A practitioner would put together a treatment plan that could include a course of acupuncture treatments and an herbal formula tailored to address your specific experience of depression," says Rosa Schnyer, L.Ac., licensed acupuncturist in Tucson and a research specialist in the University of Arizona's psychology department.

Chinese medicine doesn't focus on treatment of specific diseases but on trying to balance the life force, or chi, says Schnyer. And it doesn't separate psychological from physiological symptoms. So it wouldn't be necessary for a licensed acupuncturist to attribute your lethargy directly to depression, anxiety, or fatigue. Instead, the acupuncturist would try to understand how your personal experience of fatigue, combined with other symptoms, affects your life and would design a treatment to correct this imbalance.

The acupuncturist would select certain points along the surface of your body and insert small, fine needles to supplement what is empty and drained and to correct obstruction and blockage in the areas where the energy is stagnant. In addition, she may create an herbal prescription and make dietary and lifestyle recommendations.

Even with treatment (whether through medication, psychotherapy, or alternative treatments), it can take a few months to recover from depression or anxiety disorders. In the meantime, nurture yourself and let family and friends help you. "It's a shame to let depression go untreated," says Dr. Chambliss. "The majority of people who seek help will show dramatic improvement in a relatively short time."

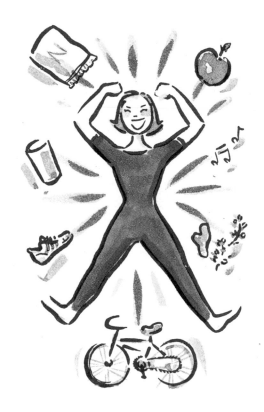

PART THREE

Energy
Chargers

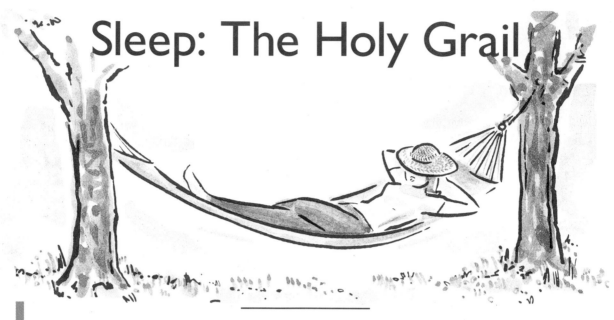

Sleep: The Holy Grail

It's 5:00 P.M. and Carolyn is anxious to leave the office. If she can get home early, she just might get to bed at 9:00 instead of midnight. Suddenly, her boss pops into her office, needing help with some memos for a meeting that night.

Her stomach churns. "I was here late last night. And the night before," Carolyn mutters as she grudgingly plops her bags on the floor and restarts her computer. "When will I ever get any rest?" she asks herself.

Bleary-eyed and exhausted, she plods through the assignment, finally dragging herself home at 7:30 P.M. All she can think of is crawling into bed and getting some sleep.

But first she has to eat, review her son's homework, clean the kitchen, and call her mom. By the time she dots the last "i" and crosses the last "t" on Michael's book report, it's nearly midnight. Desperate to get some shut-eye, Carolyn pops a sleeping pill and calls it a night.

Sleep Defined

Sleep experts recommend that we get at least 8 hours of sleep each night. Yet the average woman from ages 30 to 60 sleeps only 6 hours and 41 minutes a night during the workweek. No wonder we fantasize about a good night's sleep more often than a dip in a hot tub with Harrison Ford.

Like food, clothing, and shelter, sleep is something that we can't live without. It's considered an altered state of consciousness that restores us physically and emotionally. And it is as essential to our long-term health as daily exercise, says Kathy Sexton-Radek, Ph.D., a sleep medicine specialist and professor and chair of the psychology department at Elmhurst College in Illinois.

Researchers aren't sure how or why sleep renews us, but they do have some ideas. Sleep lowers our body temperatures, decreases oxygen consumption, and slows our heart rates and metabolism (the rate at which we burn calories) 5 to 25 percent. These changes may force our bodies to conserve energy overnight so we feel rejuvenated in the morning, says Suzanne Woodward, Ph.D., an expert on women and sleep and assistant professor of psychiatry at Wayne State University School of Medicine in Detroit.

Another theory is that sleep gives our brains a much-needed rest from the flurry of daily activity, says Margaret Moline, Ph.D., director of the sleep-wake disorders center at New York Presbyterian Hospital–Weill Cornell Medical Center in White Plains and New York City. It's like a Zamboni for our brains, clearing away the detritus of the day much like the giant machine clears the pitted ice of a skating rink. If our brains didn't have the opportunity to sleep, we wouldn't be able to concentrate or think as clearly, she says.

Sleep is vital to learning, too. In a study of 27 people examining one night's sleep, researchers found that those who slept about 8 hours and got enough deep, slow-wave sleep in the first 2 hours of slumber and at least 2 hours of rapid eye movement (REM) sleep in the early morning had an easier time learning and retaining information compared to those who didn't get that quality of sleep.

It's also important for emotional balance. When we get enough restful sleep, we're less likely to snap at our husbands, yell at our kids, or kick our pets. We're also less sluggish. In fact, missing as little as 2 hours of sleep every night for a week sends our levels of fatigue, confusion, and anxiety skyrocketing and causes mood swings, according to researchers from the University of Pennsylvania School of Medicine.

WOMEN ASK WHY

Why do I sometimes wake up with a headache?

Most morning headaches are triggered by tension or stress, which increases blood circulation in the brain, causing you pain. Even though you're relaxed while you sleep, those 7 to 8 hours aren't enough to undo the chronic tension experienced during the day.

Fatigue is another factor. Researchers surveyed 113 chronic headache sufferers, about half of them women, and 110 healthy participants, and found that those who endured ongoing tension and migraine headaches 1(especially the women) were more tired than those who didn't. Part of the reason was that those with headaches didn't sleep as well.

Chronic headaches can interfere with falling asleep and staying asleep. And the fatigue you experience the next day often makes the pain even worse, creating a vicious circle.

There's also a link between morning headaches and high blood pressure. Women with high blood pressure may wake up with a pulsating head pain known as a hatband headache. Because their blood is more apt to clump, their blood vessels have to dilate to make way for the bunched-up blood cells. This repeated expansion of the blood vessels throughout the night can cause a morning headache.

Another possibility is sleep apnea, a common sleep disorder characterized by loud snoring and brief interruptions in breathing while sleeping. The lack of oxygen and changes in blood pressure that result can cause a headache.

Experts consulted
Kathy Sexton-Radek, Ph.D.
Sleep medicine specialist
Professor and psychology department chair
Elmhurst College
Illinois

Suzanne Woodward, Ph.D.
Expert on women and sleep
Assistant professor of psychiatry
Wayne State University School of Medicine
Detroit

The reason is that sleep loss causes daytime sleepiness, which creates a struggle to stay awake, alert, and motivated enough to do anything that requires energy. And that has a negative effect on our mental health.

When you think of the perfect good night's sleep, you might imagine fluffy pillows, a cozy blanket or comforter, sweet dreams—and no alarm clock to startle you into wakefulness in the morning.

But there's a lot more to catching some z's than you might think. Soon after you crawl into bed, you begin a complex but fascinating journey that takes you through four stages and two distinct types of sleep: REM and non-REM.

Usually occurring about five times during the night, REM is that part of the sleep cycle where we dream, subconsciously fantasizing about winning the lottery and buying that mansion in Maui. Our brain waves hit warp speed as if we were awake. Our eyes bounce back and forth like Ping-Pong balls, and we actually get a mini-cardiovascular workout as our hearts beat faster and we breathe harder. "It's like stepping on the accelerator while your car engine is running to give it more gas," says Dr. Sexton-Radek. But even though our brains and bodies are "active" during REM sleep, it is still restful sleep. And everyone experiences it—even those who swear they don't dream.

We spend about 25 percent of the night in REM sleep. The rest is non-REM sleep, which occurs in four stages. Each stage of the non-REM

DEMONS IN THE NIGHT

If you're snoozing for 8 hours and still don't feel rested, you may have a sleep disorder. Here are some of the most common ones that may be contributing to your fatigue. If you suspect that you have any of these conditions, talk to your doctor right away.

Sleep Apnea

What is it? The second most common sleep disorder after insomnia, sleep apnea strikes 2 percent of middle-age women. The most common form is obstructive sleep apnea, which usually occurs when the throat muscles and tongue relax during sleep, causing the soft palate at the base of your tongue and uvula (that small fleshy tissue hanging in the back of your throat) to sag and partially block the airway. If you have this type of sleep apnea, you can stop breathing as few as 5 or as many as 100 times an hour while sleeping.

Central sleep apnea occurs when your brain fails to send certain signals to your diaphragm and chest muscles to initiate breathing. As a result, you wake up several times a night to catch your breath. Mixed apnea is a combination of obstructive sleep apnea and central sleep apnea.

What are the symptoms? Sleep apnea results in brief interruptions in breathing while sleeping, loud snoring, snorting, gasping for air, daytime sleepiness, irritability, morning headaches, and impaired thinking. Depression, high blood pressure, heart attack, and stroke are the more dire consequences.

What is the treatment? The most effective treatment is continuous positive airway pressure (CPAP). You wear a mask over your nose that's connected to a machine that pumps pressurized air in to keep your airway open during sleep. There are also several dental devices that prevent your tongue from sliding backward. Surgery may also be used to increase the size of your airway, but the procedure is only 30 to 50 percent effective.

Narcolepsy

What is it? Narcolepsy is a chronic neurological disorder that affects about 1 in every 2,000 people. Although it has no known cause, sleep experts suspect an abnormality in the chemistry regulating sleep and wakefulness.

What are the symptoms? Signs of narcolepsy include overwhelming daytime sleepiness; sleep attacks with or without warning; cataplexy, which are brief episodes of muscle weakness or paralysis triggered by strong emotional reactions such as laughter, anger, or fear that may last a few seconds to several minutes; sleep paralysis, which is a temporary inability to talk or move when falling asleep or waking up; and hypnagogic hallucinations, which are vivid, frightening, dreamlike images that occur while falling asleep or upon awakening.

What is the treatment? For daytime sleepiness, there are prescription drugs that stimulate the central nervous system, such as modafinil (Provigil), dextroamphetamine (Dexedrine), methamphetamine (Desoxyn), and methylphenidate (Ritalin). For cataplexy, there are antidepressants and other drugs, such as fluoxetine hydrochloride (Prozac), clomipramine (Anafranil), and imipramine (Tofranil). Many of these antidepressants work by suppressing REM sleep, thus limiting or eliminating episodes of cataplexy.

Restless Legs Syndrome (RLS)

What is it? This sleep disorder causes unpleasant sensations in your legs and sometimes in your arms.

What are the symptoms? You have creepy, crawly, tingly feelings in your legs that often compel you to walk, stretch, give yourself a massage, or perform knee bends for relief. Daytime sleepiness, fatigue, and difficulty falling asleep and staying asleep are also common.

What is the treatment? Mild RLS symptoms are usually relieved by regular exercise, massage, hot baths, heating pads, ice packs, or eliminating caffeine. Moderate to severe cases call for prescription medications from any one of the following drug classes: dopamine agents like pramipexole (Mirapex) and pergolide (Permax); benzodiazepines like clonazepam (Klonopin); and opiates, including codeine and oxycodone hydrochloride (M-Oxy).

part of the cycle is necessary to help replenish our physical and mental energy, sharpen our memory and ability to learn, and restore us emotionally. If we skip a stage or fail to remain in any particular one long enough, we wake up bone tired and cranky. All of the stages work in sync to help refresh and energize us.

- Stage 1. We enter this phase of non-REM sleep when we first fall asleep. A light doze, it's a transition between wakefulness and sleep during which our muscles relax. Our brain wave activity is similar to when we're awake, because we're not really asleep. It lasts a mere 1 to 7 minutes, starting the cascade of sleep.
- Stage 2. During this stage, our brain wave activity and body mechanisms begin to slow as we move into a slightly deeper sleep. This is what sleep experts actually call "sleep." Again, we're in this stage for 1 to 7 minutes.
- Stages 3 and 4. Although they are defined as separate stages, sleep experts still lump these two stages together because the differences between them are so slight. Known as delta, or deep, sleep because of their association with slow brain wave patterns, it is during these deeper stages that the immune system is at its best, reacting with a surge of energy to produce white blood cells that fend off bacteria and viruses. "That's why if you get enough rest during a cold or flu, you're more

Nine times out of 10, we are already tired before we get into the car; we just don't know it. A quick spin to the store usually won't tell us how tired we are, but driving for an hour or more definitely will. Driving is a boring activity that provides very little physical stimulation.

And if you're sleep-deprived and driving between the hours of 2:00 and 4:00 P.M., toothpicks may not be able to keep your eyes open. During those hours, your circadian rhythm, which determines how alert or drowsy you are throughout the day, dips. That's where the phrase "afternoon slump" comes from. This is the time of day when driving can be the most dangerous.

Drowsiness slows reaction time, decreases awareness, and impairs judgment, which can lead to traffic accidents. The U.S. National Highway Traffic Safety Administration (NHTSA) estimates that approximately 100,000 crashes annually are attributed to drowsiness. Here's what you can do to stay alert while on the road.

- Pull in to a convenience store parking lot or gas station the moment you start to feel sleepy. Get out of the car, stretch your legs, buy some coffee, drink up, and then take a nap for 20 minutes while giving the caffeine a chance to kick in.
- Plan to drive during the times of the day when you are the most alert. Avoid driving during your body's "downtime."
- Schedule a break every 2 hours or every 100 miles. Stop sooner if you get tired.
- Share the driving with a friend. You'll have someone to talk to, and you'll be able to rest up while your friend drives.

Expert consulted
Joyce Walsleben, R.N., Ph.D.
Director of the Sleep Disorders Center
Research Associate Professor
New York University School of Medicine
New York City

apt to fight the infection," says Dr. Sexton-Radek. Along with REM sleep, these two stages are the most restorative because this is when our bodies turn on the switch for many of our necessary functions, including the release of hormones and neurotransmitters.

When we first fall asleep, we go through non-REM stages 1 and 2 and then have our first REM. After that, we go through non-REM stages 1 through 4 and then have our second REM. The entire pattern is repeated throughout the night. In all, we typically have five REM episodes that usually last 4 to 12 minutes each, but can last up to 30 minutes. So if we sleep 8 hours a night, we get 30 minutes to 2 hours of REM sleep; the rest is non-REM.

The 10 Commandments of Sleep

There are things we do (or don't do) that affect how quickly we fall asleep and how well we sleep. We call them the 10 Commandments of Sleep, and following them should lead to blissful rest, energized mornings, and sweet dreams.

1. Thou shalt not drink alcohol or caffeinated beverages within 4 to 6 hours of bedtime. A nightcap before bed may help you conk out faster, but it can shorten the time you spend in the deeper stages of sleep and cause you to wake up several times during the night. It can also cause nightmares and early-morning headaches. One reason for the middle-of-the-night awakening is that your nervous system becomes aroused as your blood alcohol levels drop.

As for caffeine, it stimulates the brain. So don't be surprised if you find yourself staring at the ceiling in the wee hours if you had an after-dinner cup of coffee. Colas, chocolate, cocoa, and certain prescription drugs also contain caffeine. Moderate daytime use usually doesn't interfere with sleep, but if you have trouble falling asleep or staying asleep, cut caffeine out completely, Dr. Woodward says. While most people's systems clear the caffeine from a cup of coffee in 3 to 5 hours, others need as many as 10 hours.

2. Thou shalt not smoke cigarettes within 4 to 6 hours of bedtime. Like caffeine, nicotine stimulates the central nervous system. It interferes with falling asleep and staying asleep by increasing heart rate, blood pressure, and adrenaline levels, says Amy Wolfson, Ph.D., co-chair of Women in Sleep and Rhythms Research (WISRR) at the College of the Holy Cross in Worcester, Massachusetts.

3. Thou shalt not nap for longer than 30 minutes. The urge for that midafternoon snooze is associated with your body's internal biological clock. Between 2:00 and 4:00 P.M., a drop in body temperature occurs, which usually causes you to feel sleepy, says

WOMAN TO WOMAN

She Has Shift Work Down to a Science

Claire Dodds, 32, a registered nurse at the University of California–San Francisco Medical Center makes the tough transition between working nights and days with relative ease. Here's her story.

As a clinical nurse, I work the day shift 16 weeks a year and the night shift the remaining 36 weeks. When I work nights, I'm at the hospital from 7:00 P.M. to 7:30 A.M. three evenings in a row, then I'm off for 4 days. After the first two nights, I go to bed at 9:00 A.M. and get up at 5:00 P.M. When I come home from the third night, I hit the sack at 9:00 A.M. and set my alarm for 2:00 P.M. Then I immediately force my body back into a day schedule. I feel jet-lagged, groggy, and disoriented for the rest of the afternoon, but I deal with it because it happens only once a week, and it enables me to go to bed around 10:00 P.M. that night and wake up to a normal day schedule.

To switch from a daytime to a nighttime schedule, I get up before 8:00 A.M. and jog 3 miles. The aerobic exercise makes me just tired enough to take a nap from 3:00 to 5:00 P.M., which is just enough rest to recharge my batteries before I report to work. If I don't exercise, I'm not tired enough to nap, and that makes the transition difficult. I also stop drinking coffee at 4:30 P.M. when I work days, and at 4:30 A.M. when I work nights.

The key to handling shift work successfully is having the ability to manage your anxiety about being overly tired and possibly making a mistake. Just a little anxiety keeps me alert enough that I won't make an error. It takes some planning and preparation to get enough rest. But once I figured out the formula that works for me—and stuck to it—I didn't have any problems.

Terri E. Weaver, R.N., Ph.D., associate professor at the University of Pennsylvania School of Nursing and a sleep researcher at the Center for Sleep and Respiratory Neurobiology at the University of Pennsylvania School of Medicine,

HOW IN THE WORLD DO THEY SLEEP?

Sleeping in a Sleep Disorders Clinic

Night after night, Kathy Allwein of Fleetwood, Pennsylvania, struggled to breathe while she slept. And she snored loudly. Her husband complained, but Allwein dismissed his comments.

Some mornings on her way to work, Allwein, 38, a licensed practical nurse, fell asleep at the wheel and drove off the road. Luckily, she never had an accident or hit anybody.

She wound up in the office of an ear-nose-and-throat specialist who referred her to the sleep disorders center at Reading Hospital and Medical Center, where she works. Doctors suspected sleep apnea, a disorder that causes your throat muscles and tongue to relax during sleep and block your airway, and recommended an all-night evaluation.

Allwein arrived at the sleep lab at 9:00 P.M. with her pajamas, toothbrush, and pillow.

Technicians spent an hour preparing Allwein for the night ahead. They attached a series of thin wires to her body to monitor brain wave activity, keep tabs on her sleep stages, track breathing, and detect movement. They also put a strip under her nose to monitor airflow.

She dozed off around 11:00 P.M. as the video camera rolled and the machines in another room monitored her vital signs. At 5:30 A.M., a technician woke her to remove the wires and allow her to get dressed.

Her doctors' suspcions were confirmed: Allwein had severe obstructive sleep apnea. They prescribed continuous positive airway pressure (CPAP). Today, she sleeps with a mask that's connected to a machine that pumps air into her nose to keep her airway open.

Reflecting on her overnight stay in the sleep clinic, Allwein says, "I was very comfortable. I had no problems falling asleep. In fact, I felt like I was in my own home."

Allwein says that she now has much more energy because she's getting a good night's sleep. She's awake from the time she gets up between 5:00 and 6:30 A.M. until she goes to bed between 10:00 and 11:00 P.M.

both in Philadelphia. A 20- to 30-minute nap works wonders if you didn't get enough shut-eye the night before.

One Swedish study found that eight participants who were deprived of sleep and then allowed to take a 30-minute midafternoon nap the next day reported feeling more alert. They performed better on certain tests than when they weren't permitted to take a nap. As seen in this study, naps can help make up for lost sleep. "If you slept for 7 hours last night but need 8 hours to feel your best, a half-hour nap can help put you back on track," says Dr. Moline. "But it won't make up for a 5-hour sleep deficit accrued the prior week."

Further, it's important that you take the nap in the afternoon. Snoozing too late in the day will make you less sleepy at your normal bedtime. And don't doze more than 30 minutes. Nap longer than that, and you'll fall into the deeper stages of sleep and feel even groggier when you wake up. Choose a room for your nap that is dark and quiet. If you nap regularly, do it at the same time, Dr. Moline says. Just be aware that those who nap on a regular basis often sleep less at night and can become sleep-deprived if they start missing their naps, she adds.

4. Thou shalt not exercise within 3 hours of bedtime. As you wind down in the evening, your body temperature falls to get you ready for sleep. Aerobic exercise and weight training do just the opposite. They raise your temperature, boost your heart rate, speed your breathing, and increase levels of the stimulating hormone adrenaline. This prevents you from falling asleep at your normal bedtime, says Dr. Weaver.

It's best to exercise in the morning because that helps you sleep better at night, notes Dr. Weaver. Researchers don't know why, but they suspect that expending a burst of energy early in the day tires the body out just enough so that sleep comes more easily at night.

5. Thou shalt not sleep in on weekends. Changing your sleep patterns on the weekends resets your internal clock. "Hitting the sack late on Friday and Saturday night, and then sleeping in on Saturday and Sunday morning will prevent you from getting to sleep at your normal bedtime. So you'll wake up tired on Monday morning," says Dr. Weaver. The corollary to this commandment: Thou shalt go to bed at the same time every night and get up at the same time each day.

6. Thou shalt not lie awake in bed for more than 15 minutes. If you can't fall asleep, chances are you'll watch the clock, toss and turn, and become anxious. That will make falling asleep that much more difficult, says Dr. Woodward. The better alternative is to get up, leave your bedroom, and do something relaxing like reading or watching television. Keep the lights dim and

THE BEST WAY TO WAKE UP
IN THE MORNING

When your alarm clock goes off, you:
a. Hit the snooze button (for the fourth time)
b. Hide your head under your pillow
c. Toss your alarm clock across the room
d. Spring out of bed and start your morning

Unless you answered "d," you certainly could use some more get-up-and-go. This morning makeover comes from a survey of 22 women who share the tricks that give them the most energy.

Don't be alarmed. Several respondents said they wake up every day without the aid of an alarm clock. The key is to go to bed and get up at the same time every day (including weekends). Use an alarm only when you need to get up early, such as when you're catching a 4:30 A.M. flight.

Shy away from snoozing. If you're not ready to stash away your alarm clock for good, resist the temptation to hit the snooze button. Many of the women who do use an alarm clock feel more awake if they skip the snooze.

Wake up with nature. One woman starts her day with a dose of Mother Nature. "Before I turn off the bedroom lights at night, I open the window shades and the window. I love to wake up to fresh air, the rising sun, and the sounds of birds," says Molly Brown, 42, of Allentown, Pennsylvania.

Shed some light. If you're a city dweller, you can still get the benefits of light without being roused by traffic noise. Get yourself an alarm clock that simulates the sunrise by gradually lighting up the room. These are available from Visionweaver for about $156. For more information, write to them at PO Box 891, Bellingham, WA 98227.

Make like a cat. Did you ever notice that your feline (or canine) always stretches after waking from a nap? Several women say stretching wakes them up and leaves them feeling more energized.

Get up on the right side of the bed. Try starting your day on a positive note by reading an inspirational quote, poem, or scripture. Keep a poem-a-day book or a calendar with inspirational sayings on your bedside table.

the noise down, and make sure that whatever you read or watch doesn't excite you. Return to bed only when you feel drowsy.

7. Thou shalt not bathe less than 2 hours before bedtime. Whether you take a cool shower or soak in a hot bath, you can alter your body temperature. Remember that a natural dip in temperature helps cue your body that it's time to sleep. "Bathing too close to bedtime may throw off that natural cue," Dr. Woodward says.

8. Thou shalt not use your bed for anything other than sleep or sex. Reading, watching television, or doing office work in your bedroom can make it more difficult to fall asleep because it leaves you feeling alert, which is not the best emotional state to be in when you finally turn out the lights. "You want to associate your bedroom with tranquillity and calm, not with tension or entertainment. Reading the last chapter of a murder mystery or becoming aggravated at the evening news may keep you awake," says Dr. Moline.

9. Thou shalt design thy bedroom for rest. Flip through any department store catalog and you're bound to find the picture-perfect bedroom that you wish you had in your own home. Notice that there are no computers, fax machines, or televisions crowding the view. And everything matches. You can create the same environment.

First, ditch the hardware, software, and boob tube, and consider purchasing a color-coordinated bed ensemble that includes a comforter, duster, pillow shams, and matching sheets. The

WOMEN ASK WHY

Why doesn't my husband's snoring keep him awake?

That's a question spouses often ask. And it's no wonder, since more than 30 percent of all people snore. Most snorers are overweight men, but women catch up with them somewhere around menopause.

A few people who snore hear themselves in the light stages of sleep. But usually, it's just not on their radar screen. He doesn't hear it because he's asleep. You hear it because it's keeping you awake.

When you sleep, the muscles that open your throat relax. As you breathe, air still passes easily through your throat on the way to your lungs. If you snore, your muscles may relax too much, or your jaw may be smaller than normal. Those around you hear the vibrations of your soft palate (the fleshy part at the back of the roof of your mouth), uvula (which hangs from the soft palate), tongue, and tonsils. It sounds like a flag flapping in the wind. Some people's snoring can be heard in other rooms of the house or even by the neighbors.

Excessively loud snoring may be a sign of a more serious condition such as sleep apnea, in which those relaxed throat muscles briefly stop your breathing, awakening you for a few seconds. The pattern may go on all night. You won't remember waking up, but you may be overly tired, irritable,

matching linens will help calm the setting for sleep. Buy draperies to match, and make sure they have blackout linings to keep the room as dark as possible when it's time to sleep, says Charlotte Thompson, president and owner of Charlotte Thompson and Associates, an interior design company in Dallas. Look for shades and drapes with blackout linings at any window treatment retailer that offers custom drapes.

headachy, forgetful, or accident-prone during the day. And your partner may notice that your snoring is interrupted by gasps as you stop breathing and awaken.

There are things you can do to still get sleep while sharing a room with a snoring partner. First, go to bed a half-hour before your snoring partner. The snoring only bothers you when you're trying to fall asleep. If you're asleep first, you probably won't notice it.

You could also sew a pocket onto the back of his T-shirt and fill it with a couple of tennis balls or walnuts in the shell to prevent him from lying on his back. He'll snore less if he's on his side since the soft structures of his throat won't slide backward.

In addition, encourage him to lose weight. Obesity makes snoring worse.

Keep him away from alcohol within 4 hours of bedtime, and tell him to avoid sleeping pills, sedatives, and antihistamines. All of those things can slow breathing and worsen snoring.

When all else fails, try the time-honored "elbow technique."

Expert consulted
Nancy Fishback, M.D.
Sleep Disorders Center
Sentara Norfolk Hospital
Associate professor of medicine
Eastern Virginia Medical School

Select calm, soothing shades from the blue and green color families. Reds, oranges, and yellows tend to stimulate rather than relax you, says Thompson. Opt for incandescent or halogen lighting instead of fluorescent. Halogen is closer to natural light, which is softer on the eyes.

Consider aromatherapy. Use relaxing, soothing scents like lavender, bergamot, chamomile, vanilla, and sandalwood in your bedroom. Place one drop of essential oil on a handkerchief and sniff, or dab it on your sheets; put five drops in some bathwater and soak; or put four drops in a pan of hot water and inhale before you go to bed. If you experience any skin irritation, discontinue using the oil.

10. Thou shalt dress appropriately for bed. Wear whatever is comfortable for you: a silk negligee, a flannel nightgown, a cotton T-shirt. Or sleep in the buff. But keep in mind that your body temperature drops prior to falling asleep, rises during the night, then falls before you awake. So always think lighter rather than heavier when choosing pajamas. If you have perimenopausal symptoms such as hot flashes and night sweats, wear cool cotton pajamas, Dr. Woodward suggests.

The Ins and Outs of Sleeping Pills

If you haven't slept well for a few nights, popping a sleeping pill to cure your insomnia seems the logical thing to do. But before you reach for that bottle tonight, here's what you should know about the safety and effectiveness of sleep medications.

Over-the-counter (OTC) brands. The medications that you can buy at your drugstore may not be the best choices to help you get a good night's sleep. They contain the antihistamine diphenhydramine, which is found in many allergy, cough, and cold medicines. It causes drowsiness, but it also

THE IDEAL MATTRESS

If you lived in the days of the Roman Empire, the Renaissance, or the 16th century, your mattress would have been stuffed with hay, wool, straw, or feathers. Today, thanks to technology and manufacturer ingenuity, there are futons, water beds, and several other kinds of mattresses that provide the illusion of floating off to dreamland when we crawl under the covers.

To find the one that's right for you, test-drive a few at a bedding store. Spend at least 20 minutes lying on your back, your side, and your stomach to determine whether the mattress is too hard, too soft, or offers great support, says Mary Ann Keenan, M.D., director of neuro-orthopedics in the department of orthopedic surgery at Albert Einstein Medical Center in Philadelphia.

Firm. If you experience back pain from time to time or if you have arthritis, a firm coil mattress with a soft surface is the way to go, says Pamela Adams, D.C., a chiropractor and yoga instructor at Magnolia Chiropractic in Larkspur, California. You'll get great support for your back, and the soft surface will cushion your hips, knees, and shoulders. If you can't find one with a soft surface, place a piece of foam that is 2 inches thick over the mattress and then add a mattress pad, Dr. Adams suggests.

Even if you've never had any aches and pains before, chances are you'll develop them if you invest in a soft mattress. They're bad for your back and neck, and they make it difficult for you to get out of bed without straining your arms and shoulders, says Dr. Keenan.

Foam. Foam mattresses can support your back just as well as firm coil varieties. The quality of a foam mattress is measured in density. A mattress with a 34-pound compression ratio (a measure of firmness) may do the trick, but always let your back decide. For a firmer feel, try a mattress with a higher ratio. The drawback is that over time, the pressure and heat of your body may cause changes in the foam that affect the mattress's ability to give you the support you need, says Dr. Keenan.

Water. Unlike solid mattresses, water-filled beds conform to your exact shape and give your body customized support. That's okay if you don't have any aches or pains and don't mind feeling like you're on a boat every time you change positions. For people with arthritis, the problem isn't the surface but the bed itself. A water bed can be difficult to get into and out of, especially in the morning, when joints are sore and stiff, notes Dr. Keenan. A water bed is also not good if you have a problem with motion sickness.

Air. Air mattresses are great as long as they're filled with enough air to make them firm. These mattresses work best for those who are prone to bedsores and other skin irritations because they can't turn themselves over in bed. While the mattress is firm, the surface is soft enough to prevent abrasions on the skin, says Dr. Keenan.

In addition to choosing the correct mattress for your needs, the position you sleep in can affect how rested you feel the next morning. "Sleeping on

dries nasal passages and other mucous membranes. Some also provide the pain reliever acetaminophen, which you don't need if you're not in pain, says Joyce Walsleben, R.N., Ph.D., director of the Sleep Disorders Center and research associate professor at New York University School of Medicine in New York City.

In addition, you can develop a psychological dependence on OTC sleeping pills and build up

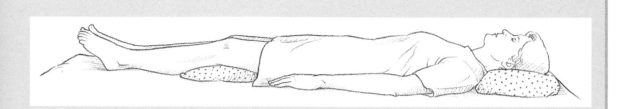

your back is best," says Darin P. Mazepa, D.C., a network chiropractor and founder of Vitality of the Lehigh Valley, a holistic healing center in Emmaus, Pennsylvania. Just make sure your pillow supports your neck so that your head is in line with the rest of your body. This helps keep your spine in alignment. You can place a pillow under your knees to relax your lower-back muscles and to sustain your body's natural curves. Put your arms at your sides, not above your head. Sleeping with your arms up works your shoulder (trapezius) muscles all night and may cause muscle tightness and pain throughout the day. "Try standing with your arms raised above your head for 20 minutes," says Dr. Mazepa. "Imagine doing that for 8 hours."

If you prefer to sleep on your side, lie on your side with your knees bent and your pillow under your head, not your shoulder. To keep your spine in alignment, the pillow should be thick enough so your head is in line with the rest of your body. Place a pillow between your knees or thighs (whichever is more comfortable) so your upper hip and leg form a straight line and are parallel with your lower hip and leg. The pillow prevents you from putting stress on the gluteus muscles in your butt and on the iliotibial (IT) band, a tract of ligaments, tendons, and other tissues that stretches from above your hip to just below your knee.

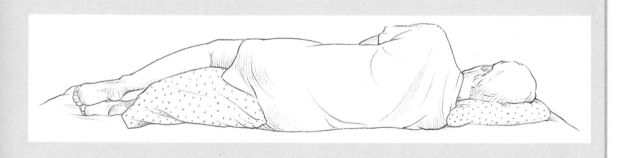

a tolerance, so you'll need to take more to get the same effect. Other side effects include disruption of sleep and memory loss. They can also make you feel drowsy and hungover the next morning.

Prescription sleeping aids. These may be a better choice, says Dr. Walsleben. They're best used for short-term treatment of insomnia and for specific circumstances, such as during times of grief, loss, or illness.

WHY CAN'T YOU SLEEP?

Ask yourself the following questions. If you answer yes to one or more of them, you need more shut-eye, and you may want to talk about your sleep habits with your doctor.

1. I have too much on my mind to fall asleep.
2. I can't go back to sleep when I wake up during the night.
3. I can't relax because I constantly worry.
4. I don't feel rested in the morning even when I've slept for 8 hours.
5. Sometimes I'm afraid to close my eyes and go to sleep.
6. I wake up too early.
7. It takes me more than 30 minutes to fall asleep.
8. I am stiff and sore in the morning.
9. I feel irritable when I can't sleep.
10. I seem to dream all night long.

➤ Non-benzodiazepines. Associated with the fewest side effects, this class of drugs includes zaleplon (Sonata) and zolpidem (Ambien). Approved by the FDA in 1999, Sonata sends you off to sleep within 30 minutes and won't cause drowsiness or that "hungover" feeling the next morning. It can be taken at bedtime or later in the evening after you've tried to fall asleep on your own, as long as you have at least 4 hours remaining in bed before you get up, says Dr. Walsleben. It's best used if you have difficulty staying asleep. Side effects are rare, but some people have reported headaches, drowsiness, and dizziness.

Unlike Sonata, Ambien stays active within your body for 7 hours instead of 4. So as long as you take it at bedtime with plans for getting at least 7 hours of shut-eye, you'll feel refreshed and energized the following morning. Both drugs are to be taken for no longer than 2 weeks.

➤ Benzodiazepines. This is the most frequently prescribed class of sleeping pills, and it includes a group of mild tranquilizers called triazolam (Halcion), estazolam (ProSom), and temazepam (Restoril). ProSom is best taken when you plan to sleep for at least 8 hours. Halcion and Restoril should also be taken only at bedtime.

Each drug varies in how fast it starts working and how long it remains active in your body once you've taken it. The longer it stays active, the more likely you'll feel groggy the next day. Halcion, for instance, starts working within 30 minutes and stays in your body up to 5½ hours. ProSom and Restoril take effect within 2 hours and remain active 8 to 15 hours.

Side effects include confusion, depression, light-headedness, dizziness, clumsiness, fainting, mood changes, increased dreaming, nausea, vomiting, drowsiness, grogginess, and weakness. These drugs shouldn't be taken longer than 2 to 3 weeks, and you must be weaned off them gradually to prevent side effects associated with withdrawal symptoms.

Food: The All-Day Energizer

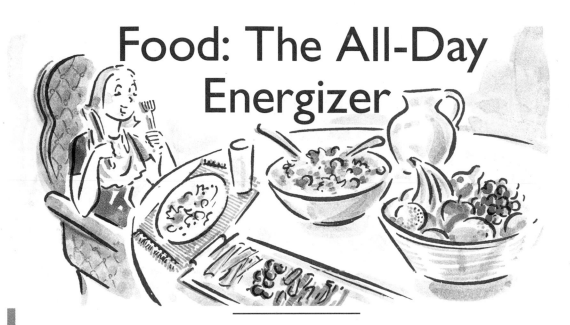

It's another Monday morning, and Carolyn is up at 6:00 A.M. As usual, she feels groggy, light-headed, and weak. Her brain is humming about as well as a cotton-stuffed piccolo.

Still bleary-eyed even after her shower, she stubs her toe on a stool in the kitchen. Aggravation adds to fatigue as she pours the kids' cereal and orange juice in between feeding the dog and loading the dishes from last night's late-night ice cream fest into the dishwasher.

There's no time for a real breakfast of her own, so she brews a pot of coffee strong enough to cut diamonds, pours it into her travel mug, and grabs a chocolate-covered doughnut for the road.

By the time she gets to the office, the caffeine and sugar have kicked in and she has enough energy to get through the first three items on her to-do list. But by 10:00 A.M., she's dragging again, so she joins her coworkers at the office coffeepot for another cup of brew and a slice of crumb cake that someone brought from home.

Lunch is a fast-food bacon cheeseburger, fries, and soft drink devoured in the car as she hits the dry cleaner, video store, and library. By 2:00 P.M.,

however, she can barely keep her eyes open, so she grabs another cup of coffee and a candy bar.

As soon as the clock strikes 5, Carolyn hits the door. With practice for both kids and a stop by her mom's, plus the fact that Ben is out of town again, dinner tonight will be late—and takeout—because even if she had the time, she really doesn't have the energy to cook.

It's a classic catch-22 situation: We're too tired to eat right, but unless we eat right, we won't have the energy we need, and if we don't have the energy we need, we won't eat right . . . you get the picture.

"If you're not eating a nourishing diet, you're just not going to run at your peak optimal level," says Phyllis Woodson, R.D., a registered dietitian at the Strelitz Diabetes Institute and in the division of maternal-fetal medicine at Eastern Virginia Medical School in Norfolk. Woodson counsels women about their eating habits, many of whom, she says, complain of fatigue. There's no surprise there, when you consider the following:

➤ Up to 39 percent of premenopausal women have low iron levels. While a full-blown de-

WOMEN ASK WHY

Do energy bars work?

Originally designed to enhance athletic performance by providing a slow release of complex carbohydrates, energy bars are now marketed for just about everyone, fueling a $160 million industry. But do they deliver?

Steve Hertzler, R.D., Ph.D., assistant professor of medical dietetics at Ohio State University in Columbus, decided to answer that question. He and his students at Kent State University, where he formerly taught, compared a bar that derives 70 percent of its calories from carbohydrates to a bar that derives 40 percent of its calories from carbohydrates. Both promised to enhance athletic performance in endurance events by moderating blood sugar.

They compared the blood sugar levels of 12 volunteers, including 10 women, after participants ate pieces of the bars, four slices of white bread, or 1½ candy bars, each containing 50 grams of carbohydrates.

The result: Only volunteers who ate pieces of the 40-percent bar experienced the long-term, moderate increases in blood sugar known to boost performance in endurance athletes. While the 70-percent bar and candy bar both initially raised glucose levels sharply, that was followed by a sharp decline in blood sugar, which saps energy.

Dr. Hertzler suggests that the sample of the 40-percent bar kept blood sugar levels steadier because it also contained more protein (34.8 grams versus 11.9 grams) and fat (17.4 grams versus 2.4 grams) per piece compared to the high-carbo bar. This combination helped balance the sugar.

Energy bars won't necessarily provide harried moms or office workers with a burst of energy, says Dr. Hertzler. But when we miss an occasional meal, a moderate-carbohydrate bar may do the job.

Nonathletes interested in a moderate sugar boost might as well eat a granola bar—a box of which costs about the same as one energy bar.

ficiency, or anemia, causes fatigue and general weakness, research suggests that even levels not low enough to be classified as anemia may impair performance.

- Nearly half of all women in the United States get less than the recommended Daily Value of vitamin B_6, a member of the B-complex family of vitamins responsible in part for peak mental and physical performance.

- In one study of 350 healthy women conducted at Arizona State University in Tempe, researchers found that 30 percent had low blood levels of vitamin C, another key fatigue-fighting vitamin.

With our nonstop lifestyles, says Baltimore dietitian Colleen Pierre, R.D., it's easy to mistake hunger for fatigue and vice versa.

"We're rushed," Woodson says. "We're at the computer, we're in our cars, we're on our cell phones." When it comes to what we're eating, she says, a lot of women "are just sort of winging it."

To understand food's impact on energy, consider the definition of the word *calorie*. Calories are not just the reason you've gone up two dress sizes in as many years; they're also a measure of the potential energy in food.

Like the wood that feeds a fire, the calories in food fuel every part of our bodies, from our brains to our muscles. For peak energy, we have to use high-quality fuel. That means a balance of vegetables, fruits, whole grains and pastas, lean meats, low-fat dairy products, and small amounts of fats. And research suggests that how we combine those foods may be just as important for energy as the foods themselves. Even the size or timing of our meals may affect our concentration, energy levels, and sleep.

Eat Already

Before we even begin with what and when we're eating, however, we need to make sure we're eating. "I see it a lot," says Pierre, who has interviewed women around the country about their eating habits. "Women go all day without eating. Or they eat as little as they can."

Not eating starves our brains, which makes concentration difficult, writes Pamela Smith, R.D., in her book *The Energy Edge*. That's because to function properly, our brains need the energy that comes from glucose, which comes from our food. Without it, fuzziness often translates into fatigue.

So we come home, ravenous and weary, and binge on whatever is convenient: cookies, cakes, pepperoni pizzas. Worried about the pounds that come with this out-of-control eating, we continue to avoid food the next day.

And forget about getting a balanced diet, with enough fruits, vegetables, whole grains, fiber, vitamins, and minerals. Only about 17 percent of us eat the recommended five or more fruits and vegetables a day.

Repeated nutritional skimping, whether for months or even years, leaves us chronically tired, irritable, prone to headaches, or moody, and sets us up for serious illnesses ranging from diabetes to heart disease to cancer. It's akin to putting inferior fuel in our cars. As every good mother would say: Eat already!

But don't eat too much. Because the heavier we are, the more energy we require just to move—in fact, to function—every day.

"Carrying extra weight is a drag," says Pierre. Think about hauling a couple of 20-pound dumbbells up three flights of stairs. Imagine how exhausting it would be to carry them around all day. That's about how it feels to weigh an extra 40 pounds.

In one study of more than 40,000 women, researchers found those who gained 5 to 10 pounds were less able to perform routine daily tasks, such as vacuuming, than women who lost similar amounts of weight.

Being overweight can drain us even while we sleep. Our lungs are forced to work harder, and fatty tissue in our throats can keep us from getting plentiful doses of energizing oxygen.

So the key, as any nutritionist worth her calorie counter will tell you, is those two bastions of nutritional health: balance and moderation.

Basic Beginnings

The best place to begin is with breakfast. Unfortunately, only one in four of us starts there, says Elizabeth Somer, R.D., in her book *Food and Mood: The Complete Guide to Eating Well and Feeling Your Best*. And of those who *are* eating breakfast, one-third eat this most important meal of the day away from their homes, and often in their cars.

"The grab-and-go approach has made it even tougher to find a healthy breakfast," notes a report by the Center for Science in the Public Interest (CSPI), a nonprofit Washington, D.C., group that monitors supermarket and restaurant foods. "Most take-out breakfasts are nutritional nightmares."

CSPI likely would call that doughnut Carolyn grabbed as she ran out the door dessert for breakfast, since its prime ingredients (sugar and fat) do nothing for long-term energy.

With that one palm-size piece of fried cake, Carolyn is getting one-fourth of her entire day's quotient of fat, one-fifth of all the calories she needs in a 24-hour period, and unhealthily large dollops of artery-clogging saturated fat and cholesterol. What she is *not* getting is a balanced mix of stick-to-her-ribs fiber, cell-building protein, and all-important, start-the-day-right vitamins and minerals.

"Breakfast is the worst time to be eating a doughnut," says Linda Barnes, R.D., a registered dietitian in Virginia Beach, Virginia. "After you eat a doughnut, you don't feel good."

If only Carolyn had reached for the bran cereal. In one British study, eating cereal in the morning put volunteers in a better mood, enabled them to perform better on a spatial-memory test, and resulted in their feeling calmer at the end of the tests than those who didn't eat cereal. Another study showed less fatigue in people who ate a low-fat, high-carbohydrate breakfast (like a high-fiber cereal with fat-free milk) than in those who ate any other combination of fat and carbohydrates.

Sugar as Energy Snatcher

Carolyn's doughnut is loaded with nearly 8 grams of sugar, which sets her up for a nutritional crash-and-burn around 10:00 A.M. Forget the myth about sugar boosting energy (and sending kids careening off the walls). While sugar (also known as glucose)

WOMAN TO WOMAN

She Changed Her Eating Habits, Gained Energy, and Lost Weight

For years, Norma Cusick, 57, of Allentown, Pennsylvania, ushered her nine children to school and various extracurricular activities, cooked, cleaned, and volunteered outside her home. But she had little time for formal exercise, and often found herself munching on the kids' high-fat, high-calorie snacks rather than on fruits and vegetables. When her youngest son was about to graduate from high school, Cusick decided to change her exercise and eating habits. She lost pounds and gained muscle and energy.

I grew up in Brooklyn, New York, where walking is a way of life. Everyone walked to school, the stores, and the theaters. It kept us fit.

When my husband, Richard, and I moved to just outside Allentown 27 years ago, with four children and one on the way, we discovered suburban life. Everyone drove to get where they were going, and there were few sidewalks.

By the time we had nine children, we were so busy that walking was all but forgotten. I encouraged the children to participate in sports and to attend the local theater, which often meant driving them to and from events. My active walks had turned into sedentary drives, so I was sitting a lot more, and I felt lethargic. It was as though I didn't have a plan for the day, no purpose for myself. Plus, walking had been my favorite stress reliever, so the worries of the day sometimes sliced into my sleep time.

Our eating habits changed, too. When my children were young, we always ate dinner together. It was a time for sharing, for being a family. And I cooked from scratch, with lots of fresh vegetables and fish. But as the children grew older and their schedules became more varied—a game here, a practice there—it was difficult to schedule meals together. When the microwave came along, we could pop foods in and pop them out in minutes any time of the day. The fast-food drive-thru, where we grabbed burgers and fries, became a necessity. We had more potato chips, candy, and other junk food in the house than we did fruits and vegetables.

Something else was different, too. The 138 pounds I usually weighed when pregnant had become my normal weight. I'm 5-foot-3, and I had always started my pregnancies around 125 pounds. I was on the go, but didn't have as much energy as I used to. The extra weight not only sapped my energy but also lowered my self-esteem.

About 2 years ago, when my youngest son was about to graduate from high school, I decided to return to a healthier routine. Richard and I began walking together in the evenings twice a week, for 60 to 90 minutes. Soon, my thighs were thinner and I felt more vigorous as I went about my day. I was more enthusiastic about the tasks that lay ahead, whether buying groceries or attending a volunteers' meeting.

Then I started a weight-training regimen and a high-fiber, low-fat eating plan. The plan required me to eat at least three vegetables and two fruits daily, along with extra fiber and soy. I started cooking with healthy foods like spinach, broccoli, carrots, and fish again. Richard even followed the "diet" with me.

Today, I'm still following the routine. Every morning, I train with weights for about 30 minutes before I do anything else. When the weather is good, I walk. I don't use a headset, so walking is a quiet time for me. And that energizes my mind. All of my stresses just drain away. I noticed a difference within a few weeks of starting the program, and now I'm more toned than ever. I weigh 132 pounds (I've lost 6), but I went from fat to muscle. I was almost up to a size 12, and now I wear an 8 petite.

Training with weights and walking in the morning puts me in a good mood that sets the time for my whole day. I feel invigorated, and that energy feeds on itself. I can do whatever I need to do, because I've taken care of myself. When I hit that pillow at night, I'm sound asleep. And during the day, I just want to be out there, living fully, because I look and feel good.

does initially boost our blood sugar levels (and therefore makes more energy available to our cells), the effects disappear quicker than a week's pay at an amusement park.

Sugar releases all of its energy at once into our bloodstreams, causing our blood sugar levels to spike. This increases levels of the hormone insulin, which pushes the sugar into our blood cells. The glucose is immediately absorbed and just as quickly disappears, and our blood sugar levels drop, often ending up lower than they were before we ate the doughnut or candy bar. The dizziness, headache, and fatigue that may follow comes from low blood sugar. In one study at Kansas State University, researchers gave 120 women either 12 ounces of water or drinks sweetened with either aspartame or sugar. Within 30 minutes, those who drank the sugar-sweetened brew were sleepiest.

Sugary foods contain few nutrients. So if we fill up on sugar, we crowd out the vitamins, minerals, antioxidants, and other food components that help us feel and look good. No wonder Carolyn is reaching for the crumb cake at 10:00 A.M.

If she'd munched a whole wheat, low-fat bran muffin with a banana, however, she would probably be just fine until lunch. Complex carbohydrates like that muffin burn more slowly. Therefore, no quick blood sugar spike and resulting crash follow. They keep us going and going like little battery-powered bunnies.

WATER, NATURE'S ENERGIZER

We could survive a month or more without eating, but we couldn't last a week without water. Yet we are a nation on the verge of dehydration. In a survey of 3,000 people, participants reported drinking an average of 37 ounces, instead of the 64 ounces a day we need to not only remain healthily hydrated but also to wash away fatigue.

Poor hydration can zap mental alertness and physical performance because water transports nutrients, carries away waste, and hydrates cells throughout our bodies. Without it, our blood thickens and becomes more difficult to pump. The extra work involved in pumping this sludgy blood can cause our energy levels to plummet.

"To maintain energy, you need water," says Barbara Gollman, R.D., a Dallas nutrition consultant and spokeswoman for the American Dietetic Association. And we don't just need it when thirst strikes. By that time, our water levels are depleted enough to drag us down. One small study of cyclists showed that performance dropped when they lost as little as 2 percent of their weight in fluids.

The standard recommendation is to drink at least eight 8-ounce glasses daily. You need more if you exercise, take certain medications such as diuretics for high blood pressure, are ill, drink alcohol or caffeinated beverages (including coffee), or simply if it's hot outside, says Linda Barnes, R.D., a registered dietitian in Virginia Beach, Virginia.

But you're not stuck with water. Milk, juices, soups, fruits, and vegetables all contain fluid. And while most decaffeinated beverages replenish your fluids, stay away from caffeine and alcohol, which drain your water stores. Or, quaff an extra cup of water for each cup of coffee or glass of wine you drink. You'll know you're getting enough water if your urine is straw-colored, not bright yellow.

If you don't like the taste of water, try flavored waters, or puree melon chunks or peach slices in a blender with buttermilk, crushed ice, and a touch of ginger or cinnamon to taste.

Fatiguing Fat

A chocolate-covered doughnut contains a significant amount of fat, and most of it is the truly-bad-for-our-hearts trans fats, which are created when hydrogen is whipped into liquid vegetable oils to make them solid. Trans fats are extremely unhealthy; studies show that they significantly increase the risk of developing coronary heart disease.

Plus, too much fat slows us down and robs us of energy by creating a kind of sludge in our bloodstreams, says Smith. Our bodies are so busy digesting and storing excess fat that our blood circulation actually slows down, reducing the delivery of oxygen to our cells.

You don't want to avoid fat entirely, however. We need it to transport vitamins and produce hormones, and at 9 calories per gram (compared to 4 per gram for carbohydrates and protein), fat packs slowly digested energy that gives our meals staying power.

Carolyn also should have had more protein at breakfast, such as a glass of low-fat milk or a cup of yogurt. Protein helps stabilize energy levels by working with carbohydrates and fats to regulate blood sugar, says Smith.

"There's a symphony effect with all of them being there together that moderates blood sugar," says Barnes.

Eating for Energy: Breakfast

A simple but healthy breakfast can be ready in 5 minutes, Somer says. A slice of vegetable pizza served with a large glass of orange juice fuels us through the morning as well as a bowl of cereal.

In fact, vitamin C, which is found in oranges, cantaloupe, and other fruits and juices, is a proven energy booster. When we're short on this critical vitamin, fatigue is one of the first symptoms to appear. One reason may be that vitamin C helps our bodies absorb iron, a mineral that carries energizing oxygen to our cells. One 8-ounce glass of orange juice more than meets our daily requirements for vitamin C.

To get a balanced, energy-boosting start to your day, the CSPI suggests these strategies.

- Stuff half a whole wheat pita with ½ cup of low-fat cottage cheese and sliced peaches, pears, or banana.
- Roll up a tortilla with a scrambled egg and some salsa. (For a quick scrambled egg, spray a microwave-safe bowl with cooking spray, mix one egg and 1 tablespoon of fat-free milk, and microwave on high for 90 seconds.)
- Melt a thin slice of low-fat cheese over a sliced tomato on a whole wheat English muffin.
- Stir ½ cup each of plain low-fat yogurt and orange-pineapple-banana juice with ⅓ cup of

COFFEE: ENERGY SAPPER IN A MUG

If you've been feeling a little run-down lately, the culprit may be as close as that mug full of steaming coffee. While this caffeine-spiked beverage can give us a morning jolt, chase the fuzzies from our brains, and keep us going through a marathon meeting, it can also send us crashing later in the day.

Caffeine delivers its jolt by blocking a sedating nerve chemical called adenosine. Caffeine's stimulating effects kick in within 30 minutes of that first cup, leaving us not only more energetic but more focused.

But caffeine-rich beverages and foods have a downside. Within hours of that first cup, we feel sluggish and muddle-headed as our bodies react to mild caffeine withdrawal.

The caffeine in coffee may zap us in other ways, too. It's a diuretic, so it depletes the body of water. If we become dehydrated and our muscles and cells don't function properly, we feel fatigued. Caffeine also inhibits our absorption of certain vitamins and minerals, such as iron and calcium, which are important for optimal health and energy. And it can interfere with our nightly rest, leaving us more drained the next day, says Nancy Fishback, M.D., of the Sleep Disorders Center at Sentara Norfolk Hospital and associate professor of medicine at Eastern Virginia Medical School.

Limit your intake of caffeine to about 300 milligrams a day, Dr. Fishback says. That's one to three 5-ounce cups of your run-of-the-mill cup of coffee. Beware that specialty brews served up at coffee bars may pack as much as 550 milligrams of caffeine in one serving. Add the caffeine in some prescription and over-the-counter drugs, and you may be headed for caffeine overload, says Dr. Fishback.

In one study, people who followed a caffeine-free, sugar-free diet for 2 weeks reported feeling less tired. When they added those ingredients back into their diets, 44 percent reported that their fatigue returned as well.

If you want to cut your caffeine habit, go at it slowly because giving it up abruptly is likely to cause headaches. Try mixing half decaffeinated coffee and half regular coffee in your morning brew. Or, try some of the newer "light" coffees, which contain less caffeine.

INDIVIDUALIZE YOUR EATING-FOR-ENERGY PROGRAM

We all have different schedules, dietary needs, and likes and dislikes. Here are some tips for eating for energy under special circumstances.

I need to feed my family, and we don't like the same foods. It may be tempting to pop a few frozen dinners into the microwave and put one in front of each family member, depending on likes and dislikes. But read the labels. Many frozen dinners are packed with sodium and fat, but few vegetables, says Jayne Hurley, R.D., senior nutritionist at the Center for Science in the Public Interest (CSPI), a nonprofit Washington, D.C., group that monitors supermarket and restaurant foods.

Instead, try one of the frozen meal kits in a bag. The consumer group sampled them and found that many are lower in fat and sodium, are easy to fix with just a little water or oil, and taste terrific. What's more, these dinners have a decent number of energy-boosting vegetables, Hurley adds. So you and your family get a hot, tasty meal, along with vitamins A and C, fiber, and more.

I eat out frequently. You're given "a million bad choices" nutritionally when you eat out, Hurley says. That's even truer if you're pulling up to the fast-food window. A study by researchers at the University of Memphis and Vanderbilt University showed that women who ate out more than five times a week consumed more energy-sapping calories, sodium, and fat than women who ate more meals at home.

Restaurants seldom make nutritional information available, but some have "light" menus. Order from them if you can, Hurley says. Ask to have your food grilled, baked, or blackened instead of fried; try sandwich wraps enclosing fresh veggies; and nix the cheese, unless you opt for the low-fat variety. And watch out for salad dressings. They can turn an otherwise nutrient-rich, low-fat meal into a high-fat, high-calorie, energy-draining nightmare. The typical chef or Caesar salad with dressing contains more than half the fat women need in a day, Hurley says.

I'm very overweight. If you're overweight, you may deprive yourself of nutrient-dense fruits, veggies, and grains, says Linda Barnes, R.D., a registered dietitian in Virginia Beach, Virginia. You may feast on cakes, cookies, ice cream, french fries, and other fried foods—or hardly any food at all. Either way, there's little fuel to keep you going. Your metabolism slows in an involuntary attempt to head off starvation. Your energy level drops like an elevator with a cut cable.

sliced banana and a half-dozen fresh or frozen blueberries. Freeze overnight.
➧ Combine ¼ cup of low-fat ricotta cheese with ½ cup of applesauce and a dash of cinnamon. Sprinkle with granola cereal.

Eating for Energy: Lunch

Regardless of how healthy breakfast was, our blood sugar and energy levels still begin to lag about 4 hours later. It's time for lunch.

There would have been nothing wrong with the fast-food burger Carolyn gulped for lunch—if she had added a salad or a couple of pieces of fruit; ordered the burger without the heavy sauces, double cheese, and bacon; skipped the fries; and substituted a glass of water or low-fat milk for the sugary, nutritionally desolate soft drink.

For lunch carries with it its own smoking gun: the postlunch slump. To a certain extent, we're going to feel a bit drowsy in the early afternoon

You can give yourself a jump start. Along with energy-enhancing exercise, such as a walk around the block and dusting the furniture to your favorite CD, aim for balanced meals and a few less calories each day.

Here's a trick: Draw an imaginary line down your plate, says Colleen Pierre, R.D., a registered dietitian in Baltimore. Fill half of the plate with vegetables such as broccoli, spinach, asparagus, and green beans. On one-quarter of the plate, put nutrient-dense starches, such as brown rice, whole wheat couscous, and whole grain pastas. On the other quarter, put lean red meat, chicken, or fish.

Keep a food diary for a few days, Barnes suggests. By giving up a mere 200 calories a day (a pat of butter and a half-glass of wine, for example), you can lose 1 pound a week. Since that wine glass is half-full, simply add some ice and enjoy, she says. And, yes, you can snack.

Losing weight slowly and steadily will keep you from feeling calorie- and energy-deprived, Barnes says. Your metabolism will be humming, and so will you.

I'm an athlete. To sustain the energy they need, endurance athletes such as marathon runners may get about 60 percent of their calories from nutrient-rich carbohydrates, about 15 percent from lean proteins, and the rest from fat, says Pierre.

Here are some tips for athletes from nutritionist Pamela Smith, R.D., author of the book *The Energy Edge*; and Steve Hertzler, R.D., Ph.D., assistant professor of medical dietetics at Ohio State University in Columbus.

- Drink a glass of water an hour before you work out and another one about 15 minutes before. Drink water during your workout, too.

- Many sports nutritionists recommend sports drinks rather than water, often because athletes may prefer the taste of the high-carbo drinks and simply drink more, Dr. Hertzler says. Look for drinks with 6 to 10 percent carbohydrates.

- Eat a high-carbohydrate snack like crackers, a slice of whole grain bread, or a banana 60 to 90 minutes before exercising.

- Follow your workout with some protein, such as chicken or milk, and carbohydrates, such as fruits, juices, baked potatoes, or grain products (brown rice, pasta, bagels, bread). And drink about 2 cups of water for every ounce of weight lost. (Step on the scale before and after the workout.)

regardless of what we eat, because of our circadian rhythms. But what we eat can worsen their effects. This is where balance comes in.

If you chow down on something like fettuccine Alfredo, chances are you'll be drooling all over your expense reports by 2:00 P.M. That's because you've just eaten a meal composed almost entirely of carbohydrates and fat. Carbohydrates aren't all bad. In fact, they're our best source of energy, found in everything from candy bars and soft drinks to beans, fruit, and vegetables. It's only when we eat too many carbos, eat the wrong kinds, or eat them alone, without a bit of protein, that we gain weight or feel sluggish.

Additionally, eating more than 1,000 calories at any meal forces our bodies to work harder just to digest them. Just think about the ubiquitousness of the post-Thanksgiving snooze.

Every time we munch something like a bagel, a big plate of pasta, or that huge holiday feast of turkey, mashed potatoes, stuffing, and gravy, our brains produce a neurotransmitter called sero-

FATIGUE-BUSTING RECIPES

APRICOT BREAKFAST PARFAITS

Are you looking for a fun, delicious way to jump-start your day? This dish provides rib-sticking complex carbohydrates (granola), protein (yogurt), and vitamin-jammed fruit (apricots).

- 1   cup low-fat granola (without raisins)
- 8   ounces fat-free plain yogurt
- 8   large apricots, pitted and thinly sliced
      Ground cinnamon

Place 1 tablespoon granola in each of four parfait dishes or glass dessert bowls. Add 2 tablespoons yogurt to each dish, spreading to make an even layer. Divide half of the apricots among the dishes. Sprinkle lightly with the cinnamon. Place 1 more tablespoon granola in each dish.

Divide the remaining 4 ounces yogurt among the dishes. Top with the remaining apricots and the remaining ½ cup granola, dividing evenly among the dishes.

Serve immediately, or cover and chill for up to 2 hours.

Makes 4 servings.

BLACK BEAN CONFETTI SALAD

The staying power of beans will help keep your blood sugar levels steady for hours, avoiding the spike-and-crash effects of simple carbohydrates like pasta and sugary snacks. Try this for an energy-enhancing lunch.

- 2   cans (15–19 ounces each) black beans, rinsed and drained
- 1   small red bell pepper, finely chopped
- 4   scallions, thinly sliced
- 2   tablespoons chopped fresh cilantro
- 2   tablespoons white wine vinegar
- 1   tablespoon extra-virgin olive oil

In a large bowl, combine the beans, pepper, scallions, cilantro, vinegar, and oil. Toss to coat well. Let stand for 15 minutes to allow the flavors to blend. You can prepare this salad up to a day in advance. Cover and refrigerate if not serving immediately. Bring to room temperature before serving.

Makes 4 servings.

WESTERN-STYLE DRUMSTICKS

This dinner recipe is packed with protein to give you a second wind for all your evening activities.

- 1   tablespoon paprika
- 1   tablespoon Worcestershire sauce
- 2   teaspoons packed brown sugar
- ½   teaspoon ground red pepper
- ½   teaspoon onion powder
- ¼   teaspoon celery seeds
- 8   chicken drumsticks

Preheat the broiler. Coat a broiler pan with cooking spray.

In a small bowl, combine the paprika, Worcestershire sauce, brown sugar, pepper, onion powder, and celery seeds to make a thick paste. Using your fingers, gently loosen the skin from the drumsticks and spread the paprika mixture evenly under the skin, covering as much of each drumstick as possible. Place the drumsticks on the broiler pan.

Broil 6" from the heat for 8 to 10 minutes per side, or until a thermometer inserted in the thickest portion registers 170°F and the juices run clear. Remove the skin before serving.

Makes 4 servings.

tonin, which has a calming effect. If we eat too much of a serotonin-boosting food, however, that calmness morphs into catatonia.

But add a bit of protein to smaller meals—by substituting clam sauce for the cream sauce on that pasta, for example—and you can curtail serotonin's sleepy-time effects. That's because most proteins (meat, dairy, legumes and beans, fish) boost our brains' supplies of dopamine and norepinephrine, neurotransmitters shown to enhance alertness and energy. One British study showed that protein actually moderated the effects carbohydrates had on serotonin.

That's why most experts suggest combining small amounts of protein, fat, and carbohydrates at meals. In fact, in one study of 18 volunteers (15 of them women), those who ate a lunch of balanced carbs, protein, and fat were less drowsy, uncertain, and muddled (and more cheerful) than those who ate lunches tipping the scales in terms of fat or carbohydrates.

A hamburger on a bun meets the basic balance requirements; it's a good mix of protein (the burger), carbohydrate (the bun), and not too much fat.

But there's a major player missing: fruits and vegetables. Not only do they provide a plethora of vital minerals and vitamins, but researchers are now discovering they also contain hundreds of phytonutrients, like lycopene, lutein, carotenoids, and indoles, that appear to have tremendous effects not only on our energy levels but also on our overall health.

Unfortunately, most women don't even come close to getting enough fruits and veggies. On average, we eat about 3.6 servings a day—one apple, ½ cup of string beans, and a glass of orange juice—well below the 5 or more servings that most nutritionists recommend we eat. And french fries don't count.

Think yellow, orange, dark green, and leafy.

"Vegetables are the Cadillacs of your food," Woodson says. "If you're not tapping into vegetables, it's to your detriment." Here are some ideal lunches.

- Have a small bowl of canned, low-fat minestrone soup and 2 ounces of turkey on whole wheat bread with lettuce and mustard, along with 8 ounces of fat-free milk.
- Eat a tossed salad with ¼ cup of canned, drained kidney beans, 1 ounce of low-fat cheese, and 3 tablespoons of low-fat dressing. Serve with two slices of sourdough bread and sparkling water.
- Make a peanut butter crunch sandwich (2 tablespoons of peanut butter mixed with 1 tablespoon of wheat germ and 2 teaspoons of honey, spread on multigrain bread) and serve with 1 cup of fresh strawberries and 8 ounces of fat-free milk.
- Have 3 ounces of extra lean roast beef on a whole wheat roll with tomato, lettuce, and mustard, along with one piece of fruit and 1 cup of raw cauliflower florets, sliced carrots, and broccoli.

Snacking Success

One way to keep fatigue and mental fogginess at bay is to eat minimeals every 2 to 3 hours. In a study conducted at Tufts University in Medford, Massachusetts, healthy older women (average age 72) ate meals of 250, 500, and 1,000 calories. Their blood sugar levels rose and then rapidly returned to normal (as desired for sustained energy) only after the 250-calorie snack.

But candy bars, cookies, or chips aren't the best choices for that midafternoon snack. You should follow the same parameters for your snacks as for the rest of your meals: a mix of protein, carbohydrates, and fat with minimal amounts of fats and processed sugars.

SNACKING FOR ENERGY

Try these more healthful alternatives to the typical fat-, sugar-, and caffeine-laden choices.

Instead of . . .	Try . . .
A doughnut and coffee	A fruit-filled, whole grain cereal bar and a piece of fruit, or a piece of raisin-cinnamon toast topped with mashed banana and a sprinkling of chopped walnuts, and flavored green tea
A chocolate, caramel, and nut candy bar and a soda	A few slices of lean ham, a dozen fat-free whole wheat crackers, and 1 cup of orange juice or bottled water
Three chocolate chip cookies and coffee	Orange slices dipped in fat-free chocolate syrup, or half a cantaloupe with 6 ounces of low-fat lemon yogurt and decaffeinated tea
A wedge of chocolate mousse cheesecake and a postdinner glass of wine	Three fig bars and a cup of warm fat-free milk flavored with almond extract and topped with nutmeg
A small bag of potato chips and a diet soft drink	One large pear and bottled water, ½ cup of dry whole grain cereal, and ½ cup of dried fruit or ½ cup of trail mix
A bowl of premium chocolate ice cream with peanuts and chocolate sauce	Low-fat ice cream or frozen yogurt topped with sliced bananas or fresh blueberries

And watch the calories in snacks. "We've lost sight of portion size," says Jayne Hurley, R.D., senior nutritionist at the Center for Science in the Public Interest. Our cookies, cakes, and beverages are bigger than ever. "I call them sweets on steroids." In one CSPI sampling, a popular cookie purchased at a shopping mall contained 750 calories and 48 grams of energy-stealing fat.

So think about how much food you normally eat during the day, and divide it into smaller portions, says Barnes. If you brought a tuna sandwich, yogurt, and apple for lunch, eat the apple and sandwich at lunchtime and save the yogurt for an afternoon snack.

Eating for Sleep

What we eat soon before bedtime can come back to haunt us worse than a bad job performance.

Caffeine and alcohol can disrupt both the quality and duration of sleep. Even a chocolate peppermint can mean a 2:00 A.M. wake-up call. Eaten within 2 hours before you go to sleep, caffeine and alcohol can cause gastric reflux during the night, says Nancy Fishback, M.D., of the Sleep Disorders Center at Sentara Norfolk Hospital and associate professor of medicine at Eastern Virginia Medical School. Your stomach acid churns and rises, splashing into the top of your esophagus or throat, waking you up with a burning, upset stomach or chronic cough.

Forget the cake, ice cream, and other rich foods or big meals before bedtime too, Dr. Fishback says. Because rich, sugary foods wreak havoc with our blood sugar levels well into the night, they also disrupt our sleep. All of those carbs raise blood sugar, and in comes insulin to flush out the sugar. When blood sugar falls, we may feel hungry enough to wake up and stumble to the refrigerator.

If you must eat within 2 hours of bedtime, try an ounce of low-fat cheese, a cup of low-fat yogurt, or a hard-cooked egg. Add a half-dozen whole wheat crackers or a piece of fruit, and a small handful of macadamia nuts or an avocado. Sometimes, however, there's just no avoiding that late night meal. In that case:

- Wait an extra hour or so before going to bed, so your food has a chance to digest. That way, you're less likely to make that nasty gastric reflux worse.
- Raise the head of your bed by putting bricks under the legs of the bed so you're propped up. This may keep those gastric acids from waking you in the night.

Carolyn Revisited

Carolyn decided to visit a nutritionist to find out if her diet could be a cause of her fatigue. Two months after a complete nutritional makeover, she's feeling much better. She is sleeping better, has more energy during the day, and has even dropped a few pounds. Here is a sample of the energy-revving nutritional plan Carolyn adopted.

Breakfast: 1 slice of whole wheat bread, 1 ounce of low-fat cheese, and an apple

Midmorning snack: Five whole-grain crackers and a cup of fat-free strawberry yogurt

Lunch: 1 pear, 1 baked potato with 1 teaspoon of butter, 2 to 3 ounces of grilled chicken, 2 cups of fresh spinach topped with raw carrot slices, broccoli, mushrooms, and fat-free salad dressing

Midafternoon snack: $1/2$ cup of plain yogurt mixed with 1 tablespoon of all-fruit raspberry jam

Late-afternoon snack: $1/2$ cup of trail mix that Carolyn makes at home and stores in a resealable plastic bag. The mix: 1 cup of unsalted dry-roasted peanuts, 1 cup of unsalted dry-roasted shelled sunflower seeds, and 2 cups of raisins

Dinner: 1 cup of vegetable soup, 1 cup of cooked cauliflower, $1/2$ cup of brown rice, 3 ounces of lean fish sautéed in 1 teaspoon of canola oil, and 1 cup of raw carrot sticks

A few hours before bedtime: $3/4$ cup of toasted-oat cereal and $1/2$ cup of fat-free milk

Vitamins and Other Supplements

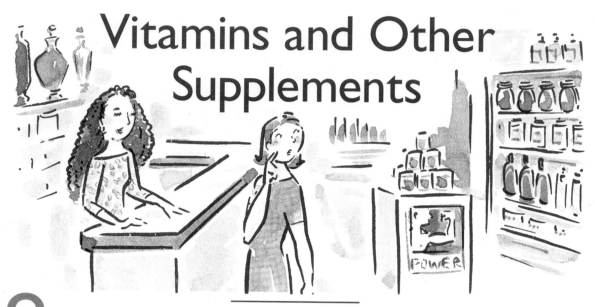

On her way home from work, Carolyn has a few rare minutes to spare. She has, almost blessedly, missed the usual traffic snarls.

Running down the list of errands she could fit into those precious bits of time, she notices the little health food store she drives past almost daily. Maybe it's time to stop in. She used to take a multivitamin, along with a few milligrams of iron. Somehow, the bottles got pushed to the back of her kitchen cabinet along with the outdated spices. Surely her vitamins are outdated by now, too. She zips into the parking lot, figuring it won't take more than a few minutes to choose a multivitamin.

Inside, she quickly spots the vitamins and minerals, but she isn't prepared for what she sees. On one side, the shelves are stacked with multivitamins and single vitamins like E, C, and B_6. There are vitamins with minerals such as iron and zinc, and minerals in bottles of their own. There are natural products, synthetic products, and chelated products. Doses range from micrograms to milligrams and more.

On the other side of the aisle hangs a sign: FOR ENERGY. Underneath are dozens of other supplements, including the hormone melatonin. Carolyn thinks that one has something to do with sleep. But some of those other names: NADH, coenzyme Q_{10}, alpha lipoic acid? They sound like something straight out of chemistry class.

Desperate for something to help her fatigue, Carolyn debates whether she should try one of the multis or just grab an armload of supplements and hope for the best. Instinctively glancing at her watch, her muscles tighten. She has to pick up the kids and get dinner on the table—fast. She leaves the store empty-handed and more confused than ever. Even shopping for vitamins is a physical and emotional drain!

Nearly half of us pop dietary supplements, according to a survey by the National Center for Health Statistics and the Centers for Disease Control and Prevention. Among the most common reasons for taking them are to increase energy and to improve performance. And we're willing to pay to do it: We spend up to $10 million on supplements every year.

We're also reaching for plenty of products beyond the typical multivitamin, says Barbara MacDonald, N.D., a naturopathic physician in Portland, Oregon, who specializes in women's health. "I've had people come in with suitcases full of supplements," she says. When she helps her patients sort through the boxes and bottles, about three-quarters get tossed. Some may contain ingredients that are inappropriate for them, such as the stimulant herb ephedra (also known as ma huang). Others just don't suit a woman's needs.

It's okay to supplement, Dr. MacDonald says, but first you need to talk with your doctor about other causes of fatigue, such as a thyroid condition and depression. (For more on these conditions, see Exhaustion Only a Woman Could Know on page 21 and Energy and Emotions on page 92.) Then, you need to think about what you're trying to accomplish, she says, instead of reaching for the supplement of the moment.

In fact, many of us can benefit from vitamin, mineral, and other dietary supplements beyond even the popular herbals, says Richard A. Kunin, M.D., a nutritional specialist in San Francisco. He believes that many women have marginal deficiencies of vitamins and minerals that go undetected in standard blood tests or physical examinations.

That's because too many of us simply aren't eating right, Dr. Kunin says. We're on perpetual diets, skimping on calories and

THE BASICS

The Food and Drug Administration doesn't regulate dietary supplements like vitamins and minerals, which means they also don't approve them for safety or efficacy. But there are a few things you should look for when you're shopping for supplements.

Daily Value. Listed on labels of vitamins and minerals, Daily Values are general guidelines set by the Food and Nutrition Board of the National Academy of Sciences to help avoid over- or undersupplementing. It's best to talk to a registered dietitian or a nutritionally savvy physician before you customize a supplement plan that exceeds label recommendations.

USP. Found on vitamin and mineral labels, USP stands for United States Pharmacopeia and is an indication that the product is pure and contains the listed nutrients. Also look for an expiration date to be sure the product is still potent.

Brand. In most cases, it doesn't matter whether you buy a name brand or generic product, says Mary Ellen Camire, Ph.D., professor of food science and human nutrition at the University of Maine at Orono. It also doesn't matter if the supplement you're buying is natural or synthetic. Folate, one of the B vitamins, is one exception, however. We absorb and use the synthetic form more easily.

Fillers. Some women may be allergic or sensitive to stabilizers, starches, cellulose, and additives in supplements, which is why Barbara S. Silbert, D.C., N.D., a naturopathic physician in Brookline, Massachusetts, recommends that her patients avoid them.

Chelated. A product labeled as "chelated" simply means that the mineral is bound to another substance to hasten its absorption. There is little evidence, however, that chelated materials work better, and they can cost up to five times more than unchelated products.

Frequency of dosage. Take your supplements with or after a meal to slow their breakdown and to boost absorption, says Joanne Larsen, R.D., L.D., a registered dietitian in Seattle.

missing out on many nutrients. To compensate, Mother Nature dials our energy production too low. "Vitamin and mineral deficiencies are characterized by a drop in energy production, a sense of malaise, and fatigue," Dr. Kunin says. We may not develop full-blown deficiencies or related diseases, such as scurvy from too little vitamin C, he says, but we won't feel at our best, either, especially when we're running from sunup to sundown.

Think of supplements, then, as a nutritional insurance policy, says Mary Ellen Camire, Ph.D., professor of food science and human nutrition at the University of Maine at Orono. They're not replacements for a poor diet or lack of exercise, however. Foods contain many beneficial nutrients that science is only beginning to understand.

Still, many products are safe to try, Dr. Kunin says. If you combine them with other energy-boosting strategies, such as exercising, rooting out sources of stress, and eating a balance of fresh vegetables and fruits, whole grains, fish and lean meats, and dairy products, you may be able to leave fatigue in the dust.

You should also take a break from supplementing for a couple of days or a week every 3 to 6 months, says Barbara S. Silbert, D.C., N.D., a chiropractor and naturopathic physician in Brookline, Massachusetts. Your body gets used to the supplements and they may not work as well. And check with your doctor regularly to be sure you're not getting too much of any one product or missing or masking other health problems.

Managing with Multis

Thirteen vitamins and more than three dozen minerals help you turn food into energy and the tissues that compose your body. They each work in slightly different ways, however, and you need them in varying amounts to feel your best every day.

Unless you're eating at least 1,600 calories a day, you probably aren't getting all the nutrients you need for optimal health from your food, especially during your childbearing years, says Joanne Larsen, R.D., L.D., a registered dietitian in Seattle.

One of the simplest, safest, and least expensive ways to supplement is with a multivitamin/mineral combination that contains 100 percent of the Daily Values set by the Food and Nutrition Board of the National Academy of Sciences, Dr. Camire says.

In general, says Dr. Camire, look for a product that contains at least vitamins A and C, the B-complex vitamins, and minerals such as calcium, chromium, copper, iron, manganese, selenium, and zinc.

How much? Dr. Kunin says that it is safe to take up to 10 times the Daily Value for most vitamins, and double the DV for all minerals except iron, magnesium, and potassium. "For many people," he says, "the recommended amounts are not enough." Talk to your doctor about the amount that is best for you, however.

Betting On the B-Complex

When it comes to energy, the B-complex vitamins—thiamin, riboflavin, niacin, B_6, B_{12}, folic acid, pantothenic acid, and biotin—are most often linked to peak mental and physical performance. You get the B-complex vitamins in beef, chicken, and other animal foods, and in whole grains, such as breads and cereals. They help you turn carbohydrates into the blood sugar that fuels your cells, muscles, and brain.

And each one works a bit differently, says Dr. Camire.

Vitamin B_6, for instance, helps form neurotransmitters, the nerve chemicals that send messages to your brain. B_{12} makes red blood cells that contain iron-dense hemoglobin and deliver energizing oxygen to your cells. Folic acid, or folate, makes amino acids, the building blocks of life-sustaining protein.

Suboptimal levels of the Bs may contribute to fatigue, but they're difficult to assess through standard blood tests. "The science isn't there yet," says Dr. Camire. In one study, 12 people with untreated chronic fatigue syndrome had lower levels of B_6, riboflavin, and thiamin than did 18 healthy people.

We also need more Bs as we age. For example, as the years go by, your body absorbs less B_{12} even when you eat foods rich in it. If you are a vegetarian or eat little meat, you're also at risk for lowered B_{12} levels. Deficiencies can lead to pernicious anemia, where you don't make the red blood cells you need and, as a result, feel headachy and miserably fatigued.

Then there's folate, or folic acid, which is vital to energy stores. "Lots of folks run low on folate, unless they take it in a vitamin," Dr. Kunin says. Even the Food and Nutrition Board has upped its recommendation for folate to 400 micrograms. Folate helps our bodies make new cells, and it works with B_{12} to form hemoglobin. We can also develop anemia if we get too little folate. And women of childbearing age should take folate even before they become pregnant because studies show that it helps prevent neural tube defects such as spina bifida in the early stage of pregnancy.

How much? The Bs work together like a well-rehearsed orchestra, so choose a multiple-B product that supplies 25 to 100 percent of the Daily Value for each vitamin. To offset anemia, Rebecca Wynsome, N.D., a naturopathic physician in Seattle, sometimes gives B_{12} injections to patients with diminished levels of the vitamin. The injections deliver the vitamin more quickly than a capsule or liquid sold in health food stores does. For others, she recommends supplementing with at least 50 milligrams each of B_{12}, riboflavin, B_6, and niacin. This is higher than the Daily Value for niacin (35 milligrams), so check with your doctor. Too much niacin may cause flushing, itching, and other side effects.

C: The Energy Vitamin

The benefits of vitamin C extend far beyond boosting your immune system. It's a powerhouse for fueling you through your day, Dr. Kunin says. Along with a host of other attributes, vitamin C makes a substance in your body called carnitine, which your muscles need to burn fat for energy.

Vitamin C also is a potent antioxidant that boosts your immune function and energy by enabling your adrenal glands, which sit atop your kidneys and regulate the stress hormone adrenaline, to work properly, says Dr. Wynsome.

You get vitamin C in fruits such as oranges and in vegetables, including broccoli. But studies show that only about 17 percent of us eat the recommended five fruits and vegetables needed daily for optimal health and vigor.

When you're low on C, "it shows up in very short order as malaise and a lack of energy," Dr. Kunin says. In a study of 400 healthy people (350 of them women) conducted by researchers at Arizona State University in Tempe, 30 percent showed levels of vitamin C low enough to cause fatigue. Another 6 percent had levels indicative of vitamin C deficiency.

How much? Many nutritionally oriented physicians, including Dr. Kunin and Dr. Wynsome, recommend up to 1,000 milligrams daily, even more under conditions of physical stress and illness. The safe upper limit set by the Food and Nutrition Board is 2,000 milligrams. Try dividing your dosage in two to keep blood levels of C steady all day. One possible side effect of such high doses is diarrhea. Cutting back on C, without cutting it out, can help.

Minding Your Minerals

Choosing vitamins is as easy as A-B-C. But choosing minerals is a bit trickier, says Larsen. That's because minerals are more dependent on one another for their actions. If you take too much of one, you may tip another out of balance. Feast on zinc, for example, and you may lower your levels of copper. Gulp down iron tablets daily, and your zinc levels may sink.

Yet minerals are also critical for good health and energy. They repair your tissues and bones, ferry oxygen to your cells, guard your nervous system, and even help your muscles contract. Select a multivitamin with minerals, and follow the Daily Value on the label, suggests Larsen. Here are some of the key players on the energy field.

Iron. If you're going to pump iron in the gym, or even haul that load of laundry up and down the stairs, iron is a must. It's part of the hemoglobin in your blood, helping to taxi oxygen to every cell and muscle within you, including your brain. Menstruation and a tendency to avoid calorie-dense red meat put women at risk for low iron levels. If you get too little iron, you become pale, tired, and listless.

Premenopausal women need 18 milligrams of iron a day. At menopause, however, look for a multivitamin with no more than 9 milligrams of iron. Too much iron can lead to cardiovascular and other problems. Meats, fish, and poultry contribute the most iron, but legumes,

enriched grain products, and eggs are also good sources. If you eat little or no meat, you may need an iron supplement, so check with your doctor. If your doctor recommends an iron supplement, the most common form is ferrous sulfate. You should avoid taking more than 18 milligrams a day unless a blood test indicates that you're anemic.

Copper. This mineral helps you store and release iron so your oxygen-ferrying blood can fuel your tissues and muscles. Copper is abundant in fish and shellfish, legumes, nuts, peanuts, raisins, soybeans, and spinach. But Dr. Kunin says 7 out of 10 of us don't get enough. When he prescribes copper supplements to his patients, "many of them wake up more alert and some bound out of bed," he says.

Look for a multi with a Daily Value of 2 milligrams of copper, but no more than 9 milligrams, the safe upper limit set by the Food and Nutrition Board. Beware when buying: One study shows that many multis contain a copper compound, called cupric oxide, which your body doesn't absorb. Look for copper sulfate, or cupric sulfate, on the label.

Zinc. Found in every cell in your body, zinc has garnered headlines in recent years as a cold treatment and possible player in improving short-term memory. But zinc might also help on the energy front by smoothing out the highs and lows in your insulin and blood sugar levels. A shortage can leave you feeling sluggish, fatigued, or lethargic. And zinc, which is most abundant in meat and oysters, is the one mineral you're most likely to lack.

Studies show that exercising hard over long periods depletes your zinc stores. Long-term endurance training such as running significantly lowers zinc levels in women and men even when they're not running and can result in decreased endurance.

When choosing a multi with zinc, look for 15 milligrams, the Daily Value. The safe upper limit is 30 milligrams.

Magnesium? Maybe. When your diet is less than perfect (sound familiar?), you may not get enough magnesium. It's found in green vegetables, nuts and seeds, cooked dried beans, and whole grains, but in tiny amounts. So getting enough from food alone is difficult.

Magnesium turns food into energy and keeps your muscles and nerves humming on even the most harried of days. One study of 16 healthy men who were deprived of sleep and then asked to exercise on stationary cycles showed that those given 100 milligrams of magnesium performed better than those who received none.

Diuretics, some antibiotics, and some cancer medicines increase your loss of magnesium, as does excessive alcohol use.

When shopping for magnesium in a multi, choose one with 100 milligrams; few have more than that. The Daily Value is 400 milligrams and the safe upper limit is 700 milligrams, but more than 350 milligrams in a supplement may cause diarrhea. To get more than 350 milligrams without the uncomfortable side effects, try eating more magnesium rich foods.

As with other minerals, it is possible to get too much magnesium. If you have heart or kidney problems, check with your doctor before supplementing.

Chromium. You may have heard about chromium, as it has gained quite a reputation as a weight loss aid. Although study results are mixed, people who take chromium supplements often say that they're more energetic, says Harry G. Preuss, M.D., professor of medicine at Georgetown University Medical Center in Washington, D.C.

That may be because chromium, found naturally in foods such as apples, sweet potatoes, brewer's yeast, and molasses, helps you burn carbohydrates for fuel. Doctors suspect that it also helps keep your insulin and blood sugar levels in check, so you're less likely to feel shaky or fatigued on the blood sugar roller coaster.

Dr. MacDonald often recommends 200 micrograms a day of chromium picolinate, the form your body absorbs best. The Daily Value is 120 micrograms, and the safe upper limit is 1,000 micrograms. But check with your doctor before choosing a supplement with more than 200 micrograms.

Supplement Savvy

Beyond the alphabet soup of vitamins and minerals on the store shelves, you almost need a dictionary or encyclopedia to interpret some of the labels on the newest supplements marketed to the fatigued masses. These products have varying claims to fame: Some say they build strength or muscle, while others promise to reenergize your days or help you sleep better at night.

There are no Daily Values for these latest over-the-counter supplements, however, so start with a quality health food store or ask a nutritionally oriented physician for advice, says Dr. Silbert. If you self-supplement, follow product labels carefully for dosages.

CoQ$_{10}$

Coenzyme Q$_{10}$, or ubiquinone, is an antioxidant that occurs naturally in your body and is an essential part of the mitochondria, or energy centers, in your cells. In the mitochondria, it creates adenosine triphosphate, or ATP, the fuel

ANEMIA VERSUS LOW IRON

For 3 to 5 percent of women in the United States, that knocked-down, dragged-out feeling is caused by iron deficiency anemia, which occurs when we don't have enough iron to make hemoglobin, the blood cells that deliver energizing oxygen to our muscles, lungs, and brains. Symptoms include pale skin, headaches, and so little energy that we often have trouble getting out of bed in the morning.

But research shows that you don't have to be anemic to suffer the consequences of low iron. Another 8 to 10 percent of women are probably borderline anemic, says Jere Haas, Ph.D., director of the division of nutritional sciences and professor of maternal and child nutrition at Cornell University in New York. That means they experience depleted iron reserves but not full-blown anemia.

These suboptimal stores of iron go undetected by standard hemoglobin tests and generally are ignored during physical checkups, says Dr. Haas. Yet they can drain us without our even knowing it. Deficiencies come on slowly, with no clear symptoms. A woman with marginal iron deficiency likely works harder and comes away more tired than a woman whose iron stores are optimal, Dr. Haas says. So you may just notice that lately, the routine activities of life, such as cleaning up after the kids and mowing the lawn, have become more draining.

If you suspect that you're marginally iron-deprived, ask your doctor for a hemoglobin test. If your levels are 13.5 or below, ask for a serum ferritin test, which counts iron in the liver and more precisely detects marginal levels.

your cells run on. Though most people aren't deficient in CoQ_{10}, levels of the antioxidant do decline with age.

The energy spin comes from studies suggesting that combining CoQ_{10} and a high-potency multivitamin/mineral supplement may help women with chronic fatigue syndrome (CFS).

In heart patients who may be deficient in CoQ_{10}, the supplement seems to work by improving the heart's ability to contract and use oxygen. Because it's an antioxidant and energizer, Dr. Silbert sometimes prescribes CoQ_{10} to help women overcome fatigue from cancer and its treatments.

How much? CoQ_{10} is sold as capsules or soft-gels of 10 to 200 milligrams. Dr. MacDonald recommends 30 milligrams a day, particularly for athletes, to replenish energy stores. There are no known side effects. Discuss supplementation with your doctor if you are taking the blood thinner warfarin (Coumadin).

NADH

Preliminary studies on NADH, or nicotinamide adenine dinucleotide, suggest this supplement may rekindle energy for women with CFS or even the garden-variety I'm-just-tired kind of fatigue, says Dr. Preuss. Like CoQ_{10}, the supplement is a coenzyme—a vitamin-like molecule that boosts your metabolism (the release of energy from your food). Also like CoQ_{10}, NADH contributes to the high-grade cell fuel ATP.

In a preliminary study at Georgetown University School of Medicine in Washington, D.C., 26 women with CFS took 10-milligram capsules of NADH or a placebo daily for 4 weeks. Thirty percent of those taking NADH reported renewed vigor, compared to 8 percent of those who took a placebo.

Though the study was small and more work is needed, it was a significant finding, says Dr. Preuss, one of the researchers. Chronic fatigue syndrome is "the worst of the worst fatigue," he says. So the study holds promise, even for those of us who just need a jolt around the middle of the afternoon.

How much? Women with CFS should consult a physician before taking NADH. Otherwise, try one 10-milligram capsule once a day, preferably with food. Some women report feeling better after about a week, Dr. Preuss says.

The supplement is considerably more expensive than a vitamin tablet, he notes. But it appears safe, with no known side effects. Nervousness and loss of appetite have been reported in the first few days of supplementation, and the supplement may cause stomach upset.

If you're looking for an even better pick-me-up, Dr. Preuss suggests taking CoQ_{10} along with NADH. Try one for about a month, and then add the other. Or, take them together.

Alpha Lipoic Acid

Did you ever wonder where a 2-year-old gets her energy? It comes from alpha lipoic acid. Unfortunately, by the time you're 40 or 50 (and trying to deal with that 2-year-old daughter or granddaughter), your supplies are sorely depleted. Yet without this mighty antioxidant, you wouldn't have enough energy to push the buttons on your remote control, let alone master those calendars jammed with activities and obligations, says Bert Berkson, M.D., Ph.D., author of *The Alpha Lipoic Breakthrough*.

Alpha lipoic acid helps metabolize carbohydrates, fats, and amino acids, jump-starting everything from your brain to your toes. It also keeps other energy-providing antioxidants like vitamin C and vitamin E in your body longer.

You get alpha lipoic acid from many foods, including liver, broccoli, and spinach, yet they don't contain much of the acid. You would need to put away 200 pounds of spinach to take in one-third of the recommended daily amount. "You really need to supplement if you want the high energy you need," Dr. Berkson says.

The acid appears to be safe, says Dr. Berkson, but he suggests talking to a nutritionally oriented physician or nutritionist before trying it. Look for capsules or tablets from Germany or Italy, which Dr. Berkson says are of the highest quality.

How much? Try a 100-milligram tablet three times a day, preferably with meals. Prepare to feel an energy boost in about 10 days. Women with diabetes can safely supplement with 600 to 1,000 milligrams a day, says Michael Janson, M.D., author of *Dr. Janson's New Vitamin Revolution*. But make sure you tell your doctor.

One caveat: Lipoic acid supplements may lower B-complex vitamin stores, so if you're taking it, supplement with a B-50 complex.

Carnitine

Carnitine powers the inner engines of your cells, called the mitochondria, by carrying fatty acids across the cell membranes so they can be burned for fuel. Carnitine can be found in avocados, red meat, and dairy products, but your body also makes its own supplies. The trouble is that production fizzles as you age. Research shows that carnitine supplements may safely enhance your physical performance, Dr. Janson

JUMP START

Drink

Get up, fill a glass with water, and drink it down all at once. Dehydration is one cause of fatigue.

says. There also is evidence that it may benefit people with CFS.

How much? For general fatigue, Dr. Janson suggests 1,000 milligrams of carnitine daily, divided into two doses. It's most often sold as tablets. Do not take the "D" form because it may cause muscle weakness. Doses above 2,000 milligrams may cause mild diarrhea.

DHEA

Dehydroepiandrosterone, or DHEA, is a hormone produced by your adrenal glands. "It's the bank account of energy," says Dr. Wynsome, who sometimes prescribes DHEA along with cortisol, another hormone related to energy, if salivary tests show that a woman's levels are depleted. When you're drained of these hormones, you may indeed be exhausted. And your levels drop as you age.

But Dr. Wynsome does not recommend over-the-counter DHEA supplements for women because DHEA is a precursor to the hormones estrogen and testosterone. When you take DHEA without a physician's guidance, your body may churn out too much estrogen or testosterone. That could increase your risk of breast cysts, and even cancer, Dr. Wynsome says. And too much of the predominantly male hormone testosterone in women may cause facial hair and acne.

So stay away from it, says Dr. Wynsome, unless you're under a doctor's care.

Melatonin

More than 20 million Americans turn to melatonin each night in hope that it will bring them slumber. The irony is that there's no clear evidence that the supplement, often a synthetic version of the hormone you produce in your pineal gland, actually helps you get a better night's sleep, says Nancy Fishback, M.D., of the Sleep Disorders Center at Sentara Norfolk Hospital and associate professor of medicine at Eastern Virginia Medical School.

The tiny pinecone-shaped gland in your brain goes into production around dusk, sending melatonin into your bloodstream. The melatonin reaches peak levels around 2:00 A.M. and is critical to a sound night's sleep. And it can help with jet lag, Dr. Fishback says, by adjusting your internal timekeeper, known as your circadian rhythms. "But no one knows what an effective dose is," she says.

One pilot study of eight hospital patients in intensive care, where sleep deprivation is common, showed that melatonin treatments improved both the duration and quality of sleep and may help reset the body's internal clock.

But Dr. Fishback says the research isn't strong enough to recommend that you turn to melatonin supplements when you're tossing and turning at night. "It will probably be an important drug someday," she says, "once more is known about its actions." You should take melatonin only under the supervision of a knowledgeable medical doctor because it may lead to adverse effects with many medical conditions. It may also interact with prescription medications.

Creatine

Popular with athletes bent on building muscle and enhancing performance, creatine comes from animal foods such as meat and fish. Ninety-five percent of it gets tucked away in your muscles, where it mixes with phosphate and becomes a backup source for ATP.

Creatine can provide quick bursts of energy for running or strength training, according to a report from Tufts University in Medford, Massachusetts, and supplements may reduce muscle fatigue so that you can exercise longer. But it probably won't do much if you're looking for a burst of midafternoon energy, even if you're at the gym, says Melvin H. Williams, Ph.D., professor emeritus of exercise science at Old Dominion University in Norfolk, Virginia, and coauthor of *Creatine:*

The Power Supplement. And there are potential side effects.

One survey of college baseball and football players at the University of Washington in Seattle who used creatine showed that they experienced muscle cramps, diarrhea, and weight gain when they regularly took doses beyond the recommended 2 to 5 grams daily. And nine male baseball players who took creatine as part of a study at Old Dominion University gained 5 pounds in just the first week.

The bottom line, says Dr. Williams, is that if you're interested in serious strength training, creatine may be worth a try. But forget about it for a daily energy boost.

Moving Into Energy

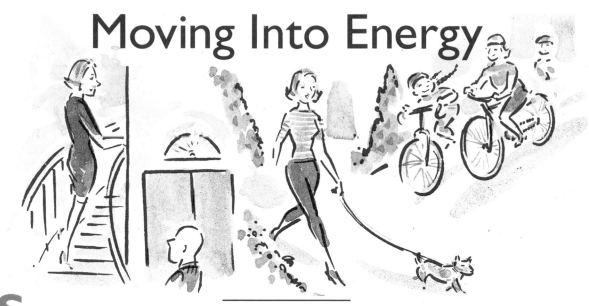

Some days, I barely have the stamina to drag myself to bed at night," Carolyn confides to her best friend, Beth, as they sit in a restaurant near their offices. They are indulging in a rare, relaxing lunch instead of munching on french fries in front of their computers.

"You should join my aerobics class," Beth says.

"Ha!" Carolyn laughs. "Getting through the day is enough of an effort. Why would I want to tire myself out even more?"

"You would be surprised how much more energy you have when you work out," her friend replies.

Carolyn wonders if Beth is right. Could going to an exercise class make waking up in the morning easier? Could lifting weights make her energy slump less noticeable? She doesn't know how she would fit it into her schedule, but she likes the idea of using exercise to let out some of her tension and stress.

A week later, during a particularly exhausting afternoon at work, she calls Beth. "Where do I sign up for your aerobics class?"

Carolyn has the right idea. Moving more really will give us more energy to do those things

that seem so hard: dragging ourselves out of bed before the sun comes up, carrying an overflowing laundry basket up the stairs, surviving a stressful day at work.

Whether it's a formal aerobics class or a heart-pumping dig in the garden, exercise not only helps our bodies by burning fat and strengthening our bones and muscles but also stimulates our metabolisms, improves our sleep, helps us avoid illness and chronic disease, and keeps us mentally healthy.

You know that drained feeling you get when you're fighting a cold or the flu yet continuing to do the million other things you do every day? If you exercise, you're less likely to get sick in the first place because your workouts wake up your immune cells, which attack and kill bacteria and viruses. And because working out keeps you healthier overall, you'll have more energy in every stage of life. Researchers say the decline in health that occurs between the ages of 30 and 75 is only partly due to aging. It can also be blamed on lack of exercise.

The problem for most of us is that being told to exercise is like being told to eat our Brussels sprouts. We know it's good for us, but it's hard to swallow. Less than 10 percent of Americans exercise 4 times a week, and fewer women than men get a regular workout.

In a survey of 2,002 people, more than half of them women, 23 percent said that nothing—not their doctor's advice, pleading from family, or access to workout facilities—would increase their physical activity. Among those who start an exercise routine, half quit within a year.

Maybe we stop because we think the only purpose of exercise is to help us lose weight. When we don't drop 10 pounds after a month of aerobics, we throw in the towel.

We're also more confused than ever about what it means to be in shape, says exercise physiologist and personal trainer Risa Olinsky, owner of Classic Fitness in Maplewood, New Jersey. Too often, we think that fitness equals a sculpted body, but size has nothing to do with it, she says. She knows slender women with low fitness levels and overweight women with strength and endurance.

We also need to get over feeling like we haven't had a good workout unless we're completely exhausted. Exercise should give us a pleasantly tired feeling, not make us want to collapse on the couch.

Many of us also view exercise as boring. But ask us to walk the beach, play volleyball with friends, or go dancing, and we jump at the opportunity because then it's not exercise, it's getting in touch with our bodies in ways we truly enjoy.

Once you begin to feel your own energy and strength, it's hard to let go. Ask 49-year-old

---

MOVING TOO MUCH

There is such a thing as exercising too much, says certified personal trainer Jana Angelakis, owner of PEx Personalized Exercise in New York City. If you're so sore the next day that you can hardly move, you're working too hard. Getting sick is another sign that you should cut back on your workouts. Knowing when to stop means you're listening to your body, so you won't hurt yourself, and you'll stay healthy and energized. Here are a few more red flags.

- Your performance has decreased.
- Your form and technique have deteriorated.
- You need more recovery time than usual.
- You experience a loss of appetite.
- You feel fatigued or nauseated during workouts.
- You get headaches during workouts.

If you experience such symptoms as undue breathlessness, light-headedness, chest pains, and an irregular heartbeat, you could just be overdoing it with exercise, but you should consult a physician to be sure.

Martha Coopersmith, founder of the Bodysmith Company, a personal-training firm in New York City. She runs 15 to 20 miles a week, works out twice a week with her own trainer, and knows her own strength, which usually lets her do anything she has to.

She views exercise as something we're meant to do, and she's right. In fact, research suggests that we're actually hardwired for it. We have a control center in our nervous systems that regulates our energy. This keeps a balance between the calories we take in and the energy we expend. After taking in more calories, we naturally want to move. And when we move more often, we gain better health, strength, and confidence.

"For some people, exercise is like religion," Coopersmith says. "It's something they believe

THE ALEXANDER TECHNIQUE

Some women relieve tension with a massage, others with a trip to the chiropractor. And some find the root of their tension and use take-home skills to relieve it every day through the Alexander Technique, an educational method that aims to correct the alignment of your head, neck, and spine as you sit, stand, and move.

The technique was invented more than 100 years ago by actor F. M. Alexander when he cured his vocal problems by studying his own movement. He learned that the relationship between the head, neck, and spine is the "primary control" in our posture, breathing, and movement. Once they're aligned correctly, we release muscle tension, our upper bodies expand, and we breathe more easily.

"Some of my clients tell me they'd rather attend a session with me than get a massage," says Hope Gillerman, a certified Alexander Technique teacher in New York City and spokesperson for the American Society for the Alexander Technique.

We develop habits of strain and tension from physical and emotional stress: Sitting in front of a computer for too long, bending our necks while we're on the phone, not getting enough exercise or sleep, or feeling overwhelmed by work and home responsibilities. As a result, we overuse our neck muscles, Gillerman says, which pulls our heads down and compresses our spines, causing poor posture, excess tension, and loss of muscle tone.

"Tension is the warning sign that we have to adjust something," Gillerman says. "The Alexander Technique teaches people to listen to that signal and adjust it themselves."

During a session, Gillerman watches the student move and then guides her head into a better alignment as she stands, bends, walks, and talks. While the student lies on a padded table, Gillerman subtly moves her head and limbs, encouraging her to release tension. Throughout the session, she instructs the student to think about her body in a new way in order to replicate these experiences on her own.

At first, the new posture could feel unfamiliar, Gillerman says. If you're in the habit of tilting your head to the left and she helps you adjust it to an upright position, you might swear you're now tilting it to the right. But a glance in the mirror shows that it's straight.

Because the teacher continually shows you what better posture is, it doesn't take long for you to feel less tense. Tension makes you feel heavy and sluggish, Gillerman notes. Once you have better posture and more relaxed muscles, you'll feel lighter and more energized.

Costs range from $50 to $80 per individual session. Gillerman suggests starting with 10 sessions, but the length of study is up to the individual practitioner and student.

To find a certified practitioner, contact the American Society for the Alexander Technique at (800) 473-0620 or log on to their Web site at www.alexandertech.org.

in, it gives them a sense of calm, and they can always rely on it to make them feel better."

Studies support the anecdotal evidence. A small study of cancer patients suffering from fatigue found that aerobic exercise clearly reduced their exhaustion and gave them more energy for daily activities. Another study found that people with CFS who regularly exercised felt more energized than those who didn't.

Although her clients are usually skeptical at first, Olinsky says that they usually tell her they feel more energetic once they start a workout program. After a few weeks of walking and lifting weights, they report feeling more rested in the morning and less drowsy in the evening. "When you start exercising, you realize that you have energy you didn't know you had," Olinsky says.

AMAZING ENERGY

Epic Journey

Laura Geoghegan, along with Mark Tong, rode a tandem bike 20,155 miles from London, England, to Sydney, Australia. The trip started on May 21, 1994, and ended on November 11, 1995, and was the longest bike journey on record to date.

Exercise's Edge

It's hard to believe that tiring ourselves out actually gives us more energy, but here's how it works. When we do a significant amount of aerobic activity and lift weights, our muscles adapt and increase in size. Our cardiovascular system, which transports blood, becomes more efficient and improves the delivery of oxygen, which makes it easier to get up and go when we have to. We also produce more of the hormone testosterone, which is necessary to build and maintain muscle. The more muscle tissue we have, the higher our metabolisms.

If you think of metabolism as the flame of a gas stove that is always lit, food is fuel for the fire and exercise is the control valve. Every time we turn up the heat by walking or jogging, our bodies work to provide more energy for the workout by breaking down carbohydrates and fats, delivering oxygen to our tissues, and storing more glycogen and triglycerides in our muscles. Over time, the cycle becomes more efficient, and we feel like we have more energy. Also, simply being stronger makes it easier to get through the day.

After age 40, we begin to lose 6 to 8 percent of our muscle every 10 years. The good news is that it takes only 2 months of strength training (40 minutes, three times a week) to get back 20 years' worth of muscle. If you can't lift weights that often, you'll benefit from even a fraction of that time.

Exercise's Calm

Besides all the physical benefits, a great workout just makes us feel good. And when we feel good, we have the energy to accomplish our day-to-day tasks—and then some. After exercise, our muscles are more relaxed and we get a better night's sleep. When it's time to get up in the morning, we feel more refreshed.

During the rest of the day, we often have to deal with difficult situations, such as traffic jams, working overtime, and arguing with the kids to get their homework done. Confronting these circumstances may cause physiological reactions, known collectively as the fight-or-flight response: perspiration, accelerated respiration, and increased heart rate and blood pressure. When our bodies' systems return to normal, we can be left feeling both emotionally and physically drained.

When we exercise regularly, a similar physiological reaction takes place—our heart rate increases, we perspire, and so on—but when we're finished exercising, we're not left with that

WOMAN TO WOMAN
More Exercise, Less Sleep

Janice Saeger, a 50-year-old senior marketing associate in Wescosville, Pennsylvania, credits exercise for her energy, health, and confidence. But most important, running, biking, and strength training enable her to do more today, like keeping up with a stressful job and completing projects around the house, than she could 20 years ago. And she accomplishes it all on only 6 to 7 hours of sleep a night. Here's how she does it.

I've gradually increased my fitness level in the last 12 years, and it's given me more energy than I ever imagined. When I started a walking program in my thirties, I could do only a half-mile before I needed a rest. But over the years, I built up my endurance and fitness, first with that walking program, then by adding strength training and biking. Now, I've started running instead of walking, and I can go for 30 minutes without stopping. That's five times the distance I could only walk 20 years ago.

These workouts keep me up and going from 5:00 A.M. until as late as 11:00 P.M. I take on tough projects at work and deal with a packed schedule all day. Even so, when I come home, I have energy left to tend to my flower beds and vegetable garden and to plant a new tree or bush instead of collapsing on the couch.

As long as I exercise, I'm not tired during the day. But if I skip a workout, I notice a big change in my energy level. One Saturday, I didn't exercise at all and I was so sleepy that afternoon that I needed a nap. I didn't do my usual workout the next day either, and by 1:00 P.M., I was falling asleep on the couch. I put on my sneakers and went for a run and was full of energy for the rest of the day.

The best part is that once our bodies are conditioned to respond in this way, they'll do so in response to a variety of stimuli, not just in response to exercise. So when we're faced with a difficult situation, chances are we won't feel as exhausted and will regain our energy more quickly. Exercise can even be better than meditation in getting rid of anxiety. Studies show that during exercise, our brains release endorphins, the feel-good hormones that produce the runner's high you've heard about. Consistently exercising also increases levels of resting hormones, such as serotonin, dopamine, and acetylcholine. When levels of these hormones are higher, it's easier for us to relax because they keep our heart rates and blood pressures low.

The mind-body connection that exercise provides probably also has something to do with our improved physical feeling. When we use our muscles, we're focused on putting one foot in front of the other, breathing rhythmically, or doing the aerobic moves correctly, and our minds clear. Along with the release of endorphins, that results in a heightened state of alertness when we're finished exercising. It might even be as good as psychotherapy in lessening depression, and it can also enhance our creativity and imagination.

Finally, exercise gives us control, which is something we don't always have in the rest of our life. We control our health and fitness when we work out regularly. *We* control how far we walk, how long we swim, or how fast we run. *We*

wiped-out feeling that often lingers after a stressful day. Instead, we feel calm and even rejuvenated because regular exercise trains our bodies to handle the physiological reactions better (our hearts get stronger, and our respiratory systems function more efficiently) and to recover from them more quickly.

define what success feels like, whether it's a 5-minute mile or bench-pressing our weight. That sense of control spills over into the rest of our lives, providing us with more confidence and thus with more energy.

An Energy Plan

The official recommendation from the Surgeon General is to exercise 30 minutes on most or all days of the week. But working out doesn't have to equal traditional exercise, and it doesn't mean you have to do it for 30 minutes continuously. In fact, all you may need to do is increase the time you already spend on certain activities, such as dancing.

Figure in your fitness level. If an aerobics class is just too much for you to jump into right now, start with lower-impact activities such as walking and gardening. You might be surprised to learn that many of the things you do every day provide you with the same workout as walking or aerobics. In a half-hour, a 150-pound woman burns 136 calories walking briskly, 221 calories doing aerobics, and 272 calories playing singles tennis. Compare that to the following activities, which are based on the same 150-pound woman doing them for a half-hour. Although the number of calories you burn isn't the issue—you're trying to increase energy, not lose weight—burning a certain number of calories ensures that your metabolism goes high enough to provide increased energy.

WOMEN ASK WHY

Why do I yawn after exercise?

You've probably been told that you yawn after exercise to bring in more oxygen, but that's not true. Your blood cells are 98 percent saturated with oxygen already, so there's no reason to saturate the last 2 percent. Yawning also has nothing to do with how tired you feel or how much sleep you've had. The truth is, no one knows what function yawning serves, but we do know what causes it: hormones.

Yawning seems to be controlled by your parasympathetic nervous system, which is responsible for your resting state. Whenever you're at rest, you secrete hormones such as dopamine, serotonin, and acetylcholine that keep your blood pressure and heart rate low. When these hormones are predominant, you're more likely to yawn.

When you exercise, the relaxation hormones are suppressed so your heart rate and blood pressure can rise. Energizing hormones such as epinephrine and adrenaline kick in. But once you stop moving, your body quickly changes gears again, and you get a surge of relaxation hormones, which is why you tend to yawn after exercise.

Expert consulted
Kara Witzke, Ph.D.
Associate professor and exercise physiologist
Norfolk State University
Virginia

- Shoveling snow: 204 calories
- Outside carpentry (such as building a fence): 204 calories
- Scrubbing the floor or mowing the lawn: 187 calories
- Dancing to disco, country-and-western, or polka music: 187 calories
- Gardening: 170 calories
- Trimming shrubs with a power trimmer: 119 calories

(continued on page 148)

THE ENERGY WORKOUT

All forms of exercise give you more energy. But for optimal energy, you need a program that combines cardiovascular activity, strength and toning exercises, and stretching. Try this general fitness workout designed by exercise physiologist and personal trainer Risa Olinsky, owner of Classic Fitness in Maplewood, New Jersey.

Be sure that you're working at the right level by rating how you feel on a perceived exertion scale of 1 to 10. One is the easiest, such as how you feel when you're sitting and watching television, and 10 is the hardest, such as how you feel sprinting up-hill. Work at a perceived exertion level of 5 or 6.

Not every exercise is right for every person; listen to the messages that your body sends you. Check with a health care professional if you have individual limitations, like back or knee problems that may affect your ability to do these exercises.

Cardiovascular fun. Work in 30 minutes of cardiovascular fitness every day by choosing an activity that you enjoy. You might try singles tennis, cross-country skiing, swimming, a brisk walk with a friend, or inline or ice skating. Start out at a comfortable speed, and gradually increase your intensity within 5 minutes. You should break a light sweat and be slightly breathless but still able to hold a conversation.

Strength training. Always start your strength workouts with a 5- to 8-minute cardiovascular warmup. This will increase your heart rate and muscle temperature, which prepares your muscles to work harder. You will need a few sets of dumbbells, in weights ranging from 3 to 10 pounds. The weight you use will depend on your fitness level and the body part you're working. Different muscle groups require different weights: Your biceps (the front of your upper arms) might need a 5-pound dumbbell, while your triceps (the back of your upper arms) might require only 3 pounds.

Do your strength-training workouts 2 or 3 days a week. Your muscles need time to rebuild and adapt to the stress you've placed on them, so leave at least a day between each workout.

Use weights that you can lift slowly and steadily but that are too heavy to lift more than 15 times. Lifting lighter weights won't build muscle. When you're able to do more than 15 reps, you can either add a second set at the same weight, with a 30- to 45-second rest in between sets, or you can increase the weight slightly and maintain a one-set program. Move at a comfortable pace without stopping too long at the top or the bottom of each movement. Exhale during the lift phase of the repetition.

Stretching. Stretching boosts your energy level and helps prevent injury by releasing the tension you've placed on your muscles during the workout. Be sure to stretch after your workout because your body is most pliable then.

Stretching Exercise

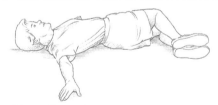

Cooldown Stretch

Lie flat on your back and bend your knees so that your feet are flat on the floor with your toes pointing forward. With your arms extended outward and your palms facedown on the ground, inhale deeply. As you exhale, slowly drop both knees over to the left side, keeping your feet on the floor, your shoulders on the ground, and your knees together. Hold for 30 to 45 seconds; then return to the starting position. Repeat to the right side.

Strength-Training Exercises

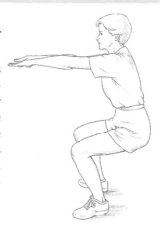

Squat ▶

Stand with your feet slightly wider than shoulder-width apart and your toes turned slightly outward. Keep your shoulders back and extend your arms forward for balance. Looking straight ahead, slowly bend your knees and drop your hips toward the floor as if you were sitting on a stool. Stop when your thighs are parallel to the floor and your knees and toes are at a 90-degree angle. Be sure that you don't tuck your seat as you lower yourself; don't let your knees pass your toes. Return to the starting position, being careful not to lock your knees. Keep your feet flat on the floor throughout the movement. To intensify this exercise, hold a dumbbell in each hand and keep your arms at your sides.

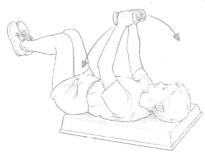

◀ Chest Fly

Lie on your back on a flat bench, a piano bench, a step bench, or a narrow ottoman. Bend your knees so that your lower legs are parallel to the bench, or place your feet flat on the floor on the sides of the bench. Allow your spine to relax without arching it or pressing it down. Hold a dumbbell in each hand above your chest. Your palms should be facing each other. Inhale and slowly open your arms to the sides, with bent elbows, until you feel a slight stretch across your chest, but do not go so far that you lose control of the weights. Do not straighten your arms; you should be able to see your hands in your peripheral vision. Exhale as you return your arms to the starting position.

Overhead Press ▶

Stand with your feet shoulder-width apart. Hold a dumbbell in each hand with your arms bent and the dumbbells at your shoulders. Keep your arms close to your body. Take a deep breath; with your palms facing either away from you or toward each other, press the weights straight over your head, exhaling as you press up. Do not lock your elbows or lean back as you lift. Inhale as you lower the weights back to the starting position.

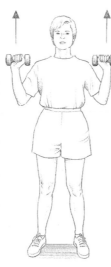

Row ▶

Put your left knee on a bench or the seat of a sturdy chair and bend so that your back is straight and parallel to the floor. Rest your left hand in front of you on the bench. Hold a dumbbell in your right hand and extend your right arm toward the floor. Pull

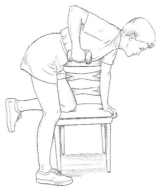

your right hand up until it almost reaches your armpit; keep your arm close to your body and your elbow pointing toward the ceiling. Lower your arm straight down toward the floor and repeat. Switch hands and repeat with your left arm.

ENERGIZING STRETCHES

These stretches can be done sitting in any chair. They should be held between 15 and 30 seconds, with deep breathing throughout, says exercise physiologist and personal trainer Risa Olinsky, owner of Classic Fitness in Maplewood, New Jersey.

Stretch your neck and shoulders. Sit erect on the edge of your chair and look straight ahead. Lace your fingers behind your head as if you were lying back in the sun, and take a deep breath. Exhale, slowly tuck your chin into your chest, and gently press your head down and forward. Inhale as you lift to the starting position. Repeat three times.

Stretch and relax your back. Sit on the edge of your chair with your feet hip-width apart and flat on the floor. Let your arms relax at your sides. Take a deep breath and tuck your chin into your chest. Exhale and slowly roll forward until your chest is resting on your thighs (as if your body were folded in half). Breathe deeply from this position and, as you exhale, uncurl your back to the starting position. Repeat three times.

Wake up fatigued arms, neck, and shoulders. Straighten your right arm and cross it over the left side of your body at shoulder height with your palm facing back. With your left hand, hug your right upper arm, gently pressing it against your body. Keep your right elbow slightly bent. Breathe deeply. Repeat with your left arm.

Loosen tight hamstrings and calves. Sit erect at the edge of your chair, with your feet flat on the floor. Extend your right leg straight out in front of you, keeping your heel on the floor and flexing your toes toward the ceiling. Relax, place both hands on your left thigh, take a deep breath, and lean forward as you exhale. You will feel a stretch in the back of your right leg. Repeat with your left leg.

Choose a variety. For the energy that comes from strong muscles, endurance, and flexibility, you need strength training, stretching, and aerobic activity. Women who skip strength training and work only their cardiovascular system eventually lose upper-body strength. The big question is, "Will strength training make my muscles bulky and unattractive?" The experts' answer is a resounding no. Here's the proof: Marilyn Monroe, a feminine icon in her own right, lifted weights.

Promise yourself half. If you really think you can't make it through the entire 30 minutes of exercise, tell yourself you'll walk, swim, or skate for just 15 minutes. Chances are, once you get going, you'll keep going. Even if you don't finish the entire 30 minutes, at least you started—and maybe you'll do more the next day.

Break it up. If you don't have 30 minutes, break up your workout into three 10-minute walks throughout the day, or add activities such as walking to work, taking the stairs, and parking as far away from the door as possible. "You can even work while you work out," Coopersmith says. "I put a problem in my head before I go running. By the end of my run, I often have a solution."

Please your personality. If you like the outdoors, hike in the summer and cross-country ski in the winter. If you like exercising in privacy, pop an aerobics tape into your VCR. If you enjoy being around others, join a

Researchers found that women usually work out longer and burn more calories doing these kinds of activities because their motivation comes from simple enjoyment instead of weight loss.

walking group. If none of these please you, think about what you liked to do as a kid, Coopersmith suggests. If you loved roller skating, try inline skating. If you were a gymnast, join an adult gymnastics class. Chances are, you'll still enjoy doing it.

To recruit others for your workout, start a morning, lunch, or evening walking group with friends or coworkers; organize your own sporting events with neighbors; or set up a volleyball net or play soccer at your next picnic.

Get the beat. Put together a tape of songs that move from a slow to a fast beat for your walk. The opportunity to listen to great music will probably get you out of the house. Once you get moving, Barry White will warm you up and Gloria Estefan will help you step up the pace.

Put on the pressure. Sign up for a charity walk, or join a sports team. When you have a specific goal, no matter the size, you're more likely to stick to your workouts.

Buy some toys. So it won't be the Red Ryder BB gun that Ralphie got in *A Christmas Story*—getting some toys for yourself might just get you moving. You might try a heart rate monitor when you walk, a medicine ball for your strength work, a stability ball for abdominal crunches, resistance bands to work your arms and legs, or a chin-up bar in the doorway of a room in your home.

TEAM ENERGY

Loraine Frey, 39, used to sit and watch her daughters play soccer. Now, her daughters watch her play.

Frey joined Super Soccer Moms, a soccer league and clinic in Columbia, Maryland, where she learned footwork, how to kick hard enough to pass the ball to teammates, and even how to hit the ball with her head. The adrenaline of the games, her new confidence, and her increased fitness level have given her tons of energy that she didn't know she had.

"A lot of us felt like we were always driving our kids places and watching them have a great time," she says. She wanted to have some fun of her own, and she found it in Super Soccer Moms, complete with laughs and bruises. It gives her a chance to play a team sport, an opportunity women of her generation never really had.

Before soccer, Frey's exercise routine included walking and lifting weights. After she started playing, she realized that exercise for exercise's sake can be boring. Soccer involves competition, camaraderie, and the challenge of making the goal. She still lifts weights and walks, but now she does it to stay in shape for soccer. She has even started jogging—again, for soccer. She's determined to increase her speed, endurance, and overall fitness, all for the love of the game.

Her teammates feel the same way. "Soccer is a different type of energy," says 38-year-old Cindy Ardinger, another member of Super Soccer Moms. "Before soccer, I never pushed myself this hard when I exercised." Now Ardinger can lift weights and play tennis for a longer period of time than she could before she started playing soccer.

That extra effort comes with loads of energy. After her Tuesday-night games, Ardinger says that she has more energy than on any other day of the week. She even wakes up on Wednesday mornings totally energized for a new day. By the weekend, she's craving another night of soccer.

Frey admits that as she approached 40, she worried that she was too old to be as physically active as soccer requires. But after joining Super Soccer Moms, "I realized that I can actually improve my fitness level. I'm not too old to learn, my body isn't falling apart after all, and I can push myself to my limits."

TAKE TWO BARBELLS AND CALL ME IN THE MORNING

To reduce your risk of disease in the future, it's important to be more active now. We're already at risk of developing osteoporosis, which results from the natural loss of bone mass after age 30. Weight-bearing exercise, such as weight lifting, step aerobics, walking, and even gardening, puts tension on our muscles and bones and forces our bodies to compensate by increasing bone density as much as 8 percent a year. Among women over 60, those who are physically active have fewer bone fractures than those who don't exercise at all. There are other ways that staying active helps us avoid disease.

- Exercise reduces the risk of breast cancer among pre- and postmenopausal women.
- Moderate to intense exercise for a half-hour helps lower blood glucose levels and blood pressure, decrease insulin resistance, improve cholesterol levels, decrease body fat, and prevent type 2 diabetes.
- Brisk walking, jogging, swimming, biking, aerobic dance, and racket sports improve the way your blood clots, lowers blood levels of artery-clogging triglycerides, and raises levels of HDL ("good") cholesterol, thereby lowering your risk of heart attacks and heart disease.
- Researchers suspect that exercise lowers your risk of stroke.
- Exercise reduces your risk of some forms of cancer, such as colon cancer and cancers related to obesity.
- Strength training not only maintains your bone density and builds muscle but also improves your digestion and lowers LDL ("bad") cholesterol levels.
- Stretching and abdominal crunches help prevent back pain.

Overall, the benefits add up. Studies show that regular exercise can add years to your life.

Take the dog with you. Taking Rover on your walk not only provides you with good company, but he might come to rely on the workout so much he'll give you that extra nudge on days you try to skip.

Train Swede-style. In Sweden, they take the routine out of exercise with an interval training technique called *fartlek*. Go as fast as you can for as long as you feel comfortable, then slow down. When the urge hits, do whatever keeps you moving and having fun, even if it means skipping for 30 minutes. You'll be more motivated to finish your workout when you're having fun. This type of interval training also increases your fitness level, which helps give you more energy.

Change the scenery. If you're tired of walking by your neighbor's pink flamingos day after day, try hiking in the woods or walking around the mall.

Congratulate yourself. Don't let small achievements go unnoticed; they're proof that you're making progress. Thank yourself for working out when you're less tired after grocery shopping or when you can walk, garden, or play tennis longer than usual.

Finding Energy the Alternative Way

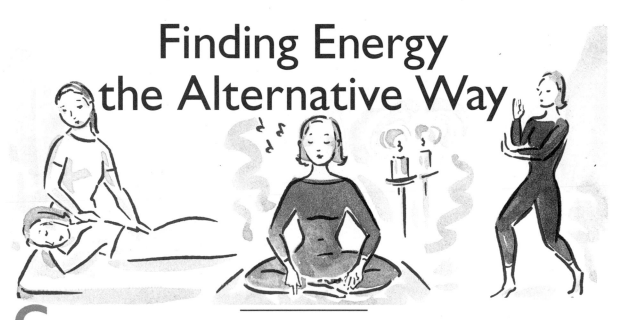

Carolyn stares blankly at her computer screen. While her eyes are fixed on the cursor, her mind ticks off the endless to-do list that dominates her every waking moment: Stop at the grocery for peanut butter on the way home, print out a fall release schedule of new software, order prescriptions for her mother, mend Michael's soccer uniform . . .

"Hey, are you still on this planet?" Carolyn's head snaps toward the voice. It's her coworker Beverly, delivering an inventory printout. Beverly always has a spring in her step and a sparkle in her eye, even though her job is just as demanding as Carolyn's and she has three kids. What's her secret?

"Yoga," is Beverly's answer. She took it up 10 years ago when her children were small and her fatigue was overwhelming. It gave her time away from the whirl of life and a chance to recharge. Plus, it was great for her muscle tone. "You should try it," she tells Carolyn.

But Carolyn isn't sure that yoga is for her. Her mental image of a yoga class is a New Age salon filled with lithe Gumby-like creatures contorting themselves into impossible poses. Beverly as-

sures her that isn't the case and scribbles the name of her yoga teacher on Carolyn's notepad. "What can you lose by trying a few classes?" she calls as she turns to go. With fatigue threatening to become the defining feature of her life, Carolyn decides that she's ready to try anything, even yoga.

She's not alone. Alternative health treatments like yoga have gained wide acceptance in the United States largely because these techniques seem to work when more conventional methods don't. The number of Americans using alternative therapies such as massage, herbs, vitamins, energy healing, and homeopathy rose from about 33 percent in 1990 to more than 42 percent in 1997. And in the 1990s, Americans spent more than $27 billion on these therapies—more than we spent out of pocket for hospital costs.

Alternative therapies may tend to be better for chronic conditions like fatigue, allergies, and stress because they treat the root cause of the illness rather than just the symptoms, says Mark Stengler, N.D., director of natural medicine at Personal Physicians clinic in La Jolla, California,

TAP INTO YOUR ENERGY

The thymus, which is one of the endocrine glands, is located behind your breastbone. It's large in your infancy and starts shrinking after puberty, which results in a slow decline of immunity throughout adulthood. Some naturopathic physicians believe that the thymus plays a large role in your energy levels because two of your body's energy meridians run through it.

By tapping your breastbone firmly—21 times is the recommended number—you may be stimulating your thymus and releasing energy-enhancing energy, according to Chinese medicine theory. "Don't pound your chest like Tarzan," says Mark Stengler, N.D., director of natural medicine at Personal Physicians clinic in La Jolla, California, and associate clinical professor at the National College of Naturopathic Medicine in Portland, Oregon, but do tap decisively with the tips or flats of four fingers, or with a loose fist.

associate clinical professor at the National College of Naturopathic Medicine in Portland, Oregon, and author of *The Natural Physician*. For instance, if you have mild allergies, rather than suggest you pop a decongestant, a naturopathic physician would evaluate your digestive system, where mucus and histamines are made, then propose a treatment plan aimed at correcting the problem underlying the stuffiness in your head.

Approaches differ, yet all alternative therapists suggest that good health depends upon a natural energy balance of all of your body's systems, known as homeostasis, says Dr. Stengler. Every cell has a perfect energy balance, he says, just as the body as a whole has a perfect energy balance. Too much stress disrupts this equilibrium and can cause all kinds of illness. Most alternative medical theories are based on the concept that vital life energy, called chi in Oriental medicine, flows throughout your body along invisible zones called meridians. Balanced, freely flowing chi generates good health, says Dr. Stengler, while sluggish, blocked, or overstimulated chi is a sign of poor health.

"Chi flows through the body like blood," he says. There is an electrical charge to your body, and treatments used for hundreds of years that strengthen and balance energy flow have been shown to improve health. Exactly how these treatments work is still a mystery. But the same can be said for some facets of conventional medicine.

As for chi's relation to energy, "we each experience energy in our own way, but one thing is certain: Energy flows," Dr. Stengler says. "It circulates consciously and unconsciously throughout the body on physical, emotional, and mental levels."

One sign of the popularity of alternative therapies is their accessibility. You need look no further than the nearest YWCA or health club for yoga classes. Chiropractic offices are nearly as common as gas stations. And even corporate offices bring in massage therapists for on-the-job treatments.

Although their popularity has exploded in just the past decade, most alternative therapies have ancient roots. Interest may have brought them back into the public consciousness, but when it comes to finding energy the alternative way, "everything old is new again."

Yearn for Yoga

Yoga stems from Hinduism, one of the oldest religions on the planet. A discipline that engages your mind as well as your body, yoga's roots go back about 5,000 years. Many women practice yoga to find personal meaning in life and in the process gain energy, vitality, and an improved sense of well-being.

Yoga is about the balance of your physical, mental, and spiritual states. Its purpose, according to yoga philosophy, is to get your physical body under control so that the more perfect "inner you" can emerge. Yoga practitioners learn to breathe properly and strengthen their bodies through postures known as *asanas*.

"Because yoga connects the body and the mind, it tends to energize women more than aerobics does," says Dawn Braud, an exercise physiologist and director of the fitness center at Woman's Hospital in Baton Rouge, Louisiana. Unlike other forms of exercise that involve only your body, yoga's psychological aspect encourages you to mentally release your burdens and give your mind a chance to recharge as well.

Yoga is also a stress reducer, which makes it an ideal workout. "What the mind has forgotten, the body remembers," she says, but after the deep relaxation of yoga, those stressors melt away and leave you refreshed.

The beauty of yoga is that it is so different from our on-the-go lives. There is no multitasking here. Instead, yoga rooms are quiet and serene; the art requires mindful concentration to get the poses right. As a result, says Braud, most women leave a yoga class feeling lighter, a little less burdened.

At the core of yoga philosophy is the belief that we have three bodies: the physical body; the astral body, or mind; and the causal body, or pure spirit, which can be reached through meditation. While each can function separately, they

---

WASHING YOUR WAY INTO ENERGY

Hydrotherapy is an age-old form of healing that uses water to relieve stress and tension. Using a handheld showerhead, run warm water up and down your arms and legs for 15 seconds, followed by 15 seconds with water that is as cool as you can comfortably stand. (Cold water is too shocking and stimulating to your system.)

The warm water soothes and relaxes you, while the cool water stimulates your immune system, says Mark Stengler, N.D., director of natural medicine at Personal Physicians clinic in La Jolla, California, and associate clinical professor at the National College of Naturopathic Medicine in Portland, Oregon. The contrast between warm and cool improves your circulation and provides overall stimulation. Continue this alternating shower for 5 minutes, and you'll feel a spike in your energy level.

If you have access to a hydrotherapy clinic, Dr. Stengler suggests that you try a total-relaxation treatment, where showers and tubs with high-powered jet sprays will wash away tension from your stressed-out muscles. Initially, you may feel a bit tired from your aqua-pummeling, but within a few hours, you'll experience a marked energy rebound.

---

are intimately related, so to know your whole self, you must develop an awareness of all three. When you do, you reach a state of self-actualization where, yogis say, you'll realize your profound connection to the universe and its abundant energy.

The beauty of yoga is in its versatility: You can focus on the physical, the psychological, the spiritual, or a combination of all three. Unlike traditional forms of exercise, which tend to be goal-oriented, yoga is a process. Your awareness is focused on what you're doing and how it feels. With the "happy pose," or triangle, for example, your focus is on the stretch in your legs, chest, and arms.

To do this pose, stand with your legs about 3

THE SOUND OF ENERGY

Music touches the core of our souls. Its power transcends language, cultures, and generations. Soothe a cranky baby with a lullaby. Put on a CD of upbeat tunes to crank up your energy level.

The record of the therapeutic effect of sound dates back to the writings of Plato and Aristotle. The modern discipline of music therapy began after World War I, when community musicians went to government hospitals to play for thousands of veterans to ease their physical and emotional trauma from the war. The patients' responses to the music prompted the doctors and nurses to ask the hospitals to hire musicians. Today, music is used in many hospitals to alleviate pain, induce sleep, and counteract apprehension or fear.

A pounding beat isn't the only way to recharge your energy cells, according to music therapists. Any style of music can jazz you up or help you get rid of stress, as long as it's a sound you like.

And you don't have to be just a passive listener. Making music can also boost your energy and reduce stress. So the next time you need a lift or a little relaxation, try some rhythmic drumming or heartfelt singing. You may be surprised by how good it makes you feel.

Too often, women are intimidated by the idea of an exercise class, believing that they're not fit enough to even join. Not so with yoga, says Braud. "You can start at any level of fitness, and yoga will meet you where you are." As you improve with practice, you graduate to more difficult postures.

Unlike many exercise classes, where you learn a routine and repeat it, yoga is an ongoing learning process. You learn a pose, then refine it, moving to more challenging variations as you advance. And "yoga is not about looks," Braud says. Classes are filled with people of all shapes and sizes. A totally non-judgmental discipline, "yoga has you focus inside," she says, "and you can be in any body to do that."

Realizing the benefits of yoga requires some dedication. Braud recommends working out three to five times a week for 20 to 30 minutes. Within that brief time, the meditative aspect of yoga can put you back in touch with who you are, both emotionally and spiritually. "In today's society, we tend to become disconnected from our minds and spirits," she says, "which makes us far too vulnerable to other peoples' expectations, one of the biggest energy drainers around."

Holistic health centers and YWCAs are good places to find yoga classes. Or check out www.yogasite.com, which has a state-by-state directory of teachers. This site also lists workshops and retreats across the United States. To receive general information on choosing a yoga instructor, send a self-addressed stamped envelope (with postage for 2 ounces) to the

feet apart, with your right foot pointed forward and your left foot comfortably turned out. Bend from your waist to the left, resting your left hand on your left ankle or calf, and extend your right arm straight up over your head. Feel the stretch in your neck as you look straight ahead or up to the sky. As you hold this pose, notice how strong your legs feel against the ground and the way your chest opens up, bringing in energizing oxygen. Keep your body in the same plane. Your left hand may never reach your ankle, but that's okay. With conventional exercise, you fail if you miss your goal. With yoga, you succeed simply by trying.

American Yoga Association at PO Box 19986, Sarasota, FL 34276, or check out their Web site at www.americanyogaassociation.org.

Massage In the Energy

Strong fingers knead the tops of your shoulders, then glide up your neck. The tension in your taut muscles begins to dissolve, and before long, the soreness that's been lurking at the base of your skull starts melting away. As the pressing and stroking continue, stress evaporates from every muscle group, leaving you limp with relaxation.

There are approximately 100 different methods of massage therapy, the majority performed with various hand strokes. Massage has been an element in Traditional Chinese Medicine for more than 4,000 years. It has also, in some form, been part of Western healing since the fourth century B.C., when the Greek physician Hippocrates endorsed it.

There's no denying that massage feels exquisite. But it also has healing and energizing properties that are gaining widespread acceptance as scientists document the effects of touch through biochemical changes in the brain and body, says Donna Mack, R.N., director of the Center for Health and Restoration at Mercy Medical Center in Baltimore.

Blood chemical tests of patients done before and after massage show an increase in T-cells, which bolster the immune system, and endorphins, your body's natural painkillers and de-

ENERGY MEDICINE

Simply put, any form of touch is energy medicine, says Donna Mack, R.N., director of the Center for Health and Restoration at Mercy Medical Center in Baltimore.

"When you give somebody a hug, it makes them feel better. Just in that moment, your intentions become energy. You want that person to feel better. There is a very real transfer of energy that can be quite therapeutic."

Practitioners of energy medicine believe that the human body is composed of various energy fields and that we get sick when the energy in those fields is blocked, unbalanced, or otherwise disturbed.

Therapists use a variety of techniques to balance and release the body's flow of energy. Most place their hands either on or near the patient's body. Treatments like "healing touch" or Reiki operate on the belief that a trained practitioner can feel or sense a person's energy field. By altering rips or blockages in that person's energy field, practitioners say that they can help a patient relax or heal.

Any form of touch changes your energy, as your body and the therapist's experience an energy exchange, says Mack. Nurses and other healers have always known intuitively that the way people are touched can speed the healing process. The difference today, she notes, is that scientists are beginning to quantify the effect.

Several alternative therapies, such as homeopathy and acupuncture, are based on energy and the ability to rebalance it for healing. Naturopaths can read a patient's life energies through a computerized biofeedback device that determines the type of stressors (like pesticide exposure or clogged internal organs) that are causing ill health. Reams of anecdotal reports indicate that these treatments work, but conventional science cannot yet say why.

stressors, says Monica Haynes, R.N., a certified massage therapist at the Center for Health and Restoration at Mercy Medical Center.

Apart from manipulating muscles to relieve stress and promote relaxation, massage therapy helps to energize people through touch. "Touching is an intimate act," says Haynes. Whether you're rocking a baby or giving someone a hearty handshake, "when we touch another person, something happens between us." Massage therapists know that touch can convey the therapeutic emotions of caring and concern, and some believe that touch can help release blocked emotions, allowing the patient's body to renew itself.

At the very least, the total relaxation that massage affords allows your body to repair the daily damage done to it by stress, Mack says, noting that most women come to her center seeking stress reduction. "As energetic as our lives are today, we get sapped of energy, largely through stress. Massage allows women to go into a very deep state of relaxation, and from that state, their bodies can heal and reenergize themselves."

Whether you prefer traditional European methods or some form of Oriental manipulation, all types of massage can take you to that healing state of relaxation. In Mack's opinion, Swedish massage, the type most commonly performed, works best for stress reduction. Its long, gliding strokes tend to promote a more nurturing, loving massage, she says, more so than a treatment-type massage that pinpoints a particular discomfort. "You can tell that a woman's stress has been dramatically reduced when she steps out of a massage room looking like a limp dishcloth," says Mack. And although it sounds counterintuitive, such deep relaxation is actually quite energizing.

WOMEN ASK WHY

Why do I feel like I'm losing my memory when I'm tired?

The short answer is that your brain isn't getting the fuel it needs. When you're tired, you tend to breathe shallowly and sluggishly, which means your brain isn't receiving the full supply of essential oxygen it needs. The less oxygen you take in, the less your brain cooperates, opting to keep critical functions going and dropping elective operations like memory.

Ideally, you should be taking 18 deep, lung-filling breaths a minute. If you're fatigued, you're more likely to be inhaling only 10 times a minute, breathing shallowly through your upper chest.

If you feel like your memory is slipping, stop and practice focused breathing for 5 minutes. Breathing is largely driven by your unconscious, but you can override it and learn to take in more oxygen.

Try diaphragmatic breathing, fully filling your lungs by inhaling through your nose and exhaling through your mouth. Most people tend not to use their diaphragms when they breathe, breathing only from their upper chests. Whenever possible, you should breathe through your nose because the fine hairs in your nostrils help filter out toxins.

There are other ways to get oxygen into your lungs. Try breathing from your lower abdomen: Exhale deeply several times and feel your body relax as oxygen rushes in. Roll up the windows while you're driving and sing as loudly as you can for as long as you can. Anything that gets the air going in and out properly is going to kick-start your energy and your memory.

Try this breathing exercise. Sit comfortably in a straight-back chair or lie on a relatively flat surface. Place your right

Many hospitals and health clubs have massage therapists on their staffs. The American Massage Therapy Association (AMTA) can refer you to a qualified therapist in your area.

hand over your belly button and your left hand over your sternum. Allow yourself to exhale just a bit longer than usual, then inhale fully. Imagine filling your belly up with air like a balloon, allowing your diaphragm to contract or move downward. Your right hand should move out, but your left hand should move as little as possible. After a brief natural pause, exhale again, extending your exhale a bit longer than usual. Repeat.

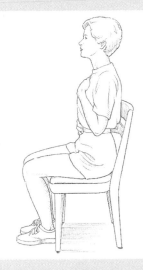

This exercise helps you learn to breathe more deeply, lower in your lungs. Start with one round of 3 to 4 minutes each day. Add rounds as you feel ready, until you are doing two or three a day.

Expert consulted
Mark Stengler, N.D.
Associate clinical professor
National College of Naturopathic Medicine
Portland, Oregon
Author of The Natural Physician

You can call AMTA's "Find a Massage Therapist" national locator service at (888) 843-2682, or visit its Web site at www.amtamassage.org/findamassage/locator.htm.

Reflexology: Fonts of Energy in Our Hands and Feet

Grab your big toe. Press your thumb firmly into the bottom tip and hold for 90 seconds. Repeat with the opposite foot, and in a few minutes you should feel your weariness lifting. Believe it or not, pressing the flesh in certain areas of your feet and hands—following a system of alternating pressure techniques called reflexology—may reduce fatigue, leaving you refreshed and alert.

Your bioelectrical energy, or chi, flows in meridians throughout your body. Every organ falls along one of these meridians, which end at the tips of your fingers and toes. According to the healing art of reflexology, which dates back to at least 2330 B.C., the soles of your feet and palms of your hands represent a map of your body; applying pressure to the right point on these extremities sends an energy signal that stimulates a specific organ such as the brain. Anything that unblocks the energy meridians into the brain will quickly increase energy, says Marcia Aschendorf, N.D., a naturopathic physician in Cincinnati and executive director of the International Academy of Naturopathy. This signal also clears any blockages that stop chi from circulating freely throughout your body, strengthening and balancing your body's flow of vital energy.

"Reflexology can quickly alleviate fatigue by restoring mental alertness and reducing tension," says Dr. Aschendorf. When people wring their hands because they are sad or overwhelmed, they are instinctually employing a form of reflexology, bringing energy into the body in times of distress. She notes that people often unconsciously do whatever their bodies need to feel better.

The brilliance of reflexology is that you can practice it on yourself in any setting whenever your energy starts lagging. She recommends these energizing exercises that you can do yourself.

+ For a quick energy burst, bring your hands together, fingers straight, as if you were praying, then flex the fingers of both hands so that the tips are touching with your palms a few inches apart. Tap your fingertips together for 3 to 5 minutes. Be sure to tap the tips, not the pads, of your fingers for maximum energy stimulation. Your fingertips and the ends of your toes correspond to the brain, which controls vital life functions. Triggering the brain reflex restores vitality by directing your body to breathe more efficiently and by stimulating mental electrical exchanges.

+ Make a "butterfly" with your hands by placing one thumb on top of the other, with your palms facing away from your body. Curl the fingers of the top thumb's hand over onto the fleshy part of your other hand under your thumb. Wherever the middle finger of your top hand falls, apply firm pressure on the opposing hand's thumb mound, pulling it slightly, as though you were milking a cow. Do this for 90 seconds, then reverse your thumbs and repeat. This exercise stimulates the adrenal reflexes, which govern your heart, lungs, and kidneys, thus boosting your energy. You can perform a variation of this exercise in your car when you're at a stoplight by pressing the fleshy mound of your palm below the thumb into the steering wheel. Hold the pressure for

several seconds, then release. Tapping your fingertips on the steering wheel helps, too.

To find a reflexologist in your area, log on to the Reflexology Association of America's Web site at www.reflexology-usa.org.

The Healing Powers of Homeopathy

This 200-year-old system of holistic healing, which is based on the idea that "like cures like," claims to stimulate your body's own recuperative

---

JOURNALING FOR ENERGY

There's something strangely invigorating about putting pen to paper in a personal journal, says Judy Lin Eftekhar. "This blank page is just for me. I can say whatever I think without fear of being misunderstood. It's incredibly freeing."

Between a full-time job in the engineering school at the University of California, Los Angeles, her 5-year-old daughter, her husband, and her home, Eftekhar doesn't have much time for herself. But every morning, she rises a half-hour earlier than the rest of her family to sit in her kitchen with a cup of tea and pour out her feelings into her journal. This is her time, her place.

She writes spontaneously about the highs and lows of her life. "If something is upsetting me, it doesn't drag me down by doing battle in my subconscious and unconscious mind all day if I get it down on paper," she says. If something is really bothering her, she'll write about for several days in a row until it loses its power over her.

The tone of her writing varies from day to day, from complaining and whining to being very appreciative and positive. Airing her victories and grievances in this truly private format is "like talking to someone and having them listen nonjudgmentally."

Journaling also helps her prepare for the day. "If I miss it, I'm out of whack mentally," she says, "not to mention tired and blue, too."

Jennifer Wortman agrees. Quiet, centering experiences are what give her more energy, says the San Diego public relations account executive, who has been keeping a journal for most of her life. "It's important to take time for yourself, to disconnect from the craziness of the world." She notes that she has more energy to give when she feels grounded.

When you write in your journal, you're never judged, there's no controversy, and life is what you make of it. For one golden portion of the day, "there's no worrying about what people think of you," she says. "That judgmental aspect of society takes away energy. In your journal, it doesn't exist."

Wortman's time for her truest self comes in the evening when she plays classical music and writes in her journal by candlelight. She thinks of her journal as her best friend because it serves as a laboratory for decision making, reflection, and personal growth. Even when recounting some less-than-thrilling event, she tries to stress the positive and find the life lesson in every experience.

"I see journal keeping as a way of being accountable to myself," she says. Many women today hurdle through their lives on autopilot and it becomes too easy for things to slip by. Taking time to sort through her thoughts allows her to see the themes and patterns in life, to learn from her mistakes, and to realize that today's catastrophe is really no big deal. All of this frees her from the stress of the day, enabling her to face tomorrow fully charged.

powers with remedies that contain extremely small amounts of substances which, in larger quantities, would produce the very symptoms they're meant to treat.

A few conventional therapies, such as allergy desensitization and immunization, follow this same "law of similars," but because homeopathic remedy extracts are so highly diluted, the FDA does not require them to undergo safety testing. The FDA estimates sales of homeopathic remedies at around $201 million, and they are growing 20 percent a year.

Paradoxically, homeopaths say that the more dilute a homeopathic remedy is, the greater its potential to cure. The highest potency, or most dilute, homeopathic remedies contain virtually none of the active substance, so their demonstrable efficacy seems to defy known laws of chemistry and physics. No one knows why it works, says Dr. Stengler, beyond the belief that an extract's vibration provokes the cell structure to return to normal.

"Everything in nature works on a frequency," he says. "Think of your body as one big cell that receives energy vibrations; homeopathy seeks to reestablish its system of harmony."

While there are general homeopathic remedies available in health food stores, Dr. Stengler says that the most effective treatments are specific to the individual. If you're dragging through the day, a homeopath or naturopathic physician should evaluate the cause and suggest a treatment uniquely for you.

Before prescribing remedies for new patients, homeopaths conduct in-depth interviews designed to determine basic physiological and psychological characteristics. These mind/body characteristics, called typologies, are important factors in prescribing the right remedy, especially for chronic conditions.

The two basic types of remedies are single remedies and combination remedies. Single remedies, which contain one active substance, are generally the most effective. Combination remedies, with two or more active substances, are designed to offer the greatest relief to the greatest percentage of sufferers. Each active substance is intended to alleviate a distinct symptom, with some overlap built in to ensure a higher rate of success.

Potency is indicated by a standard code. A

WOMAN TO WOMAN
Spirituality Energized Her

Anyone who meets Selma Schuerman remarks on her energy. At 88, she personifies pep. Schuerman walks at least 2 miles every day, gardens, bakes, and works with a community-outreach program in rural Smiley, Texas. But when she was 45, Schuerman found herself slogging through the day, fatigued by the challenges of life. Then she began a spiritual journey that filled her life with energy and joy. This is her story.

Struggling in an unhappy marriage, knowing my life had a void that needed to be filled, I began studying Christian Science and found my spiritual home. I came to realize that God would provide everything I needed, but first I had to tune in to Him. Rather than feeling sorrow over what was lacking in my life, I began to know a sense of peace and the security of plenty.

I began rising early to study Christian Science lessons and the Bible for 2 hours or so before my "real day" began. It didn't take me long to realize that this meditative period was the "realest" part of my day, giving the other 22 hours vitality and focus. If I skipped my studies, I found that the day didn't go as well and I wasn't as energetic. Little things would annoy me unduly. I needed the balance that spiritual insight gave me.

Not long after my journey began, my step felt lighter and my thoughts clearer. To my delight, I found that I could teach four 2-hour sewing classes a day, plus three classes on Saturday, without feeling exhausted. I had more than enough energy to run my household, work with the church, and socialize with friends.

My marriage never really improved, but because my thinking did, the relationship no longer drained my energy. Getting my mind right gave me boundless energy. It was like tapping into an eternal circuit. When people ask me where all my energy comes from, I tell them it comes from God.

Homeopathy is frequently used to treat fatigue and stress, says Dr. Stengler. If you can't wait to see a practitioner, here are some remedies he recommends for most women.

Arsenicum. Good for mental and physical exhaustion, especially when symptoms of anxiety are present. Arsenicum is an extremely dilute form of arsenic, which is extracted from metals like iron and cobalt, then finely ground and weakened by mixing with larger and larger amounts of milk sugar. Typically, health food stores sell 30C tablets. Take two tablets twice a day.

Gelsemium. Specific for feelings of drowsiness and fatigue, especially when your muscles ache as well. This is the diluted preparation of yellow jasmine. Take two 30C tablets twice a day.

Phosphoric acid. Best used when you're so fatigued you may not be able to get out of bed, or if you have a strong craving for carbonated beverages. This is the homeopathic dilution of phosphoric acid, the same ingredient that makes soft drinks fizzle. Take two 30C tablets twice a day.

Ferrum Phosphoricum. Good for low energy caused by iron deficiency anemia. This remedy is made from a compound of iron and phosphorous, either of which can be deadly in large enough amounts; the minerals are diluted with milk sugar to make them nontoxic. The most widely sold formulas are 6X; take three tablets three times a day. Your doctor should monitor you with blood tests to make sure your anemia is improving.

number indicates the number of dilutions performed and a letter indicates the ratio of each dilution. The letter "X" stands for a 1:9 dilution, while "C" indicates a 1:99 dilution.

If you try an over-the-counter homeopathic remedy, don't take it within 30 minutes of drinking coffee because the coffee may cancel out any positive effects. For the same reason, it is best not to touch a tablet; shake it into the lid of its container, then drop the tablet under your tongue. If you're using a liquid remedy, shake the bottle first.

To find a homeopath in your area, you can contact the National Center for Homeopathy at (703) 548-7790 or visit their Web site at www.homeopathic.org. State licensing requirements vary, although most require some type of medical training.

Flower Essence Energy

If you want to enjoy vigorous, blooming health, Dr. Stengler suggests flower essences, which counteract those negative emotional reactions that zap your energy. A specially prepared liquid concentrate made by soaking flowers in pure spring water, each flower essence treats a specific emotion such as stress or anxiety. Developed more than 70 years ago by homeopathic physician Dr. Edward Bach, flower essences are said to contain specific plant energy that affects the energy balance of the person taking them.

Two to four drops of an essence, taken in a glass of water or dropped under your tongue, may reset your body's emotional equilibrium, says Dr. Stengler. By restoring homeostasis, your body's natural energy balance, flower essences restore vitality and prevent negative feelings from leading to physical illness, he says.

Dr. Bach distilled 38 separate essences. He also created an emergency combination of flower essences that he called Rescue Remedy, which Dr. Stengler suggests every woman carry in her purse. When we're faced with sudden bad news or a stressful event, this liquid remedy may help us face the distress and emotional rebound from it by reducing fear and nervousness, two major energy siphons, he says.

Rescue Remedy contains five flower essences: impatiens (to allay impatience and irritability), star of Bethlehem (to relieve the aftereffects of fright, grief, or shock), cherry plum (to keep fear of losing control and other irrational thoughts at bay), rock rose (to calm feelings of terror or sudden alarm), and clematis (to treat daydreaming and lack of interest in the present).

Flower essences are generally safe to use under the tongue, to swallow, to apply to the skin, and to use in the bath. Avoid getting them in your eyes, and don't apply them to mucous membranes or abraded skin. Most flower essences contain alcohol as a preservative, so if you're sensitive to alcohol, check with your doctor before using them.

Energizing Fragrances

Freshly baked apple pie. Lavender in full bloom. The powdery smell of a newborn. Certain smells make us smile, or feel good. That positive feeling is at the core of aromatherapy, which uses fragrant concentrated plant extracts, known as essential oils, to soothe the mind, restore balance within the body, and treat a variety of symptoms, including fatigue.

Aromatherapists believe that essential oils work on the emotions because the nerves that enable you to smell are directly linked to your brain's limbic system, which governs your emotions. Practitioners say that the active components of essential oils give each a unique therapeutic quality. The scent of lavender, for example, is calming, while thyme is strongly stimulating. These are some energy-enhancing aromatherapy remedies.

Citrus oils. The scents of orange and lemon have antidepressant and uplifting qualities, providing a pick-me-up when you have flagging energy.

Peppermint. This scent is invigorating and good for fatigue and depression. Three drops is the most you should use in your bath, and you should avoid getting it near your eyes. Also, do not use peppermint at the same time as homeopathic remedies.

Frankincense. This scent is stimulating and elevating to the mind. It's also soothing to the spirit.

Rosemary, geranium, and basil. All three oils are energy boosters. Rosemary has a powerful effect on the nervous system, so it's not recommended if you have hypertension or epilepsy. Don't use more than three drops of basil oil in your bath, and avoid it altogether if you're nursing.

Not every energizing scent works for every person, Dr. Stengler cautions. "Scent is very individualized. What may elevate one person's mood and energy levels may drive another person crazy."

To find an essential oil that will help raise your energy, Dr. Stengler suggests that you just sniff and note your reaction. If you draw back from a scent, it's not for you; if you draw closer, it's a good one.

Essential oils can be used externally in many ways, but you should never apply them directly to your skin or swallow them. During pregnancy, use half the recommended amount and don't use them at all on infants and small children. Store essential oils in dark bottles, away from light and heat, and out of the reach of children and pets. When you find an energizing scent, put a few drops on a cotton ball or a wad of tissue and tuck it into your bra. Your body heat will cause the scent to radiate upward for a constant energizing aroma.

To keep up your energy at work or home,

HOW IN THE WORLD DO THEY SLEEP?
Famous Sleepers through History

Have you ever slept in on a weekend and woken up feeling like you had slept forever? Compared to some people throughout history, you hadn't even come close.

Take Charlemagne of the 9th-century Holy Roman Empire. Because of insomnia-ridden nights, he was known to nap for 3 hours after his midday meal. French mathematician Abraham de Moivre was reported to have slept 20 hours a night (and day) as he neared his death in 1754. And sleep researcher Peretz Lavie reported on 19th-century women and adolescent girls who slept for days or months on end—there was even one who slept for a year.

Consider fiction's legendary sleepyheads. Washington Irving's hero Rip Van Winkle imbibed a charmed drink and woke up 20 years later. He spent the remainder of his days as a makeshift historian, telling willing listeners what life was like 2 decades earlier. And who can forget Sleeping Beauty, who spent 100 years in an ageless, enchanted sleep, only to be awakened by her charming prince?

But if you've ever felt like you just didn't get enough sleep, you're in for some competitive (and powerful) company.

place a few drops of essential oil on a light bulb ring, which heats the oil and diffuses the scent throughout the area. You can also use essential oils in a relaxing bath or energizing foot soak. No matter what you choose, your energizing oil will alleviate fatigue and invigorate your entire body, Dr. Stengler says.

Visualize Your Energy

Unlike teenagers, your mind will believe anything you tell it. So if you spend all day thinking about how exhausted you are, you'll be exhausted. But if you let go of those negative

While running Great Britain, former Prime Minister Winston Churchill, who slept little, once chided a younger colleague who complained of fatigue, "I have never been tired in my life." Margaret Thatcher, another former Prime Minister, reportedly slept only 3 to 4 hours each night. It was said that President John F. Kennedy worked in the Oval Office until the wee hours of the morning and then awoke just a few hours later at 7:30 A.M.

Short sleepers in history were at no loss for creativity, either. Inventor Thomas Edison required less than 4 hours of sleep per night, often napping on a couch in his workroom only when he felt fatigued. He considered 8 hours of sleep "excessive" and a symptom of weakness and stupidity. Edison's competitor, Yugoslavian electrical engineer Nikola Tesla, inventor of the wireless radio, scoffed at Edison's sleep habits: Tesla reportedly slept only 2 hours each morning.

Fellow inventor and 15th-century artist Leonardo da Vinci was said to have worked almost continuously by napping 15 minutes every 4 hours (a mere 1½ hours per day) and not sleeping at all at night. Painter Salvador Dalí was rumored to have napped in a chair while holding a spoon over a tin plate. When he drifted into sleep and dropped the spoon, the clatter would wake him, and he would feel completely refreshed.

thoughts and emotions, and see yourself sparkling with energy and always up for life's next challenge, you'll eventually start feeling that way, says Edie Raether, a psychotherapist in Raleigh, North Carolina. That's the key to visualization: If you conceive it and believe it, you can achieve it.

"If you're not capitalizing on this power to gain more energy and a better life, you're wasting a tremendous natural resource," says Raether. But don't think in terms of letters or words. Like a small child, your mind comprehends pictures far better than words. When you visualize what you want, you must provide a clear blueprint—marching orders that your unconscious mind can put into effect.

Visualization is actually a means of gaining control over our lives, she says. Too often, we move through our lives reacting to events, trapped in a perception of being overwhelmed, and that can drain our energy.

The miracle of visualization is that it speaks the language of the body. The most dramatic illustration of its power has come in the battle against cancer. Anecdotal evidence collected over the past 30 years has brought visualization into the mainstream mix of cancer treatment. The American Cancer Society says that imagery may help cancer patients because it promotes relaxation and reduces stress. It can't cure the disease, but it is an important technique that helps the mind influence the body in positive ways.

You should practice visualization at least once a day, Raether says, or more often if possible. And you have to dispense with the negative before you can put in the positive. "You can't plant a beautiful garden in a weed-infested patch."

Begin by sitting or lying in a relaxed posture with no physical stress on your body. Close your eyes and breathe easily. Empty your mind of everyday thoughts. Forget about the leak under your car, the braces your 13-year-old needs, and the silent treatment you've been getting from your boss. This is much more challenging than it sounds.

Focus on your breathing. As you feel yourself entering a relaxed, trancelike state, begin visualizing. It should involve all of your senses: See it, smell it, taste it, touch it, and hear it. "Bombard your sensory systems," says Raether. "Sensory details activate neuron centers in the brain. The more brain activity there is, the more real the visualization becomes."

See yourself spring out of bed, tingling with anticipation at the glorious day stretching before you. The sun wraps you in a warm glow of energy. Your spine is straight and your stride is confident as you effortlessly pluck the perfect outfit from the closet. You personify energy itself as you visualize yourself moving through the day, poised and in control.

Don't limit yourself; use your mind like a telephoto lens to magnify your goal and see it bigger, bolder, and brighter. If you want enough energy to rise at 5:00 A.M., work out for an hour before going to the office, distinguish yourself in your profession, help your kids with their homework, cook a healthful dinner, and then get romantic with your life partner, you have to think big.

Meditate On Energy

Many cultures recognize the calming, therapeutic effect of quiet contemplation or meditation, which asks you to stop, let go, and passively observe the experience of life, says Raether.

Meditation is a self-directed practice for relaxing your body and calming your mind. It is a free-flowing experience, she says, like spontaneous artwork. As you relax into meditation, you enter an altered state of consciousness, sending your brain into a resting but conscious state. Detaching helps you to disconnect from the stressors of normal life, allowing your body to truly rest and recharge.

Although meditation seems simple, keeping the usual stream of conscious thoughts from flowing through your mind takes practice. Thoughts of dirty dishes and your children's science projects will pop up, dragging you back to the real, exhausting world. When other thoughts intrude, Raether suggests that you take notice of them, then let them go.

Meditate in a quiet place with as few distractions as possible. Sit quietly in a comfortable position, preferably with your back straight. Focus your mind on your breath, on a silently repeated sound, or on a stationary object like a flower or a candle flame. As you focus your mind, allow all other thoughts to float away, gently refocusing as many times as necessary.

Practice for 15 to 20 minutes twice a day if possible. Meditating at the same time every day helps reinforce the habit, Raether says. Many people who practice meditation say that the relaxation and focus provided by regular sessions positively affects every aspect of their lives, especially their energy levels. Several studies show a decrease in blood pressure among people who meditate regularly.

Brush Up Your Energy

It may sound ridiculous, but the act of brushing your dry skin first thing in the morning can give you an instant energy lift. It not only feels great but also stimulates the sensory nerves of your peripheral nervous system (the nerves and ganglia outside your brain and spinal cord), energizing your entire body, says Dr. Stengler. It may also improve your circulation and lymphatic flow (the clear fluid that transports white blood cells), thus strengthening your immune system. Further, sloughing off dead skin cells may help speed your body's expulsion of toxins through perspiration. Many of Dr. Stengler's clients who practice daily skin brushing report fewer ailments such as headaches, colds, and flu.

To start, you'll need a natural-bristle body brush, the type available in any bath shop. Start out with medium-soft bristles because if the bristles are too stiff and hard, they will scratch your skin, but if they're too soft, they'll be ineffective. Once you get used to brushing, you can move on to slightly firmer bristles.

You can choose either short- or long-handled brushes, but a long-handled brush makes it much easier to reach your back. And don't share with your loved ones. Think of this brush as you do your toothbrush—for personal use only, says Dr. Stengler. Be sure to clean your brush every few weeks with soap and water and allow it to air dry.

Starting with your feet and ankles, brush upward in quick strokes, working your way up your calves and thighs. Brush up your torso, then up your arms from your fingers to your shoulders. Every stroke should be directed toward your heart, Dr. Stengler says. You should concentrate your brushing on the lymphatic areas of your body—your inner thighs, behind your knees, under your arms—to give those glands a little extra stimulation, encouraging the expulsion of toxins. Brush the entire surface of your body except for your face and breasts because the tissue in those places is too delicate for brushing.

The whole process should take no more than 3 minutes, yet leave you revved and reenergized. If you shower in the morning, do your body brushing in advance, says Dr. Stengler, so that any cells left behind are washed away. Some women dry brush their bodies before bed, finding it a good way to relax at the end of the day.

Be Thankful and Energize

A grateful attitude can make a huge difference in your everyday energy levels, says Raether. In fact, there's an emerging school of thought

JUMP START
Get the Light

If you're trapped in an office building all day, it's no wonder that you may be dragging. Fluorescent lights have an energy-draining effect on most people. Recharge your energy by walking around outdoors in the sunlight for 10 minutes.

among psychologists that promotes the power of optimism. "Positive psychology" explores how affirmative human feelings affect life satisfaction. The first positive psychology summit was held in January 2000, with the theme "Building a Positive Human Future."

Rather than feeling burdened by your responsibilities, be grateful for them. Be thankful for the mess after a party because it means that you have friends. Rejoice in the piles of laundry and ironing because it means that you have a family to nurture. Revel in the lawn that needs mowing and the gutters that need cleaning because it means that you have a home. Work at viewing your daily rounds as a privilege, not drudgery. "The more you practice gratitude, the more positive your life will become and the more energy you will have," Raether says.

And while you're at it, laugh a little. It's impossible to be uptight when you're in the midst of a belly laugh, says Raether. Your body is totally free of anxiety and stress, which builds up your energy stores. So try to see things in a humorous light as much as you can. As some psychologists say, "Comedy is tragedy, plus time." Turning today's catastrophe into a giggle will make you a more energetic person.

Play and Creativity

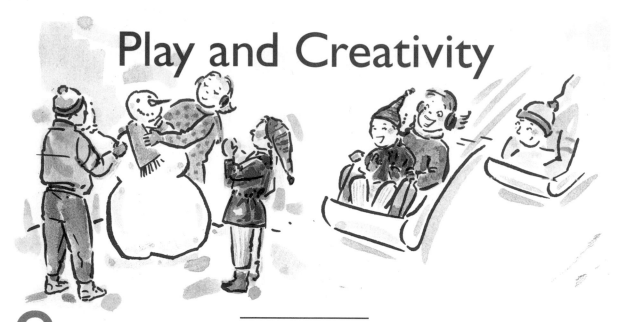

One sunny Sunday in February, Carolyn and her neighbor Jean take their kids to the park for a morning of snow tubing. Carolyn plans to sit at the top of the hill and supervise, but when Jean takes off on a tube, whooping her way down the slope as the kids yell encouragement, Carolyn just has to follow.

Off she goes, with her hair streaming, her eyes tearing, and a few delighted shrieks of her own. Her ride lasts 30 seconds, but her sense of exhilaration lingers as she hauls her tube up the hill for another run. And another. And another. By the end of the afternoon, Carolyn has taken dozens of runs. And while she's physically exhausted, she feels more energetic than she has in weeks. She's learned a powerful lesson: Play isn't just kid stuff. And it can be extremely energizing.

It's true that children are masters of play. Whether they're into Lego towers, elaborate tea parties, or skipping rocks across a pond, children view the world as a vast playground, and play as vital to life as breathing.

As grown-ups, however, our playground shrinks. Balancing the checkbook takes precedence over checkers, and cleaning house is more important than playing house. An anthill, once a thing of mystery and awe, is now just a sign to reach for the insect spray. We lose touch with what it means to play—to do something for no payoff or purpose other than to have fun. Worse, the less we play, the less we use our creative energies. It's true that "all work and no play make Jane a dull girl."

Women may be particularly "play deficient," says Lenore Terr, M.D., clinical professor of psychiatry at the University of California, San Francisco, and author of *Beyond Love and Work: Why Adults Need to Play*. All that working, mothering, and nurturing make it hard to stay awake, much less play.

But if we want more zing in our lives, more spring in our steps, more light in our eyes, and more fire in our bellies, we must make time to swing on the jungle gyms of our minds. Therein lies vitality, the unseen generator of mind, body, and spirit.

Are We Having Fun Yet?

Play is not just an activity. It's a state of mind. And while there's virtually no research on adult

Why do babies and teenagers need so much sleep?

The obvious reason is to recharge. Have you ever tried to keep up with a 2-year-old? If you did exactly what they did, you would be exhausted in 30 minutes, and they would still be going strong. Then again, they take a nap every afternoon.

But that's just the beginning, according to Jodi A. Mindell, Ph.D., associate professor of psychology at St. Joseph's University in Philadelphia, and author of *Sleeping Through the Night*. A lot happens both hormonally and metabolically while kids sleep. For instance, they secrete growth hormone. They may need more sleep in order to grow.

Kids even appear to need more of different types of sleep. For instance, we typically spend only 20 to 25 percent of our sleep in the rapid eye movement (REM), or deep-sleep stage, while a newborn spends about 50 percent in REM sleep. Some researchers suspect that babies need more of this dream sleep so their brains will grow.

All theories aside, what we do know is that the younger you are, the more sleep you need. On average, adults require 8 hours of shut-eye. Teenagers need a little over 9 hours. Toddlers need 10 to 12 hours of sleep at night, and 1½ to 3 hours during the day. And newborns need 15 to 18 hours in any 24-hour period.

Insufficient sleep can stifle memory, decision-making skills, and creativity. So if kids stay up past their bedtime for several days, they can become totally lost in the classroom.

Also, when kids don't get enough sleep, parents suffer. "When you treat a child's sleep problem, very often the parents become less depressed, experience fewer marital problems, and function better on the job," Dr. Mindell says.

Signs you're dealing with a sleep-deprived child include crankiness, irritability, and extreme moodiness. If she thinks something's funny, she gets silly; if a task seems daunting, she becomes easily frustrated. Children who aren't getting enough sleep may become anxious or introverted.

If you suspect that your child isn't getting enough sleep, Dr. Mindell suggests asking yourself these questions.

1. Does she meet the sleep need for her age group?

2. Does she wake up on her own in the morning?

3. Given the same bedtime, does she wake up at the same time on weekends as she does on weekdays?

4. Does her behavior remain the same if she gets more sleep at night?

If you answered "no" to any of these questions, your child may need more sleep.

play, the few scholars who do study it say that it is, quite literally, soul food. "Play is a refuge from ordinary life, a sanctuary of the mind, where one is exempt from life's customs, methods, and decrees," says Diane Ackerman, Ph.D., visiting professor at the Society for the Humanities at Cornell University in Ithaca, New York, and author of *Deep Play*. "Play always has a sacred place, some version of a playground, in which it happens. This place may be a classroom, a sports stadium, a stage, a courtroom, a coral reef, a workbench in a garage, or a church or temple."

With so many playgrounds available to us, it

seems a crime against femininity to deny ourselves the chance to zip down the slide. But if you need reasons to play, then just read on.

Play energizes. When we're intensely focused on our play—building a Victorian dollhouse, cooking an elegant gourmet meal, digging in our gardens—we're transported into a heightened and pleasant mental state called flow. When we're in flow, we forget ourselves. Time doesn't exist. We *become* our play: There is only *this* wood, *this* sauce, or *this* dirt. We emerge from our trances refreshed and reenergized.

Play calms. While exercise and meditation are time-honored stress busters, a brief bout of either physical or mental play can be just as effective. Studies on the play habits of laboratory rats suggest that play may help rodents withstand environmental stressors—and that it may serve the same function in people, Dr. Ackerman notes.

"The parts of the brain that are thought to regulate play in rats are very similar to what we see in the human brain," says Steven Siviy, Ph.D., associate professor of psychology at Gettysburg College in Pennsylvania. Rats who play as juveniles tend to deal better with social stressors (such as confronting other rats) as adults. So it's possible that play makes rats—and people—more adaptable and flexible, qualities that function as built-in stress buffers.

Play feels good. "When people play, there is a sense of good-humored, spirited, even sparkling pleasure," says Dr. Terr. One woman, a writer and personal trainer in her late twenties,

HOW IN THE WORLD DO THEY SLEEP?

How do women in long-distance competitions sleep?

"I sleep in a sled with a furry team member," says dogsledder Dee Dee Jonrowe, who has competed in the world-famous Iditarod dogsled race for 18 consecutive years, finishing second in 1993 and 1998. Temperatures on the more than 1,100-mile trail through Alaska can drop to 100°F below zero. So Jonrowe, who sleeps in her sled most days, pulls a pup into her sleeping bag for warmth. For the 9- to 10-day race, Jonrowe runs her dogs for 6 hours and rests them for 6 hours. During their downtime, she must feed her 16 teammates, mend their cuts, fix any damaged equipment, and make her own dinner. That doesn't leave much time for sleep. She typically gets 1 to 2 hours of sleep every 8 hours. Sometimes, during the last 3 days of the race, she doesn't sleep at all. "Everybody has one talent, and mine is the ability to go without much sleep and still make good judgment calls," she says.

"I sleep wedged into my bunk," says Dawn Riley, who completed two 32,000-mile, round-the-world races formerly known as the Whitbread (now called the Volvo Around-the-World Race) in 9 months. Riley and her crew typically worked and slept in 4-hour shifts. The roughest sleeping conditions were in the Antarctic Ocean. "You're chronically cold, wet, and dodging icebergs," says Riley. She slept in a bunk with a pulley system that wedged her into the bed, preventing falls during rough seas. Around the doldrums of the equator, however, the problem is the opposite—it's too hot to sleep. "It's more than 100°F, and you have to keep all the hatches closed so the water doesn't get inside," she says. If she's lucky, she finds some shade on deck in which to take a nap.

says she loves to play so much that she's structured her life around it. "I compete in and write about sports as an excuse to play."

Some of us return to our childhood "play-

"I sleep anywhere I can," says extreme runner and United Airlines pilot Janine Duplessis. She finished the toughest human-powered race ever—the Iditasport Extreme—running and snowshoeing the entire 1,100-mile Iditarod Alaskan trail in 41 days. She traveled from 8 to 30 hours before stopping to rest, sleeping only an hour or two a day for the first 2 weeks, 6 to 8 hours during the final 2 weeks. She bedded down under the stars on 7 nights—twice in 30-below temperatures. Frost accumulated as she slept, so when she woke, it looked as if it had snowed inside her tent. Other lodging arrangements included an assortment of primitive shelter cabins that had no running water but offered much-needed shelter from the cold and wind. On one occasion, she slept for a mere half-hour before everyone else started getting up. "I had to get up, too, so that I wouldn't miss the free breakfast of a packet of instant oatmeal and coffee."

"Sleep? What's that?" jokes mountain biker and young mom Kathie Evingson, top finisher in the Iditasport 100, a 100-mile bike race through the Alaskan wilderness. In 1999, she finished in less than 17 hours without a wink of shut-eye. "Having two children under the age of 4 was great training in sleep deprivation and pushing myself to my limits," says Evingson. But in 2000, with two kids sleeping through the night and less endurance training than the previous year, exhaustion hit like a brick wall 15 hours into the race and 12 miles shy of the finish. "The finish line could have been 2 miles away and it wouldn't have mattered. I couldn't go any farther," says Evingson. She laid her sleeping bag on hard-packed snow, took off her boots, and crawled in. Six hours later, she awoke refreshed and reenergized. After a few cookies and some hot chocolate (the breakfast of champions), she pedaled to the finish.

Now, she knows that her play breaks make her happier, more well-rounded, and more vital. So she's rediscovered the pleasures of running through sprinklers, riding the shopping carts at the grocery store, and sliding down stair banisters.

The Golden Rules of Play

If you haven't played in a while, you may not know where to start. Should you buy a hula hoop? Ride a roller coaster? Relax. It doesn't matter what you do, as long as you approach play with the right mind-set. These guidelines will help define the rules of the game, whatever your game is.

Make play dates—and keep them. "You must consciously decide to play," says Dr. Terr. So as silly as it may seem, schedule regular play periods into your appointment book.

"My vision is for all adults to dedicate at least 1 percent of their lives to play," says David Earl Platts, Ph.D., founder of David E. Platts and Associates, a management training, personal coaching, and counseling firm in England. "In practical terms, that's 15 minutes a day, or less than 2 hours a week."

Look to your past. Can't think of a thing that seems like fun? Think back to how and what you played as a child. "You'll find clues as to what would be fun for you now," says Dr. Terr. Maybe you loved playing with dolls. "You might collect dolls, make doll houses, or fix old dolls," she says. If you were the tomboyish type, consider signing up for the local women's softball or basketball league.

grounds" later in life. "I had to get over the idea that every minute of my life had to be productive," says Annette Bunge, Ph.D., a professor of chemical engineering in Golden, Colorado.

One woman remembers how she loved to play "pioneer" as a girl, creating her Wild-West world with Lincoln Logs, dolls, and a little cast-iron stove. "Now that I'm grown, I've created my own little homestead on 1 acre, with chickens, bunnies, a greenhouse, gardens, and a woodstove," she says. "I guess some people never grow up."

Another woman remembers the joy of coloring as a child. When she was in college, she began to experience stress. She remembered a friend's mother telling her that coloring helped with stress. "I still color," she says. "I find that I'm able to completely forget everything else. And when I'm done, I feel better."

Stay in the moment. To truly play, you must be able to put reality on temporary hiatus. No composing a mental shopping list while you build that cute birdhouse you found in a crafts magazine. "If we don't live in the moment, how can we play with the moment?" says Sister Anne Bryan Smollin, Ph.D., executive director of Counseling for Laity in Albany, New York, and author of *Tickle Your Soul: Live Well, Love Much, Laugh Often*.

"I know I'm playing when I don't care about anything other than being in that exact moment. When I play with my dog, I stare at her, rub her belly, and run around the backyard with her. When I'm doing that, I can't imagine anything else being that fun. But then we turn on the sprinkler," says one woman.

Nix the I'm-not-good-enough thoughts. Maybe you're worried that you won't play well.

WOMAN TO WOMAN
She Pieced Together Her Life with a Pin

When Sue Snyder signed up for a jewelry-making class, she learned much more than how to make key chains. This 44-year-old business manager for two major cycling magazines fashioned her passion and discovered the hidden artist within.

It was the summer of 1999, and I'd had it. I didn't know what I needed, but I did know that my job wasn't completely giving it to me. With a career counselor's encouragement, I wrote down five things I would like to do. Half the list consisted of things I knew I'd accomplish, like learning four new words a day and reading certain books. The other half were goofy things that interested me but I never thought I'd do, like learn sign language, sing in a choir, become a massage therapist, and take jewelry and pottery classes.

I didn't do art. My husband and oldest daughter were the artists in our family; I drew stick figures on napkins. Instead, I bought word-a-day tapes (and listened to them for about a week), read my books, and crossed each item off my list as I achieved it.

But I wasn't about to sign up for the art classes—until a pottery studio, the kind where you paint premade vases, mugs, and plates, opened up near my home. One warm Saturday night in August, I went there by myself, picked out a serving platter, and painted a multicolored fish I had seen in a magazine. I was so caught up in painting the details of the fish that 3 hours passed before I knew it.

Perhaps you would like to paint but can't draw a straight line, or play volleyball but are embarrassed to try.

Fear of ridicule or failure kills playfulness dead, says Bernie DeKoven, a former toy designer and author of *The Well-Played Game*, who now gives presentations on how to make work and play more fun.

When I brought the platter home, my family loved it so much that they displayed it in the front window. (My friends were so jealous.) For them to say my work was cool just blew me away. I think that's what made me sign up for the jewelry class.

My first project was to design a pin that told a story about my life. When I talked about it with an art director at work, she described me as linear, that I liked things in order. That's all it took. I immediately knew what to make.

I cut out five silver bars representing five areas of my life: exercise, career, creative interests, family, and friends. Then I cut out squiggly lines in gold, for the ups and downs in my life. I made a moon, cut it in half, and placed the pieces off center on the squiggles. The half-moons were my husband and I—sometimes we're together; sometimes we have separate interests. Then I added two stones—one off to the side and one in the middle—to represent my two daughters.

That pin demolished any insecurities I had about my artistic ability. Instead of lying awake at night worrying about my job or family, I was thinking about what I'd make next: rings, key chains, and necklace pendants. The whole time I worked on the jewelry, I thought about the person I was making it for, the times we'd spent together, and what they'd like. I could sit there for hours and never think of anything else. It was playtime for me.

Little did I know that a course in jewelry making would teach me so much about myself. I realize now that as long as my job enables me to do the things I enjoy after work, I can deal with the corporate world during the day.

Ready, Set, Play!

A patient in Dr. Terr's practice found a stuffed animal in a cabin that she rents. "Weasel" has been her constant companion ever since.

Since the woman is a frequent traveler, Weasel has been to a great many places. He's washable, serves as a pillow on planes, and sits on the bed of every hotel room she stays in. People talk to him, and he talks back. Someday, this young woman executive says, she's going to write a children's book about him.

This is a woman who has given herself permission to play. And if she can talk to a stuffed animal, you can approach play as a vast frontier filled with opportunities to revitalize your life.

Looking for new ways to play? Consider the ideas below for inspiration. But try anything and everything, from crossword puzzles and word games to kayaking and swing dancing. Trying different types of play can help you define who you are as well as what you might like to be. Just as it did when you were a kid.

Turn Your Job into a Playground

Say you've never painted before and you want to give it a try. Great! But you also think that the fruit bowl on your canvas must look exactly like the fruit bowl on your table. That's not fun; that's frustration. Painting becomes play when you tune into the "dance" between what you intend the painting to be and what it winds up being, says DeKoven. "That's the fun of it!"

- Buy a Nerf gun (they're about $10 at discount stores) and encourage your fellow coworkers to do the same. Institute a new work ritual: Welcome new employees with an all-in-fun "ambush."
- Buy a small basketball hoop and a Nerf basketball (available at your local toy store) and place it in a quiet corner, away from

others' workspaces. When you hit your midafternoon energy slump, round up a few coworkers for a 15-minute game of Nerf basketball.

- Buy yourself an Etch-a-Sketch and give yourself a daily artistic challenge. You might try to do a semirecognizable self portrait in 5 minutes, "sketch" an item on your desk, or simply squiggle to your heart's content.

- Post one silly to-do item on your appointment calendar. At 11:15 A.M. on Wednesday, write, "Save world from meteor." At 2:58 P.M. on Thursday, "Disassemble computer; replace gerbil; reassemble computer." You get the idea.

- Buy a yo-yo that comes with an instruction booklet. When you're bored or stressed out, practice "walking the dog" for 10 minutes.

Barbie and Beyond: Playing with Kids

- Color with your kids. Make a game of who uses the most colors, who stays within the lines the best, or who comes up with the best special effects with glitter pens or puff paints.

- On hot days, run through a sprinkler with them, or soak one another with water balloons or huge water guns.

- Stage a play, complete with props. Let the Cinderella or the Wicked Witch in you come out.

- Play Barbie (even if your child is a little too old). Pull out the old dolls and dress them for a party. Spend long minutes deciding on

the perfect ensemble. Have Barbie flirt with Ken or ogle G.I. Joe.

- Take your kids to the zoo or aquarium. It's fun to experience the pleasure of a child's delight and awe. Don't have a kid? "Rent" one for a day from a friend and live in her world. Take her to the zoo and impersonate animals, pick apples to make applesauce, or make murals out of household junk.

TOP 10 WAYS TO HAVE A RELAXING VACATION

1. Let the kids help plan. There'll be less moping and complaining at tour sites if they agree with the vacation agenda. Also, stay at hotels with a swimming pool for the kids and a spa for you. Try to find activities for them that don't require your presence, so you can have some time to yourself or with your husband. Or, you and your husband alternate who gets to sun by the pool and who gets to cart the kids around.

2. Leave the laptop and cell phone at home. Just leave a phone number where you can be reached with a trusted neighbor or one person at work in case of an emergency, with strict instructions not to give it out. Resist the urge to check your voice mail. Don't even buy a newspaper. You want to feel as if you're living in a special world for at least these few days.

3. Spend within your means. Hawaii is beautiful, but it's a lot nicer if you can actually afford to buy food while you're there. Make sure you choose a destination or tour package that you can afford so you're not concerned about out-of-pocket expenses like meals and souvenirs.

4. Reserve the basics. Don't wait until you reach your destination to find a hotel or rent a car, especially if you're traveling with four or more people. You may end up with a single room or a compact car. Book everything in advance to reduce any possibility of anxiety-provoking uncertainty. While you're at it, buy your museum and transport passes, too.

5. Pin your kids. Nothing is more stressful than losing a kid in a strange town or country. Before leaving your room each

day, pin your hotel's business card to the inside of your child's clothing—preferably to a layer he won't strip off and possibly lose.

6. Learn the local currency and some key phrases. Find out the approximate equivalent of $10 in the local currency so you can make quick conversions while shopping. The exchange rate may change while you're away, but at least you'll have a general guide. Consider carrying a book of key phrases, which can help with ordering food and finding help.

7. Watch for warnings. While traveling abroad, work with a travel agent to avoid problems related to local customs and to receive forewarning of major holidays that may make it difficult to get basic services. Before you leave for your vacation, ask your agent about any travel warnings related to your destination, and be mindful of potential health hazards related to food- or water-borne diseases. (It's always a good idea to avoid the water in most foreign countries.)

8. Leave your itinerary behind. You'll have greater peace of mind if you leave an itinerary with someone who is watching your house and checking your mail. By taking this step, you'll know that if any problems arise, someone can reach you.

9. Be flexible. It's good to have a plan, but keep in mind that the world won't end if you don't follow it exactly.

10. Vacation after your vacation. Arriving home late Sunday night only to get up early for work the next morning can smother your newfound vacation zen. Instead, plan to come home on a Saturday so that you have a day to unpack, settle in, and enjoy feeling relaxed before heading back to the office.

Make a Play Date with Your Mate

- Rent a convertible for a day and go for a long drive on a country road. Take a blanket and an armful of your favorite CDs. Stop at roadside antique stores. Rent a canoe for an hour. Continue on your merry way.

- Challenge your man to a game of strip poker. (If you're pathetic at cards, wear lots of layers to prolong the fun.) Or drag out that dusty game of Twister—the loser buys dinner.

- Go grocery shopping together and ask him to give you a ride on the shopping cart. The disapproving stares of other grown-ups as you careen down aisle 7 are priceless.

- Play the "name game" on car trips. You name a famous person. Your partner then has to come up with a celebrity whose name begins with the last letter of the name you gave. "My husband and I can play this for up to 7 hours," says one woman.

Reenergizing Ways to Play with Friends

- Organize book-group dinner parties with meals from the month's novel. For example, if you're reading *Bridget Jones's Diary*, make shepherd's pie and smoothies (served with chardonnay, of course).

- Start "e-mail jousts" at work. One-upping each other's witticisms is a great way to get your creative juices flowing and to stay connected. Or challenge your friends to compose a haiku on a particular topic, such as Spam.

- Cajole your mom, sister, neighbor, and a few good friends and coworkers into meeting at the bowling alley every Wednesday night. Have everyone buy a bowling shirt, and have your names stitched on them.

CREATE A HOME SPA

Although it would be nice to escape to one of those exclusive spas by the sea or in the desert, it just isn't financially realistic for most of us. The next best thing is to create a spa in your own home. Laura Hittleman, beauty director of Canyon Ranch in the Berkshires Health Resort in Lenox, Massachusetts, tells you how to create your own weekend spa.

Preparation

1. Send your husband on a 2-day trip with his pals and let your kids stay with their friends or grandparents. This weekend is all about you; it's time to indulge your senses.

2. Do all of your shopping and prep work before your weekend begins so that everything is as simple as possible. Buy a bouquet of your favorite flowers. (Ask the florist for extra petals; you can use them in your bath.)

3. Get rid of clutter. Hide piles of bills and anything else that could stress you out.

4. Cover your furniture with white sheets and throw a few big pillows on the floor.

5. Unplug the television and phone and open your windows so that you can hear the sounds of nature. If you live in a city or it's below freezing, play a CD of nature sounds or soothing music.

6. Surround yourself with objects and images that give you strength, such as photos of your family.

7. Post a picture of a place you've always wanted to visit on the wall where you can see it from your bathtub.

8. Turn off all overhead lights. Dim the lamps, or try a colored light bulb. Light lots of candles.

Pampering

Try each of the following at least once over the weekend.

1. Hot oil treatment: Warm ¼ cup of olive oil with three to five drops of your favorite essential oil, such as geranium, tea tree, or peppermint. Massage the oil into your scalp and cover with a plastic cap. Leave it in your hair for 30 minutes, then shampoo.

2. Bath fit for a queen: Pour ½ cup of milk under running bathwater; wrap a sliced orange in cheesecloth and squeeze under the running water to release the orange oil; and soak. Add a relaxing essential oil like lavender or vanilla extract to your bathwater, or put five to six drops in a light bulb ring.

3. Facial: Chill ¼ cup aloe gel. Break open a vitamin E capsule into a small bowl and add ½ teaspoon of vanilla extract. Whip together with aloe until frothy, and smooth over your face. Leave it on for 10 to 15 minutes and then rinse with a warm washcloth. Place warm, moist chamomile tea bags on your eyes while you relax with the facial.

4. And the rest: When you're finished soaking, towel off with a big fluffy cotton towel. Pull your hair back, slip on loose cotton clothing, and give yourself a manicure and pedicure. If you don't have cuticle cream, use olive oil. Cut off any hangnails and buff your nails.

Dining In

1. Dine on a variety of fresh seasonal fruit and vegetables, fresh fish or chicken, hearty whole grain bread, and a light starch like couscous or rice. Have sorbet with sliced fruit for dessert.

2. Walk around all weekend with a large bottle of spring water always in your hand so that you drink as much water as you can.

- If there's a wildlife sanctuary near your home, take an all-day hike with a friend. Pack a fabulous lunch, and bring binoculars.
- If you sew, propose to some fellow needleworkers that you stage a weekly quilting bee or sewing circle.

Eight Ways to Play Solo in 10 Minutes or Less

- While you wait in the checkout line at the store, ponder playful questions, such as "What if people could fly?" or "What if men could give birth?"
- Pick up two oranges. Try to juggle. Juggle badly. Try three. Juggle even more badly. Giggle. Start over. Repeat.
- Go fly a kite. Literally.

JUMP START

Dance

Put on some music and dance around the room.

- Borrow your kids' Legos and try to build your dream house.
- Learn by heart a poem you've always loved.
- If it's summer, do some quick-and-dirty gardening before you take your morning shower.
- If there's snow on the ground, make a snow angel. Don't get up immediately; look up at the clouds and see what they remind you of.
- Walk in the rain. Wear a pair of old sneakers so you can jump in a mud puddle if you feel like it.

Energy for Everything: A Year Later

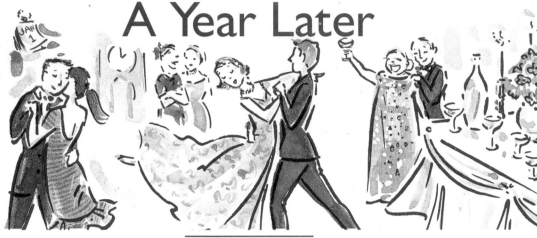

It's 9:30 P.M., and Carolyn is nestled in a warm bath, thinking. It's been a year of change and renewed energy. She's filled her office with plants and the rejuvenating aroma of citrus. She's eating breakfast every morning and taking a walk every evening. She's started on a small dose of supplementary estrogen to help with some of her perimenopausal symptoms, joined a women's soccer team for fun, and chucked 15 years' worth of clutter from her house.

Of course, life occasionally knocks her off-course, and her newfound vitality flags. That's when she must struggle to honor her Bill of Rights. Inspired by that bone-deep fatigue of a year ago, it is still posted on her refrigerator at home and on her computer at work. But those times are fewer and farther between. She's learned to live by what she's come to call Carolyn's Credo: I Can't Do It All, and I Won't. (If she were artsy, she would embroider it on a throw pillow.) She knows that a little self-care today is worth a ton of energy tomorrow.

The only hurdle she has left is to bring what she's learned about peak vitality in everyday life to her energy "problem areas"—the holidays, the annual family vacation, the back-to-school maelstrom, the occasional business trip, and Monday mornings. (Like the backs of her arms, Carolyn's morning routine still needs some toning.)

Let's give Carolyn a hand for changing her life, and a parting gift to send her on her merry way with all the gusto she deserves: top time management and organizational experts who can help Carolyn plan, prepare, and execute the special events in her life with the flair of a five-star general planning a major campaign—with energy to spare as well as joy. After all, joy is one of the most powerful energy generators there is.

In the Eye of the Holiday Hurricane

Only a few years ago, Carolyn happily hummed "White Christmas" as she signed and mailed cards, baked cookies, decorated the house and tree, and prepared her annual holiday dinner for 24.

But with a full-time job and two kids with a

full calendar of social obligations, her holiday mood, along with her best-laid plans and preparation, has turned distinctly Scrooge-like. That may be because the holidays bring out her inner Martha Stewart. The house must be immaculate at all times, the gifts must be painstakingly matched to their recipients (with elaborate wrapping), and the holiday dinner must be remarkable. (Last year's theme was *A Christmas Carol*, with stuffed goose and plum pudding.) The endless round of church and school events, recitals, open houses, and eggnog parties also exhausts her.

Stephanie Winston, a well-known time-management expert and author of *Getting Out from Under: Redefining Your Priorities in an Overwhelming World*, has one word for Carolyn: delegate. "Carolyn is the coordinator of this effort," says Winston. "But that doesn't mean she has to do it all herself. Her job is to get it done."

Her first executive decision should be to give herself two days to rest and regroup after Thanksgiving. Then it's time to tackle her holiday plans.

The most energy-conserving approach is the "Christmas countdown," says Winston. She suggests that Carolyn make a list of each and every task, group them by week (week 1 being the week of Christmas Day), and attack them with all the zeal she usually reserves for end-of-season sales.

Four weeks before Christmas, she

WOMEN ASK WHY

Why does time seem to speed up as we grow older?

Our perception of time is part of our consciousness, the internal model of the universe that we use to represent the world to ourselves. But not everything our senses perceive enters our consciousness. Generally speaking, unusual, unexpected, and interesting events make it in, while routine, expected, and unimportant ones don't.

Take driving. Most of us have had the experience of being on the road and suddenly realizing that we've driven miles without noticing. Those miles may have been so uneventful that our brains didn't bother to put our perceptions into our short-term memories. Or they may have been so routine that our brains handled the driving while our consciousness was occupied with other thoughts.

As we grow older, more things turn out just as we expect. (And some of us get better at ignoring the things we don't want to see.) So our brains have fewer unusual and unexpected events to put into our consciousness. And our perception of time runs event to event, rather than second to second. So perceiving fewer events in the day means that the day—and time—passes faster.

On the other hand, it might be argued that time can also speed up if our lives are full of activities that are so interesting, so much fun, or so exciting that we focus just on them, and we don't notice the passage of time. It just zooms by.

Yet another possible answer is that as we grow older, we become more aware of our mortality. When we're young, we feel as though time will go on forever. But once we enter middle age, many of us suddenly become aware that time (for us) has a definite end point. We begin to perceive time not as running on forever but as something that comes in a box and is given out one to a customer.

Expert consulted
Martin C. Young, Ph.D.
Adjunct professor of philosophy
El Camino College
Torrance, California

might decorate the house and mail cards. Three weeks before, she might bake cookies and freeze certain holiday dinner dishes so she can pop them into the oven on Christmas Day.

At any time during the countdown, she can take off from work to tackle her most time-consuming tasks, whether shopping for gifts, baking, or cleaning. To reward herself, she should schedule relaxation breaks, such as a half-hour of reading and an hour of a soap opera.

She should also nix the complicated holiday menu and stick to old-time favorites, says Stephanie Denton, president of Denton and Company Professional Organizers in Cincinnati. Why should she knock herself out creating a menu from *Food and Wine* magazine when what her family probably really wants is a simple ham or turkey with all of the traditional fixings?

If Carolyn hasn't purchased her gifts throughout the year ("You're going to be at the mall anyway," says Winston), she should start her shopping no less than 3 weeks before.

To streamline her shopping, Carolyn should decide on a gift theme, says Denton. She should buy one specific type of item—books or beautiful picture frames—for friends, coworkers, and Great-Aunt Ida, while spending her energy on choosing special gifts for her family.

Right before and after the holidays, Carolyn might give *herself* a gift: 1 day of maid service. Or, she can call the placement office at a local high school or college, who will "undoubtedly find students who are willing to do a day of cleanup to make a few bucks," says Winston.

PETS GET HOLIDAY STRESS, TOO

Fido or Fluffy may not have to brave Thanksgiving dinner at your in-laws' or the holiday crowds at the mall, but pets can experience just as much holiday stress. Changes in routine, a houseful of unfamiliar relatives, or the loud merrymaking that accompanies your annual eggnog party can be upsetting for pets, says Alan Beck, Sc.D., director of the Center for the Human-Animal Bond at Purdue University in West Lafayette, Indiana.

Stressed-out pets send clear behavioral signals, says Dr. Beck. They often refuse to eat, and they nip or growl (even a usually gentle dog or cat), have "accidents," or engage in compulsive behaviors. A dog may begin to chew his foot (or that very expensive pair of shoes), run in circles, or lick his lips, while a cat may lick or scratch endlessly.

The most common cause of pets' holiday stress is topsy-turvy holiday schedules. For example, taking a few days off to entertain your out-of-town relatives, then returning to work, can trigger fierce separation anxiety. "Whereas you used to be able to say goodbye at the door, they'll start to scratch at the door and whine," says Dr. Beck. Fortunately, they'll stop once your schedule is back on track.

To help ease your pets' jangled holiday nerves, try these guidelines, advises Dr. Beck.

- Keep cats and birds in a quiet, closed-off room during your in-laws' visit or holiday shindig. They'll feel much calmer and safer.

To cut down on her chronic "event fatigue," Carolyn should sit her family down at the kitchen table and have each choose one event or outing that he or she would like the whole family to attend, says Denton. Jocelyn might pick her school Christmas pageant; Michael, a night on the ski slopes; Carolyn, an open house hosted by close friends of the family; and Ben, his boss's annual Christmas party. By turning down a few invitations, Carolyn's holiday whirl becomes that much less draining. As a bonus,

❥ Before company arrives, put your dog in a quiet room. Introduce him to guests after you've hugged at the door, offered refreshments, and put away coats. Fluffy will probably want to stay there for the duration.

❥ Be sensitive to your pets' reaction to loud, galloping children and infants—especially crying infants. "Many dogs are agitated by a baby's crying," says Dr. Beck. "They can become aggressive and nip—not the baby, but the caretaker. The crying triggers a kind of protective instinct."

❥ If your dog begins to growl or display other negative kinds of behavior, distract him: Give him a treat or a toy and gently lead him to a quiet room. This way, he isn't punished for his bad behavior. He's rewarded for not following through on it.

❥ Keep your schedule as normal as you can. Dogs, in particular, are more upset by changes in routine. So try to feed and walk them at the usual times.

❥ Protect your pet's delicate innards from well-meaning guests. Put a well-labeled bowl of cat or dog treats on the table or buffet along with the cheese puffs. This way, if Grandma really needs to nurture, she can offer a treat that won't make your pet sick.

Our pets are always there when we're tired and stressed, "so it's nice for us to return the favor," says Dr. Beck. "If you're sensitive to your pet's needs, you can both have a good time."

she'll have more energy to spend time with those she cares about the most—her family.

The On-the-Fly Dinner Party

With her go-go-go schedule, Carolyn has enough trouble putting food—real food, not takeout—on the table as it is. So it sends her over the edge when Ben calls her on Wednesday to tell her that he's bringing home clients for dinner on Thursday. Simmering with resentment (which just saps more of her energy), Carolyn takes a half-day off to shop, cook, and clean. As a result, the meal is perfect and the house is spotless—and Carolyn is a furious wreck.

Carolyn's preparations are costing her precious time and energy, says Audrey Lavine, president of the New York chapter of the National Association of Professional Organizers in New York City. She needs a lesson in the fine art of winging it with flair. "This is no time for Carolyn to cook from scratch," she says. Her advice is to buy as much of the meal as she can at a gourmet or specialty food store. "They offer beautifully prepared food that she can take out of the plastic containers and put on her own china."

The night before the party, Carolyn could buy a big pan of lasagna and a *tiramisu* from a specialty Italian store and round out the meal with a salad and garlic bread, purchased at lunchtime or after work. Ben could also buy a bottle or two of good red wine on his lunch hour. This is in no way cheating, says Lavine. "Plus, the expense of purchasing dinner is worth what it would cost her in stress to do it herself."

If Carolyn prefers to cook, she should stick to simple, familiar dishes, says Lavine. Keeping it basic reduces her workload—and the possibility of disaster. "This is not the time for Carolyn to make Beef Wellington or a souffle-type dish that will fall when she closes the oven door."

On her way home from work, Carolyn could pick up a simple bouquet and candles from any supermarket to give the table a festive look. In the warmer months, if she has a garden, she could have Jocelyn pick some homegrown blooms. "I've seen people take wild-flowers from their gardens, rip off the petals, and scatter them by each place setting," says Lavine. "This makes a lovely table decoration and is less expensive than a floral arrangement."

As for cleaning, Carolyn may want to zero in on the rooms the guests are most likely to use and call in the reinforcements. She might take on the kitchen and dining room while Ben tackles the bathroom and the kids dust, vacuum, and declutter the living room.

There's no doubt that impromptu guests are unnerving. But when they're knocking on your door, you need to focus more on hospitality and less on the "shoulds," says Lavine. "You don't need to prove you're Martha Stewart. If you put a plate in front of someone and it has tasty food on it and it looks nice, and your house is welcoming and relatively clean, they won't care how you did it."

Can This Vacation Be Saved?

Carolyn has made a vow: This year, she is going to come home from the family's annual vacation rested and refreshed, rather than wanting to crawl into bed for a week of recuperative pillow-clutching, because her vacations are usually exhausting. Carolyn chooses the destination; organizes the itinerary; arranges to have the dog walked, the plants watered, the house watched, and the mail stopped; and cleans the house before leaving. The rest of the family simply shows up.

Once on vacation, they have the nerve to complain. Last year, the kids whined that they

WOMAN TO WOMAN

She'd Had Enough of Holiday Travel

Imagine driving 960 miles with two small boys in a minivan stuffed with kid paraphernalia and gifts to visit relatives during the holidays, and then driving 671 miles back. For 6 very long years, that's what Denise Herich, 35, her husband, Chris, and their kids did. Until last year, when the account supervisor from Germantown, Maryland, said, "Enough!" This is her story.

My husband and I would take our two boys (now ages 3 and 6) on this incredible journey. From Germantown, we would drive to Harrisburg, Pennsylvania, to visit my mother and her husband, my sister and her husband, and my father and his wife (thankfully, they're only 10 miles down the road from one another). After a few days, we would hop into the minivan, which was stuffed with a mind-boggling load of toys and gifts, and set out for Chris's mother's place in Lake Geneva, Wisconsin. We would spend a very cramped New Year's in her two-bedroom condo, then drive to the suburbs of Chicago, where his sisters and their husbands live. Finally, we would make the 15-hour drive back to Washington, D.C., and arrive home in time for work the next day.

The trip wasn't too bad when it was just Chris and me. We figured that our parents were older and weren't going to come to our place. The problem was, after we had kids, we still felt as if we had to go to our parents.

As the holidays approached, my stress level would start

were bored. (In a fit of insanity, she had decided that they would visit a slew of historic landmarks and botanical gardens.) Ben grumbled that he would rather be fishing. Carolyn wishes that her family would just up and leave for 2 weeks so that she could lie in the backyard and work on her tan, read trashy novels, and sip white wine.

Carolyn needs to make her family vacation a bona fide family vacation. That means involving them in the planning and prep work—and in

climbing. For one thing, the trip took a full day of preparation—dismantling the high chair and shoving it into the minivan, emptying toys out of the playpen because that had to be the baby's makeshift crib, and cramming the van full of gifts. It was extremely tiring, as was sitting in the car for all those hours. But I have to admit that the kids were pretty well-behaved.

Last year, I finally said, "Let's have everybody come to our place." I had just started my current job and I simply could not handle the stress of the trip along with the stress of a new job. But I also wanted to start my own holiday traditions, like having my kids go to bed on Christmas Eve knowing that Santa would come down *their* chimney. (My kids would always ask, "How does Santa know we're at Grandma's?")

I expected a guilt trip from my parents, but I was pleasantly surprised that they were supportive, as was the whole family. In fact, everyone said that they had been waiting for me to speak up.

The Harrisburg, Lake Geneva, and Chicago contingents all came, which was wonderful. And I really enjoyed doing all the decorating and the cooking myself. It wasn't tiring; in fact, I had a lot more energy this year. Maybe it was because I could sleep in my own bed.

So we now have a compromise. Everyone will come to our place for the holidays, and we'll visit them during the summer, when we don't have to cope with toting a ton of stuff and driving in bad weather.

while Ben wants to head to a lake to camp, fish, and loll in a hammock. Jocelyn votes for New York City, and Michael says he doesn't care because it will all be boring anyway. After an hour of brainstorming, they might agree to vacation in a lush resort in the Poconos in Pennsylvania. Carolyn can sun and relax; Ben can fish and loaf. They'll take a 3-day jaunt to Manhattan to shop and see the sights. Michael may even decide that it would be cool to see Greenwich Village and to stand in front of MTV's studio window in Times Square.

Carolyn should also divvy up the grunt work involved in planning a vacation. She can make the reservations, stop the mail and newspaper delivery, and ask a neighbor to keep an eye on the house while they're gone. Ben can take the car in to be serviced a week before they depart and arrange to have the grass mowed. Michael and Jocelyn can enlist a neighbor to water the plants and walk and feed the dog. And everyone can help clean the house the day before they leave so that they aren't greeted by the awful sight of clutter and loads of dirty laundry when they return.

Here are some more tips to ensure that your vacation will recharge your batteries rather than drain them.

Hang out alone. Plan to do some things by yourself on your vacation. Read that special book or your favorite magazines, meditate, take quiet walks, or just watch a beautiful sunrise. Spending quality time by yourself helps recharge your emotional batteries. Begin planning some of those private times before your vacation, and let your family know how important this time is to you.

sharing the fun of picking the destination. She should assemble the family and have each member tell what they would like to do, says Catherine G. Braun, a success coach and founder of InterPersonal Coaching in Port Washington, New York. Then the family can brainstorm potential destinations that give everyone a taste of what they crave.

Say Carolyn wants to go to a Caribbean resort for 2 weeks of sun, sand, and spa pampering,

Keep your expectations in check. "Don't expect a vacation to relieve all of your stress and fatigue," says Braun. "If you do, the vacation itself will become stressful because you'll feel that you have to have a good time if it kills you."

The Back-to-School Blitz

Each year, on the 3rd weekend in August, Carolyn embarks on a task she especially dreads: taking the kids shopping for their back-to-school wardrobes. On Saturday morning, she hauls them to the mall, fighting the crowds of equally harried mothers as well as her children, who plead for $95 sneakers or $50 pants that look as if they've been rescued from the town dump. They rush from store to store, Carolyn grimly ferreting out polo shirts and jeans for Michael and tops and skirts for Jocelyn. They leave when they're so burdened with bags that they can barely walk. Thank goodness that's done, thinks Carolyn—until next year. Now she just has to figure out how to get Jocelyn to after-school piano lessons and field hockey games, and Michael to soccer practice and saxophone lessons, all of which start in 2 weeks.

Rome wasn't built in a day, and neither are two kids' back-to-school wardrobes. The first order of business is to shop for one child at a time, one week at a time. But before she wastes energy carting them to the mall, Carolyn should talk to her kids to find out what's hot this year, says Braun. Based on their input, she should make a list of what they need versus what they want.

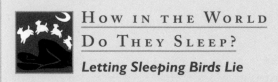

HOW IN THE WORLD DO THEY SLEEP?
Letting Sleeping Birds Lie

For 30 years, sleep researchers have known that birds often sleep with one eye open and half their brains awake, a state known as unihemispheric slow-wave sleep (USWS). Until now, what they haven't known is why.

Research conducted by Niels Rattenborg, Ph.D., a postdoctoral fellow in the department of psychiatry at the University of Wisconsin at Madison, suggests that birds have a good reason for this behavior: They're literally keeping an eye out for predators.

Dr. Rattenborg and his current colleagues at Indiana State University in Terre Haute took groups of four mallard ducks, each in its own clear plastic case, and lined them up in a row. They predicted that if birds do indeed engage in USWS to watch for predators, the ducks on the ends of the row—vulnerable on one side—would keep one peeper peeled more often than the ducks in the center would, and that they would direct the open eye away from their mates and toward an approaching attacker.

Videotapes and electroencephalographic (EEG) records of the ducks' brain waves proved the researchers right. Ducks

The day of the expedition should be a celebration as well as an opportunity for bonding. "Carolyn can make a day of it with her kids," says Braun. "They can shop for an hour or an hour and a half, have lunch, and shop for another hour or two." The lunch break is a great opportunity for Carolyn to talk with each child about goals for the upcoming year as well as get a bead on their extracurricular activities.

Another option is to set a budget, give the kids a credit card with strict instructions to remain within that budget, and send them off to do their own clothes shopping. The kids learn

on the end of the row, at the highest risk of meeting with fowl play, spent 150 percent more time in a state of USWS than those in the center. And at least 85 percent of the time, the birds on the edge slept with one eye open, directed away from the group and toward potential predators.

Which means that sleeping ducks aren't necessarily sitting ducks.

The only other animals that exhibit USWS are some sea mammals, such as dolphins and seals (so they can return to the surface of the water for air while they're "sleeping"), notes Dr. Rattenborg.

But why don't all animals sleep this way? After all, the Donald Ducks and Flippers of the animal kingdom aren't the only animals vulnerable to attack. Dr. Rattenborg can only guess. "There may be something fundamentally better or more efficient about sleeping with the whole brain at one time."

While it's dangerous to relate animal studies to human behavior, there may be a link between birds' ability to be "half-asleep" and sleepwalking in people, says Dr. Rattenborg. "Some sleep disorders, such as sleepwalking, may occur when some parts of the brain are awake, while other parts remain asleep," he says. "It is conceivable that these disorders are a vestige of the ability to sleep with one eye open."

Michael and Jocelyn's teams. By making a few phone calls, she can cut her shuttling duties in half. But before she picks up the phone, she needs to think of her work schedule; it's no good agreeing to drive a carload of kids on Wednesdays if she has a weekly 2-hour strategy meeting that day.

What about the rare times that Jocelyn has an important piano recital at the same time that Michael has a crucial soccer game that might send his team to the tournament? Carolyn shouldn't even consider attending both; driving across town and fighting late-afternoon traffic will leave her drained and resentful. "She'll also be sending dangerous messages to her children: That she can do it all, and that they matter more than she matters," says Braun. "Everyone in the family is important." Instead, Carolyn should call her kids together and ask them which event they think she should attend. "You would be surprised at how fair and generous kids can be."

The Business-Trip Tango

Carolyn travels on business two or three times a year and loves it. Sure, it can be draining meeting clients or attending conferences, but she also gets a reprieve from her household's morning rush and has those precious postbusiness hours to luxuriate in the tub or command the remote. What she doesn't love is the prep work. She invariably waits until the night before she leaves to pack her bag, so she often brings too much or too little and forgets the right shoes and accessories. Jet lag can drain her for the first 2 days. And Ben is no cook; she winces at the

responsibility, and Carolyn avoids the fights and the whining and can use that time for a massage. If you would rather not give your child a credit card, give her cash instead.

While she's buying notebooks and pencils for the kids, Carolyn should also purchase a large wall calendar. She should hang this family calendar in the kitchen and tell her kids that they're responsible for penciling in their commitments. "This way, Carolyn has an overview of her kids' schedules and can plan accordingly," says Lavine.

Carolyn should also make carpooling arrangements with the moms whose kids play on

JUMP START

Make plans to do something endearingly strange or new once every 2 weeks. Check out an upscale billiard hall. Attend a poetry reading at the local arts house. Crash a sixth-grade school play in a neighboring town.

thought of her family eating out of paper sacks for 3 to 5 days. But jetting off on business doesn't have to drain your energy, as long as you know how to travel smart, says Denton.

Carolyn's trips will be off to an energizing start if she buys one simple, inexpensive item: a freestanding clothing rack. The weekend before her trip, Carolyn can arrange her wardrobe on it, placing shoes underneath and draping belts, scarves, and other accessories over the outfits themselves. At a glance, she'll know what to bring and what to weed out. Then she can pack and go.

For a weeklong trip, "Carolyn can get away with two suits and a couple of blouses, sweaters, or twinsets," says Denton. She can wear one suit with a sweater one day and the skirt or pants with a blouse or twinset the next. "Sometimes I buy both the pants and the skirt to a suit, so I can pack just one suit," says Denton. "I can get three or four outfits out of it." As a bonus, there's no need to pack multiple pairs of shoes.

Carolyn can also keep an array of sample-size toiletries packed and ready to go in her suitcase (along with hose, bras, and underwear). And when she gets makeup samples—tiny lipsticks or blushers or moisturizers—they should go straight into her toiletry bag.

To combat jet lag, Carolyn should shift her mealtimes and bedtime by 1 hour at a time (earlier if she's flying east, later if she's flying west) 2 or 3 days before she leaves. "She should also try

to sleep on the plane if she's flying west so that she can stay up later and get to bed at the right time," says Denton.

If Carolyn isn't comfortable letting her family subsist on takeout, she can prepare two meals and freeze them the weekend before she leaves. "She should prepare enough so that there are leftovers of each meal. That way, she can cover 4 days with two different dishes," says Denton. "They can pick up a pizza on the 5th day."

Ending the Monday Morning from Hell

Despite her newfound energy, nothing but absolute, blood-freezing panic will get Carolyn out of bed on Monday morning. This panic hits when she pushes the snooze button for the eighth time and sees that it's 7:10 and she has to leave the house by 8:00. She spends a frenzied hour showering, selecting and ironing an outfit, and gathering her laptop, briefcase, and outgoing mail from the third-floor study. She usually makes it out the door by 8:20.

Winston sympathizes with Carolyn's predicament because many of her clients are in the same boat. Carolyn must call a family meeting to address the issue, hammer out a morning routine for everyone, and stick to it. Here are some of her suggestions.

Move the alarm. Since Carolyn is helpless in the face of her alarm's snooze button, she should put her alarm clock across the room so she'll have to get out of bed to turn it off. If she has a radio alarm clock, she can turn it to the station she hates the most. It's a cruel but effective method: Imagine being assaulted by the musical stylings of a hard-rock band at 6:30 A.M.

Stagger wake-up times. To avoid bathroom gridlock, Carolyn and Ben should be in the bathroom by 6:45 A.M., Michael by 7:15, and Jocelyn by 7:45. (Yes, Carolyn should consider showering with Ben. What better way to squeeze in some more face time together?)

Go on autopilot. After she rises, Carolyn's Monday morning should run on autopilot. There should be no decisions about what to wear, since she'll have picked out her outfit on Sunday night (and ironed it, if necessary). And since Michael and Jocelyn are both old enough to iron, they'll have their own standing Sunday-night dates with the ironing board, too.

Get preset for takeoff. The whole family should set their backpacks, briefcases, and other paraphernalia by the door before they turn in. This eliminates Monday-morning gnashing of teeth over a forgotten notebook, field hockey stick, or computer disk.

Pick a place. Carolyn won't forget to mail her bills and birthday cards or have to hunt for her car keys if she keeps all out-the-door items in a small basket on a table close to the front door so she'll be sure to pick them up on her way out. If she's a particularly tough case, she can put them right in front of the door so she'll have to step over them to get out.

If Carolyn is smart, she'll use this Sunday-night checklist every night of the week, says Winston. "If she commits to a morning routine, she'll save precious time, cut down on stress, and conserve her energy."

AMAZING ENERGY

Energy That Endures

Being 67 years older than her classmates didn't stop Doris Eaton Travis from completing her bachelor's degree in history at age 88. She is the University of Oklahoma's oldest graduate and is working toward her master's degree in Liberal Arts. And that's not all this energetic former member of the Ziegfeld Follies dancers does to foster her enduring talent and spirit. She still keeps in shape by dancing. At an AIDS benefit in 1998, she danced the same routine she had performed 79 years earlier.

Index

Underscored page references indicate boxed text. **Boldface** references indicate illustrations.

A

AARP, 8, 78
Acupuncture, 88, 155
Adenosine triphosphate (ATP), 135–36
Adrenal glands, 30, 95
Adult day care, 79
Advanced sleep phase syndrome, 31
Aging, 30–31, 177, 185. *See also* Eldercare
Alcohol, 18, 97, 108–9
Alexander technique, 142
Allergies, 82–83, 87
Alpha lipoic acid, 137
Alternative health treatments
  acupuncture, 88, 155
  aromatherapy, 43, 161–62
  attitude, positive, 165
  Chinese medicine, 101–2
  chiropractic, 87
  exfoliation, 164–65
  flower essences, 161
  homeopathy, 155, 158–60
  hydrotherapy, 153
  journaling, 19, 158–59
  massage, 155–57
  meditation, 164
  music therapy, 43–44, 154
  naturopathy, 152, 155
  popularity of, 151–52
  reflexology, 157–58
  spirituality, 101, 160
  touch therapy, 70, 155
  visualization, 162–64
  yoga, 151–55
Alzheimer's Association, 78
American Association of Homes and Services for the
    Aging, 78
American Association of Retired Persons (AARP), 8, 78
American Massage Therapy Association (AMTA),
    156–57
American Society for the Alexander Technique,
    142
American Thyroid Association, 29
Amino acids, 133

AMTA, 156–57
Anemia, 136
Anticonvulsants, 98
Antidepressants, 85, 96, 98, 99
Antihistamines, 83
Antimalarial drugs, 90
Anxiety disorders, 96
Aromatherapy, 43, 161–62
Arsenicum, 160
Art classes, 170–71
Assisted-living facility, 79
ATP, 135–36
Attitude, positive, 165
Autoimmune hypothyroidism, 29

B

Back-to-school preparations, energy for,
    182–83
Balanced life, 4, 37–38, 52
Basil oil, 162
Baths, sleep and, 112
B-complex vitamins, 132–33
Bed, sleep and, 36–37
Benzodiazepines, 98–99, 116
Bipolar disorder, 97
Birth control pill, 22, 26
Blood sugar levels, 118, 134
Blood tests, 28
Board and care facility, 79
Body clock, 15–16, 17
Body temperature, 19–20, 20
  during sleep, 14, 16, 23, 113
Breakfast, 123–24
Breast cancer, 88–89
Breathing exercises, 18, 156–57, **157**
Burnout
  eldercare and, 76–78, 80
  slump vs., 38
  work and
    company strategies for, 44
    factors causing, 36–39
    preventing, 39–42
    signs of, 38–39

Business trips, energy for, 183–84
Buspirone (BuSpar), 99

C

Caffeine, 97, 108–9, <u>123</u>
Calendar, household, 57
Calories, 118, 125
Cancer, breast, 88–89
Carbohydrates, 125, 127
Caregiving, parental. *See* Eldercare
Carnitine, 137–38
CFS. *See* Chronic fatigue syndrome
Children, 58–59, <u>71</u>, 166, 172
Chinese medicine, 101–2
Chiropractic therapy, 87
Christian Science, <u>160</u>
Chromium, 135
Chronic fatigue syndrome (CFS), 81–85, <u>82–83</u>, <u>84</u>,
    136
Circadian rhythms, 11–13, 15–16, <u>17</u>, 18–20
Citrus oils, 43, 161
Coenzyme Q₁₀, 135–36
Coffee, <u>123</u>. *See also* Caffeine
Cognitive behavioral therapy, 85, 98
Color, energy and, 42, <u>54</u>
Computer work, fatigue and, <u>40</u>
Continuing-care retirement communities, <u>79</u>
Continuous positive airway pressure (CPAP), <u>106</u>,
    <u>110</u>
Cooking, 60–63, <u>62–63</u>
Copper, 134
CoQ₁₀, 135–36
Corticotropin releasing factor (CRF), 95–96
Cosleeping, <u>50–51</u>
Counseling, 85, <u>95</u>, 98
CPAP, <u>106</u>, <u>110</u>
Creatine, 138–39
Creativity. *See* Play and creativity
CRF, 95–96
Cycles of energy, 11

D

Dance, <u>175</u>
Daylight Saving Time, <u>17</u>
Death, depression and, <u>94–95</u>
Decorating, interior. *See* Feng shui
Dehydration, <u>83</u>, <u>138</u>

Dehydroepiandrosterone (DHEA), 30–31, 138
Depression
    alcohol and, 97
    battling, <u>94–95</u>
    caffeine and, 97
    death and, <u>94–95</u>
    fatigue vs., 93
    hormones and, 94–96
    light and, <u>100–101</u>
    sleep and, <u>23</u>
    treatments for, 97–102
    types of, 96–97
    in winter, 18, <u>100–101</u>
    women and, 93–94
DHEA, 30–31, 138
Diary, energy, 19, <u>158–59</u>
Dietary fat, 90–91, 122, 127
Dining out, <u>124</u>
Dinner, 59–63, <u>62–63</u>
Divorce, <u>68–69</u>
Downtime, <u>3</u>, 8–10, <u>8</u>. *See also* Relaxation
Dreams, <u>16</u>
Driving, 18–19, 59, <u>108</u>
Dry eyes, <u>40</u>
Dual-career families, 4
Dual roles, 36–37
Dysthymia, 97

E

Eating patterns, 119–20, <u>120–21</u>
Echinacea, <u>83</u>
EEG, 94, <u>182</u>
Eldercare, 75–76
    burnout and, 76–78, 80
    long-distance, <u>76</u>
    options for, <u>79</u>
    resources for, <u>78</u>
    support groups for, 80
    women and, 8, 73–75
Eldercare Locator, <u>78</u>, <u>79</u>
Electroencephalograph (EEG), 94, <u>182</u>
Emotions, 92–93, 105. *See also* Depression
EMS, 87
Endocrine glands, <u>152</u>
Endorphins, <u>52</u>, 144
Energy, exceptional, examples of, <u>4</u>, <u>9</u>, <u>19</u>, <u>72</u>, <u>143</u>,
    <u>185</u>
Energy bars, <u>118</u>

Eosinophilic myalgia syndrome (EMS), 87
Epworth Sleeping Scale, 6–7
Essential oils, 43, 161–62
Estrogen, 22–23, 26–27, 29
Exercise(s)
    breathing, 18, 156–57, **157**
    calming effect of, 143–45
    for energy, 143
    excessive, 141
    fartlek, 150
    fitness level and, 145
    food and, 125
    health problems, preventing with, 150
    hormones and, 144
    in managing
        chronic fatigue syndrome, 85
        depression, 99–100
        lupus, 90
        osteoporosis, 150
    metabolism and, 143
    selecting, 145, 148–50
    sex as, 53
    sleep and, 110–11, 144
    stairs, using for, 58
    strengthening, **146**, **147**, 147
    stretching, **146**, 146, 148
    team, 149
    women and, 140–43
    work and, 40, 41
    workout for energy, **146–47**, 146–47
    yawning after, 145
    zinc and, 134
Exfoliation, 164–65
Exhaustion. *See* Fatigue
Expectations, managing, 47–49, 182
Eyestrain, 40

F

Fartlek (interval training), 150
Fatigue. *See also* Chronic fatigue syndrome (CFS)
    acute, 27
    caffeine and, 123
    causes of, 82–83
    chronic, 27
    computer work and, 40
    Daylight Saving Time and, 17
    depression vs., 93
    DHEA and, 30–31

    diagnosing, 26–27
    doctor's visit for, 84
    driving and, 18–19, 108
    as epidemic, 2
    eyestrain and, 40
    food allergies and, 87
    headache and, morning, 18, 105
    hormones and, 21–22
    inactivity and, 31, 41
    light and, 100–101, 165
    memory and, 156–57
    menopause and, 21, 24–28
    menstruation and, 21–24, 22, 95
    pregnancy and, 90–91
    productivity and, 19
    prolonged, 27
    relationships and, 19
    thyroid gland and, 28–30
    tongue tickle and, 77
    water intake and, 138
    women and, 2
Fat. *See* Dietary fat; Overweight
FDA, 131, 159
Female fatigue syndrome (FFS), 2
Feng shui
    in home, 46–47
    at work, 42–43, **43**
Ferrum Phosphoricum, 160
FFS, 2
Fibromyalgia, 85–88
Fibromyalgia Network, 86
Fight-or-flight reaction, 96
Fitness level, 145
5-hydroxytryptophan (5-HTP), 87
Flower essences, 161
Folate, 133
Folic acid, 133
Food(s). *See also specific types*
    allergies, 87
    for athlete, 125
    breakfast, 123–24
    carbohydrates, 125, 127
    cooking, 60–63, 62–63
    dietary fat and, 90 –91, 122, 127
    dining out and, 124
    dinner, 59–63, 62–63
    eating patterns and, 119–20, 120–21
    energy and, 40, 118–19, 120–21, 124–25
    exercise and, 125

Food(s) (cont.)
   lunch, 124–25, 127
   protein, 127
   recipes, fatigue-busting, <u>126</u>
   sleep and, 128–29
   snack, 127–28, <u>128</u>
   sugar and, 120–21
   women and, 117–19
   work and, 40
Food and Drug Administration (FDA), <u>131</u>,
      159
Frankincense oil, 162
Friends, 69–70, 173, 175
Fruits, 127
Fun. *See* Play and creativity

G

Gamma-linolenic acid (GLA), 90–91
Gelsemium, 160
Generalized anxiety disorder, <u>96</u>
Geranium oil, 162
GLA, 90–91
Globulin, 27
Glucose, 120–21
Guilt, <u>3</u>, 65

H

Hashimoto's thyroiditis/disease, 29
hCG, <u>90</u>
Headache, morning, 18, <u>105</u>
Health problems. *See also specific types*
   breast cancer, <u>88–89</u>
   chronic fatigue syndrome, 81–85, <u>82–83</u>, <u>84</u>, 136
   fibromyalgia, 85–88
   lupus, 88–91
   preventing, exercise for, <u>150</u>
Heart disease, lupus and, 90
Hemoglobin, 134, <u>136</u>
Herbal therapy, 43, 87, 101, 162
High blood pressure, <u>105</u>
Holidays, energy for, 176–79, <u>180–81</u>
Home
   children in, 58–59, <u>71</u>
   cooking and, 60–63, <u>62–63</u>
   dual-career families and, 4
   family sleeping habits and, <u>50–51</u>
   feng shui in, <u>46–47</u>

   household chores and
      outside help for, 63–64
      sharing, 50–51
      tips for, 49–54
      women and, 47–49
   men in, <u>55</u>
   organizational skills and, 54–58, <u>56–57</u>
   relaxation and, 59–60
   respite from, <u>48–49</u>
   spa, <u>174</u>
   technology and, managing, <u>60–61</u>
   transition from work to, 59–60
   women in, 6–8, 45–46
Home health care, <u>79</u>
Homeopathy, <u>155</u>, 158–60
Hormones. *See also specific types*
   depression and, 94–96
   exercise and, 144
   fatigue and, 21–22
   measuring levels of, <u>28</u>
   sex, <u>52–53</u>
   stress, 22–23
Hormone replacement therapy (HRT), <u>24</u>, 27
Hot flashes, 21, 24–26
Household chores
   outside help for, 63–64
   sharing, 50–51
   tips for, 49–54
   women and, 47–49
HRT, <u>24</u>, 27
Human chorionic gonadotropin (hCG),
      90
Hydrotherapy, <u>153</u>
Hypericum, 101
Hyperthyroidism, 29–30
Hypothalamus, 95
Hypothyroidism, <u>27</u>, 28–29
Hysterectomy, energy and, <u>25</u>

I

Immunosuppressive drugs, 89–90
Inactivity, fatigue and, <u>31</u>, <u>41</u>
Infants, <u>167</u>
Infections, <u>83</u>
Internet, managing time and, <u>61</u>
Interpersonal therapy, 98. *See also* Therapy
Interval training technique, 150
Intimacy, 67. *See also* Sex

Iodine, 29–30
Iron, 134, <u>136</u>

J

Jet lag, <u>14–15</u>, 15
Job dissatisfaction, 37
Journaling, 19, <u>158–59</u>

K

Kelp, 29

L

Larks (morning people), <u>12–13</u>
Laughter, energy and, 40
Lavender oil, 161
Learning, sleep and, 105
Light
    depression and, <u>100–101</u>
    energy and, 13–14, <u>47</u>
    fatigue and, <u>100–101</u>, <u>165</u>
    lupus and, 90
    seasonal affective disorder and, 18, <u>100–101</u>
    therapy, 18
    at work, 43
Love, sustaining, <u>70</u>
Lunch, 124–25, 127
Lupus, 89–91

M

Magnesium, 135
Mail Preference Service (Direct Marketing
    Association), <u>56</u>
Manic-depressive illness, 97
Massage, 155–57
Mattress, sleep and, <u>114</u>
Meals. *See* Cooking; *specific meals*
Medications. *See specific types*
Meditation, 164
Melatonin, 14–15, 138
Memory, fatigue and, <u>156–57</u>
Men, <u>55</u>, 65. *See also* Relationships
Menopause, 21, 24–28
Menstruation, 21–24, <u>22</u>, 95
Metabolism, 20, 23, 28–29, 143
Milk, lupus and, 91

Mind-body connection, 144, 159
Minerals, 134–35, <u>136</u>
Monday mornings, energy for, 184–85
Mother-daughter relationships, 68–69. *See also*
    Eldercare
Multivitamins, 85, 132
Music therapy, 43–44, <u>154</u>

N

NADH, 85, 136–37
NAHC, <u>78</u>
Napping, <u>35</u>, 109–10
Narcolepsy, <u>106–7</u>
National Alliance for Caregiving, 8, <u>78</u>, 80
National Association of Area Agencies on Aging, <u>78</u>
National Association of Geriatric Care Managers, <u>79</u>
National Association for Home Care (NAHC), <u>78</u>
National Association of Professional Organizers, 64
National Center for Homeopathy, 161
National Citizens' Coalition for Nursing Home
    Reform, <u>79</u>
National Family Caregivers Association, 75, <u>78</u>, 80
National Institute on Aging, <u>78</u>
National Mental Health Association, 93
Naturopathy, <u>152</u>, <u>155</u>
Neurally mediated hypotension (NMH), 83
Nicotinamide adenine dinucleotide (NADH), 85,
    136–37
Nightmares, <u>16</u>, 18
Night shift work, 16, <u>109</u>
NMH, 83
Non-benzodiazepines, 116
Nonsteroidal anti-inflammatory drugs (NSAIDs), 86,
    90
Norepinephrine, 96
NSAIDs, 86, 90
Nursing home, <u>79</u>

O

Obesity, snoring and, <u>113</u>
Obsessive-compulsive disorder (OCD), <u>96</u>
Omega-3 fatty acids, 90–91
Opt-Out Service, <u>56</u>
Oral sex, <u>53</u>
Organizational skills, 54–58, <u>56–57</u>
Orgasm, <u>52</u>
Osteoporosis, <u>150</u>

Overactive thyroid, 29–30
Overweight, 113, 124–25
Ovulation, 22. *See also* Menstruation
Owls (evening people), 12–13, 17
Oxytocin, 52–53

P

Panic disorder, 96
Peppermint, 43, 162
Perfectionism, 36
Pets, holiday stress and, 178–79
Phosphoric acid, 160
Photoreceptors, 14
Physical activity. *See* Exercise
Physical rhythms. *See* Body clock; Circadian rhythms
Pill, the, 22, 26
Pineal gland, 14
Planner, personal, 57–58
Play and creativity
    advantages of, 166–69
    alone, 175
    art classes, 170–71
    with children, 172
    children and, 166
    dance, 175
    with friends, 173
    guidelines for, 169–71
    home spa and, 174
    new, trying, 184
    relationships and, 173, 175
    with spouse/partner, 173
    vacation, 172–73
    at work, 171–72
PMS, 95
Pregnancy, fatigue and, 90–91
Premenstrual syndrome (PMS), 95
Productivity, fatigue and, 19
Progesterone, 22–24, 22
Protein, 127
Psychodynamic therapy, 98
Psychotherapy, 85, 95, 98
Psychotropic drugs, 99

R

Rapid eye movement (REM) sleep, 23, 24, 94,
    105–7
Reflexology, 157–58

Relationships
    with children, 71
    divorce and, 68–69
    energy and, 65–68
    fatigue and, 19
    with friends, 69–70
    give-and-take in, 68–72
    intimacy and, 67
    mother-daughter, 68–69
    play and creativity and, 173, 175
    romance in, 70–71, 70
    saying "no" and, 66–67
    sex and, 65
    solitude and, 67–68
    with spouse/partner, 70–71, 70
    stress and, 66
    talking and, 29
    women and, 65–68
    at work, 40–41, 71–72
    yes-woman syndrome and, 66–67
Relaxation
    breathing exercises for, 18, 156–57, **157**
    in home, 59–60
    in managing
        chronic fatigue syndrome, 85
        depression, 101
    with spouse or partner, 70
    at work, 41–42
Religion, 101, 160
REM sleep, 23, 24, 94, 105–7
Rescue Remedy, 161
Restaurants, eating at, 124
Restless legs syndrome (RLS), 107
Rest. *See* Sleep
RLS, 107
Romance, 70–71, 70
Rosemary oil, 162
Routine, erratic, 15–17

S

SAD, 18, 100–101
S-adenosyl-L-methionine (SAM-e), 86–87
St. John's wort, 87, 101
Saliva test, 28
SAM-e, 86–87
Schedule, irregular, 15–17
Seasonal affective disorder (SAD), 18, 100–101
Selective serotonin reuptake inhibitors (SSRIs), 98, 99

Serotonin, 22–23, 96, 125, 127
Sex, _53_, _55_, 65
Shift work, 16, _109_
Siesta, _35_
Single mothers, dilemma of, _3_
Sleep
    adequate, 17–18
    aging and, _30–31_
    alcohol and, 97, 108–9
    allergies and, _82–83_
    baths and, 112
    bed and, _36–37_
    body temperature during, 14, 16, _23_, 113
    caffeine and, 108–9
    Daylight Saving Time and, _17_
    defined, 104–6
    depression and, _23_
    deprivation, _6_
    disorders, _31_, _106–7_, _110_
    dreams and, _16_
    emotions and, 105
    exercise and, 110–11, _144_
    experiment, 12–13
    families and, _50–51_
    famous people and, _162–63_
    food and, 128–29
    headache from, 18, _105_
    hormone replacement therapy and, _24_
    importance of, 104–5
    infants and, _167_
    jet lag and, _14–15_, 15
    learning and, 105
    mattresses and, _114_
    measuring need for, _6_, _7_, _116_
    medications and, _82–83_, _99_, 113–16
    menstruation and, 23–24
    napping, _35_, 109–10
    phases of, _23_, _24_, 94, 105–7
    position for, _114–15_, **115**
    on sailboat, _168–69_
    scale, _6–7_
    shift work and, 16, _109_
    smoking and, 109
    snoring and, _112–13_
    on space shuttle, _74–75_
    stages of, 107–8
    stress and, 18
    teenagers and, _167_
    tips for, 18, 108–13
    unihemispheric slow-wave, _182–83_
    waking from, _111_
Sleep apnea, _105_, _106_, _110_, _112_
Slump, burnout vs., 38
Smoking, sleep and, 109
Snacking, 127–28, _128_
Snoring, _112–13_
Socializing, 100. _See also_ Relationships
Solitude, 67–68, 175, 181
Spa, home, _174_
Spirituality, 101, _160_
Spouses, 70–71, _70_, 173
SSRIs, 98, _99_
Steroids, 89
Strengthening exercise, _146_, **147**, _147_
Stress
    fight-or-flight reaction and, 96
    holiday, 177–78, _178–79_
    hormones, 22–23
    managing, with
        Alexander technique, _142_
        breathing technique, _18_
    relationships and, 66
    sleep and, 18
    work-related, _39_
Stretching exercise, **146**, _146_, _148_
Sugar, 120–21
Sunlight. _See_ Light
Supplements
    alpha lipoic acid, 137
    carnitine, 137–38
    coenzyme Q_{10}, 135–36
    creatine, 138–39
    DHEA, 31, 138
    kelp, 29
    labeling of, _131_
    melatonin, 14, 138
    NADH, 136–37
    St. John's wort, 101
Support groups, 80, 85
Systemic lupus erythematosus, 88–91

T

Technology, managing, _60–61_
Teenagers, _71_, _167_
Testosterone, 26–30, 138
Therapy, 85, _95_, 98
Thymus, _152_

Thyroid gland, <u>27</u>, 28–30
Thyroid-stimulating hormone (TSH), 29
Time
   aging and, <u>177</u>
   Daylight Saving Time, <u>17</u>
   energy experiment and, 12–13
   management, <u>5</u>, 41, 59, <u>60 –61</u>
Tongue tickle, fatigue and, <u>77</u>
Touch therapy, <u>70</u>, <u>155</u>. *See also* Massage
Travel
   business, 183–84
   holiday, <u>180–81</u>
   jet lag and, <u>14–15</u>, 15
Tricyclic drugs, 85, <u>99</u>
TSH, 29

U

Underactive thyroid, <u>27</u>, 28–30
Unihemispheric slow-wave sleep (USWS), <u>182–83</u>
United States Personal Chef Association, 64
USWS, <u>182–83</u>

V

Vacations, <u>172–73</u>, 180–82
Vegetables, 127
Visionweaver, <u>111</u>
Visualization, 162–64
Vitamins. *See also* Supplements
   B-complex, 132–33
   labeling of, <u>131</u>
   multivitamins, 85, 132
   vitamin C, <u>83</u>, 123, 133–34
   women and, 130–32

W

Water intake, <u>83</u>, <u>122</u>, <u>138</u>
Windstar Solutions (minivan), <u>5</u>
Women
   childless, 37–38
   depression and, 93–94
   downtime and, 8–10, <u>8</u>
   dual-career families and, 4
   eldercare and, 8, 73–75
   energy solution and, 10
   exercise and, 140–43
   fatigue and, 2

   food and, 117–19
   in home, 6–8, 45–46
   minivan and, <u>5</u>
   mother-daughter relationship and, 68–69
   relationships and, view of, 65–68
   single mothers, <u>3</u>
   vitamins and, 130–32
   at work, 2, 4–5, 34
Work
   aromatherapy at, 43
   burnout and
      company strategies for, 44
      factors causing, 36–39
      preventing, 38–42
      signs of, 38–39
   business trips and, 183–84
   computer, <u>40</u>
   contemporary workplace and, 34–38
   dissatisfaction with, 37
   energizing environment at, 42–44
   exercise and, 40, <u>41</u>
   feng shui at, <u>42–43</u>, **43**
   food and, 40
   inactivity at, <u>41</u>
   light at, 43
   music therapy at, 43
   play and creativity at, 171–72
   quitting, <u>44</u>
   relationships at, 40–41, 71–72
   relaxation at, 41–42
   shift, 16, <u>109</u>
   siesta and, <u>35</u>
   stress related to, <u>39</u>
   transition to home from, 59–60
   visual stimuli at, 43
   women at, 2, 4–5, 34
Workaholic syndrome, <u>38</u>
Workout for energy, **146–47**, <u>146–47</u>

Y

Yawning after exercise, <u>145</u>
Yes-woman syndrome, <u>66–67</u>
Yoga, 151–55

Z

Zinc, 134–35

The New Gnosis. 269

Shamans and the Spiritual Future 274

Mystical Pluralism 277

Final Considerations: A New and Better Way? 279

Notes 282

Index of Names 318

Index of Subjects 322

ACKNOWLEDGMENTS

A large number of people have contributed in important ways to this project. The following individuals deserve special thanks. I want to thank the students in my Senior Seminar class at Hope College over the past fifteen years whose comments in response to early drafts of the manuscript helped me think through a number of issues. There are too many of them to mention by name, but Brian Boersma, John Brandkamp, Timothy Cupery, Daniel Foster, Christopher Poest and Pamela Van Putten have been particularly instrumental in encouraging me along the way. Another student, Jon Adamson, helped a great deal with early research.

Many friends and colleagues have shown constant interest in this project as well. My friend Russel Hirst encouraged me, suggested important themes that shaped several chapters, and responded to early drafts of the book. Marc Baer made helpful suggestions about how to frame the discussion of these issues and directed me to important resources. Richard Poll and Deirdre Johnston also provided a number of useful sources. Peter Payne allowed me to test some of my ideas in talks before his InterVarsity graduate student groups at the University of Michigan. Linda Koetje helped a great deal in preparing the manuscript for the publisher. Gary Deddo and the editorial staff at InterVarsity Press, as well as their outside readers, provided encouragement and made important suggestions about how to present my case. Research grants from Hope College allowed me to devote several summers to writing and research.

I am indebted to a number of writers and scholars as well, again, too many to name individually. However, several deserve special mention. Richard Noll's work on Carl Jung, and Carl Raschke's scholarship on gnosticism were especially helpful in forming my thinking about the origins and direction of contemporary spiritual movements. James Sire's remarkably practical book *The Universe Next Door* has been a helpful guide to my thinking about worldviews in general, while C. S.

Lewis's *The Abolition of Man* was a constant and prophetic reminder of the seriousness of the issues under discussion in the following pages.

One's family always bears the brunt of such a time-consuming enterprise. My children, Daniel, Stephen, Laura and Alicia, have been extraordinarily willing to endure my distraction and even my absence as I worked on the manuscript. Special thanks to Stephen for his help with the index. Finally, my wife, Janet, has provided constant encouragement through the long process of writing and rewriting.

1

INTRODUCTION

A Changing View of the Spiritual World

We are only at the threshold of a new spiritual epoch.

CARL JUNG,
"The Difference Between Eastern and Western Thinking"

These modern movements may be harbingers of a newly dawning and more adequate myth and spirituality.

JOHN P. DOURLEY,
The Illness We Are

We are persuaded that gradually, in religious thought as in the sciences, a core of universal truth will form and slowly grow to be accepted by everyone. Can there be any true spiritual evolution without it?

PIERRE TEILHARD DE CHARDIN,
The Future of Man

We are at the dawn of a new consciousness, a radically fresh approach to our life as the human family in a fragile world. . . . Perhaps the best name for this new segment of historical experience is the Interspiritual Age.

WAYNE TEASDALE,
The Mystic Heart

The idea of changing culture is important to me, and it can only be done in a popular medium.

JOSS WHEDON,
creator of Buffy the Vampire Slayer

Harvard graduate and former Green Beret Gary Zukav, a frequent guest on the *Oprah Winfrey Show*, is just one of dozens of popular writers currently promoting an emerging new spirituality. Zukav confidently anticipates nothing less than the "birth of a new humanity," which even now is apparent in "new perceptions and new values" including the insight that "the Universe is alive, wise, and compassionate." Members of the new humanity are currently participating in "a learning process" that is contributing to "the evolution of our souls." Zukav's books are part of his effort to "serve the needs of the emerging multisensory humanity," for which "current social structures" are inadequate. Thus, these outdated structures "are dissolving" while Zukav and a growing number of like-minded individuals are busily "creating their replacements—seven billion of us, together."[1]

Zukav's *The Dancing Wu Li Masters*, winner of an American Book Club award in 1979, explored the intersection of quantum physics and emerging spiritualities. Like many contemporary writers on spiritual topics, Zukav finds in science a key to human spiritual awareness and development. Science is no longer confined to only physical phenomena, but is the source of a new theology. In his bestselling *The Seat of the Soul* (1989) Zukav writes that the "discoveries of science illuminate both inner and outer experiences," that is, both "physical and nonphysical dynamics."[2] Science has even suggested a new understanding of God, not as the personal Deity of the Judeo-Christian tradition, but as "conscious light" and "Divine Intelligence" that animate, not a single entity, but the universe itself.[3]

The individual spiritual seeker exercising innate rational power is central to the new spiritual views. "The intellect is meant to expand perceptions, to help you grow in perceptual strength and complexity."[4] At the same time, the spiritual seeker may acquire hidden knowledge from "nonphysical Teachers," or spirit entities equipped to assist the process of spiritual evolution to higher levels of awareness. The capacity to "communicate consciously with a nonphysical Teacher, is a treasure that cannot be described, a treasure beyond words and value."[5] Such guidance is crucial, for the "advanced or expanding mind" does not find answers "within the accepted understanding of truth." The old paradigms do not take into account the most important fact about the human race—its continuing evolution.[6] "Our species is evolving," writes Zukav, and this evolutionary process will result in a species that is "more radiant and energetic," more "aware of the Light of its soul," and

more capable of communicating with "forms of Life that are invisible to the five-sensory personality."[7] Many members of the human race already exhibit some of these signs of ongoing evolution, and further progress is assured under the guidance of both science and "spirit Teachers."

Gary Zukav is just one example of dozens of writers and media celebrities who have helped both to shape and popularize a medley of religious ideas that I will be referring to throughout this book as the New Religious Synthesis. Such public religious advocates have had enormous influence in the past fifty years, and the audience for their ideas grows steadily. Zukav's books alone, for example, have sold in excess of five million copies worldwide and have been translated into sixteen languages. His appearances on the *Oprah Winfrey Show* have made his ideas available to an estimated twenty-two million viewers.

The new spiritual outlook Zukav and many other talented advocates are promoting stands in sharp contrast to its predecessor, the Judeo-Christian worldview. Proponents of this ancient and venerable worldview have long insisted that it is, not a human discovery, but rather a revelation from a living and personal God. For this reason I will be referring to the tradition emerging from the pages of the Old and New Testaments as the Revealed Word. What I take to be the fundamental, and fundamentally opposed, components of two perspectives currently competing for the Western religious mind—the New Religious Synthesis and the Revealed Word—will be set out in detail below.

So substantial has been the shaping influence of the New Religious Synthesis on contemporary religious thought that it has now displaced the Revealed Word as the religious framework of a large and growing number of Western people. This powerfully persuasive synthesis blends strands of religious thought that began to appear, or reappear in Western religious writing around 1700. Over the past three centuries, and under the guidance of scores of gifted public advocates working in a number of genres and media, the New Religious Synthesis has now successfully colonized Western religious consciousness. The intriguing migration of these provocative ideas from the fringes of religious exotica to Western spirituality's Main Street is the story told in this book.

"One cannot but feel," wrote the famous scholar of religions Joseph Campbell in 1989, that there is a "universally recognized need in our time for a general transformation of consciousness."[8] In a similar fashion, Marilyn Ferguson maintained in her bestselling *The Aquarian Conspiracy* (1980) that scientific and spiritual breakthroughs

would soon "thrust us into a new, higher order" of consciousness.[9] As noted in the quotations at the opening of this chapter, the enormously influential psychoanalyst Carl Jung remarked more than seventy years ago that the Western world was "at the threshold of a new spiritual epoch."[10] In apparent agreement, Catholic lay brother Wayne Teasdale has written that "we are at the dawn of a new consciousness, a radically fresh approach to our life as the human family in a fragile world."[11] Though he is deeply concerned about some of its implications, historian of religion Carl Raschke has also noted the recent emergence of a "new religious consciousness."[12] Have we, in fact, now entered a new spiritual era?

For many Westerners, the long-prophesied new spiritual age certainly has arrived. The Revealed Word and its busy, personal God have faded into our collective spiritual memory, and bright new spiritual commitments encourage fresh religious thought. The New Synthesis appears less rigid and systematic than a worldview, less august and enduring than a tradition. And yet, its basic components are considerably more integrated than the simple "toolbox" of religious ideas that French scholar Daniele Hervieu-Leger referred to in 1999 as characterizing the contemporary religious mind.[13] This emerging outlook provides a new theological hypothesis for a dawning age, a user-friendly alternative to the doctrinally insistent Revealed Word. For the spiritual seeker, the New Religious Synthesis has become the Other Spirituality.

In the following pages I want to explore just how this massive transformation in Western spiritual thought has occurred, taking as my focus the work of public religious advocates. At this juncture in the religious history of Western culture, it also seems timely to ask what is gained and what is lost in the dramatic shift now occurring from one spirituality to another. I will begin with the assumption that, in a society accustomed to the free and public exchange of ideas, it takes a great deal of time and enormous effort to replace that society's spiritual base with a wholly new one. After all, two major tasks are involved: dismantling the old view by revealing its inadequacies and fashioning a new and presumably better one in its place. Thus, this act of changing Western culture's religious beliefs has meant going repeatedly before the public in broadly accessible settings and by means of popular religious media—books, speeches, magazines and pamphlets to be sure, but also movies, plays, music, radio interviews, television programs and websites.

In the following chapters I will be drawing attention to a number of authors and artists who have been important to this effort to accomplish the twin tasks of razing

the Western world's old spiritual edifice and publicly constructing a new one in its place. What follows, however, is not a comprehensive catalog of the efforts that brought either task to completion. Rather, I have chosen what I take to be representative examples of spiritually influential works from a three-hundred-year-long public persuasive process. Some of the works selected are quite famous and their impact widely recognized. Others were well known in their own day but are now virtually forgotten. In such cases it has seemed to me that the work's influence has nevertheless persisted in the public mind as beliefs, ideas, assumptions, convictions and images. While not including a number of major milestones of religious thought because their influence seems to have been greatest among scholars, I do focus attention on several important intellectual figures who possessed the rare talent for impressing both their academic colleagues and the wider public.

I have been asserting that a massive shift in Western religious attitudes has taken place. Perhaps some basic evidence of such a change is in order before considering the historical sources and impact of the New Religious Synthesis on our religious thought. Even a brief survey of events on the recent Western religious stage suggests that something like a fundamental shift in spiritual assumptions has transpired, almost without our noticing it.

SPIRITUAL CHANGES: A NEW AGE OF BELIEF?

Observers of the religious scene have for some time now noted that an extraordinary redefinition of fundamental religious belief has occurred in the West and that the resultant spiritual transition has been stunning in its rapidity, scope and impact. A decade ago journalist Michael D'Antonio wrote that "sociologists at the University of California, Santa Barbara estimate that as many as 12 million Americans could be considered active participants [in alternative spiritual systems] and another 30 million are actively interested."[14] Perhaps 1,000 to 2,000 new religious movements have arisen in the United States alone in the twentieth century, and few of these are rooted in traditional Judeo-Christian theological assumptions.

The diverse manifestations of the emerging spirituality "obscure its size and its impact on the larger society." Nevertheless, that impact is felt "in public schools, hospitals, corporate offices, and the popular media."[15] And, we might add, in politics. The pervasiveness of alternative spiritualities forcefully confronted Americans with revelations that Ronald and Nancy Reagan sought advice from an (expensive) astrologer and that Hillary Rodham Clinton solicited contact with Eleanor Roosevelt

through the offices of psychic researcher Jean Houston. Spirituality, it seems, is no longer confined to the sanctuary and the synagogue, but has now moved into the lecture hall and the classroom, the movie theater and the surgical theater, the corporate office and the Oval Office.

In his book *Spiritual Marketplace: Baby Boomers and the Remaking of American Religion* (1999) Wade Clark Roof suggests that, unlike old established religious denominations, "popular religious culture is more diffused, less contained by formal religious structures." The evidence for a new Western spirituality includes "widespread belief in angels and reincarnation; the appeal of religious and quasi-religious shrines, retreat centers, and theme parks; interest in metaphysical and theosophical teachings; prosperity theology and 'possibility thinking'; and large proportions of Americans reporting mystical experiences." At the level of popular belief, Roof concludes, "we observe an eclectic mix of religious and spiritual ideas, beliefs, and practices."[16]

The success of this "eclectic mix" of ideas is not due to its being "institutionalized," that is, propagated and maintained by formal organizations. Rather, these once exotic but now commonplace notions have pursued a different route into public consciousness. "They persist," writes Roof, "largely as a result of loosely bound networks of practitioners, the publishing industry, and the media." Even the names of many new religions practiced by Westerners are not widely recognized by either government record keepers or scholars in religion. Roof's examples of the new spiritual systems existing just off official radar screens include "the paranormal, Neo-Paganism, astrology, nature religion, [and] holistic thinking," often collected under broader headings such as "New Age, or New Spirituality."[17]

Wayne Teasdale applauds this new Great Awakening noted by D'Antonio, Roof and many others, finding it marked by such positive signs as greater "ecological awareness," a recognition of "the interdependence of all domains of life and reality," as well as "a deep, evolving experience of community between and among the religions." Teasdale writes that more and more of us are becoming aware that "the earth is part of the larger community of the universe."[18] He adds that "each of these shifts represents a dramatic change," and that "taken together, they will define the thought and culture of the third millennium." Teasdale recommends dubbing the new religious era the "Interspiritual Age," and he maintains that new "awarenesses" will profoundly affect all areas of our personal and social lives.[19] "All of these awarenesses are interrelated, and each is indispensable to clearly grasping the greater shift taking place, a shift that will sink roots deep into our lives and culture."

Remarkably, Teasdale believes the new spirituality is "preparing the way for a universal civilization." The basis of this new, universal civilization will be what Teasdale terms "perennial spiritual and moral insights, intuitions and experiences." Moreover, "these aspects of spirituality will shape how we conduct politics and education, how we envision our economies, media, and entertainment; and how we develop our relationship with the natural world."[20]

No assessment of a sea change in religious perspective could be more sweeping than is Teasdale's. Is he overstating the case? Perhaps, but certainly interest in new spiritualities is extraordinarily high if we are to judge by one rough indicator of public interest—book sales. Teresa Watanabe, writing for the *Los Angeles Times*, notes that "sales of religious books skyrocketed 150% from 1991 to 1997, compared to 35% for the rest of the industry." She adds, "Ingram Book Co., the nation's largest book distributor to retail markets, reported a cumulative growth in religion titles of nearly 500% from June 1994 to the third quarter of 1996, an additional 40% increase in 1997, and a 58% rise in the first quarter of 1998."[21] And these figures do not reflect the enormous sales of books on spiritual themes that are ostensibly devoted to business success, medicine and healing, relationships and science.

Clearly, spiritual books sell, as do spiritually oriented seminars, movies and an extraordinary array of personal spiritual products ranging from clothing to candles. However, the beliefs energizing this vast cultural phenomenon are not those of the Revealed Word perspective that held sway in the West for most of two millennia. In fact, our basic spiritual assumptions have changed so dramatically in the past fifty years that sociologist of religion Robert Wuthnow notices nothing less than a "transformation of American spirituality."[22] Wuthnow remarks that "a majority of the public has retained some loyalty to their churches and synagogues, yet," he adds, "their practice of spirituality from Monday to Friday often bears little resemblance to the preachments of religious leaders."[23] Similarly, historian of religion Philip Jenkins has written recently of the New Age phenomenon that "the vast majority of people holding New Age beliefs do not identify themselves as representing a distinct denomination, but describe themselves as Unitarians or Jews, Methodists or Catholics."[24]

It is relevant to note here that self-professed belief in astrology, reincarnation and a non-personal divine energy characterizes upwards of 30 percent of Americans, and these concepts are viable spiritual options for many more. One popular astrology website created for Time Warner Electronic Publishing attracts 1.3 million visitors every month. Another similar site, AstroNet, established with the support of America

Online, attracts an astonishing 300,000 visitors each day.[25] Thus, though church and synagogue attendance remains strong, this fact may not accurately portray the spiritual convictions and practices of millions of Americans and Europeans. Wuthnow writes that whereas "95 percent of the U.S. population claims to believe in God," the nature of that divinity is defined in widely divergent ways.[26]

It seems that the God (or gods) in whom many today believe is not the biblical Yahweh, even for self-identified members of traditional faiths.[27] D'Antonio notes that millions of devotees of new religious systems still "consider themselves Christian, Jewish, Muslim" because they "hold to much of their old religious identity" while at the same time "adopting any number of . . . ideas about health, politics, psychology or spirituality" from new spiritual movements.[28] D'Antonio sees this mixing of spiritualities as "enriching." Whether enriching or simply an expression of spiritual wanderlust, the evidence of spiritual experimentation in the contemporary West is present virtually anywhere one cares to look. Whence this new spiritual orientation?

BESTSELLERS AND BLOCKBUSTERS: SPIRITUALITY GOES PUBLIC

As might be expected when assessing such a massive change in public attitudes, several explanations have been advanced to account for this seismic shift in Western spiritual attitudes. Some observers subsume all of the observed changes under the heading the New Age movement, and find its sources in the experiments of the hippie culture of the 1960s and 1970s. However, the spiritual changes afoot in the West are broader than even the broadest definitions of a so-called New Age movement. By the same token, to emphasize the drug, rock and spiritual experimenta tion subculture of the 1960s as the principal source of a new Western spiritual paradigm is to risk overlooking the long historical development of the Other Spirituality and to isolate it within a relatively small and easily dismissed subculture.

A longer historical view reveals that major spiritual changes have been afoot in the Western world for some time and that they correspond roughly with scientific advances, corrosive biblical criticism and rising awareness of other faiths on the part of Westerners. Thus, a second explanation of sweeping religious change in Europe and the United States is that it reflects an attempt to "fill the spiritual vacuum" created as Christian assumptions inexorably disintegrated under pressure from cultural pluralism, Enlightenment criticism of the Judeo-Christian tradition and the staggering successes of modern science. This common explanation of re-

cent religious change has merit; the loss of a cherished and ennobling understanding of transcendence leaves one longing for a substitute. But this account's inactive root metaphor of a vacuum being filled distracts attention away from the concerted and highly successful efforts of a host of skilled advocates who have for more than three centuries actively and persistently promoted alternative spiritualities in broadly public settings and through powerful popular media.

Because I have been placing such heavy emphasis on religious advocates as agents of spiritual change, it may be helpful to illustrate their important role by considering several recent examples of their work. Surveying these cases of public spiritual advocacy does reveal that a large number of Western people have indeed been seeking answers in the spiritual realm by moving outside the boundaries of what I have termed the Revealed Word. But this survey also indicates, I believe, something more—that the public spiritual advocate has also functioned importantly to suggest the direction and the destination of our vast cultural quest for spiritual satisfaction.

Spirituality's surprising successes. In the 1980s many commentators noted the stunning popularity of actress Shirley MacLaine's accounts of her spiritual journeying in books such as *Going Within* and *Dancing in the Light*.[29] "God lies within," she taught, "and therefore we are each part of God."[30] It is estimated that fifty million viewers watched her television special based on the book, *Out on a Limb*, the central message of which was the divinity of the individual. "MacLaine's books," writes one observer, "have introduced millions to psychics and channelers, healers and spirit guides."[31] At the same time her captivating narratives made a persuasive case for a new worldview standing in direct opposition to the Revealed Word.

Numerous earlier writers in the genre of the personal spiritual narrative paved the path to MacLaine's astounding popularity. For example, the drug-enhanced mysticism and magic of Carlos Castaneda's phenomenally popular *The Teachings of Don Juan* series, beginning in 1968, fascinated and often convinced college-aged readers that there was more to the spiritual world than the church had suggested.[32] Castaneda's appealing stories related what he claimed were actual experiences under the tutelage of a Mexican shaman named don Juan, a medicine man and sorcerer who taught him how to use hallucinogenic plants to acquire "wisdom, or knowledge of the right way to live."[33] Through arduous training involving intense inner exploration, Castaneda learned the powers and secrets of an alternative spiritual world.

In the nonfiction realm, works like Marilyn Ferguson's *The Aquarian Conspiracy* (1980) set about "challenging our old assumptions" which are "the air we breathe,

our familiar furniture."[34] Ferguson argued that the prevailing Western paradigm, founded on the Judeo-Christian worldview, had run its course. A new way of thinking about nature, the divine and human potential had arrived. Ferguson celebrated a growing "conspiracy" of the spiritually informed, a massive collaboration that was changing the way we thought about spiritual matters. *The Aquarian Conspiracy's* dust jacket confidently announced that "a great, shuddering, irrevocable shift is overtaking us. It is not a new political, religious, or economic system. It is a new mind—a turnabout in consciousness in critical numbers of individuals."

Indeed, even a cursory glance at recent artifacts of popular culture suggests that something *was* overtaking us as the twentieth century ended. James Redfield's New Age adventure story, *The Celestine Prophecy*, turned down by publishers but successfully promoted by its determined author, made *The New York Times* bestseller list 165 consecutive weeks starting in 1994. Again, Redfield's path into the public mind was prepared by works like Richard Bach's proto-New Age bestseller *Jonathan Livingston Seagull*—the simple story of a seagull with a profound faith in his capacity to overcome personal limitations. Bach's book sold a surprising three million copies in the mid-1970s. In the cinematic realm, George Lucas's staggeringly successful *Star Wars* movies recently have marketed a decidedly non-Western religious philosophy to their audiences of millions worldwide. Similarly, phenomenally popular television series such as *The X Files* have recently attracted highly receptive, mainly younger audiences as the programs explore alternative understandings of the spiritual realm.

Witches and goddesses. The "great, shuddering, irrevocable shift" in spiritual attitudes has been equally apparent from various cultural vantage points. Many ancient religious traditions, for example, have recently been refurbished and popularized for a new generation of spiritual seekers. Contemporary reworkings of pre-Christian pagan religions, including Wicca, goddess worship, Native American religions, Druidism and the worship of ancient Norse gods are enjoying great popularity. Carol P. Christ writes, "One of the most unexpected developments of the late twentieth century is the rebirth of the religion of the Goddess in western culture."[35] The goddess being worshiped was, in some cases at least, quite close to home. Ms. Christ writes, "I found God in myself, and I loved her fiercely."[36]

One prominent proponent of the goddess revival was the cultural anthropologist Marija Gimbutas, author of *The Language of the Goddess*. Gimbutas hoped for a return to a tradition far older than the Judeo-Christian, a faith she calls "Old Euro-

pean."[37] "We are still living under the sway of the aggressive male invasion [of Europe] and only beginning to discover our long alienation from our authentic European Heritage," which, Gimbutas contends, was "nonviolent," "earth centered" and "gylanic," that is, making no social or political distinctions between males and females.[38] Similarly, Barbara Walker urges a Western "return" to goddess worship. Her book, *Restoring the Goddess,* calls on women and men to leave the patriarchal religion of the Revealed Word, and to embrace a Nature-centered religion that worships Gaia—the spirit of the earth—as Goddess. Walker finds that goddess worship is more "an evolution than a revolution" in religious thought.[39]

In a similar vein, Akasha Gloria Hull's book *Soul Talk* explores a "new spirituality [that] has arisen among black women."[40] For Hull, spirituality involves "conscious relationship with the realm of the spirit, with the invisibly permeating, ultimately positive, divine, and evolutionary energies that give rise to and sustain all that exists." Though the new spirituality of African American women may draw upon "traditional Christian religions," Hull affirms that it also "freely incorporates elements popularly called 'New Age'—Tarot, chakra work, psychic enhancement, numerology, Eastern philosophies of cosmic connectedness, and others."[41]

Relearning goddess worship has been linked to a striking revival of interest in a related pre-Christian spiritual tradition. Books on witchcraft, both fiction and nonfiction, move briskly from the shelves of the largest bookselling chains. Von Braschler, director of trade sales for the largest occult publishing house, Llewellyn International of St. Paul, Minnesota, states that the "typical reader" of books on witchcraft "is a very young woman in her teens." So intense is the interest in these books that "more than half of the 100 titles that Llewellyn publishes revolve around Wiccan themes."[42] Estimates of actual practitioners of the pre-Christian, nature-based spiritualities known generally as Wicca or witchcraft range up to 1.5 million.[43] Popular teen websites such as Bolt.com direct their mainly female visitors to a wide array of links dealing with witchcraft and the occult.[44]

An example of the many popular books in this genre is Phyllis Curott's *Book of Shadows.*[45] Rejecting what she calls "the Church's crusade to suppress the Old Religion of the Goddess and to establish religious hegemony," Curott writes that she is contributing to "a renaissance of a pre-Hebraic, pre-Christian, and pre-Islamic Goddess worship" through her advocacy of witchcraft.[46] She asks, "How can we rediscover the sacred from which we have been separated for thousands of years?"[47] Old spirituality is suddenly new again.

This is the message of Ashleen O'Gaea's *The Family Wicca Book* as well. Noting that in "pre-patriarchal primal cultures . . . the first human beings were cooperative and gentle with each other," O'Gaea shows families how to return to the Old Religion of our ancient ancestors.[48] Wicca develops around honoring the Great Mother, but acknowledges a large number of gods. It also teaches reincarnation and incorporates rites, spells and holy days from early European tribal groups. With chapters including "Raising Children to the Craft," O'Gaea instructs parents on how to teach basic witchcraft to their children. "Our life as a family of witches is full and satisfying," she writes. "Wicca permeates our lives, enriches our lives, guides our lives."[49] O'Gaea claims that Wicca is gaining wide acceptance, and that growing numbers of covens of practicing witches now meet in many American cities.

Of course, no discussion of the renewed interest in witchcraft and magic can exclude the current international sensation, J. K. Rowling's Harry Potter series. With four books and two movies in release at this writing, the Potter phenomenon is unparalleled. The four books have been translated into two hundred languages, and sales are now in excess of $110 million. The first of the Harry Potter movies, *Harry Potter and the Sorcerer's Stone*, smashed box office records in its first week of release with ticket sales of more than $97 million. After only twenty days in theatres, box office receipts were well in excess of $220 million, putting the Potter movie on a trajectory to match the enormous success of George Lucas's *Star Wars* blockbusters. Though controversy has raged around the witchcraft themes in Rowling's literary and cinematic stories, the public has found little reason to resist the appeal of these captivating supernatural tales created against a backdrop of magic.

Hidden Judaism, emerging Buddhism. This rising tide of interest in "new" religious traditions with ancient roots is not limited to disaffected Christians fleeing Protestantism and Catholicism for refreshingly unfamiliar spiritual territory such as goddess worship and Wicca. Rabbis David A. Cooper and Leibl Wolf, among many others, have successfully revived interest among upwardly mobile American, Australian and European Jews in the ancient mystical Jewish teachings of the kabbalah. Cooper's *God Is a Verb* and Wolf's *Practical Kabbalah* offer popular, simplified treatments of a highly complex and traditionally secret system of textual interpretation.[50] But Yahweh and the increasingly popular deity of kabbalah—an impersonal force known as Ein Sof—appear to be two different entities.

Of course, ancient Eastern traditions have shaped the new spirituality even more dramatically than have ancient Middle Eastern ones. Buddhist influence is evident

virtually everywhere on the contemporary cultural scene. Rodger Kamenetz's book *The Jew in the Lotus* affirms the relevance of Buddhist thought and practice for modern Jews.[51] Motivational seminars emphasizing elements of Buddhist thought attract hundreds of thousands of business leaders at great cost by promising power, peace, mystical experience and business success. As early as 1985, John Heider's *The Tao of Leadership: Leadership Strategies for a New Age*, popularized for the business community the teachings of fifth-century B.C. Chinese sage Lao-Tzu.[52] The book taught executives "how to govern or educate others in accordance with natural law." Among the foundational principles of this natural law are "I am one with everything else" and "all creation is a single whole that operates according to a single principle."[53]

Buddhist thought has received a boost from perhaps the most popular person in contemporary America, Oprah Winfrey. Through her television program, website and magazine, Winfrey has introduced her audiences to a variety of new spiritual approaches. The August 2001 edition of *O: The Oprah Magazine* features an upbeat interview with the Dalai Lama. Oprah asks if "there wasn't part of you that had always known you were different?" The Dalai Lama replies, "Sometimes I do feel that, yes, I may feel some effect of previous lives. . . . I have had glimpses of memory from past lives in which I identify with those from, in some cases, one or two centuries ago. I once had the feeling that I may have been in Egypt 600 years ago."[54]

The Dalai Lama himself has had an inestimable impact as a proponent of Buddhist values and practices in the West. One of the nation's most popular business books in 1999 was the Dalai Lama's *Ethics for the New Millennium*, selling more copies than popular books for executives by Bill Gates and Stephen Covey. The Dalai Lama's book resided near the top of *The New York Times* bestseller list for nine weeks, and "was listed as that paper's number two business book for six weeks."[55] In fact, the Dalai Lama has produced a steady stream of popular books for Western readers over the past several years. His recent titles include *Transforming the Mind*, *The Art of Happiness* and *The Path to Tranquility*.[56] Even the Dalai Lama's mother has become an author of note with her recent release of *My Son: A Mother's Story*, which is edited by her grandson, Khedroob Thondup.[57] Of late, the Dalai Lama's spiritual perspective has received a crucial assist from Hollywood as well. A host of recent popular movies including *Seven Years in Tibet* and *Kundun* have presented Buddhist ideas in a sympathetic and persuasive fashion to millions of viewers.

Has all of this emphasis on the wisdom of the Buddha had any particular effect in the traditionally Christian United States? By one estimate, the number of

American adherents to some aspect of Buddhist teaching now exceeds ten million. This number represents an incredible increase from the estimated 200,000 Buddhists residing in the United States in 1960, most of them Asians living in California or Hawaii.[58]

Spiritual science and scientific religion. On the contemporary religious scene, spiritual insights arise nearly as often in the arena of science as in that of religion. Fritjof Capra helped to popularize the idea that science reveals the spiritual nature of the physical universe in books such as *The Tao of Physics* (1975) and his 1982 bestseller, *The Turning Point*.[59] In his recent book *The Web of Life*, Capra contends that science proves that "living nature is mindful and intelligent." Thus, there is no need to maintain the old notion of a specially created universe with "overall design or purpose."[60] Similarly, the notion of "self" or individual identity, a mainstay of Western metaphysics, has yielded to Buddhist-inspired scientific thinking. "The Buddhist doctrine of impermanence includes the notion that there is no self," he writes. "Cognitive science has arrived at exactly the same position . . . our self, our ego, does not have any independent existence."[61]

The New Science often has arrived at conclusions paralleling Eastern religious thought, such as the illusional nature of physical matter. Thus for Fred Alan Wolf the new physics demonstrates that "reality is not made of stuff, but is made of possibilities that can be coherent so that possibility forms into matter" under the direction of consciousness, including even human consciousness.[62] He declares that new scientific findings suggest that "the universe is being created in a dream of a single spiritual entity," and that each individual human consciousness may reflect that entity. "Are we the dreamer?" he asks.[63] Another physicist, Amit Goswami, contends that "science proves the potency of monistic philosophy over dualism—over spirit separated from matter."[64] That is, for these writers science disproves the Judeo-Christian notion of a personal God existing distinctly separate from his creation.

This trend toward spiritualizing science continues in books by a host of contemporary writers working the New Science beat. Examples include Gary Zukav's *The Dancing Wu Li Masters: An Overview of the New Physics* and, more recently, Fred Allen Wolf's *The Spiritual Universe: How Quantum Physics Proves the Existence of the Soul*.[65] Capra and Wolf are physicists who claim that the findings of a spiritualized science will be crucial to the next wave of religion in the West. In several important respects this "new wave" actually reflects a return to ancient spiritual traditions. Similarly, in *The Aquarian Conspiracy*, Ferguson presented her readers nothing less

than "a startling worldview that gathers into its framework breakthrough science and insights from the earliest recorded thought."[66]

Turning this idea of a spiritualized science on its head, some anthropologists are now suggesting that we look to the spiritual world for scientific insights. In his essay, "Shamans and Scientists," Canadian anthropologist Jeremy Narby reports a fascinating encounter between three molecular biologists and a shaman residing in the Peruvian Amazon.[67] Each of the biologists voluntarily enters a drug-induced trance under the guidance of the shaman, and each puts several questions to various entities encountered in this state. For instance, one of the scientists specializing in reproductive research asked the spirit guide, "was there a key protein that makes sperm cells fertile?" The answer he received was, "No, there is not a key protein. In this organ there are no key proteins, just many different ones which have to act together for fertility to be achieved."[68]

Narby comments that "in interviews conducted in their respective laboratories four months after the Amazonian experience, the three biologists agreed on a number of key points. All three said that the experience of ayahuasca shamanism changed their way of looking at themselves and at the world."[69] Moreover, all three scientists said they are "planning to return to the Amazon at some point" to pursue further understanding of how shamanism might contribute to scientific knowledge.

Psychology, psychiatry and medicine: insight, healing and alien voices. A sharp tension between science and religion often characterizes public debates about educational policy. Surprisingly, many of today's popular religious works suggest a different picture—the alleged spiritual wasteland of the sciences is, on closer inspection, replete with oases to refresh the spiritual seeker, deep pools furnished by hidden and unstaunchable springs of religious insight.

It is perhaps less surprising that psychology, psychiatry and medicine have recently provided alternatives to traditional Western religious thought for the modern thirster after spiritual truth. For instance, popular psychoanalyst Mark Epstein, in books such as *Buddhism and the Way of Change: A Positive Psychology for the West* and *Going to Pieces Without Falling Apart: A Buddhist Perspective on Wholeness* presents a Buddhist approach to psychology and counseling. Epstein affirms that "within psychotherapy lies the potential for an approach that is compatible with Buddhist understanding, one in which the therapist, like the Zen master, can aid in making a space in the mind."[70] Far from occupying the fringe of psychotherapeutic practice, the *Chicago Tribune* has written that "Epstein is on the cutting edge of change as psycho-

therapy and spirituality, once antagonistic, move toward a rapprochement."[71]

These particular spiritual springs started flowing early in the twentieth century. Carl Jung, a founder of psychoanalysis, introduced ancient Gnostic and Eastern religious thought to Western psychoanalytic theory and practice. Richard Noll argues in *The Jung Cult: Origins of a Charismatic Movement* that Jung's ideas are steeped in the gnostic teachings that Jung so admired. He is today a more potent influence in counseling circles than is Sigmund Freud, and Jung reading groups meet across the Western world to cultivate spiritual insight.[72]

Navigating rather more alien waters, Harvard professor of psychiatry John Mack attributes shamanic religious insight to the scores of UFO abductee claimants that he has counseled. His original alien abduction book, *Abduction: Human Encounters with Aliens*, was a bestseller.[73] More recent titles include *Secret Life: Firsthand, Documented Accounts of UFO Abductions* and *Passport to the Cosmos: Human Transformation and Alien Encounters.*[74] Mack insists that we must study and heed the spiritual truths being taught us by extraterrestrial visitors through their abductee messengers.

Helen Schucman (1909-1981), a professor of medical psychology at Columbia University's College of Physicians in New York City in the late 1960s and early 1970s, also asks us to listen to the spiritual wisdom of voices from beyond. She and colleague William Thetford, disillusioned with traditional psychological and psychiatric techniques, began to seek "another way." Over a period of three months, Schucman claims to have experienced a virtually uninterrupted flow of "highly symbolic dreams and descriptions" as well as "strange images." For seven years from 1965 through 1972 "a Voice" attributed to Jesus Christ delivered to her a long series of messages which she dictated to Thetford.

The result of this lengthy process of spiritual wisdom transmission was the ponderous bestseller *A Course in Miracles.*[75] The wild popularity of this channeled mix of advice and spiritual insight is indeed surprising to any objective observer who has attempted to wade through its nearly incomprehensible prose. Nevertheless, that humans possess divinity, that sin is an empty concept, that the creation is an illusion, that we save ourselves from spiritual darkness, that "there is not past or future," that "birth into a body has no meaning," that sickness is the result of faulty thinking, and that death is "the central dream from which all illusions stem" are all repeated themes.[76]

This sort of approach to the mind and its latent powers has driven the phenomenon of schools for psychic development. In January 2000 the Associated Press

reported "a nationwide surge in facilities known as enlightenment schools and metaphysical institutions." These schools include The Advanced Metaphysical Studies Center in New York, The Berkeley Psychic Institute and the College of Metaphysics in Clearwater, Florida. Students learn to "develop their psychic abilities" and "read the thoughts of others." The Berkeley Psychic Institute has taught classes in "meditation, healing and intuition" to more than 100,000 students over the past twenty-five years.[77]

The body as well as the mind is a subject of interest to practitioners of alternative spiritualities. "Alternative medicine," healing practices often based on a spiritual paradigm rivaling the traditional Western worldview, has now become as popular as more conventional medical treatment with the general public. In 1999, Americans spent as much money out of their own pockets on alternative medical products and services as they did on conventional medical treatments. To satisfy this vast market, numerous authors have advocated healing techniques ranging from "visualizing" health to deep massage. Medical students today are encouraged, and sometimes required, to explore the possibilities in alternative healing techniques such as therapeutic touch, while prominent medical schools have now established centers for the study of the mind-body healing connection. Ruth Walker of *The Christian Science Monitor* reports that "the trend toward inclusion of some form of spiritual practice in healthcare appears to be accelerating." She adds that "this year, 72 medical schools—well over half of those in the United States—have offered some kind of course on spirituality and healing. This represents an increase from only three such courses in 1992."[78]

Works devoted to alternative healing have steadily increased in popularity. Books by authors such as Yale surgeon Bernie S. Siegel, author of *Love, Medicine, and Miracles* and *Peace, Love, and Healing*, have sold millions of copies and occupy dozens of feet of shelf space in book stores. Other prominent figures in the alternative medical field include Indian physician Deepak Chopra, author of *The New York Times* number one bestseller *Ageless Body, Timeless Mind*, and Andrew Weil, author of *Spontaneous Healing* and many other related titles. Journalist Peter Fenton has retrieved the medical secrets of the East for Western readers in his popular book *Tibetan Healing: The Modern Legacy of Medicine Buddha*.

Meditation techniques derived from Eastern religious practices and physical regimens such as yoga have become an integral part of the stress reduction for millions of Westerners. Readers of Stephen Cope's *Yoga and the Quest for the True Self*

learn how to employ ancient Hindu religious exercises to alleviate modern Western consumerist stress. And the *Tantric Toning* videotape series brings Hindu insights to physical training for the aerobically inclined.

Finally, we might note that neurologist and Zen practitioner Dr. James H. Austin has suggested that our study of the sources of altruism and other "higher motives" in the human brain might be guided by the insights of ancient Zen masters. "Perhaps we would be advised to begin our searching for their subtler, deeper networks in the limbic system, thalamus, basal ganglia, and brain stem," he writes. "Indeed, there will always be multiple levels of interpretation of Master Chi-chen's statement, 'The way upward is by descending lower.'"[79]

TALKING ABOUT SPIRITUALITY

Though goddess worship, the New Science, Buddhist-inspired motivational seminars, UFO abduction reports, spiritually oriented psychology and alternative medical practices may seem at first glance to have little to do with one another, each phenomenon reflects changes in the Western world's basic spiritual orientation. It is my view, as noted above, that such phenomena also betoken a concerted and successful effort on the part of a large number of spiritual advocates, including writers, speakers and performing artists, to open new religious pathways in the Western mind.

Shaping a society's thinking on an important topic such as religious belief is a complex process involving many sources, pressures and influences. One often-neglected but important force shaping our spiritual views is public religious discourse, that is, the many ways we communicate about and seek to persuade one another regarding spiritual matters. Public religious discourse includes speeches, essays, fiction and nonfiction books, self-help manuals, television programs, movies, plays and other forms of communication about religion. Such communication often is intentionally persuasive, and the success of this persuasive effort is particularly likely when similar messages are encountered repeatedly in various media—print, film, music, television, magazines and so on.

Spiritual advocates engaged in public religious discourse have constituted a powerful force shaping Western religious thought since their first prominent public appearance around 1700, and that shaping influence has continued unabated to the present day. Popular books, widely circulated periodicals and public lectures carried religious ideas in the eighteenth century. To these were added mass circu-

lation magazines and the enormously popular American public lecture circuits in the nineteenth century. Movies, popular music, radio and television and other mass media provided additional avenues for disseminating religious ideas in the twentieth century. Advocates of religious ideas—believing and skeptical, orthodox and heterodox—have exploited each medium as it has appeared. That is to say, advocates engaged in public religious discourse have never simply *reflected* what the public was thinking. They have also persuaded us, changed our minds, shaped our views of what is true or false, right or wrong, assumed or questioned in religion.

In the following chapters I highlight some of these persuasive efforts on behalf of a particular set of religious ideas constituting the New Religious Synthesis. Most of my examples are from the print media, especially books, both fiction and nonfiction. Books have remained a constant source of public discussion of religious ideas since 1700, and books have been the characteristic medium of Western contention over religious ideas. I have also included a number of tracts and pamphlets, some popular movies, several speeches, one or two plays and the occasional television program. The works examined by no means exhaust the important public statements on spiritual themes in the modern period. Rather, they are merely representative examples, occasionally odd ones, of important efforts to persuade the reading and viewing public to new ways of thinking about spiritual matters. This synthesis of concepts now constitutes a widespread framework for understanding ourselves and the spiritual world.

THE REVEALED WORD AND THE NEW RELIGIOUS SYNTHESIS

I referred earlier to two comprehensive spiritual views or systems. One I have termed the Revealed Word, the other the New Religious Synthesis. It may be helpful at this point to outline these perspectives. Some readers will take issue with my characterization of the principal components of either system, but the following overviews will at least serve to express in general terms what I intend by these labels. Subsequent chapters will clarify the contours and expand on the content of each perspective.

Religious thinking is a trait of virtually all human beings. For much of the last two millennia that thinking in the Western world typically has been informed by biblical presuppositions, even when biblical *piety* was notably absent. And yet, the working religious assumptions of many, perhaps most, Western people today are

not the assumptions of what I have called the Revealed Word. Though it would be difficult to achieve agreement on the point even within the Christian community, the following tenets provide a recognizable sketch of the Revealed Word perspective. I recognize that not all Christians at all times have accepted this entire set of beliefs. With the exception of the reference to Jesus Christ as God incarnate and the authority of the Christian Scriptures, many orthodox Jews would affirm these propositions as well, though certainly disparity of belief marks the Jewish community as it does the Christian. The following, then, are a reasonable approximation of the commitments making up the spiritual perspective I have called the Revealed Word, the spiritual outlook dominant in the Western world until relatively recently.

The Revealed Word. I will begin with the very notion of a word from God, which is, not surprisingly, at the center of the Revealed Word view.

1. *The supernatural authority of the Judeo-Christian Scriptures.* The Bible is taken to be divinely delivered and thus uniquely authoritative as a source of religious truth. The Scriptures record messages delivered to humanity by God through various means—prophetic utterance, the traditions and wisdom of Israel, the life and teachings of Jesus of Nazareth. The Revealed Word perspective is based on this written record. Where the record relates events, including miraculous events, these are usually assumed to be historical and not symbolic or mythological.

2. *A personal, creating and wholly other God.* The traditional attributes of God present him as all-knowing, present everywhere and all-powerful. That this God is also personal is assumed in these attributes, meaning that he possesses traits of a personality—thoughts, motives, emotions and the capacity to form relationships. This personal, all-powerful God is credited with creating the physical and spiritual worlds ex nihilo or out of nothing. Moreover, he remains "wholly other," neither contained in nor equivalent with the created order.

3. *God's creation of the human race.* Assumed in the concept of God's creative activity is his creation of the human race. However, it needs to be noted that the Revealed Word alleges that the human race is a special creation of God, the only part of the creation said to bear "his image." This commitment to the special creation of the human race has historically been taken to imply that humans are not a product of strictly natural processes.

4. *An intervening God.* The Revealed Word affirms that God's activity includes

involvement in the lives of individual human beings. On occasion, this intervening God communicates directly with human beings and at other times miraculously alters the ordinary course of cause and effect. Though this personal and active God invites address and petition through prayer, this does not imply that the divine is a power at the command of human beings.

5. *Humankind's Fall.* The human race experienced a Fall into sin early in its existence, a consequence of the earliest humans' refusal to recognize a divinely mandated limitation on their activities. This Fall carried with it various catastrophic consequences, including spiritual confusion, a state of spiritual separation from God and the inevitability of physical death.

6. *Jesus Christ as God Incarnate.* The historical figure of Jesus Christ uniquely manifested God in human form. Jesus is a revelation of God's nature in a person and the only human being ever to express fully the divine nature. Moreover, the death and resurrection of Jesus Christ are uniquely redemptive of fallen humanity. These events are the sole provision by God for the salvation of the   human race.

7. *Human destiny and divine judgment.* The Revealed Word insists that the destiny of the human race is to be determined by God. Neither the present earth nor the human race exists indefinitely. A final judgment of the human race will occur, and each individual human being will be held accountable for the life lived. It should be noted that the Revealed Word perspective maintains that each human lives only one life.

The New Religious Synthesis. As already noted, the past three centuries have witnessed a stunning shift in Western religious thinking away from the tenets outlined above. For many of us a new set of religious commitments has now replaced the fundamental claims of the Revealed Word. The following are, I will maintain, the basic components of this New Religious Synthesis. This alliance of available, complementary spiritual commitments constitutes the background assumptions currently shaping much of our contemporary religious thought. Moreover, at every critical juncture these new presuppositions pose a dilemma: either the New Synthesis correctly describes reality or the Revealed Word does. But on no crucial point can both systems be true at the same time. Here, briefly stated, are the components of the Other Spirituality.

1. *History is not spiritually important.* History as a record of events in space and time has no particular significance to the spiritual understanding or progress of the

individual human being or of religious communities. In fact, history as traditionally understood may be a hindrance to spirituality by tying people to local beliefs, particular places and individual teachers. Records purporting to be spiritual histories, the prime example being the Bible, are not principally historical. Rather, such sacred texts are largely symbolic, allegorical or mythic.

2. *The dominance of reason.* Reason—also mind, consciousness, intellect, awareness or imagination—is the divine characteristic in humans. It is virtually unlimited in its potential for development through scientific study, mystical experience and evolution. Reason is the principal means for human apprehension of spiritual truth, with the most substantial spiritual insights coming to those with the greatest awareness, the most highly evolved consciousness or the most capacious reason.

3. *The spiritualization of science.* Science, the empirical study of the material universe, is the principal instrument reason employs to acquire spiritual knowledge. Science is both the source and the test of theology—it discovers new spiritual truths and confirms what has long been known to human beings through certain spiritual traditions.

4. *The animation of nature.* Nature is infused with a divine spirit, consciousness or life force. Physical nature is thus alive with divine energy or soul. In short, nature is divine. This fact about physical nature warrants its study by science as a source of spiritual knowledge.

5. *Hidden knowledge and spiritual progress.* Knowledge is the key to spiritual insight and human progress. Such knowledge comes by means of reason employing science, but it may also come through certain individuals specially gifted to understand and directly experience the spiritual realm. Spiritual knowledge, then, is the special preserve of extraordinarily gifted individuals including some scientists, but also a new class of shamans, mediums between the physical and spiritual realms. Because this spiritual knowledge is not immediately accessible to all people, it is, at least initially, hidden or secret.

6. *Spiritual evolution.* Human beings are destined to realize unimaginable spiritual advancement through a process of spiritual evolution. Spiritual evolution is not simply change, but advancement that occurs incrementally over time. The eventual result of this process of spiritual evolution will be actual human divinity. Through science, the means of directing and hastening this process is now within our grasp.

7. *Religious pluralism as rooted in mystical experience.* The only universal religious experience is the mystical experience. Thus, mysticism provides a basis for reli-

gious pluralism, for the uniting of disparate spiritual traditions around common mystical insights. There is a steadily increasing awareness of this fact within each religious tradition.

GOALS OF THE STUDY

This book examines certain representative and highly influential statements that have contributed to a radically new way of thinking about religion in the West. These statements have contributed importantly to the twofold public activity of religious criticism on the one hand and spiritual invention on the other. My goal is to trace the historical trajectory in popular religious discourse of a set of religious ideas that, though once considered exotic or even heretical, now hold sway in the Western religious mind. I hope not only to clarify the sources and interconnections of the ideas making up the New Religious Synthesis, but also to assess the implications of our new spirituality for human happiness. After all, the goal of true spirituality ought to be contributing to our fulfillment, freedom and contentedness as people. Thus, the concluding chapter offers my own assessment as to which system—the New Religious Synthesis or the Revealed Word—is a preferable guide to human spirituality.

The great psychoanalyst Carl Jung, himself an important proponent of a new way in religion, noted in 1933 that a new religious mind was rising in the West as Judeo-Christian thought waned correspondingly. He evaluated the situation as the simple outworking of a powerful psychic law. "I cannot take it as an accident," he wrote. "It seems to me rather to satisfy a psychological law." And what was Jung's law? "For every piece of conscious life that loses its importance and value—so runs the law—there arises a compensation in the unconscious. . . . No psychic value can disappear without being replaced by another of equal intensity."[80]

Jung was right that a fundamental shift in Western religious attitudes was occurring in the twentieth century. However, as indicated above, I do not believe the available evidence supports the notion that this change resulted from the operation of a mindless principle analogous to "the conservation of energy in the physical world." The rise of the Other Spirituality is not so much the outworking of a psychic law as the result of sustained, intentional and successful public efforts to change the Western religious mind. The next chapter surveys some spiritual movements occurring prior to 1700 that helped to prepare the ground for the long program of spiritual persuasion that followed, and of which we are the inheritors.

2

ANTECEDENTS OF THE
NEW RELIGIOUS SYNTHESIS

A Brief History of Alternative Spirituality in the West

Secrecy was a trait of all [occult organizations] and was inseparable from the very concept of esotericism, which flourishes among men who enjoy the distinction of possessing rare knowledge.
WAYNE SHUMAKER,
The Occult Sciences in the Renaissance

The human mind "reflected" a divinely ordered universe in such a way that the magus could tap the hidden powers of the universe.
HUGH KEARNEY,
Science and Change, 1500-1700

Before considering the specific persuasive efforts that toppled the Revealed Word outlook and formulated the Other Spirituality, it will be helpful to survey some important early developments that set the stage for a dramatic shift in public religious attitudes. The religious ideas that are our principal focus did not suddenly emerge in 1700, but were in many ways outgrowths of intriguing spiritual movements in medieval and Renaissance Europe. A number of social, intellectual and religious developments between 1300 and 1700 profoundly shaped subsequent Western religious attitudes, thus helping to prepare the ground for a long campaign of public spiritual advocacy.

SPIRITUAL COMMUNITIES IN THE MIDDLE AGES

A number of influential spiritual communities in medieval Europe advocated spiritual practices and doctrines that contradicted the Revealed Word perspective. For example, historian Leonard Levi writes of a fascinating medieval spiritual movement that challenged Christian thought at a time when the church enjoyed per-

haps its greatest dominance in Europe. The Free Spirits, young vagabonds who preached free love, mystical union with God, and the rejection of conventional morality, roamed across Europe in the thirteenth and fourteenth centuries. The men in the movement called themselves Beghards, the women Beguines.

Rejecting the trinitarian conception of God, Free Spirits insisted that divinity dwelled in every individual. When a person recognized this truth, she was a step closer to recognizing her own divinity. Free Spirits sought to liberate the soul from its fleshly constraints, and found conventional moral precepts irrelevant and an impediment to spiritual development. As Levi writes, "life itself was incarnation and resurrection. 'The divine essence is my essence and my essence is the divine essence,' said a Free Spirit. Another said he was 'wholly transformed into God,' so that not even the Virgin Mary could tell the difference. 'Rejoice with me, I have become God,' announced a third."[1] The Free Spirits collected their theology from gnosticism, mysticism and other sources.

Of greater concern to the medieval church were the gnostic communities spread through southern and eastern Europe. Gnosticism is the belief that secret knowledge—*gnosis*—allows certain highly disciplined individuals to transcend the limits of time and the physical body. Gnostic sects such as the Cathars, Bogomiles and Albigensians were common and influential, especially in the Balkans. Some of these groups spread even into Western Europe where the Inquisition eventually wiped them out.

These European sects reflected the typical gnostic division between masters (or *perfecti*) and the uninitiated (or *credenti*, believers). Gnostic sects attributed great power to Satan, including the creation of the world. Some taught that the cosmos reflected a struggle between a good force, associated with light and the God of the New Testament, and an evil spiritual force, associated with darkness and the God of the Old Testament. For this reason, most medieval gnostic groups rejected the teachings of the Old Testament and denigrated the God of creation.

Birth into a body was seen as either a punishment for sins during a soul's prior existence or as an opportunity for the spirit to liberate itself through *gnosis*. Gender itself was an evil consequence of the soul being embodied, and sexual intercourse often was discouraged for the same reason. Among the medieval gnostic sects of Europe, ritual suicide by starvation, called the *endura*, was also practiced. Self-imposed starvation, according to the masters, ensured a soul's advancement if an individual could not master sufficient secret knowledge to become one of the *perfecti*.

Also practiced as a sacrament was baptism into immortality by the laying on of hands by *perfecti,* termed the *consolamentum.* The Church specifically condemned this practice, leading to widespread persecution of gnostic groups. Thus, the *perfecti* dominated the lives of the *credenti,* literally holding in their hands the power of life, death and eternal blessing. Earthly life itself was considered by some groups to be hell, or punishment for sin, a fate from which only *gnosis* could provide release.

MAGIC AND THE HERMETIC TRADITION

Hermeticism is a secret magical tradition based on a set of fourteen books known collectively as the *Corpus Hermeticum* and falsely attributed to a mythical figure known as Hermes Trismegistus. The Hermetic teachings that made their way into Western Europe were based on the systems of various philosophers and teachers in Alexandria, Egypt, between A.D. 150 and 300. Even earlier Greek origins are often claimed for the ideas. Wayne Shumaker writes, "Hermeticism was basically a Greek contemplative mysticism developed on Egyptian soil. Its sources were mainly in popular Greek philosophical thought, ... but details appear to have been borrowed from Judaism, Persian religion, and, more doubtfully, from Christianity."[2]

Hermetic writings came into Europe when "a monk named Leonardo da Pistoia brought to Florence a Greek manuscript known as the *Corpus Hermeticum.*"[3] A Latin translation and tireless promotion by the enormously influential Humanist Marsilio Ficino (1433-1499) ensured the prominence of Hermetic teachings throughout Europe. Renaissance European scholars ascribed Hermetic secrets to Pythagoras, the ancient Chaldeans, the Egyptians and Zoroaster.[4] Renaissance philosophers were fascinated with the occult Greek and Egyptian teachings contained in Hermetic works. Among the most prominent of these was the handsome, brilliant and charismatic scholar, Pico della Mirandola (1463-1494). Shumaker writes, "the early support of a man who was learned, attractive, and of noble birth contributed to the system's prestige."[5] Another important Renaissance advocate was the famous speculative thinker Giordano Bruno (1548-1600).

Hermeticism emphasized mental or spiritual experience over physical; time and space are irrelevant, and history illusory. Only the interior life of the mind mattered, and God was referred to simply as *Nous* or Mind. This elevation of Mind suggested a corresponding hatred of the body akin to gnostic teaching. Mind "uses the body" to attain ever greater knowledge toward the goal of individual spiritual insight. Thus, Hermeticism often was marked by an ascetic disregard for the body, seen as

an impediment to spiritual progress that would eventually be dispensed with. The body had no real significance, and was irrelevant to the spiritual life. As various secret spiritual techniques were mastered, Mind achieved control over time, space and the body. Greek and Egyptian Hermetic teachers suggested that the soul, once liberated from the body, could be ordered from place to place instantly. "Order your soul to transport itself to India; and it is there; send it to the ocean, and it seems not to have to travel to be where you wish it. What power you have, and what speed!"[6]

A pantheistic outlook that found divinity in everything also marked Hermeticism. The *Corpus Hermeticum* repeatedly claims that "the whole world is alive" and "permeated with life." A teacher in the Hermetic book *Asclepius* asks the student, "Have I not said that everything is one and that the one is everything, inasmuch as everything was in the Creator before He created all things."[7] The general view of God is reflected in a famous formulation attributed to various medieval mystics. God is "a circle whose center is everywhere and whose circumference is nowhere." Though this statement is not found in the *Corpus Hermeticum*, followers of Hermetic teachings include it in their own writings.

Divinity in the Hermetic tradition is incapable of description in human language. Thus, the highest spiritual experience is mysticism, or direct contact with the unspeakable divine essence. Such experience is not generally accessible to human beings, but rather is the special domain of the knowing few. This sphere of the divine consciousness is referred to as Poimandres, and great knowledge and self-control are required to enter it.

Hermetic teachers embraced the idea that daemons or spirit beings exercised some control over human destiny. Through the direction of a daemon, the human soul could attain unity with the divine consciousness of Poimandres. In spiritual ascent, the "self is given over to the daemon." The adept or enlightened individual "throws himself upward toward the spheres and is purged of a different vice as he passes through each." He thus moves toward God and "at length can become a Power and enter into God."[8]

The ultimate goal of Hermetic spirituality is the individual's divinity. The Hermetic master "passes into the nature of a god as if he were himself a god; he knows the race of daemons, inasmuch as he is aware that he has the same origin with them." He is "joined with the gods by his shared divinity" and takes on divine traits such as omnipresence. "He is everything at once, and everywhere." This transition to divine status can occur during the earthly life, so that Hermetists believed that "some men

are gods."[9] Human beings possessing spiritual secrets actually control daemons (gods) by calling them into their service through occult rituals and incantations. In the *Asclepius* some highly advanced teachers are said to make or create gods.

Such knowledge is, of course, not for everyone. The Hermetic master was a person of extraordinary mental ability, physical discipline and knowledge. This collection of traits proves the presence of mind in the individual, and Hermetic writings contain "constant exhortations to secrecy" and insist "that not all men possess mind."[10] Simply put, some people are spiritually superior to others, and their superiority can be enhanced through training in spiritual secrets.

Implied in Hermeticism—Hermes himself having been a man who became a god—is spiritual evolution from lower to higher states of existence. Human beings are themselves the product of a long spiritual evolutionary process that moves from "creeping things" to fish, mammals, birds and then people. Humans can—through occult knowledge and extraordinary ability—continue this evolutionary process and become daemons, then gods, and finally planets or stars. "This," writes Shumaker, "is the upward path."[11] Thus did the Hermetic tradition seek to absorb Jesus Christ into its cosmic scheme. He is "the Lord God and the Father of every talisman [magic formula] of the whole world." Hermeticism's tradition had broad currency in Renaissance Europe, shaping even popular thinking about the supernatural. As Shumaker writes, "evidently the Hermetic influence was not limited to the scholarly world but filtered down among the populace, and that with surprising rapidity." He concludes, "a predisposition existed in all classes of society" to accept the myths and symbols of Hermeticism, a fact that "suggests vividly an intellectual temper" willing to embrace a "new gospel."[12]

KABBALAH: SECRETS IN THE PENTATEUCH

The kabbalah (also spelled cabala, kabbala and kabala) is a collection of Jewish mystical writings built around the Hebrew alphabet and numerical system, especially as found in Jewish religious writing. Two Hebrew books, the *Sefer Yetzirah* (Book of Formation) and the *Zohar* (Brightness) provide the foundation of the kabbalah, with the latter being the more important source of teachings, though the former is older.[13] Their dating and authorship are contested—some scholars believe they reflect an oral tradition dating back to the Babylonian captivity, while others find them to be the work of medieval rabbis.[14] According to some contemporary teachers of the kabbalah, these mystical teachings were derived from an-

cient Jewish sages who had traveled to India. As support, they cite Genesis 25:6, which states that "Abraham sent his sons to the east."

By one stream of Jewish lore, the kabbalah was delivered from heaven by angels in order to teach Adam, "after his fall, how to recover his primal nobility and bliss." The more common account is that Moses received these secret teachings on Mount Sinai along with the law, and passed them on to an elite group of seventy elders. Thus, kabbalah is a system intended for the personal spiritual advancement of a spiritual elite through the appropriation of secret insights. "In order to be initiated into this mysterious and sacred science it was necessary to be distinguished not only by intelligence and eminent position, but also by advanced age, as well."[15] Kabbalah has long been viewed by many within Judaism as "a doctrine of superior profundity and purity reserved solely for a small number of the elect."[16]

Kabbalistic teaching shared a low view of the body, history and the physical world with both Hermeticism and Gnosticism, two of its sources. Professor Gershon Scholem, a leading authority on kabbalah, "considers the Kabbalah to be pre-Christian and Zoroastrian in origin."[17] Shlomo Shoham, another important student of the kabbalistic tradition, writes, "both the Kabala and Gnosis regard temporal existence as an incarceration of parts of divinity in profane bodies." Thus, he finds that "the quest for participation in the *Schechina* [mystical presence of God] and in the Sophia [cosmic Wisdom] is a longing for a more benign and boundless reality that contrasts with . . . profane creation."[18] That is, the world of ordinary existence is too limited for the spiritually initiated individual. In keeping with this observation, Adolphe Franck finds the spirit of kabbalah to be mystical.[19]

Creating and controlling God. Kabbalah inverts the Revealed Word relationship of creature to creator, rendering human beings virtually divine and their place of existence a boundless and transcendent reality rather than the profane world. Human beings control and even create God rather than the other way around. In kabbalah, "activation" of God by human beings is the goal, that is, the use of a divine force for human purposes.[20] Moreover, humanity must redeem the entire cosmic order, a task that includes repairing or "mending" (Hebrew: *tikkun*) an imperfect god-force. Shoham writes that the flawed god of kabbalah "can be mended by man and only by man." This limited divinity is "entirely dependent on man for his redemption." In fact, humanity's salvation will "follow with the successful mending of divinity."[21]

Kabbalah suggests that human beings may even "destroy god, or create a new god."[22] This is desirable, for the God of the Old Testament, the God "who created

us, made us breathe, eat, reproduce, and write books; who is responsible for our historical existence" is considered to be "blind, arrogant, and merciless."[23] Space and time "were created by a vile God" who needed both to fulfill his selfish plans. It was only "because of God's needs" that "creation and man were created."[24]

Human beings "emanated from God" rather than being created by him. Our role or mission is "to mend the blemished and suffering God," an activity which gives us "meaning and purpose" by making us "a partner to God." Such a partnership "is not possible with a theistic, 'perfect' God" of the type presented by the Revealed Word tradition. Thus, God's limitations or imperfections are actually necessary in order for human beings to assume their rightful role as God's managers and healers. Under the influence of such a theology, the human ego becomes convinced that it is "a unique and exclusive center of the cosmos."[25]

To be created in God's image means only that God and the self "are identical," but with the self firmly in control. The master of kabbalah achieves "transcendence" when he can "grasp" this truth internally. The link with God "through the inner self is direct and immediate—one has only to discover that it exists."[26] Thus, mystical experience of God takes precedence over reading the record of God's activities in revelation, the latter approach to the divine being bound to space and time, and constricted by unnecessary doctrinal concerns.

Shoham concludes, "there could be no greater subordination of transcendence to man than this Kabalist conception of God." The "blemished Kabalist God resigns himself from history," leaving the "management of meaning and values in a godless history to man." God is mankind's puppet who "merely reacts" to human desire. "Man not only influences God's essence and action . . . but actually provides him with the energy for being and doing."[27] By studying and practicing the kabbalah's teachings, human beings complete the creation of an unfinished cosmos.

The kabbalah emerged onto the European intellectual scene at around the same time as the *Corpus Hermeticum*, garnering tremendous interest and exerting unusual influence on Renaissance thought. In fact, Ficino's and Pico's interest in the Hermetic writings was rivaled only by their interest in the kabbalah. Thus, magical thinking dominated much of the European intellectual scene during the Renaissance. Interest in magic greatly affected the development of science as well.

NEO-PLATONISM AND MAGICAL SCIENCE

The philosophical movement known as Neo-Platonism was founded by Ploti-

nus (A.D. 205-270) and developed by disciples such as Porphyry (A.D. 232-303). Neo-Platonism, which claimed to extend the teachings of Plato, was tremendously influential among European Humanists and other intellectuals beginning in the fifteenth century. Historian of science Hugh Kearney writes that by the seventeenth century "its influence extended to the Cambridge Platonists (more properly, the Cambridge Neo-Platonists) and their greatest pupil, Sir Isaac Newton."[28]

A magical worldview characterized Neo-Platonic thought, as it did Hermetic and kabbalistic. The cosmos was secretly coded and would reveal its secrets only to the diligent seeker after truth. Numbers, sometimes revealed by spirits or daemons, were the cosmic encryption method that needed to be broken. Thus, the Neo-Platonic philosopher held to a "mystical reverence for numbers, not a wholesome respect for practical mathematical techniques." Neo-Platonists selected objects of study on the basis of their potential for yielding personal power. This view "encouraged secrecy and an interest in the occult for its own sake by which a work of art was seen as a magical emblem or a coded message for the initiate." Scholarship became a secret enterprise to benefit a privileged elite. Drawing on an ancient Pythagorean principle, the academy's goal was "to preserve its secrets for the favored few," especially those possessing great skill in mathematics.[29]

Like Gnosticism, Neo-Platonism held that the human soul was spirit held captive in matter. This belief set the Neo-Platonists at odds with Christian teaching, which stressed the unity of the human as body and soul, the ultimate redemption of each and the conviction that the material world had been created good. Neo-Platonists looked to ancient sources such as Hermes, Zoroaster and Orpheus, all of whom taught that a divine soul animated the material universe. God was not so much a divine person as a divine energy in all things. The earth and other celestial bodies were alive with a divine spirit.

Magical science. The scientific tradition in Renaissance Europe developed around three basic approaches: the organic, the mechanical and the magical. The organic emphasized living organisms, while the mechanistic searched for mechanical metaphors to explain the universe's operation. But it is the magical tradition that may have provided the Western world with the real impetus for scientific exploration. Hugh Kearney writes that judged by strictly rational criteria "the magical tradition appears to be the least rational of the three; yet judged by its contribution to the Scientific Revolution, we may see it as the most important."[30]

At the same time, this tradition laid the groundwork for many later developments in popular skepticism and in the ascent of a new religious mind.

Neo-Platonism was important to the development of the magical tradition in science. Likewise, magical scientists sought guidance from mystical sources such as the kabbalah and the *Corpus Hermeticum*. An analogy developed between the divine mind in the cosmos and the mind of the human investigator. According to this analogy, "the human mind 'reflected' a divinely ordered universe in such a way that the magus [scholar/magician] could tap the hidden powers of the universe."[31] Thus, the scientist was "a mystic who could hear the magical music of the universe."[32] Astrology took on particular importance.

These early scientists subscribed to the view that light was the giver of all life. The sun was especially important to magical scientists, which many took to be actually divine. Stars also were divine, and the scientists' attention was directed to the night skies in a desperate search for the clues that unlocked vast spiritual secrets conveyed in the movements and harmonies of the heavenly bodies. Astrological studies were rooted in the supposed works of the famous but nonexistent ancient scribe, Hermes Trismegistus, whom we already have met. This Hermetic tradition also found the sun to be "the visible God" who "sits upon a royal throne ruling his children the planets which circle around him."[33] The connection between Renaissance science and astrology could not have been closer.

The universe's music was mathematical in nature, and in numbers lay hidden "the secrets of the cosmos." Thus, phenomena that could be mathematically decoded, including musical harmonies, deserved careful study. The mystical scientist often was an ascetic "studying the occult, within the confines of an esoteric community." Like an ancient Gnostic, he held that the material world was "the last and lowest form of being."[34]

Mystical science became a search for the single element of matter that revealed the secret structure of the whole cosmos. The earth was a microcosm of the macrocosm of all reality. The same was alleged of the human body and of the mind. The universe's structure, once understood, could be manipulated to become a source of virtually miraculous power. Because such power was sought only for personal ends, the scientist's discoveries were always carefully guarded secrets. Obscure language and codes were employed to protect secrets from rivals.

As the Renaissance progressed, interest in cosmic secrets increased. Thus, the sixteenth century witnessed a flourishing of studies such as mathematics, astron-

omy and alchemy—the search for a means of transforming common metals into gold and discovering an elixir to extend life. Mathematical direction sometimes came through guiding spirits, as in the famous case of Edmund Kelley (1559-1595) who claimed to be "following the directions of the angelic spirits" in his mathematical investigations.[35]

Bruno. Of particular importance to the rise and dissemination of the magical view of science in the Renaissance was the restive Dominican monk Giordano Bruno (1548-1600), a native of Nola near Naples. Fleeing Italy for Geneva, and Geneva for Paris, Bruno lectured widely on Copernicanism and its prospect for unveiling a vast network of cosmic secrets. Bruno believed that a new religious view that would supersede Christianity was at hand, which led to his "repudiation of orthodox Christianity, including the Bible."[36] Eventually Paris became uncomfortable for the unorthodox thinker, and he found refuge in Oxford where he frequently lectured.

European gnostics accepted Bruno's spiritual vision in which the individual "gains access to the divine directly through his own inner illumination." Carl Raschke explains that "while Catholicism required acceptance of revealed truth or 'sacred doctrine' as the first principle from which understanding follows, the new gnosticism, as represented in Bruno's writings, insisted upon *self-consciousness* as the proper window to reality."[37] For Bruno, the path to such spiritual enlightenment was scientific study of the cosmos. Robert Sullivan writes that for Bruno the study of the stars "enabled the adept to internalize the universal order and so preserved him from any fear of death."[38] This kind of liberating scientific knowledge was available only to a small number of highly talented individuals.

Bruno viewed the universe as an infinite system of planets and suns, and held that many planets were inhabited. But his opinion was rooted not so much in the observations of Galileo, from which he drew support, but in his own mystical metaphysics. According to Bruno's speculations, the mind of God or "World Soul" was diffuse throughout the universe; that is, the universe was full of the divine. Moreover, because our own reason participates in the divine reason, there is essentially no limit to human reason.

At the same time, there is no reason to think that God limited his creation of intelligent species to our own small world. The universe is filled with intelligent creatures whose reason, like ours, manifests divine reason. Numbers unlock a store of astronomical secrets, and because these secrets are at the heart of metaphysics, mathematics takes on religious significance. In fact, Bruno subscribed to the gnos-

tic and Neo-Platonic notion that "the earth and the stars were alive," and they speak to us through mathematics.[39] Bruno and other metaphysical scientists gave this originally Greek idea great currency in Renaissance Europe.[40]

Bruno's theology was at its base pantheistic and monistic: divinity is diffuse throughout the universe and all things are ultimately one thing. His defense of this position influenced other European thinkers including Spinoza, and through Spinoza a wide range of religious radicals throughout the Western world.

Brahe. Also important to the rise of the magical view of science was the Danish astronomer Tycho Brahe (1546-1601), the teacher of Johann Kepler (1571-1630) when Brahe was at Prague. Brahe treated his astronomical findings as a private treasure trove, the resources of which he would eventually employ to "build up an unchallenged position of privilege in the world of astrology."[41] Brahe pursued his studies on the model of a "mystic seeking his salvation in the night sky, and jealously guarding the results which he achieved."[42] Brahe's famous Castle of the Heavens on the Island of Hveen, a private observatory funded by King Frederick II of Denmark, became a citadel where he worked tirelessly for twenty years with tremendous success. Brahe labored hard to improve the measurement techniques employed by astronomers, and his findings were crucial to later astronomical discoveries.

But it is the object of that success that is often misunderstood. Brahe was not pushing back the veil of the cosmos for the sake of advancing science. He was, rather, peering into the secrets of the material world in order to advance his own spiritual fortunes. Brahe had a great influence on Kepler, who continued Brahe's search for the keys to the secrets of the cosmos. Kepler's work provided the foundation for the insights of Sir Isaac Newton, perhaps the last of the great magical scientists. Other similar lines of influence from magical to modern science can be traced in chemistry, biology and medicine.

Pluralism. Neo-Platonists and magical scientists advocated a broad and largely undifferentiated view of religious belief. Roland Bainton affirms that "Renaissance mystics . . . sought to discover the same set of truths beneath the symbols of many systems: in the lore of Zoroaster, the mysteries of Hermes Trismegistus, in the alluring number speculations of the Jewish cabala." There were even efforts to found a World Parliament of Religions based on this common core of mystical insight, and the hope was advanced that all nations could be united under a single religious view. Bainton writes, "tolerance became the watchword even at the expense of an emasculated Christianity."[43]

Shumaker concurs: "The Renaissance thirst for synthesis, for syncretism, was unquenchable." Bradford Verter points out that Nicholas of Cusa, a scholar close to the Pope, argued in his *De pace fidei* (1453) for "a fundamental harmony linking all faiths to the worship of a common hidden God." Marsilio Ficino suggested in 1474 that "a member of any faith who displayed the moral virtues of Jesus was properly termed a Christian." Verter adds, "here were seeds of both esoteric mysticism and theological unitarianism."[44] Ficino alleged that Neo-Platonism was compatible with Christianity, while Pico blended Neo-Platonism, Hermeticism, Christianity and the kabbalah.[45] Cornelius Agrippa, another important magical scientist, added to these "astrology, numerology, alchemy, and much else."[46] Christianity, it seemed, was compatible with virtually every philosophy or system conceivable.

The search was on for the irreducible, primitive core of all religions, for "a system of pristine and universally harmonious theology."[47] Thus it was assumed, for example, that "all of Eastern religion must have been reducible to a single pattern, which no doubt would have proved to be a gentile approximation of Christianity."[48] Thus, although Neo-Platonism and magical science, on the one hand, and comparative religious studies, on the other, might seem unrelated, the connections between them were strong and direct.

EUROPEAN MYSTICISM

Various European mystics garnered large followings between 1200 and 1700. Their writings on mystical theology and experience contributed importantly to the development of spiritual alternatives to orthodox, doctrinal Christianity. Two of the more influential mystic writers, both German, were Meister Eckhart and Jacob Böhme.

Meister Eckhart. Johannes Eckhart, often called Meister Eckhart (c. 1260-c. 1327) was the founder of German Dominican mysticism. Joining the Dominicans early in his life, he studied in Paris and returned to Germany to hold a number of positions in the Dominican order. Eckhart's basic theology was pantheistic, and he taught the gnostic idea that the human soul carried within it a divine spark. Clashing with the Church, he was condemned as a heretic by Pope John XXII.

Eckhart's troubles stemmed from his unorthodox mysticism that led to claims such as "God begets his son in the soul," so that, "as some authorities say, the soul is made equal with God."[49] Eckhart's emphasis on a divine spirit in nature, the inherent divinity of the individual and the role of contemplation in spiritual advance-

ment made him a major influence on German intellectuals in the nineteenth and twentieth centuries.

After about the age of fifty, Eckhart's major responsibility in the Dominican order was to preach to contemplative nuns in their convents. During this period of time he wrote both his *Book of Divine Consolation* and *On Detachment*. In these and other works he set out his doctrine of the soul's union with God. As one stage in the process, the soul recognizes this union. Thus the individual and God become spiritually one and the same. Eckhart's teachings tended to reinforce the notion that the individual determined what was true in religion. As R. W. Southern writes, the emphasis on personal spiritual experience and development made "institutions of religion seem less important, and, if not wrong, at least irrelevant." This theme had profound implications for public arguments against Christianity in the Enlightenment period and beyond.[50]

The last stage in Eckhart's mystical path toward union with God was called *breakthrough*. The goal of much of Eckhart's mysticism was direct contact with God or "Godhead" (*Deitas* rather than *Deus*). But this goal can easily be misunderstood. It is not at all clear that Eckhart principally sought ecstatic experience. Rather, his main objective was triumph over the restraints of conventional theology toward the expression of a radical subjectivism in religious life. For instance, Eckhart wished to break through what he saw as the limiting doctrine of the Trinity in order to make contact with the Godhead beyond, the true divine essence.

Jacob Böhme. The mystic cobbler Jacob Böhme (1575-1624) influenced many later religious writers, among them some of the advocates of a New Religious Synthesis. Much of his basic theology is set out in the book *Aurora* (1612). He was not formally educated, but he read widely, particularly the works of mystical writers such as Paracelsus (1493-1541) and Valentin Weigel (1538-1588). Böhme claimed direct divine illumination in 1600, in the midst of which he glimpsed "the Being of Beings" and "the Abyss." He claimed a similar experience again in 1610. Böhme believed the external, physical world was a projection of an inner spiritual power. For him, God was absolute but not personal. The divine is continually expanding in search of self-knowledge, a process in which human beings may participate through contemplation.

The inner spiritual world of the individual is a prototype or analogy of the outward world of the physical universe, an idea similar to Bruno's notion of similitude between the cosmos and the mind. Böhme worked out an elaborate account of the forces at

play in the natural world, and then spiritualized these forces by labeling them with names such as "love" and "the Kingdom of God." He believed that mystical insight into the material and spiritual realms could bring about harmony and peace.

For Böhme, progress toward harmony was a matter of spiritual evolution, a process through which God himself has had to pass. A flash of mystical insight (*blitz*) reveals that one may either remain in the realm of desire or transcend it through self-denial or the death of self. This process, not atonement for human sin, is Böhme's interpretation of the suffering and death of Christ. Such speculation became a major influence on the English Quakers and later Romantic writers.

Mystics like Eckhart and Böhme tended to disregard history as an account of temporal affairs to be transcended and ignored. Christ's advent, for instance, was less important as a historical event than as a stage in divine evolution. Jesus' own life is translated into "an allegory of that which must take place in the inner life." Christ as God incarnate in history is insignificant, but Christ as a metaphor for spiritual progress is highly significant. The mystical view of history also has profound implications for a view of revelation. As Roland Bainton notes, "the Bible is valuable as testimony to an experience which can arise without the book and having arisen can dispense with it."[51] Not regarding the Bible as a historical record of God's redemptive work diminishes its value as history while elevating its value as spiritual allegory.

It is often said that mystics like Eckhart and Böhme emphasized the union of the human and divine. It might be more accurate to say that they sought to move from the material realm where humanity was caught to a spiritual realm where divinity could be apprehended by the individual will. As Bainton has noted, mysticism may be compatible with Christian practice as long as it is clear that the human and the divine are, in fact, different and can never be merged. But, he writes, "if the devotee is believed to be completely merged in the abyss of the Godhead, then the subject-object relationship, the polarity of the I and the Thou, so characteristic of the Hebrew-Christian tradition, is destroyed."[52] Both Eckhart and Böhme taught such complete merging of the divine and human. The old notion was destroyed, but a powerful new notion took its place—that what is human may become divine.

HUMANISM AND THE RISE OF BIBLICAL CRITICISM

During the period running from about 1400 to about 1650, Humanism as a European intellectual movement achieved genuine stature. Many Humanist assumptions provided a foundation for a full-scale popular assault on Christian

thought that began around 1700. A deep interest in the philosophies, languages and religious ideas of the ancient Greek and Roman worlds defined Humanism, first in Italy and later in other parts of Europe. European rediscovery of classical sources had an immediate and profound impact on moral and religious thinking. "At the beginning of the Renaissance," writes historian George T. Buckley, "the classics began to be read once more as literature." As a result "the Humanists soon discovered that in Seneca and Plutarch there was a system of morals worthy to be compared with the Christian."[53]

Humanistic skepticism regarding Christianity was especially powerful at Italian universities in cities such as Florence and Bologna, but gradually spread to northern Europe as well.[54] Questions about the unique truth of Christian theology grew out of the study of writers such as the Roman politician and philosopher Cicero and the Greek physician and philosopher Sextus Empiricus.[55] The recovery of ancient philosophical and religious traditions had a major and lasting impact on the Christian consensus in Europe. In fact, historian C. B. Schmitt writes, "the recovery and the reassimilation of the ancient writings were the primary factors in the evolution of the modern skeptical attitude."[56]

Reason's rise and revelation's decline. Reason—not tradition, revelation or authority—emerged during the Renaissance as the chief criterion of religious truth. Even Jesus Christ, Sebastianus Castellio (1515-1563) pointed out, resolved questions by using his senses and his reason. Sensory evidence and critical reason increasingly were taken as sufficient for resolving religious questions. The Bible was not self-evidently true, for reason determines what is self-evident, and much that the Bible had to say was not apparent to reason. Humanists rejected claims that the biblical texts stood above the critical assessments of reason. The tension between reason and revelation was becoming starkly evident, a tension we will examine more closely in a subsequent chapter.

Increased contact with other cultures and the emerging discipline of textual criticism encouraged Christianity's comparison with other religious systems in the Renaissance.[57] Oxford scholar William Chillingworth (1602-1643) urged in *The Religion of Protestants* (1637) that "schismatics, heretics, even heathen Turks, could find that their good lives led them to salvation."[58] In the seventeenth century, English writers John Toland and Charles Blount compared various religions in search of an irreducible core of common elements. Toland, like Roman Stoics, argued that all religions have many doctrines in common. By reconstructing the "original belief

from which the separate religions were supposed to have varied" one could discover the true, rational religion of the human race.[59] Toland and many Deists affirmed a single, primitive source of all religious thought.[60]

Renaissance Humanists sought a new approach to religion built on classical sources, textual criticism, human achievement and reason. A religion of autonomous reason informed by ancient conceptions of virtue began to take shape and was advanced as a rival to the old religion of Christianity based on allegedly irrational concepts such as revelation and miracles. One's apprehension of the divine did not depend upon church authority, Christian tradition or biblical accounts. Religious belief was a personal matter for reason alone to decide.

Early biblical criticism: dismantling the Revealed Word. With the development of literary criticism and a corresponding dramatic rise in knowledge of classical languages and ancient history, the tools were in hand to demonstrate that the biblical texts themselves were open to question. Moreover, as the works of early critics of Christianity were translated into European languages, the arsenal of arguments against the faith was supplied with new weapons. Thus, Humanism provided later writers with much material for developing public arguments against Christian belief.

Of course, the Bible had come under criticism from the first centuries of the Christian church when skeptics such as Porphyry developed arguments against its doctrines and historical claims. As noted above, Italian Humanists of the Renaissance also advanced the project of biblical criticism by comparing biblical teachings to the moral teachings of Greek and Roman philosophies and by encouraging historical study of biblical texts. However, the systematic public criticism of the Bible is a more recent European development, and one that has had greater impact on scholarly *and* popular attitudes toward Christianity than has perhaps any other. The following is not a history of biblical criticism so much as an effort to identify a few important moments in the advent of a critical tradition that became particularly important in shaping religious thought in the modern period.

Benedict de Spinoza. Benedict de Spinoza (1632-1677) laid the groundwork for later biblical criticism in his most famous work, *Tractatus theologico-politicus* (1670).[61] His writings were modified by French and Dutch religious radicals to provide material for the infamous book *Traite des trois imposteurs (The Treatise of the Three Impostors)*. This scandalous work, which was condemned in both the Netherlands and France, argued that Jesus, Moses and Muhammad were frauds and the religions they established false. The book's subtitle is revealing: *ou l'Esprit d M. Spinoza*

(or the Spirit of Mr. Spinoza). In other words, the *Treatise* sought to capture the spirit of Spinoza's corrosive criticism of the Bible. Jonathan Israel, a leading authority on Dutch history, writes that Spinoza's work was "turned by a group of Dutch and Huguenot freethinkers into a potent subterranean force" against Christianity.[62]

Many of Christianity's harshest critics were drawn to Spinoza. He affirmed the supremacy of reason and argued that the only religious truths were ones taught universally. Spinoza wrote, "I determined to examine the Bible afresh in a careful, impartial, and unfettered spirit, making no assumptions concerning it, and attributing to it no doctrines, which I do not find clearly set down therein."[63] Moreover, he suggested that passages he took to be implausible were "foisted onto the sacred writings by irreligious hands," adding that "whatsoever is contrary to nature is also contrary to reason, and whatsoever is contrary to reason is absurd, and *ipso facto*, to be rejected."[64] Spinoza questioned the dating and authorship of many biblical books, particularly in the Old Testament, and advanced philosophical arguments against miracles.[65]

Spinoza sought an acid that would dissolve notions such as traditional authorship and doctrinal inspiration, thus turning biblical criticism in a "negative and destructive" direction. With the publication of the *Tractatus*, "the tools of destruction were at hand."[66] He began with the assumption that "revelation as such does not happen" and had in mind to "discuss biblical interpretation [in order] to discredit the appearance of supernatural authority."[67]

Locke and the early English tradition. The English tradition of biblical criticism extends back at least to Sir Walter Raleigh's *History of the World* (1603-1616) and was more fully developed in Lord Herbert of Cherbury's *De religioni laici* (1645) and Sir Thomas Browne's *Religio medici* (1643), in which Browne challenged such rudimentary biblical doctrines as the Fall and the curse on Adam and Eve.[68]

Late in the seventeenth century the famous philosopher John Locke (1632-1704) also encouraged critical approaches to biblical texts in his *The Reasonableness of Christianity* (1695). Locke's book suggested that the Bible is "a series of documents written at different times, the authenticity of which must often be called into question."[69] Though he sought to appear friendly to Christianity, Locke influenced many radical religious writers in the Enlightenment. Three such writers—John Toland, Anthony Collins and Lord Bolingbroke—all claimed to be his disciples.[70] J. C. D. Clark has written that Locke's "significance for the eighteenth century" was not his political theories, but introducing "heterodox theology into religious speculations."[71]

French critics. Several seventeenth-century French writers assisted the project of biblical criticism by contrasting biblical history to scientific and historical knowledge. In 1655 Isaac de La Peyrere's *Prae-adamitten* was published in which the "new knowledge" of science was contrasted to scriptural accounts. He concluded, for instance, that geographical and chronological evidence suggested that Adam was not the first man.[72] The Benedictine monk Jean Mabillon's *Acta sanctorum* (1668) "worked out the means for determining the date and authenticity of ancient documents, a cornerstone in historical method."[73]

The French priest Richard Simon (1638-1712) is often credited with having been "the direct founder of the historical-critical method."[74] His *Histoire critique du Vieux Testament* (1678) aroused tremendous controversy within the Catholic Church, and Simon was eventually expelled from his order.[75] Undaunted, he proceeded to author a series of books intending to show that the Protestant standard of *sola scriptura* was untenable as a criterion of biblical scholarship and ended only in confusion.[76] His own standards were "the evident and the rational," though he also argued that biblical interpretation must be guided by tradition.[77] As Krentz writes, during the seventeenth century "the scriptures were more and more treated like ordinary historical documents."[78]

The Reformation. The principle of *sola scriptura*, the Reformation's defining commitment, does not seem a fruitful starting point for arguments against the Bible and Christian orthodoxy. Indeed, the Reformation in northern Europe under the leadership of Martin Luther is typically associated with a return to the Bible as the standard of religious truth. However, a number of scholars have pointed out that this powerful Christian movement contributed importantly to skepticism's rise in modern Europe. Perhaps another of the Reformation's guiding principles, the priesthood of all believers, which placed biblical interpretation in the hands of the individual believer, contributed to this effect.

Of critical importance to later developments is the commitment of Reformation leaders to private interpretation of the Scriptures. "The Pandora's box that Luther opened at Leipzig," writes Richard Popkin, "was to have the most far-reaching consequences, not just in theology but throughout man's entire intellectual realm."[79] Similarly, Roscoe Pound argues that "private interpretation of the Bible" had the effect of elevating individual reason.[80] Freedom of interpretation was "a logical deduction from the right of private judgment, which was a basal principle of the Reformation," according to another historian, S. G. Hefelbower.[81]

Luther may have believed that faith was founded on rational certainties that prevented a misreading of Scripture, but thinkers less friendly to Christianity happily used his idea of personal interpretation to justify various attacks in the coming centuries. The English Deists often contended that their assault on the Bible was pursued in the spirit of reformation in Christianity.[82]

CONCLUSION

Several important spiritual and intellectual movements in Europe prior to 1700 helped to shape subsequent thinking about Christianity and alternatives to it. I have noted just a few developments that were of particular importance in preparing the way for more dramatic developments after 1700. Mystical and gnostic communities, fascination with the kabbalist tradition, humanistic studies and magical science, mystical spirituality and experiments in biblical criticism—each had a profound impact on subsequent popular thought about religious questions generally in the modern Western world. These movements often rejected traditional notions of a historically grounded revealed message from a personal God. Also important to several of these trends was a magical view of the cosmos that emphasized coded truths and an impersonal divinity. Finally, the individual's placement at the center of the spiritual cosmos marked a break with the Revealed Word tradition of a sovereign God whose power was unquestioned.

The following chapters consider several crucial components of a potent religious system that has taken shape during the modern period. Though fully formed as a popular religious view only recently, this system represents a synthesis of spiritual tendencies with deep historical roots. It is, thus, a New Religious Synthesis of often quite durable spiritual concepts.

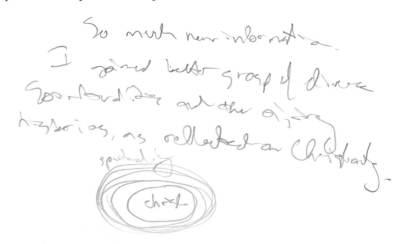

3

THE RISE OF
BIBLICAL CRITICISM

Allegory, Myth, Codes and the End of History

There are concepts in the Bible that are repugnant to the modern consciousness.
BISHOP JOHN SHELBY SPONG,
Rescuing the Bible from Fundamentalism

Carl Jung long ago pointed out, beneath the turmoil of daily activity our unconscious motivations dwell in the mythic world. Inside each of us are primal gods and goddesses.
DEEPAK CHOPRA,
The Path to Love: Renewing the Power of Spirit in Your Life

At the outbreak of the modern era, the [gnostic] system of inverse biblical exegesis was once again activated.
IOAN COULIANO, The Tree of Gnosis

The year 1727 witnessed the beginning of a strange episode in public religious debate. A professor dismissed from the faculty of Cambridge University for his attacks on the Bible—and confined briefly on the charge of mental instability—published a book with the innocuous title *A Discourse on the Miracles of our Saviour*. The book itself was, however, anything but innocuous. In *A Discourse* and the five additional discourses that followed over the next two years, Thomas Woolston systematically subjected Jesus' miracles and even Jesus himself to scathing public ridicule. Claiming that he wrote in an effort to save Christianity from those who read the Bible literally, Woolston argued that Jesus' miracles were never meant as historical accounts. They were simply allegories for spiritual truths, a point he set out to prove by first demonstrating how ridiculous the accounts were when read as history. However, Thomas Woolston's irreverence crossed a line. At the wedding

feast in Cana, for example, Jesus and Mary are "boon Companions" of drunken revelers. Jesus' reaction to Mary—"Woman, what have you to do with me?"—was "certainly the effect of Drinking." Mary knew that Jesus was "initiated in the Mysterys of *Bacchus*" when she asked him to supply more wine.[1]

Bishop Edmund Gibson warned Londoners that Woolston was a madman and a blasphemer, urged them not to read his books, and threatened to throw him in jail. But Woolston would not relent. Three more long books kept up the attack on Jesus' miracles. Thirty thousand copies were sold as quickly as they were published, and "large quantities were forwarded to the American colonies."[2] Woolston had created an international scandal, and by 1727 he was the talk of England. Clergy competed to answer Woolston in print, many reminding King George I that he "did not bear the sword in vain." Jonathan Swift himself penned verses in honor of the controversy: "Here's Woolston's Tracts, the twelfth Edition; 'Tis read by ev'ry Politician: The Country Members, when in Town, To all their Boroughs send them down: You never met a Thing so smart; The Courtiers have them all by Heart."[3] Late in 1728 Woolston was arrested and charged with blasphemy. The following year he was tried, convicted and sentenced to three years in jail and a fine of one hundred pounds.

Historians have called Woolston "clinically insane," "eccentric," "psychopathic" and an "evil genius."[4] And yet, other scholars consider him "the most influential" of all the eighteenth-century English skeptics, perhaps even the inventor of modern biblical criticism.[5] Clearly he was a skilled public advocate—clever, provocative, knowledgeable and daring. Woolston knew that by forcing a divorce between the spiritual and the historical he was inaugurating a new way of reading the Bible. He also knew that taking his new method directly to the public was more broadly persuasive than simply fomenting a debate among scholars.

Woolston's influence has been great, although his name is nearly forgotten. His insistence that the New Testament contains myth or allegory rather than literal history is now a widely accepted assumption that has been extended to a broad range of religious texts. If we fast-forward to the year 1991—two hundred and sixty years after Woolston's trial—a prominent and controversial Episcopal Bishop has just published the latest in a series of works on the Bible. Bishop John Shelby Spong's *Rescuing the Bible from Fundamentalism* reads like a seventh installment of Woolston's *Discourses*. Of Jesus' casting a man's demons into pigs who then destroy themselves by plunging over a cliff, Spong asks, "Are we drawn to a Lord who would destroy a herd of pigs and presumably a person's livelihood in order to

exorcise a demon (Mark 5:13)?" Similarly, to Jesus' cursing of a fruitless fig tree, Spong replies, "Are we impressed when the one we call Lord curses a fig tree because it did not bear fruit out of season (Matt. 21:18, 19)?" The Woolstonesque tone of Spong's criticism is unmistakable. "If the Bible is read literally, it must be said that Jesus seems to have accepted without question the language of hell employed by his religious contemporaries," which Spong takes as clear evidence of Jesus' lack of spiritual insight.[6] Jesus may be "guilty of what we today would call antisemitism."[7] The "pejorative attitudes found in Christian scriptures and even in the supposed words of Jesus . . . has led to pogroms, ghettos, segregated housing and clubs, defaced synagogues, Krystallnacht, and Dachau."[8]

Spong, like Woolston, suggests that we find the true meaning of the Bible in the "wondrous new meanings to be drawn" from a nonhistorical New Testament. Jesus himself must no longer be understood as a unique historical character, but as one among many mythical figures expressing the human desire for transcendence. Thus, "we must seek the truth that lies beneath the mythology of the distant past so that we might experience that truth."[9] Woolston wrote to save Christianity from the literalists who valued "the letter" more than "the spirit," and Spong professes the same mission. Clinging to a historical Bible means "certain death to all that we have believed."[10] The Bible's truth lies "beneath and behind" its historical façade. Reading Spong leaves one with the distinct impression that Thomas Woolston launched a new era of biblical interpretation.

During the entire modern period the Bible has been the subject of extensive, often corrosive criticism. Critics have concluded that the Christian and Jewish Scriptures are neither historically reliable nor divinely revealed. Rather, these texts are largely symbolic or mythic products of the human religious imagination. This turn away from both history and divine intervention has been justified as an effort to rescue the Bible from narrowly dogmatic literal readings, to liberate Christianity from the confines of history, or as a step toward finding the Bible's deeper, hidden meanings. But this rescue effort has also shifted the very foundations of Western spirituality. Claiming that the Bible is myth rather than history, symbol rather than revelation, now strikes many as a step toward a more personally meaningful faith. The Revealed Word tradition is now viewed as one among many efforts to express the inexpressible experience of the spiritual or "numinous." The objective history and fixed doctrine of the Revealed Word have gradually given way to mythical and metaphorical readings of the Bible as Westerners have sought and discovered a new

spirituality. This dramatic change in approach to the Revealed Word tradition has prepared Western people to embrace a wholly new spiritual orientation.

This chapter opens with a closer look at Woolston and his *Six Discourses*, the most important to the eighteenth-century attacks on New Testament history. We will then consider the rise of German biblical criticism, focusing attention on David Strauss and his enormously influential *Life of Jesus*. Two important twentieth-century statements on the Bible as symbol or code conclude the chapter. The first is Bishop Spong's *Rescuing the Bible from Fundamentalism*, one of his efforts to present the Bible as spiritual symbolism rather than historical fact. The last author considered is Michael Drosnin, whose bestselling *The Bible Code* created a sensation by claiming that the Bible's true meaning lay hidden in code.

THOMAS WOOLSTON AND THE ENGLISH DEISTS

The English Deists were a varied group of religious radicals who flourished between 1680 and 1750. Bold and effective strategists, they sought to overturn every major doctrine central to Christian orthodoxy. Among their number were the language scholar John Toland, John Locke's close friend Anthony Collins, a candlemaker named Thomas Chubb, Oxford philosopher Matthew Tindal, Cambridge professor Thomas Woolston, schoolmaster Peter Annet and the aristocrat Lord Shaftesbury.

The Deists specialized in harsh biblical criticism, the goal of which was to help their readers "think themselves out of those notions of God and religion" taught by the church.[11] Hadn't Jesus himself taught his followers to "search the Scriptures" in order to find "their true meaning"?[12] For the Deists, reading the Bible literally was a great barrier to thinking clearly about its meaning. Another approach was needed if progress toward rational religion was to be realized. The Bible could no longer be accepted as the Revealed Word. And the Deists were surprisingly successful in changing public opinions about the Bible. One prominent historian believes that "we cannot overestimate the influence exercised by Deistic thought," adding that their influence extends "right down to the present"[13]

Woolston's "Discourses." Born into a working-class family in 1670, Thomas Woolston's intellectual gifts led him to Cambridge where he specialized in the Christian church's early history. Woolston developed doubts about Christianity and as early as 1705 began questioning whether the New Testament was actually a book of history. Read as history, Jesus' miracles "imply Absurdities, Improbabil-

ities, and Incredibilities," and so "were never wrought." Woolston thus redefined the miracles as allegories with spiritual meanings, claiming he did so "to the Honour of our *Messiah,* and the Defence of Christianity."[14] A strange honor and defense this was, however. Jesus is a "magician" and a "sorcerer," and his miracles "nauseating" works of a charlatan and mere "tricks." Woolston even suggested that Jesus should have been prosecuted, even executed, for fooling the public.[15] Clearly, Woolston's persuasive tactic was to create a public scandal through such provocative language. And the approach worked as a new class of readers—often young men new to urban life—flocked to his books.

A good example of Woolston's controversial approach is found in his treatment of Jesus' healing of a blind man. Woolston rejects the eyewitness accounts because they were from Jesus' followers and thus biased. He notes that to prove the "Cure of a Disease, as of Blindness or Lameness" the testimony of "skillful *Surgeons* and *Physicians*" is required. Perhaps Jesus hid medicines from the crowd, which he then secretly used on the man's eyes.[16] Jesus was just an "impostor" passing himself off as a "miraculous Healer of Disease."[17] If we read this famous "miracle" as literally true, Jesus becomes a mere *"Quack-Doctor."*[18] Thus, Woolston dismisses the idea that this miracle occurred historically as "absurd, senseless and unaccountable."[19]

Woolston's next step is to suggest what he terms a "mystical and allegorical Interpretation of the story of this Eye-Salve" that will save *"Jesus's* divine Power."[20] As an allegory, the man's blindness is symbolic of spiritual blindness, "Ignorance, Error and Infidelity." Jesus himself is a symbol for "right Reason and Truth," which are "his mystical Names." Finally, the healing mud made of dirt and saliva represents *"perfect Doctrine,* which is Truth" that will "open the Eyes of Mens Understanding."[21] In six separate *Discourses* Woolston offered similar reinterpretations of each of Jesus' miracles.

Woolston's impact. Woolston's *Discourses* were a daring and damaging public attack on the New Testament miracles and on the whole concept of biblical history. His books sold thousands of copies in England and the American colonies, and many readers were convinced that Jesus' miracles were not to be taken seriously as historical events. Simon Browne, a Christian opponent of Woolston, commented that he was "surprised to see so many reasonable people moved to doubts by Woolston and others."[22] Bishop Gibson argued in response to Woolston that if Jesus' miracles were mere allegories, then "when the People were amazed to see the Miracles he did, they were amazed at *nothing.*"[23] However, by forcing a respected figure

like Gibson to answer his extreme claims, Woolston succeeded in making the debate appear to be contest between legitimate authorities. Gibson thus inadvertently lent credence to Woolston's claims.

Woolston not only shaped the popular religious mind of the eighteenth century, but also subsequent trends in biblical criticism that have permanently altered how Western people read the Bible. Miracles and other events in the life of Jesus, once viewed as historical, could now be read as symbolic, allegorical or mythological. Thus, the crucial Revealed Word premise of a personal God intervening miraculously in human history was undermined.[24] Similarly, religious pluralism also received a boost from Woolston's work: Christianity founded on unique historical events can stake a claim to being uniquely true, but Christianity based on myths or allegories shares this symbolic footing with many other faiths.

LESSING, STRAUSS AND GERMAN CRITICISM

Woolston sought to substitute allegorical for historical readings of the Bible and in this way rescue Christianity for a modern age. This rescued faith consisted of moral teachings supported by mythic tales. The Revealed Word with its unassailable history was refashioned into symbolic stories under a reader's interpretive control. This prepared the ground for developments in German biblical criticism between 1740 and 1850. The mythic interpretation of the Christian Scriptures would, in the decades following Woolston's highly successful court jester act, achieve a high level of sophistication.

Many German critics were influenced by English Deists like Woolston. For instance, Johann David Michaelis rejected literal readings of the Bible after visiting England in 1741-1742 at the height of the Deist controversy.[25] German biblical criticism accelerated after major works of English Deism were widely circulated in Germany.[26] While Michaelis dismantled Old Testament texts, another German pioneer of biblical criticism, Johann August Ernesti (1707-1781), focused on the New Testament documents.[27] The idea of a uniquely true Revealed Word relating divinely invaded human history would soon be rendered permanently antiquarian to the European mind.

Reimarus, Lessing and the "Fragments." Histories of modern biblical criticism usually start not with the wild-eyed English brawler Woolston, but with the staid German scholar Hermann Samuel Reimarus (1694-1768). Reimarus taught Oriental languages for a time at Wittenberg and then traveled in England where he was

influenced by Deists.[28] Respected in German intellectual circles, Reimarus's doubts about the Bible were not widely known. But he and several of his closest associates formed a secret circle of skeptics in otherwise conservative Hamburg. According to Colin Brown, Reimarus held "doubts he had long nursed about revealed religion, the historical worth of the Bible and the origins of Christianity."[29] He gradually accumulated thousands of pages of scholarly criticism of Christianity and the Bible.

A small portion of a massive, four thousand-page manuscript was published anonymously after his death. It took the form, literally, of fragments—a series of disconnected, caustic criticisms of the historicity of various Old and New Testament stories. Clearly the work of a talented and indignant opponent of Christianity, the *Wolfenbüttel Fragments* circulated widely in Germany, creating a great public controversy not unlike that created in England by Woolston's *Discourses*. Reimarus maintained an outward adherence to Christianity throughout his life, in large measure to protect his family from public embarrassment. In the *Fragments*, however, we find a skilled and knowledgeable controversialist angrily attacking the divinity of Christ and the historicity of the resurrection.[30]

Reimarus's friend and admirer, Gotthold Ephraim Lessing (1729-1781) had the *Fragments* published shortly after Reimarus's death. In order to protect Reimarus's family, Lessing falsely attributed the *Fragments* to a well-known skeptic and heretic named Schmidt. Lessing, a gifted playwright best remembered for the provocative play *Nathan the Wise*, rejected Christianity, biblical history, miracles and Jesus' divinity. An apparent pantheist, he proclaimed a "religion of humanity" founded on Reason.[31] Like Woolston, of whom he had some knowledge, Lessing held that "Christian mysteries are symbols and allegories" for spiritual truths.[32] The *Fragments* became an important foundation for later German biblical criticism.

David Friedrich Strauss. Most scholars agree that a new era in biblical criticism dawned with the publication of David Strauss's (1808-1874) *Leben Jesu* or *Life of Jesus* in 1835. This long and technical book placed imposing demands on readers. Nevertheless, *Life of Jesus* was so popular and controversial that the British romantic writer George Eliot made an English translation in 1846.[33] The book's impact was as great abroad as it had been in Germany. It "bewildered and enraged the mass of the clergy in mid-Victorian England."[34] It is no exaggeration to say that *Life of Jesus* permanently changed scholarly attitudes toward the Bible.

Life of Jesus is a massive two-volume work running to more than two thousand pages of "remorseless examination of every fact, every incident in the Gospels."[35]

Strauss sought not history but the mythological core of the Jesus stories. In the process he "etherialized the figure of Christ to the point of making his existence as a man irrelevant."[36] Rejecting all historical claims about the Christian Gospels, Strauss searched for the *mythi* or elemental mythical stories that provided the New Testament's basic materials. For his efforts Strauss was dismissed from his position at Tübingen in 1839. *Life of Jesus* created a public sensation in Germany and England in the 1830s and 1840s. What was Strauss's argument?

Myth displaces history. Strauss was testing "a new mode of considering the life of Jesus," one that would replace historical readings of the Bible. Like Woolston, he justified his work as an effort to rescue the Bible from literalists. Historical readings "had ceased to satisfy an advanced state of culture." Western people needed a "new point of view" on the Bible, which Strauss declared to be "the mythical."[37] History was old and had no future. Myth was modern and satisfied the advanced cultural mind. Strauss argued that previous biblical interpretation was based on two false assumptions. The first was "that the gospels contained a history," and the second that "this history was a supernatural one." Strauss insisted that the idea of historical content in the Gospels "must . . . be relinquished." In fact, biblical studies must begin by actively doubting that "the ground upon which we stand in the gospels is historical."[38]

The time was right for a myth, Strauss maintained, because the West had experienced "internal liberation of the feelings and intellect from certain religious and dogmatical presuppositions" that had blinded philosophers and historians. The Revealed Word was fading into the background of Western consciousness. To critics who found his rejection of history and orthodoxy "unchristian," Strauss replied that accepting such outmoded ideas was "unscientific."[39] Rejecting supernatural explanations out of hand, Strauss strategically affected a concern for the biblical tradition. "The supernatural birth of Christ, his miracles, his resurrection and ascension," he wrote, "remain eternal truths, whatever doubts may be cast on their reality as historical facts."[40] But the enduring significance of the biblical texts is ethical rather than historical. This formula—spiritual truth in the absence of historical truth—was to become an important component in New Religious Synthesis thought.

In a fashion reminiscent of Woolston, Strauss argued that to take some Gospel stories as historical was to believe things unworthy of God. He also maintained that numerous biblical accounts were never intended to be read as history. However, "the most convincing argument" for the "mythical view" is that it instantly eliminates "the innumerable, and never otherwise to be harmonized, discrepancies and chronological

contradictions in the gospel histories."[41] Like Woolston's allegorical approach, "the mythical mode of interpretation" relinquishes "the historical reality of the sacred narratives" in an effort to "preserve to them an absolute inherent truth."

Strauss was committed to the idea that the biblical writers used "historical semblance merely as the shell of an *idea*—a religious conception." The "inspiration" for these religious ideas is a "higher intelligence," but not God himself. Strauss contended that "the immediate divine agency" for religious notions like those found in the New Testament was "the spirit of a people or a community." The powerful human spiritual impulse to generate myths is, for Strauss, a *"natural* process."[42]

Much of Strauss's modus operandi is virtually indistinguishable from that of Woolston, though he presents himself as a scholar rather than as a mocking provocateur. Strauss sets before the reader an event in Jesus' life, for example, the transfiguration. He considers various interpretations advanced by scholars ancient and contemporary. Some are dismissed, others are judged plausible, the latter always pointing out impossible obstacles to a literal or historical reading. Strauss the scholar examines Greek terms used to describe an event, considering various translations and nuances. For example, the word *horama*, "vision," used by Matthew to describe the transfiguration suggests a physical event rather than a dream. Reports of the event in three of the four Gospels are compared. Apocryphal Gospels are ransacked for clues about episodes that may have given rise to the transfiguration myth. The alleged occurrence is set in its cultural and historical contexts. Thus, the two men to whom Jesus speaks—allegedly Moses and Isaiah—may be secret followers of his from the Essenes or some similar group. After his critical work is complete, Strauss's final interpretation invariably returns to the myth hypothesis. Thus, just as Woolston's caustic ridicule "cleared the way for allegory," so Strauss's more serious and sustained criticism serves a mythological interpretive scheme.

Strauss recognized, of course, that this sort of mythical criticism demolished the Revealed Word's claim to being historically grounded and uniquely true. But historical literalism was a product of ignorance to begin with, and best dispensed with. The typical Christian "knows no reason why the things recorded in the sacred books should not literally have taken place; no doubt occurs to him, no reflection disturbs him."[43] Christians find "many fictions" in other faiths, while insisting that "the accounts of God's actions, of Christ and other Godlike men contained in the Bible are, on the contrary, true." They assert, "that which distinguished Christianity from the heathen religion is this, they are mythical, it is historical."[44] These con-

clusions rest solely on the "limitation of the individual to that form of belief in which he has been educated." Such limitation "renders the mind incapable of embracing any but the affirmative view in relation to his own creed, any but the negative in relation to every other."[45] However, rational progress in religion requires Christian openness to the common foundation of all faiths—myth.

Myth and the evolution of religion. "However surprising," writes Strauss, "the Hebrew and Christian religions, like all others, have their mythi," or elemental mythical stories. From this platform Strauss launches an explanation of the origins and development of all human religions. "The inherent nature of religion," that which is "common to all religions," is their origin in myth, the source and essence of religion. Religion is, for Strauss, "the perception of truth" that is subsequently "invested with imagery." Religious communities may underestimate or overestimate the significance of their own sacred narratives.[46] Some see them as mere stories grounded in no particular spiritual insight. Others view their myths as uniquely true and historically valid. Both mistakes place the narrative outside "the proper religious sphere." The only proper understanding of religious narrative is as myth—an imaginative story bearing a transcendent truth.

Strauss developed a theory of the progressive evolution of religions around the globe. Primitives such as the Eskimos, for instance, cannot really be said to have a religion because they do not actually have any myths, only emotions. "They know nothing of gods, of superior spirits and powers," and so their "whole piety" revolves around "sentiment excited by the hurricane, the eclipse, or the magician." However, as religious sense progresses, religious ideas become more "objective." Thus, in more advanced religious systems people worship the sun, the moon, or an animal. Eventually, "a new world of mere imagination" emerges, a realm of "divine existences" whose lives and relationships are "represented only after human analogy, and therefore as temporal and historical."[47] That is, the gods take on lives of their own and are said to inhabit history. Still, all is myth. The most advanced stage of religious evolution is achieved when religious consciousness loses its specific claims to doctrines and historicity, and the reality of myth is embraced for its own sake. Because we share both common experiences and a common imagination, human myths emerge as strikingly similar stories. Thus, "mythical images" arise out of "sentiments common to all mankind." Strauss concludes that "this notion of a certain necessity and unconsciousness in the formation of the ancient mythi" is a point "on which we insist."[48]

David Strauss, then, maintained that humans create myths out of necessity, and these myths are invested with a time dimension, that is, a history. So, the wise student of religion must separate mythical history from the actual human history. However, the Revealed Word consistently fails to make this distinction, fails to recognize the crucial role of myth in religion, and thus treats biblical stories as history rather than as myth. In David Strauss the Revealed Word encounters something new—an explanation of religion that destroys religious history while celebrating the mythmaking capacity of the human mind.

The ultimate mythical insight: a new human religion. In the closing pages of *Life of Jesus*, Strauss muses on the possibility of a new view of Christ that will save Christianity for modern, scientific people. This Christology views the spirit of God and the spirit of humanity as "not essentially distinct." God produced the human mind "merely as a limited manifestation of himself." When human reason rises to a high level of sophistication, when it is "mature enough," it will realize "the truth that God is man, and man of a divine race." At this point there must appear "a human individual who is recognized as the visible God."[49] This is Christ, who lives out in his earthly life the religious evolution of the human race.

But why is this manifestation of the divine limited to one person if we all share a divine nature? Strauss's final position is that "humanity is the union of the two natures—God become man, the infinite manifesting itself in the finite."[50] This fundamental religious insight, writes Strauss, "is the key to the whole Christology." This New Christ—the divine human race—also performs miracles. We should not take more interest in "the cure of some sick people in Galilee" than we do in "the miracles of intellectual and moral life belonging to the history of the world" such as the "almost incredible dominion of man over nature."[51]

Scientific progress, then, reveals the human race to be a race of divine miracle workers demonstrating with ever greater clarity its control over the intellectual and physical realms. This great insight is the ultimate yield of Strauss's biblical criticism. In a final note, Strauss calls for clergy to be "critical theologians" who move beyond the tradition, whereby "the evangelical narratives are received as history," to the recognition that they are "mere mythi."[52] So crucial is this change of orientation that it may require ministers to appear to treat the Scriptures as history while in fact deriving from them their essential mythical sense. When the Christian church recognizes its participation in the universal mythic religious consciousness of the human race, it will finally leave behind its outdated notion of

Jesus as a single divine individual and realize the essential divinity of every human. In this way David Strauss's "scientific" biblical criticism opened the way for a new, mythically based religion of divine humanity. This new faith is now a foundational component of the Other Spirituality.

JOHN SHELBY SPONG RESCUES THE BIBLE

John Shelby Spong was born in Charlotte, North Carolina, in 1931 and grew up under the influence of Southern fundamentalism. Spong was educated at the University of North Carolina, Chapel Hill, and at Duke University. A prolific author, Spong has published more than a dozen books. In 1978, he became the Episcopal Bishop of Newark, New Jersey. During his career, Spong has been known for his strong stands against traditional doctrines of the church and for his staunch advocacy for civil rights.

As noted in the introduction, Bishop John Shelby Spong sometimes writes like a modern incarnation of the radical Deist Thomas Woolston. In literal and historical readings of the Bible Spong found a God he could not worship. "The picture of God that began to emerge from the Bible for me was neither a pleasant one nor one to which I was drawn in worship. It did not get better."[53] He provides his readers dozens of examples of God's acts by which he is "repelled" and comments that "the list of objectionable passages could be expanded almost endlessly."[54] It is not surprising, then, that in a number of popular books Spong seems determined to disabuse the public of whatever confidence it had in the historicity of the Christian Scriptures.

In *Rescuing the Bible from Fundamentalism* and *Liberating the Gospels*, Spong introduces many readers to the techniques of earlier biblical critics such as Woolston and Strauss. For example, Spong engages in ironic character assessment similar to that with which Deists provoked the British public in the eighteenth century. "Moses was a murderer," he writes, "but this was not a character flaw because his victim was an Egyptian (Exod. 2:11ff.)." Again, "Joseph was an arrogant and spoiled favorite son upon whom his father heaped lavish gifts and special favor (Genesis 37)." Finally, "adultery was said to be evil, but both Abraham and Isaac tried to pass their wives off as their sisters, even though this meant having them sexually used by Abimelech, King of Gerar (Gen. 20:1-18; 26:6-11)."[55] Such stories offend "the modern consciousness" and his own conscience.

Blaming the Jesus of history. Bishop Spong rejects biblical literalism as untenable in the modern world. "A literal Bible," he writes, "presents me with far more prob-

lems than assets." One problem is that such a Bible "offers me a God I cannot respect, much less worship; a deity whose needs and prejudices are at least as large as my own."[56] And Spong finds the historical character of Jesus of Nazareth no more appealing as presented in the Bible. One problem is that the Jesus of the Bible is often ignorant. "Jesus is presented in the Bible as believing that epilepsy is caused by demon possession (Mark 9:14-29). That is hardly a viewpoint that any of us would accept today." Moreover, Jesus reveals certain off-putting character traits. "There are passages in the Gospels that portray Jesus of Nazareth as narrow-minded, vindictive, and even hypocritical.... He called gentiles 'dogs' (Matt. 15:26).... He disowned his own family (Matt. 12:46-50)."[57]

Spong rejects the notion of biblical history when he writes, "the biblical writers had no sense at all of the sweep of historic times." But he goes a step further, calling in question the very notion of objective history. When we get down to cases, "we need to remind ourselves that even in this modern world with its technological genius, there is still no such thing as 'objective' history.'"[58] Moreover, if modern people have no objective view of history, then certainly the tribal Hebrews could not have held such a view. They inhabited the "ancient world with its narrow focus, its limited embrace of reality, its pre-scientific mind-set of miracle and magic, and its nationalistic tribal understanding of deity itself."[59] Spong rehearses a variety of scientific evidences, setting these beside the naïve and corrupted history of Scripture to convince his readers that the Bible is not a historical book. He leads his readers through a variety of critical discoveries such as the numerous sources of the Old Testament texts, problems of dating and manuscript transmission, and internal contradictions in Bible accounts.

Spong also engages in damaging psychological assessment of biblical writers. For example, "Paul's writings reveal the combination of intense levels of self-negativity covered by intensely cultivated images of superiority," he notes. "At first these forces fed Paul's devotion to Judaism at the same time that they created his defensiveness." Paul's marginal self-concept "became operative in his later devotion to and understanding of the gospel." This deeply conflicted apostle was also benighted by his cultural limitations. "Paul was not a universal man. He was indeed a man of his times. He reflected the common assumptions of his day, assumptions that time has eroded badly."[60] Paul was "uncritically part of the patriarchal system that so informed the Hebrew Scriptures." But "modern standards" reveal many of Paul's attitudes to be "not only inadequate but wrong."[61]

Spong's purposes, like his methods, seem akin to those of Woolston and Strauss. He strips Christianity of its historicity through moral critique, historical analysis, character assessment and comparison with the modern mindset. Then he revives the lifeless body of traditional Christianity through the "wondrous new meanings to be drawn" from a nonhistorical New Testament. In the process, a reinvented Christianity emerges, complete with a new understanding of Jesus. No longer a unique historical character incarnating God, Jesus is now one among many mythical figures expressing in narrative form the human desire for transcendence.

The end justifies the means for Spong, though, and courage is called for. "For those who are willing to take the journey, the stakes are high. But not to take the journey means, in my opinion, certain death to all that we have believed. So the task moves on."[62] Whether one follows Spong on his journey, or chooses to demur, the death of *historical* Christianity ensues. This, however, is a necessary step toward redefining Christianity for the modern mind.

Refitting Christianity for modernity. Spong commends to his readers a new Christianity refitted for a modern world, the Holy Grail of Woolston and Strauss as well. Rather than accepting surface historical meanings in the Bible, "we must seek the truth that lies beneath the mythology of the distant past so that we might experience that truth."[63] That truth is that God is not personal and wholly other, as the Revealed Word suggests. Rather, "God is the *Ground of Being*," the essence of existence, an idea central to New Religious Synthesis. Spong asks, "How did Jesus reflect this ground of being?" As "the Christpower we meet in Jesus," an idea quite distinct from Jesus *being* the historical Christ.[64]

Spong urges his readers to express "being" in a fashion similar to Jesus by embracing their own existence. John Spong sets history aside in order that the real spiritual truth "beneath and behind" it may emerge. This truth supports a new spirituality built on the affirmation of the self. The loss of an objective ground for religious experience renders subjective experience ultimate. "The call of Christ is an eternal call to the affirmation of that which is," and that which is, is us. "To have the courage to be oneself, to claim the ability to define oneself, to live one's life in freedom and with power is the essence of the human experience." This is what it means to express being as Jesus did. Real faith for a modern world means elevating humanity. Or, as Spong puts it, "true Christianity ultimately issues in a deeper humanism." This "deeper humanism" in turn issues in "new dimensions of consciousness and

transcendence," a conclusion strikingly similar to that advanced by Strauss at the end of *Life of Jesus*. Such is the spiritual fruit of John Spong's biblical criticism.[65]

MICHAEL DROSNIN'S *THE BIBLE CODE*

The last section of this chapter is an excursion into an unusual treatment of the Bible that may not seem to be extending the tradition of Woolston, Strauss and Spong. However, this unexpected bestseller from the late 1990s treats the Bible as bearing a message "beneath and behind" its historical surfaces, something, moreover, more important than those surfaces.

In the emerging Western spiritual view—the *Other* Spirituality—religious truth is not found in readily accessible historical texts. Rather, the truths of sacred narratives are apprehended by those prepared to ferret out their underlying allegories and myths. Of course, it takes special skill to read past the historical surfaces to deeper mythical meanings. One highly successful author has recently recommended another interpretive skill important to discovering hidden spiritual meanings in the biblical record—deciphering the complex numerical code embedded within it.

Michael Drosnin is a journalist who has worked for *The Washington Post* and *The Wall Street Journal*. On a visit to Israel in 1992 to meet with members of the intelligence community he encountered a mathematician by the name of Eliyahu Rips. Rips introduced Drosnin to the ancient idea that the Hebrew letters of the Old Testament contain a code that predicts a number of future events and describes events in the distant past. Drosnin was convinced of the hypothesis and went on to write his incredibly popular book, *The Bible Code*, a bestseller not only in the United States, but also in Germany, France, Australia, Taiwan, Korea, South Africa, Portugal, Japan and England. Drosnin, who professes no particular religious affiliation, claims in the book to lay bare the hidden messages of the Old Testament.[66] "The Bible code," he writes, "was discovered in the original Hebrew version of the Old Testament, the Bible as it was first written. That book, now translated into every language, is the foundation of all Western religion."[67] In *The Bible Code*, however, the historical sense of the biblical message is inconsequential compared to the remarkable warnings and predictions that lie hidden in various combinations of the Hebrew letters.

Reviving the spirit of kabbalah. Though Drosnin does not mention the kabbalah anywhere in *The Bible Code*, he replicates some of the approaches of the ancient rab-

bis who found hidden in the Torah a set of secret messages and spiritual truths. The secret of reading the Bible code, according to Drosnin, first came to light a mere fifty years ago. "Rips told me that the first hint of the encoding had been found more than 50 years ago by a rabbi in Prague, Czechoslovakia. The rabbi, H. M. D. Weissmandel, noticed that if he skipped fifty letters, and then another fifty, and then another, the word 'Torah' was spelled out at the beginning of the book of Genesis." Not only this, but "the same skip sequence again spelled out the word 'Torah' in the book of Exodus. And in the book of Numbers. And in the book of Deuteronomy."[68] Perhaps the rabbi from Prague was familiar with kabbalah, and was seeking just such a hidden message.

Rips pointed out to Drosnin early in their association that seeking a hidden code in the Bible has been a preoccupation of some impressive thinkers of the past. "At first I tried just counting letters like Weissmandel," says Rips. "You know, Isaac Newton also tried to find the code in the Bible, and he considered it more important in some ways than his Theory of the Universe." Drosnin adds, "The first modern scientist, the man who figured out the mechanics of our solar system and discovered the force of gravity, Sir Isaac Newton, was certain that there was a hidden code in the Bible that would reveal the future."[69] As noted in chapter two, Newton is sometimes identified as the last of the magical scientists, thinkers whose understanding of science was rooted in a worldview that elevated esoteric knowledge.

Apocalypse now. According to Drosnin, "details of today's world are encoded in a text that has been set in stone for hundreds of years, and that has existed for thousands of years."[70] Drosnin argues that what he calls the "plain text"—the ordinary, historically grounded meaning of the Bible—actually points to the deeper meaning hidden in code. For example, Drosnin writes that "crossing the words 'Bible code'" that is, literally forming a cross with this encoded phrase in the Hebrew text, "is a hidden text that states it was 'sealed before God.'" Drosnin takes this to mean that "the Bible code is the 'sealed book,' the secret revelation found in the plain text of the Bible."[71]

Drosnin's writing is drenched in contemporary apocalyptic warnings, a fact that renders his "decoding" work suspect while at the same time dramatically enhancing interest in his book. For instance, he writes near the end of the book that the Bible code predicts an imminent nuclear holocaust in the Middle East. "I felt compelled to warn both Peres and Netanyahu that the code seemed to predict an atomic attack," he breathlessly announces, "as I had warned Rabin that the code predicted his assassination." Continuing in this vein, Drosnin writes, "I never imagined that

I would ultimately find myself searching for the details of the real Apocalypse. I never imagined that the 'End of Days' would be encoded in the Bible with the current year. I never imagined that the long-known biblical prophecies of Armageddon might in some level be real."[72]

Asteroids and dinosaurs: biblical history versus coded history. Certain logical and factual problems attend Drosnin's argument about the Bible code. "The Bible code is ecumenical," he writes, "the information is for everyone." Then why were the Hebrews singled out for receiving and transmitting the code? Drosnin's reasoning on this point begs rather than answers questions. "The code only exists in Hebrew, because that is the original language of the Bible."[73] Moreover, many "predictions" Drosnin attributes to the Bible code appear to be inaccurate. The assassination of Yitzhak Rabin was, allegedly, foretold by the code. But so was a nuclear holocaust to follow—an event that did not occur.

But logic and factual accuracy are not the point of *The Bible Code*. The issue here, as in Woolston, Strauss and Spong, is the control of history. That is, Drosnin's argument that the *real* history of the Bible is a hidden history allows him to determine which historical events will occupy the foreground, and which the background. Consider, for example, a particularly odd message contained in the code—the destruction of earth's dinosaur population by a comet. Drosnin writes that "'asteroid' and 'dinosaur' are encoded together in the Bible." He explains this unexpected and surprisingly contemporary juxtaposition of terms as follows: "The name of the dragon the Bible says God fought—'Rahab'—appears in the Bible code exactly where 'asteroid' hits the 'dinosaur.'" Drosnin concludes that this "suggests that the extinction of the dinosaurs was the real slaying of the dragon, the cosmic event recalled by Isaiah: 'Was it not you who cut Rahab in pieces, and pierced through the dragon?'" Thus, God slew the dinosaurs—the dragon Rahab—for a reason.

A direct conflict between the literal biblical history and Drosnin's coded history now ensues. The opening chapters of Genesis suggest that human beings were the special creation of a personal God. However, Drosnin's coded message about an asteroid destroying earth's dinosaurs suggests a different account of human origins. "Scientists now agree that mankind would never have evolved unless the dinosaurs had been wiped out by the asteroid."[74] Thus, Drosnin's coded history teaches the evolution of the human race, albeit with cosmic assistance, while biblical history teaches special creation. Coded history is placed in the attended-to foreground, literal history the ignored background. Similarly, Woolston placed allegorical mean-

ing in the foreground and literal history in the background, while Strauss and Spong worked the same inversion with mythical and literal readings. In all four cases, the originator of the interpretive approach subjectively determines the meaning of the text, that is, decides what it "actually" says. Likewise, in all four cases the biblical text is discovered not to contain what is ordinarily understood as history.

In *The Bible Code* Michael Drosnin acts the part of a latter-day seer reading the biblical text with the aid of computer enhanced magical spectacles. And, like antihistorical critics before him, Drosnin does not find the actual history of the nation of Israel to be the principal message of those sacred pages. Rather, he finds a time-sensitive code filled with strange glimpses of the past and stunning warnings about the future. In fact, *The Bible Code* reads like a media-influenced encapsulation of stories of recent public interest, *National Geographic-meets-Newsweek*, with Drosnin as editor-in-chief. Regardless of how we understand his discovery, it is clear that traditional biblical history takes a back seat to the coded messages of the Hebrew text. Thus, *The Bible Code* represents a late twentieth-century demotion of biblical history, albeit a particularly novel one.

CONCLUSION

Throughout the modern period, the Bible as a book of history has been under a sustained, public and largely successful assault. From the early eighteenth-century Deists down to the most recent biblical critics and popular speculators, the idea that the Bible reports historical events has been questioned and even ridiculed. Nevertheless, the Revealed Word's commitment to history remains central to its conception of religion. For example, biblical scholar John Stott writes that traditional Christianity "does not rest only on a historical person, Jesus of Nazareth, but on certain historical events which involved him, especially his birth, death, and resurrection."[75]

Opponents have long recognized both Christianity's need of history and its reliance on the Bible to substantiate its claim to being historical. Thus, to attack the Bible's historicity was to attack Christianity generally. Some modern biblical criticism grows out of this specific persuasive goal. The particular school of biblical criticism emphasizing allegorical or mythological interpretations of the Bible has been our focus because this school's principal claim—that spirituality does not need history—has become an important component in the New Religious Synthesis. Connections between antihistorical readings of the Bible and the rise of a new way in religion will be developed throughout this book.

Rescuing Christianity from historical literalists has been an important justification of much modern biblical criticism. Woolston argued that he was saving Christianity from irrationality and superstition by demolishing historical readings of Jesus' miracles and rendering the accounts allegorical. On a similar line of argument, Strauss set about to prove that the New Testament incorporated myths common to many faiths, a fact obscured, he alleged, by parochial claims that the Gospel accounts were historical. The source of true religion was not a personal God's activities in history, but rather our own collective human experience. Bishop John Spong finds biblical history repulsive in many of its particulars and argues that Christianity is better off without history. Dispensing with obsolete historical claims also removes the obstacle of a personal and locally active God and opens the way to universal religious insights and experiences. Michael Drosnin finds literal history a mere carrier of coded messages, a surface that must be stripped away to reveal something more valuable beneath. That more valuable truth is an odd combination of metaphysical speculation, political prediction and recent news.

What the antihistorical critics have in common is their rejection of the Revealed Word's determined divine interventionism—the view that a personal God has been continuously and actively involved in human history. Instead, the Revealed Word's central narratives have been gradually transformed into allegories for the religion of reason, a mythic system akin to others found throughout the world, metaphors for a "new humanism," and conduits for coded messages from beyond. Correspondingly, its central figure, Jesus, is now changed from Son of God into a religious philosopher, a mythic hero, a mystic, a character in a morality play or a symbol for something more meaningful.

De-historicizing of the Bible has been strategically important to creating the New Religious Synthesis for a variety of reasons that will become more evident in subsequent chapters. Among these reasons is establishing the link between myth and secret spiritual knowledge or *gnosis*. At this point it may be sufficient to point out that severing history from spirituality renders biblical interpretation almost infinitely plastic. Subjective readings reign as history fades into the background. Moreover, the Revealed Word notion of history as the scene of God's sovereign acts is neutralized, and history itself becomes a suspect category. Events critical to the Revealed Word tradition such as Jesus' crucifixion and resurrection must also be reinterpreted, not as moments in redemptive history, but as symbolic of stages in the spiritual life of humanity or the individual.

The rise of antihistorical criticism of the Bible is just one indication that we are now, and have been for some time, in the presence of a dominant new religious view that sees no particular need for history, that in fact sees history as a problem. In the chapters that follow I will examine how this turn away from the historical path in religion is a vital component in a new spiritual view that is everywhere present in Western religious thought.

4

THE ASCENT OF REASON

Birth of a Deity

❦

The system of modern nihilism starts with a powerful substitute for transcendence,
which is belief in Reason.

IOAN COULIANO, The Tree of Gnosis

Reason . . . is God incarnate.

PETER ANNET, Lectures

❦

The fall of one god is often the precondition for the rise of another. Historian Franklin Baumer reported the strange events that took place in the famous Cathedral of Notre Dame in Paris on the morning of November 10, 1793. The cathedral was that day the site of the first, and the last, Festival of Liberty and Reason. As citizens and dignitaries of Paris entered the great church "they saw, some doubtless with astonishment, the insignias of Christianity covered up and their place taken by the symbols of a strange new religion." Baumer continues:

> Rising up in the nave was an improvised mountain, at the top of which perched a small Greek temple dedicated "To Philosophy" and adorned on both sides by the busts of philosophers, probably Voltaire, Rousseau, Franklin, and Montesquieu. Halfway down the side of the mountain a torch of Truth burned before an altar to Reason. Then ensued a bizarre ceremony.[1]

The "bizarre ceremony" involved an actress emerging onto the stage dressed in red, white and blue robes. The assembled crowd was directed to pay homage to this personification of Liberty. A little later Notre Dame was designated "the Temple of Reason."

The dramatic, almost unbelievable events at Notre Dame beg for explanation. Historian Baumer's effort focuses on a writer considered in this chapter, one of the

most famous and successful opponents of the Revealed Word tradition. The strange worship service held at the Temple of Reason in 1793 "was a symbol, first of all, of Voltairean skepticism which scored Christianity as an 'infamous thing' to be crushed . . . and replaced by a religion imbued with 'reason,' 'virtue,' and 'liberty.'"[2] Indeed, Voltaire's goal in a lifetime of activist writing was to eliminate Christian belief in Western Europe. In its place he offered the new god Reason. Reflecting on the events in Notre Dame, Carl Jung wrote, "The enthronement of the Goddess of Reason in Notre Dame seems to have been a symbolic gesture of great significance to the Western world—rather like the hewing down of Wotan's oak by the Christian missionaries. For then, as at the Revolution, no avenging bolt from heaven struck the blasphemer down."[3]

The following year, 1794, a brilliant French mathematician, the Marquis de Condorcet (1743-1794) published his *Sketch of the Progress of the Human Mind*. Condorcet argued that humanity would achieve perfection through gradual, inevitable progress guided by reason. Condorcet's "new doctrine" involved a profound belief in "the indefinite perfectibility of the human race."[4] Reason and its instrument, science, would eliminate the need for religion. Though he authored his optimistic *Sketch* while a warrant for his arrest was current and he was under sentence of death from the French Revolution, Condorcet nevertheless maintained that his own century was the great turning point in human history. According to Baumer, Condorcet believed that "in the foreseeable future, thanks to the power of reason and the discovery of new knowledge, mankind would rise to unprecedented heights, to perfectibility, in fact." Condorcet wrote, "No bounds have been fixed to the improvement of the human race." In addition, he contended that "the perfectibility of man is absolutely indefinite," and that "we are approaching one of the grand revolutions of the human race."[5]

Condorcet dubbed his new age of human perfection "the tenth epoch," mankind having already passed through nine identifiable stages of progress. The tenth epoch would be a time of world peace and scientific utopia. Food supplies would increase, wars would cease, injustice would end, disease would be vanquished, and leisure would replace labor. Condorcet referred to this perfected state of the human race as "heaven which . . . reason has created."[6] He maintained a profound aversion to the Revealed Word, the enemy of Reason—human rationality elevated to the status of a divinity. Condorcet was eventually captured by agents of the French Revolution and died in prison. Nevertheless, his hope of a human race improved by Reason never died.

This chapter explores several popular arguments for Reason as a limitless power, a virtually divine capacity, in humans. The substitution of human rationality, self-awareness, imagination or consciousness for the Revealed Word's "wholly other" deity is a critical component of the New Religious Synthesis. Reason, thus broadly defined, has been transformed into a full-fledged deity for a new spiritual age. The writers considered include the English Deist Peter Annet, for whom Reason was "God incarnate." The famous French advocate and playwright Voltaire is also considered. Voltaire advanced Reason as the antidote to the rational poison of Revealed Word theology. Though nineteenth-century Romantic writers are alleged to have rejected Enlightenment infatuation with reason, their exaltation of imagination and intellect is often difficult to distinguish in principle. We will be exploring the early Romantic writer Thomas De Quincey's arguments for what he termed Majestic Intellect.

Tracing the ascent of Reason into the twentieth century brings us to the exotic claims of the New Thought movement that held such powerful sway over the popular religious mind at the turn of the century. Mind or Consciousness—new names for the interior divinity earlier called Reason—offered healing and escape from all of our present limitations. The final section of this chapter examines novelist Ayn Rand's powerful argument that Reason prepares an elite to escape the ancient fetters of faith and to assume their rightful place as the rulers of the human race. Rand provides a fitting terminus for our pilgrimage toward the god of a new spirituality.

PETER ANNET

Englishman Peter Annet (1693-1769) trained for the ministry, but encounters with religious bigotry turned him against Christianity. Between 1738 and 1747 Annet, who made his living as a schoolteacher, created controversy in England by attacking Christianity in several popular speeches, pamphlets and books. His most controversial and successful pamphlet, *The Resurrection of Jesus Considered by a Moral Philosopher* (1744), relentlessly questioned the evidence for the central Christian miracle. In 1761 Annet began publishing a periodical called *The Free Enquirer*, a weekly collection of essays on topics of general interest with special attention to religious subjects. Annet's main purpose in this early experiment in popular journalism was to raise doubts in the public mind about the Bible.

According to Annet and other Deists, the universe follows "the rule of Reason," an omnipresent law that even a divine being cannot violate. Having thus tied his

hands and ushered him out of the cosmos, Reason took the place of the Revealed Word's God. "Reason," proclaimed Annet, is "the divinity operating within us" and our "inward illumination."[7] Adding a daring flourish to his radical claim, Annet taunted Christians by calling Reason "the only begotten son of God, the God incarnate, or God humanized."[8] Reason, not God, is "that authority . . . above all other authorities." In a new apocalypse "the dead shall rise" when they hear "the trumpet of reason." A spiritually reborn humanity will embrace Reason as "the basis of true religion."[9] But this new god—like Yahweh of old —is a jealous deity. In the new era, any "religion rebellious against Reason shall be compelled to . . . yield to the divine authority of Reason."[10] Legal sanctions and perhaps force will ensure the universal worship of Reason. In Annet's vision of the religious future, Reason replaces each member of the Trinity. Like the Father, it is "that authority . . . above all other authorities." Like the Son, "Reason is God incarnate." And like the Holy Spirit, Reason is "the divinity operating within us."

The upward fall. For Deists like Annet, the original religion of the human race was the pure and worshipful recognition of Reason's sovereignty in the universe. The first three chapters of Genesis present a rather different account of humanity's early spirituality. These passages recount the special creation of human beings by a personal God, and their subsequent tragic Fall. Relational intimacy with God was lost, and humanity was cast into spiritual darkness and rational confusion. Reason, like other capacities, fell along with the human race.

Annet, however, strategically reinterpreted the Genesis account in *The Free Inquirer* to support his spiritualized understanding of Reason. If human beings are the fallen creatures the Revealed Word makes them out to be, he asks, how is it that they find themselves in possession of the powerful faculty we call Reason? Annet advances a fascinating answer to this question in *The Free Inquirer* of November 3, 1761, a response that turns the traditional reading of Genesis on its head. The alleged Fall of Adam and Eve was not a ruinous disaster but rather a great leap forward for humanity. By asserting their independence from Yahweh, Adam and Eve gained Reason and thus became Godlike. Far from injuring human rational capacities, the Fall actually inaugurated Reason—the divine capacity for self-determination. The much-maligned serpent of Genesis was right all along—by ignoring the commands of the restrictive divinity Yahweh, Adam and Eve gained a divine quality of their own. Moses, the supposed author of Genesis, was wrong to suggest in Genesis that God would punish people for thinking on their own.[11]

The heroes of Annet's Genesis, then, are the serpent, who created a truly human race by giving us Reason, and Adam and Eve, the first rationally autonomous human beings who gained their freedom by a bold act of courage. Yahweh—if he exists at all—is a weak and malevolent deity, and Moses a purveyor of bad theology. Annet, the rationally liberated biblical interpreter, reads the story's true meaning beneath the historical surface of the text. He thus inverts the Revealed Word creation account in his effort to advance a new spiritual view that captivated audiences by the sheer exotic intrigue of its audacious inventiveness. Reason, not God, saves us and guarantees our "eternal salvation."[12] A sound moral principle will always "approve itself, to the true, genuine reason of man."[13] Thus, the worshiper of Reason follows a law higher than the constricting, arbitrary moral code of the Revealed Word. Like Adam and Eve who decided to eat the fruit of the tree of the knowledge of good and evil, only Reason's worshipers are free moral agents.

Peter Annet sought to convince his readers that Reason was a gift acquired when humans first asserted their rational independence from the Revealed Word's God. This new quality rendered human beings themselves virtually divine. Writers like Annet popularized the cult of Reason in the eighteenth century by taking the case for Reason directly to the public. These religious advocates celebrated autonomous individualism as a spiritual value, and their message was highly persuasive. In the following section we will observe how Europe's greatest skeptical writer fleshed out the practical moral implications of a religion of Reason in opposition to the irrational dictates of the Revealed Word.

VOLTAIRE AND LIBERATED REASON

Thomas Babington Macaulay has said of Voltaire (1694-1778), the most influential and prolific of all Enlightenment writers, that "he could not build, he could only tear down."[14] But there can be no question that Voltaire's irreverent wit contributed substantially to shaping the popular religious mind in the modern West. Voltaire's utter rejection of authority, his doubtfulness about all objects of reverence, his dismissal of anything claiming to stand above Reason are all marks of the serious as well as the casual intellectual of today. Among the several mottoes that sum up his life and work, one is cited perhaps more often than any other by Voltaire's biographers: "*Ecraser l'infame*," that is, crush the infamous thing. The "infamous thing" was the superstition and hierarchy of the Catholic Church, but also, by extension, the beliefs and structures of Christianity. For all of the justice implicit in his opposition

to ecclesiastical tyranny, it cannot be doubted as well that Voltaire was an ardent foe of not just church authority but Christianity itself. He commented at one time that he was tired of hearing that it took only twelve men to establish Christianity. "I'd like to prove that only one man is called for to undermine its foundations."[15] Among the passions motivating Voltaire to write, then, was his abhorrence of the Revealed Word tradition, and particularly of its tendency to limit Reason.

An enormously prolific writer, Voltaire published more than ten million words and left over twenty thousand letters. His greatest talent was as a playwright, and his works dominated French theater for more than half a century. His epic poem *Henriade*, which he considered his greatest achievement, celebrated the life of France's last liberal king, Henry IV. But Voltaire was also an able historian as evidenced by his *Age of Louis XIV*. His most lasting fame, however, derives from one short novel, *Candide*.

Voltaire's life. François-Marie Arouet, who adopted the pen name de Voltaire, was born in Paris to a prosperous family on November 21, 1694. The son of a successful legal secretary, Voltaire was sent at the age of ten to the college of Louis-le-Grand where he received an excellent classical education under the Jesuits. Initially committed to the study of law, he eventually abandoned that ambition to become a writer. As a young man he was influenced by French Deism of the type revealed in Montesquieu's *Persian Letters*, and in his twenties by the English Deism of Collins, Woolston and others. Very early in his writing career Voltaire revealed a genius for satire, often offending prominent citizens of Paris. He became a hero to many for his stand against religious fanaticism, and he vowed to "seek revenge" for acts of religious persecution and intolerance.[16]

So sharp and well aimed were his shafts that he was banished from Paris on more than one occasion. During these banishments he lived for a time in Holland, and for most of a year in the Bastille. Though often considered a perpetually smiling wit who staved off the pain of his penetrating perceptions by mocking the injustices of life, Voltaire suffered throughout his life from depression, anxiety and hypochondria. Often ill, he nevertheless lived to the age of eighty-four.

Called the most characteristic writer of the Enlightenment, Voltaire was also a great popularizer of Enlightenment ideas such as the rejection of the Bible, contempt for authority and the elevation of Reason. Voltaire's confidence in Reason was encouraged by the epoch-making work of Isaac Newton, a thinker for whom Voltaire maintained unbounded admiration. Voltaire sought not only to under-

stand Newton's *Principia* but to provide the public an accessible interpretation of it. He found in this new science a wonder and explanatory power sufficient to ground a substitute for traditional religion.

Voltaire was exiled to England in the 1720s. During this time he read the English Deists and engaged England's leading thinkers. Exposure to Deism profoundly shaped Voltaire's religious ideas. His approach to biblical criticism—dismissing miracles as fabrications, searching for contradictions, questioning the character of biblical figures—are reminiscent of Deists like Woolston. In spite of the Christian faith of his father and brother, as well as of the teachers he so admired at Louis-le-Grand, Voltaire rejected all of Christian theology.

Voltaire's influence on popular religious thought in the Western world has been great. One scholar writes, "We have . . . completely absorbed the ideas of his polemical books and pamphlets."[17] His *Lettres philosophiques* are considered the greatest single force shaping European liberal religious thought. Much of Voltaire's religious philosophy is an angry response to the great Christian mathematician Pascal (1623-1662), who died a generation before Voltaire's birth. Pascal believed passionately in both the Fall and innate human sin, two concepts Voltaire repudiated with equal passion. Such Christian doctrines enslave the mind, and come not from Reason but revelation. Ancient priests likely invented these ideas and their modern counterparts perpetuate them.

Voltaire is best remembered for his strange novelette *Candide,* a haunting and humorous story that presents the absurdity and cruelty of human life. It was originally written as an answer to Leibniz's philosophical optimism. A man highly sensitive to human suffering, Voltaire was moved by events such as the disastrous earthquake that struck Lisbon, Portugal, on October 31, 1755. The city was virtually wiped out by the quake, and many thousands of citizens died in fires while attending church services celebrating All Saints Day. How could a loving God allow such evil, particularly when so many of the victims were the devout? Voltaire posed a dilemma: Either God is not all-powerful, or he is not all good. If he is all good and allows evil to persist, he must not be all-powerful. If he is all-powerful and allows evil to persist, he must not be all good. *Candide*'s summary sentiment is Voltaire's famous maxim, "tend your own garden," but no man ever was less inclined to tend his own garden than Voltaire. Throughout his long and successful literary life he was perpetually involved in criticizing actions he thought unjust and ideas he deemed ludicrous.

"Zadig": liberating reason. Nothing occupied Voltaire's thinking more than the goal of emancipating human reason from the restrictions of the Revealed Word. His short novel *Zadig* presents a view of religion that today sounds almost contemporary. Voltaire assumes the moderate position that a reasonable person can only affirm a tentative belief in God's existence. What we can know and trust is Reason. Moreover, all established religions contain much pure superstition while at the same time each insists that it is uniquely true. Such foolish insistence on doctrinal correctness produces religious intolerance and violence. Reason leads freethinking modern people to avoid dogma and to embrace pluralism. This is the message of *Zadig*, the spirit of which has been incorporated into the New Religious Synthesis.

At the age of fifty-three, with his literary powers in full force and his freedom as a writer fully realized, Voltaire wrote this fascinating Oriental romance to convey his ideas about the place of Reason in a new religious outlook. From its first appearance in 1747 the book has been considered "among his masterpieces of light narrative."[18] More subtle and whimsical than *Candide*, *Zadig* is thus also more appealing and convincing. Theodore Besterman writes that *Zadig* was "intended to persuade with a smile."[19] A wily advocate, Voltaire chose the genre of humorous narrative to create a winsome and convincing case for Reason as the basis for religion. Besterman notes, "Voltaire's tales are carefully wrought works of art: that is, their forms fit perfectly their content and purpose."[20]

A highly sympathetic character, Zadig is the wisest of men. His adventures and misadventures tend to prove that there is no point in relying on divine providence to see one through life. Rather, one should trust Reason and hope for the best. In his elegant and captivating prose Voltaire spins a virtually irresistible tale of Zadig's life, and in the process of reading we are drawn into Voltaire's account of religion. So pleasant and accessible is *Zadig* that even today it is more likely to be required reading for French school children than is the disturbing satire *Candide*.

Zadig's full title is *Zadig, or Destiny: An Oriental Tale.* The story of Zadig is set in Babylon in the middle of the fifteenth century A.D. Zadig is introduced as a man "whose innate goodness had been strengthened by his upbringing." Voltaire adds that "despite his wealth and his youth he held his passions in check, was utterly sincere, did not always expect to be right, and made allowances for human frailty."[21] Thus, in Zadig we encounter a person of impeccable manners and character, and one who enjoys social status as well. Moreover, Zadig is just and fair-minded. "Above all," Voltaire writes, "Zadig did not pride himself on despising women and

keeping them in subjection." In addition to his other qualities, Zadig is handsome, frank, wise and noble.

Early in this elaborate tale readers learn of Zadig's suspicion of religious authorities and pompous scholars. Like a good Deist, Zadig looks to Nature and Reason, not revelation or authority, for his religious guidance. "'There is no one more fortunate,' he thought, 'than a philosopher who reads in the great book that God has spread before our eyes,'" that is, the book of Nature. "The truths he discovers are his own," that is, they come through his own reason. "He nourishes and elevates his soul. He lives in peace. No one can harm him.'"[22] Reason examining Nature discovers spiritual truth, and thus discovers the transcendent. Zadig's autonomous Reason liberates itself from the constraints of Revealed Word religion, escapes the bonds of revelation and declares unequivocally its independence.

Reason resolves religious controversy. During his days as a member of the Babylonian court, Zadig developed a reputation for Solomonic wisdom and saintly generosity. "He showed day by day the subtlety of his intellect and the goodness of his character. He was admired but he was also loved."[23] At the height of his popularity Zadig is called upon to resolve a religious dispute that "split the empire into two rigid sects" for more than fifteen hundred years. And what was the question at issue in this dispute? Just this: One of the two sects "claimed that the only way to enter the temple of Mithra was left foot first, while the other sect held this custom in abhorrence and always went in right foot first."[24]

Zadig resolves this nettlesome controversy by jumping over the threshold of the temple with both feet at the same time. He then makes a speech affirming that "the God of heaven and earth is no respecter of persons," following which an envious listener complains that Zadig has not relied sufficiently on eloquence. But, "Zadig was quite satisfied with a rational style."[25] In this episode Voltaire argues that the disputes of official religion often are ridiculous and predicated on distinctions of no consequence. Any rational observer recognizes this immediately. He also affirms that Reason is superior to the religions of the priests, the disputations of the debaters and the eloquence of the orators. Reason reigns supreme.

Reason defeats religious abuse. Through many travels, adventures and perils Zadig's reason also triumphs over brutality, bigotry and religious intolerance. Zadig challenges the Arabian practice of burning widows on their husband's funeral pyres. A widow has requested this form of death, and a defender of the practice argues: "Women have been allowed to burn themselves to death for more than a

thousand years. Which of us dares to alter a law consecrated by time? What can be more respectable than an ancient abuse?"[26] These questions sum up Voltaire's argument against religious abuses; they are brutal and persistent *because* they are unexamined by Reason.

Zadig's response reflects the belief that humanity's original religion was both natural and rational: "Reason is still more ancient." Reason is older than all religious practices, and the one source of true religious ideas at all times. Zadig convinces both the widow in question and her tribal leaders to forsake their plans. In fact, so persuasive is his argument that it eventually leads to the cessation of the practice.

Reason reveals religious unity. In one of the narrative's culminating scenes, Zadig sits down to a banquet in Egypt with representatives of several different faiths. His companions include "an Egyptian, an Indian from the Ganges, an inhabitant of Cathay, a Greek, a Celt, and several other foreigners." As the evening progresses a dispute breaks out over religious practices. An Egyptian complains that he has not been loaned money against the excellent collateral of his aunt's mummified body, while an Indian instructs Zadig not to eat a piece of chicken because "the soul of the deceased may have passed into the body of that hen." The Egyptian fails to see the problem for, he asserts, "we worship a bull but we eat it all the same." The Indian is appalled, but the Egyptian says he and his countrymen have been doing the same for over one hundred thousand years. And in this vein the argument continues with each person present defending his religion as the true one. Ridiculous claims such as that a great fish taught the human race to read or that mistletoe is sacred characterize the discussion.

Zadig listens politely to this religious babble, and is finally moved to suggest a resolution to the swirling, groundless controversy. "Gentlemen . . . you are all in agreement." Zadig's argument unfolds as follows. "'It is a fact, isn't it,' he said to the Celt, 'that you don't worship this mistletoe, but the creator of mistletoe and oak?' 'Of course,' replied the Celt. 'And you, the Egyptian gentleman, revere in the form of a certain bull the maker of all bulls?' 'I do,' said the Egyptian. 'Oannes the fish,' he went on, 'must bow before the creator of the sea and all fishes.' 'Granted,' said the Chaldean."[27] In this passage Zadig sounds one of the leading themes of Deism as well as of the New Religious Synthesis: differences among religions are superficial; what they hold in common is essential. Only the common elements in various religions can claim Reason as their source. Voltaire's "creator" of all things, however, is never quite defined.

Voltaire's intolerance and the limits of Reason. Zadig is a winsome and rational Everyman, avoiding the excesses of revealed religion while maintaining a sense of the transcendent. Voltaire has created the perfect paradigm for the religious individual for a new era, a confident and reasonable resident of the new world. Gone are the meaningless disputes over doctrine that have divided believers in various faiths, that have set nation against nation and church against synagogue. Zadig tends his own garden, but helps when he can his less rational fellow travelers still trapped in creeds outworn.

Indeed, Voltaire is said by his admirers to have "succeeded in pulling the poisoned fangs of religious intolerance."[28] However, this lifelong opponent of intolerance was, as one biographer notes, "always intolerant of Christianity."[29] Voltaire was also a notorious anti-Semite. Perhaps these contradictions in Voltaire's character are due to the fact that he was much more confident about what he sought to oppose than about what he sought to establish. Zadig, after all, has no creed. Voltaire worshiped only the god of Reason whose altar in Notre Dame his followers helped to design, a god who sharpened his famous wit but who, apparently, could not soften his heart. Writers belonging to a new century would rename Voltaire's interior god.

THOMAS DE QUINCEY

Romantic writers, like Enlightenment critics before them, substituted for the outmoded wholly other God of the Revealed Word a new interior divinity. William Covino refers to this internal power as the "magical imagination." Romantic devotion to imagination is evident in the works of Blake, Wordsworth, Coleridge, Shelley and others.[30] So thoroughgoing was the Romantics' devotion to imagination that it led some to disregard the body as its hindrance. Wordsworth attributed "Coleridge's physical decay" to his intensely interior focus and the resultant "withdrawal from the sensible world into a miraculous and improbable one."[31]

Belief that a spark of divinity animated the human soul drove Romantics' intense interest in Imagination. Moreover, the knowing devotee might nurture this inner divinity through virtual self-worship. Thus Coleridge made a "godlike representation of himself" in one of his major works, *Biographia*.[32] This section draws attention to the early Romantic writer Thomas De Quincey and to a strange and very popular book that sacralized Imagination. De Quincey, like Peter Annet, made a god of the human mind.

Opium eating. Though essayist and critic Thomas De Quincey (1785-1859) was born in Manchester, England, he ran away from home at the age of seventeen, lived in London for a time, and later attended Oxford University. By 1813 he had become addicted to opium, his use of the drug beginning with an effort to relieve severe pain in his face and head. Though his collected works run to fourteen volumes, he is remembered principally for one book based on two articles for the *London Magazine*. This book, *Confessions of an English Opium Eater*, was widely read and highly influential in the early Romantic period. De Quincey's argument helps us to understand how the cult of Reason developed in the nineteenth century.

Confessions of an English Opium Eater created a sensation when it first appeared in 1820. De Quincey's remarkable ability as a prose stylist, combined with his capacity for ushering readers winsomely into the world of London's street denizens—prostitutes, orphans, thieves—attracted readers from across a wide spectrum of the British and American public. Much of the early part of the work is taken up with De Quincey's description of unusual events from his childhood and with his ill-fated relocation to London as a student in the opening years of the nineteenth century. Through various illnesses and chance encounters, De Quincey discovered opium, a drug that would become central to his life and work. The middle chapters of *Confessions* offer an elaborate defense of opium's capacity to stimulate the mind, while the closing chapters present an equivocal lament over De Quincey's struggle to overcome the effects of his long addiction to the drug.

However, *Confessions of an English Opium Eater*, for all of its other intriguing qualities, offers the reader more than a glimpse into the drug-induced state of imaginative excitement. It also makes a religious statement, an *apologia* for the superior mind liberated from the limits of conventional social life. In this way, De Quincey's book can be read as an exaltation of Reason, the inner divinity, albeit under the influence of a powerful chemical. Opium reveals to the disciplined user a transcendent inner world of unlimited rational potential and phantasmagoric imaginative experience. In this way De Quincey prefigures later hallucinogenic writers such as Aldous Huxley.

Dreaming. In another work, *Signs from the Depths*, De Quincey wrote approvingly of what he termed "dreaming," a drug-enhanced activity in which Imagination grows unrestrained by ordinary social limitations. "Among the powers in man which suffer by this too intense life of the social instincts, none suffers more than the power of dreaming." Dreaming was crucial to this nineteenth-century wor-

shiper of Reason. After all, "the machinery for dreaming planted in the human brain was not planted for nothing." Then what is its purpose? Interestingly, De Quincey makes dreaming a means of connection to the supernatural realm. Dreaming, when guided by something he called the "mystery of darkness"—apparently esoteric knowledge that allows one to direct the dreaming mind—becomes for De Quincey a "great tube" through which one can "communicate with the shadowy," an apparent reference to the spiritual world. Of course, opium assisted this communication.[33]

In elevating dreaming, De Quincey rejected not only social convention but also, like the biblical critics, history. He proposed a new understanding of religion as free from history and rooted in what he termed "profound philosophy." Profound philosophy was an act of rational rebellion against ordinary life, conventional morality, and traditional history, a rebellion achieved only by the few truly superior minds. In this way, profound philosophy was something like the Deists' practice of freethinking, an act of extraordinary rational strength by which autonomous Reason liberates itself. William Covino comments that De Quincey wrote his *Signs from the Depths* as "a manifesto for superhumanity, an oration on the dignity of the human potential for reaching beyond [the] mundane" by employing "magical imagination" against history and society. For De Quincey, this profound philosophy constituted an "act of cultural insolence." His loathing of ordinary humanity was well known.[34]

Carrying God within: restoring the mind to its natural state. Just as the Enlightenment god of Reason was eternal and omnipresent, the Romantic's interior deity of Imagination was everlasting and infinite. V. A. De Luca writes that the devotee of Imagination "houses the infinite in his own finite corporeality," that is, carries divinity within.[35] Annet found his own thinking to mirror the movements of eternal Reason. Thus, for De Quincey as for Annet, Reason became "God incarnate." Similarly, the Romantic recognized in Imagination a divine expansion of the self. When in his dream state, "which is for De Quincey the product of an isolated, drugged, defiant, and haunted sensibility," writes Covino, "one composes the giant self."[36]

Oddly, constructing this "giant self" was enhanced by opium use. De Quincey contrasted opium's effects with those of alcohol. "The main distinction lies in this," he wrote, "that whereas wine disorders the mental faculties, opium, on the contrary, (if taken in a proper manner,) introduces amongst them the most exquisite order, legislation, and harmony."[37] Thus, opium enhanced Reason by bringing order and harmony to an otherwise inconstant, unpredictable human capacity. Opium returns

Reason to a natural, unspoiled state. As he puts the point, opium brings about "a healthy restoration to that state which the mind would normally recover upon the removal of any deep-seated irritation of pain that had disturbed and quarreled with the impulses of a heart originally just and good."[38] Annet found the elixir of freethinking to place Reason in sync with Nature. De Quincey takes the quicker and truer path to the same end; the powerful narcotic opium was a restorative medicine healing the mind of wounds inflicted by life in human society. "Opium," he writes, "always seems to compose what had been agitated, and to concentrate what had been distracted."[39]

Putting a somewhat finer edge on his description of the mind's restoration, De Quincey maintains that "the opium-eater . . . feels that the diviner part of his nature is paramount; that is, the moral affections are in a state of cloudless serenity; and over all is the great light of the majestic intellect." Opium puts one in touch with the god within, one's own rational faculties—"majestic intellect"—whose true powers have been obscured by mundane routines, obligations and fatigues. Opium achieves its effects by "greatly increasing the activity of the mind."[40] A new spiritual age dawns when profound philosophy and opium set the mind free, that is, awaken the sleeping interior god. Alluding to Christ's description of himself in the book of Revelation, De Quincey assumes the role of prophet of a new spiritual order. "This is the doctrine of the true church on the subject of opium: of which church I acknowledge myself to be the only member—the alpha and the omega."[41] De Quincey's language becomes more religious as his devotion to opium and dreaming grows. In his dream state he finds "hopes which blossom in the paths of life" and "motions of the intellect as unwearied as the heavens."[42] Reason under the influence of opium offers hope, rest, peace and even freedom from the fear of death.

De Quincey awakens an interior god possessing power to create extraordinary beauty and elevate the spirit to divine heights. He praises the virtual omnipotence of divine Reason under opium's influence. De Quincey must, then, be considered an early writer in the Western hallucinogenic tradition, the cult of employing chemical substances to enhance the power and perceptual experience of the mind. In 1922 Aleister Crowley, the infamous Victorian occultist, would follow suit with his popular and controversial work *Diary of a Drug Fiend*, and in the 1960s Aldous Huxley introduced a new generation of spiritual seekers to the possibilities of mind-enhancing drugs in *Doors of Perception*.

An elite of the mind and a new religion. De Quincey's views on the powers of the human mind incorporated a kind of spiritual elitism. "Whatever may be the num-

ber of those in whom this faculty of dreaming splendidly can be supposed to lurk," he writes, "there are not perhaps very many in whom it is developed."[43] The preoccupations of ordinary work prevent the laborer from achieving such heights of intellectual self-realization. Moreover, a certain inborn capacity is required in the greatest of minds. In order for the intellect to "dream magnificently," an individual must possess "a constitutional determination" to elevated thought.[44]

It is also true that the gift of dreaming great dreams is hindered by modern technological culture. But liberation comes by way of a new religion that replaces the Revealed Word. Amidst the din of urban culture "the brain is haunted" as if by "ghostly beings moving amongst us." This "colossal pace of advance" is not likely to be reversed, and so another remedy is needed. That remedy is "counter forces of corresponding magnitude," which meant for De Quincey the force of a new religion.[45] Guided by this new faith the great dreamer rises above the mundane tragedy of "the merely human" through extraordinary rational ability, all-conquering will power, and opium.

The great mind has a destiny to fulfill: to deliver the self from the ordinary world of people through contact with another world. The mind of the dreamer is a "magnificent apparatus" that discovers "eternities below all life."[46] For De Quincey, a new religion of the exalted Self allows access to a supernatural realm, but only to a specially gifted vanguard of the human race. They enter this realm of superawareness through secret knowledge—"the mystery of darkness"—combined with their extraordinary will power, which "forces the infinite into the chambers of the human brain." Eternity itself is within their grasp. Superior intellect, freedom from the drudgeries of daily labor, secret knowledge and extraordinary will power liberate the great minds among us from the mundane world. Reason triumphs over all of the limiting forces of life, and the human mind assumes its place as master of eternity.

The goal of De Quincey's works on opium and dreaming was to probe the great capacity of some human beings, through the exercise of "magnificent intellect," to rise above their companions. The idea of an elite of the mind has had many advocates in the modern period, Annet, Voltaire and De Quincey among them. One of the most influential recent advocates of such a view of Reason, though certainly not the subtlest or most talented, is the subject of this chapter's final section. But before turning to the works of Ayn Rand, it will be instructive to consider a peculiarly American expression of the notion of divine Reason.

AMERICAN NEW THOUGHT: MIND AS DIVINE HEALING FORCE

In nineteenth-century America, Reason's elevation was manifested in widespread interest in New Thought—the use of mental power to achieve psychological and physical healing. Ultimately, New Thought may have its origins in the animal magnetism theories of the Austrian physician Franz Friedrich Anton Mesmer (1733-1815). Mesmer taught that certain cosmic powers akin to magnetism could be harnessed for healing by the knowing practitioner.[47] He is often credited with having developed the technique of hypnosis.

The American line of descent in the New Thought movement runs from Phineas Parkhurst Quimby to his patient Mary Baker Eddy, and from Eddy to Ralph Waldo Trine, the great popularizer of New Thought philosophy in the late nineteenth century. Characteristic of these thinkers, and a host of others in the New Thought and Harmonialism tradition, is a belief in the powers of the human mind or human reason. As Stephen Gottschalk writes, these thinkers stress "the adequacy of the human mind as a source of power and meaning rather than the necessity for the radical salvation of mankind through an agency outside of the self."[48]

Quimby and Eddy. Quimby (1802-1866), a clock-maker from Belfast, Maine, practiced both mesmerism and hypnotism for a time. His observations of patients and their responses to medicines and other treatments convinced him that "there was no causal connection between prescriptions and resultant cures."[49] He concluded that healing was a consequence of patients *believing* that a medicine or other treatment was effective. As Dennis Voskuil writes, "Quimby concluded, therefore, that disease was a mental problem and that health depended upon a mental cure."[50] Quimby's metaphysical speculations upon this point led him to a striking conclusion: "He viewed man as a spiritual being who possesses an unconscious soul, which is directly related to and partakes in the divine mind."[51] Healing was a matter of understanding properly our essential divinity. This discovery Quimby dubbed the "science of healing."

Mary Baker Eddy (1821-1910) visited Quimby in search of healing in the early 1860s, and became for a time a devoted disciple. She adapted—some would say plagiarized—Quimby's basic ideas and formulated her own science of healing around an idealism that taught that illness was an error in thinking. Eddy always insisted that she had made a sharp break with Quimby and his views.[52] Quimby's ideas were also advanced by Warren Felt Evans, another former patient. In a series of books in-

cluding *The Mental Cure* and *The Primitive Mind Cure*, Evans "reiterated the basic positions of New Thought."[53]

New Thought advocates organized themselves in 1914 into the New Thought Alliance, a group that officially proclaimed "the Divinity of Man and his infinite possibilities through the creative power of constructive thinking." The group also urged attention to the "voice of the Indwelling Presence which is our source of Inspiration, Power, Health and Prosperity."[54] Mind was the indwelling divinity in human beings. As such, Mind, not the Revealed Word's God, was the source of all good things.

The Fillmores and Unity Christian School. The religion of Mind or Reason continued to develop its own distinctive theology under the guidance of Charles and Myrtle Fillmore, founders in 1889 of the Unity Christian School. The mind possessed boundless powers that were released through a practice Charles Fillmore called simply "prayer." Through prayer the skilled practitioner concentrated mental energy on a problem in such a way as to unleash the "electronic, life imparting forces" and "vibrant energies" of the "spiritual ethers" which are present also in the "cells of our body."[55] Mind was again, as with Quimby, Eddy and Evans, the sole agent of divine power.

It did not take long for religious mentalism to become the key to worldly success and even power. Prentice Mulford stands as an important example of this trend. "To think success brings success," he wrote in the 1880s. But a greedy edge bordering on megalomania begins to appear in the Mulford's religious mentalism: "Set the magnetic power of your mind persistently in the desire and *demand* the best of everything, and the best will, by an inevitable and unerring law, eventually come to you."[56]

Ralph Waldo Trine. The real popularizer of religious mentalism, however, was Ralph Waldo Trine (1866-1958). In 1897 his book *In Tune with the Infinite: Fullness of Peace, Power and Plenty* first appeared. Voskuil reports that "this book sold an astonishing one and a half million copies."[57] Trine turned "mentalism" in a direction best termed rational magic. He emphasized a technique of visualization that actually turned ideas into material realities. Through the exercise of Trine's rational techniques, the practitioner of mentalism "set into operation subtle, silent, and irresistible forces that . . . actualize in material form what is today merely an idea." Trine adds, with suggestive phrasing, that "ideas have occult power, and ideas when rightly tended are the seeds that actualize material conditions."[58] Thus, the skilled human manipulator of ideas creates reality, and the master of Reason is rendered a

divine agent. Voskuil maintains that Trine's book created "a new form of religious literature . . . that would become as common as aspirin by 1960."[59] Later proponents of Trine's mentalism included Emmet Fox and Glen Clark, who taught that "'things are thoughts' and that external reality is 'an outpicturing of our minds.'"[60]

Reason elevated to a divine status is inherent to religious and secular metaphysics ranging from the positive thinking teachings of Norman Vincent Peale to the works of New Age writers who urge their readers to create their own realities through mental projection or *maya*. The power of Reason to discover spiritual truth, to transcend earthly constraints, even to shape present reality, are now basic tenets of the New Religious Synthesis. So widely assimilated are these ideas that they have also been advocated by writers who claim no particular religious view whatever. Novelist Ayn Rand provides an important and highly influential example of just such a writer. Her morality of unrestrained egoism constitutes a luminous instance of the terminus of Reason's elevation.

AYN RAND'S ARGUMENT FOR REASON

Russian émigré Ayn Rand (1905-1982) arrived in the United States in 1926. She was highly successful as a Hollywood screenwriter, an occupation she pursued until 1943. Beginning with *We the Living* in the 1930s, Rand developed a philosophy of "enlightened self-interest" and the "virtue of selfishness." This perspective is skillfully advocated in phenomenally popular and controversial novels, including *The Fountainhead* (1943) and *Atlas Shrugged* (1957), books that continue to sell more than 250,000 copies annually. Rand achieved a degree of cultural influence enjoyed by few writers. She stated repeatedly in her fiction, as well as in nonfiction works such as *The Virtue of Selfishness* (1964), that her philosophy—a version of Nietzsche's philosophy of will—is based on regard for reason alone. The extended narrative was by far her most successful vehicle for advancing the philosophy of radical self-interest. Rand represents the twentieth-century fruition of the cult of Reason.

John Galt speaks . . . and speaks. Ultimate regard for something called Reason is powerfully portrayed in Rand's ruthless prose. John Galt, the principal character in her largest and most important novel, *Atlas Shrugged*, presents Rand's philosophy of Reason in a long speech near the end of that book. Galt's speech is perhaps the most powerful example of Rand the didactic storyteller, Rand the public advocate, Rand the popular philosopher. This famous interlude in *Atlas Shrugged* also pro-

vides a fascinating example of how Rand defines the role of autonomous Reason in reaction against the traditional moral perspective of the Revealed Word.

Some background is important to understanding the origin and purpose of John Galt's speech. In *Atlas Shrugged,* the wealthy industrialist Galt arranges for all of America's powerful and influential elite to join him in a secret enclave in the Rocky Mountains. He intends to demonstrate once and for all that the followers of Reason, a small human vanguard, are the "great ones" who make civilization possible. The speech's secondary purpose is, apparently, to convince the ordinary working drones of the world that they are parasites who make victims of their betters. At the novel's climactic moment a rapidly deteriorating nation, bereft of its most talented leaders, hears from the mighty Galt a prolonged argument for his basic philosophy of life and a harsh account of social justice.

Sacrificing Reason to faith. Despite Rand's remarkable popularity, Galt's speech reads like a rant from a self-absorbed amateur philosopher who has read Nietzsche without much power of penetration. Galt declares, "I am the man who loves his life. I am the man who does not sacrifice his love or values," by which he means that he has lived according to the rule of Reason, which for Rand is the law of complete selfishness. By taking the strong, like himself, out of the world, Galt has deprived the weak of their "victims" and thus "destroyed [their] world." The weak and poor are in their present state because they "dread knowledge."

And why have the majority of America's citizens forsaken knowledge for something lower? Rand's answer is that they have allowed the apostles of religious faith to delude them. "You have sacrificed reason to faith," Galt alleges. Consequently the masses have acted according to conventional and irrational morality. "You have sacrificed wealth to need," which constitutes a sin against Reason. John Galt makes clear, repeatedly, that for him there is no higher source of power than Reason, no greater entity than Mind. People who choose to live by Reason are "the men of the mind," an elite destined to rule.[61] Such people are not moved by human need; they find selfishness, not mercy, the highest virtue. With the great ones out of the picture, the remainder of humanity faces "a world without mind" according to Galt.[62] Speaking on behalf of the best of us, John Galt tells the rest of us, "*We do not need you*" (emphasis in original). Is this the ultimate destination of Voltaire's liberating deity, Reason? In Rand, Reason dissolves into vindictive self-importance posturing as moral philosophy.

Galt alleges that trading Reason for religious morality caused humanity's Fall.

The "scourges and disasters" of history are "brought about by your code of moral-ity." The feeble Revealed Word moral code demands love, service, charity and sac-rifice. The meek do not inherit the earth; rather they are the "incompetents on earth" who have failed to follow Reason. "Reason does not work automatically," Galt alleges. "Thinking is not a mechanical process; the connections of logic are not made by instinct." To think requires "effort," an effort the poor have not made. [63]

The Revealed Word tradition takes a severe beating in Rand's case for a new mo-rality. The despicable masses admire the old religious virtues of altruism and service, and for this they are punished. "Yes," declares Galt, "you *are* bearing punishment for your evil." [64] Their sin was to fail to follow Reason to the place it had led Galt himself. But this is an odd judgment, for Rand makes clear that following Reason is *not* within the reach of most people. The "men of the mind" are a very small elite, and Reason is the omnipotent tool of the few possessing the will to master it.

Saving knowledge. For Rand, mastering Reason is self-salvation, the gods of the religions being merely "ghosts in heaven." [65] Death is always a lurking threat, and holding on to life requires "the knowledge needed to keep it." [66] Thus, the follower of Reason seeks the special knowledge necessary to maintain and extend the life of Reason. Galt argues that one "must obtain his knowledge and choose his actions by a process of thinking, which nature will not force him to perform." [67] "Man's life" is thus "life by means of achievement." Good and evil are defined with reference to Reason. "All that which is proper to the life of a rational being is the good, all that which destroys it is the evil." [68]

Galt places this ferocious, triumphant morality of Reason in opposition to the pathetic, self-destructive morality of religion. Conventional religion preaching ser-vice and self-sacrifice "gives you *death* as your standard." [69] The founders and leaders of conventional religions are "hatred-eaten mystics who pose as friends of human-ity and preach that the highest virtue man can practice is to hold his own life as of no value." [70] Thus, Rand vehemently rejects such dictums as Jesus' proclamation that "those who want to save their life will lose it, and those who lose their life for my sake will find it" (Mt 16:25; Lk 9:24). Saving oneself in Rand's cosmos is a mat-ter of devoting oneself fully to the interior god Reason.

CONCLUSION

This chapter has explored writers who find in Reason, Mind, Imagination or Con-sciousness unlimited potential for human advancement. Elevation of Reason was a

hallmark of the Enlightenment, and Reason's central role in human spiritual life has been a theme of Western metaphysical writing ever since.

I have selected for special attention several writers who addressed a popular audience and treated some aspect of the human rational life as a substitute for either the Revealed Word or its personal God. Annet made Reason a divinity within us, the standard of human morality and the source of our spiritual life. Voltaire emphasized reason's critical qualities, its capacity to cut through the dense fog of confusion cast up by various revelations. De Quincey called attention to the intellect's imaginative dimension, making it the center of human experience and calling for its expansion through opium use. The advocates of New Thought explored the mind's capacity to heal and to otherwise alter reality. Rand made Reason the basis of ego's triumph over life's obstacles, the source of both personal success and political order, and the basis of a self-serving moral view. What each author has in common with the others is the determination to place human rational capacities, or some particular rational capacity, at the center of spiritual or moral life. Each venerates Reason, placing it figuratively, as Voltaire's followers did literally in Notre Dame, at the center of the temple of human spirituality.

The New Religious Synthesis recognizes a force, a virtual divinity, within the human cerebrum. This power of human rationality, will and creativity displaces the sovereign and wholly other God of the Revealed Word. Annet's God Incarnate, Voltaire's Reason, De Quincey's Majestic Intellect, Trine's Mind, Rand's Reason—each is an expression of rational autonomous individuality transformed into a god. The following chapter considers the public case for Reason's own creation—science—as a new source of theology. In the Other Spirituality, science reveals to Reason new spiritual truths.

5

SCIENCE AND SHIFTING PARADIGMS

Salvation in a New Cosmos

O what a world of profit and delight,
of power, of honor, of omnipotence
Is promis'd to the studious artisan!
CHRISTOPHER MARLOWE, Dr. Faustus

Do not be surprised if physics curricula of the twenty-first century include classes in meditation.
GARY ZUKAV, The Dancing Wu Li Masters

I thought of all the books I had read—and tried to understand—on quantum physics . . . the
new physics, they called it. It sounded so much like ancient Eastern mysticism.
SHIRLEY MACLAINE, Dancing in the Light

Christianity is to be found an enemy to civilization, and the struggle which modern thought and
science are compelled to conduct with it is . . . a "cultur-kampf [culture war]."
ERNST HAECKEL, The Riddle of the Universe

Auguste Comte (1798-1857), founder of the school of thought known as logical positivism, maintained "that humanity progresses through stages of thought." Each of these stages represents a rational advance over the previous one. The first stage he identified as the theological, which, as the name implies, presents God as the cause of all that exists. The second stage Comte dubbed the metaphysical, a period in our rational progress which dispenses with theological explanation in favor of more refined philosophical accounts of objects and events.

However, both the theological and the metaphysical stages in human thinking are mere stepping stones along the way to the final stage of rational progress, which

Comte called the "positivist." This is the highest achievement in human thinking, a period in which only scientific explanations are accepted as legitimate and rational. Science was for Comte the ultimate achievement of human Reason. It explained the cosmos and offered a method of controlling it. Moreover, science performed both tasks without reference to a deity.[1] Science, then, was a substitute for religion.

Comte discarded theology and enthroned Science as the sole source of knowledge, transcendence and higher experience. Comte "literally made a cult of science," and by the 1870s his many readers "invested science with power, promise, . . . even with sacredness."[2] He developed an elaborate calendar of inspirational readings from the world's great thinkers and included what can only be called holy days. "The year," wrote one observer, "is divided into thirteen lunar months, each named after some great man. Every day is dedicated to some minor celebrity—one day to the dead in general, and one day to the memory of holy women. The calendar is studded with *fete* days just like a calendar of the saints." Churches of "the Religion of Humanity" sprang up in London and other cities, and Comte himself occasionally "preached and performed marriage and burial services."[3] Comte himself, however, eventually moved from his scientific worship of humanity to the worship of his deceased paramour, Madame Clotilde de Vaux, to whom he prayed on a regular basis.[4]

If science is empirical method employed to resolve questions of physical causation, Science is that method sacralized as the sole source of saving knowledge for the human race. This chapter considers some efforts to convert science into Science, to transform a method of investigation into a source of theological insight. Science as a window on a sacred cosmos is a cornerstone of the New Religious Synthesis, the instrument of Reason in search of ever greater spiritual insight.

Joseph Ernest Renan (1823-1892), philologist, historian, director of the College de France and author of the enormously controversial *Life of Jesus* (1863), shared and helped to shape the late nineteenth-century hope in Science as a substitute for religion. "He was sure," writes historian Jacques Barzun, "that science would make all other works of the mind obsolete: philosophy, theology, literature would disappear."[5] Speaking of the Christian faith of medieval people, Carl Jung wrote in 1933 that "natural science has long ago torn this lovely veil to shreds." In the old religious view "men were all children of God under the loving care of the Most High, who prepared them for eternal blessedness."[6]

Is not Science a strictly rational endeavor intentionally denuded of such gaudy baubles that have always attended "mere faith"? Surely the picture must be more

complex. When Mary Baker Eddy invented a new religion in the nineteenth century, she called it Christian *Science*. Similarly, Philip Jenkins has noted that occult writers of the nineteenth and twentieth centuries often alleged that they were simply applying scientific discoveries to the solution of spiritual problems.[7] And physicist Amit Goswami has recently written in his book *The Self-Aware Universe* that "modern science is venturing into realms that for more than four millennia have been the fiefdoms of religion and philosophy." Consequently, "we are privileged to be a part of this evolutionary and transcendent process by which science is changing not only itself but also our perception of reality."[8] The dean of twentieth-century spiritual scientists, Fritjof Capra, arrived at the same conclusion in 1975 when he wrote that "the influence of modern physics . . . extends to the realm of thought and culture where it has led to a deep revision in our conception of the universe and our relationship to it."[9]

The following pages focus attention on several popular arguments over the past three centuries that advance Science as the pathway to a new spirituality, one prepared to replace the outdated and unscientific Revealed Word perspective. We will survey a famous eighteenth-century work that treats Science as a new source of transcendence, a nineteenth-century argument that Science opens the way for a new humanistic religion, and several twentieth-century arguments for Science as the new religion. Recently the argument about the spirituality of Science has turned decidedly in the direction of mysticism. The elevation of Science as a means of discovering a new and verifiably true spirituality is a crucial component in the Other Spirituality.

THOMAS PAINE ON THE HOPE OF SCIENCE

Thomas Paine was born January 29, 1737, at Thetford in Norfolk, England. His father was Quaker, his mother Anglican. As a young man Paine served for a time as a sailor, and later as a tax collector for the English government. Self-educated, he used the small amount of money he could save to purchase books and rudimentary scientific equipment. Paine also attended lectures in London and was particularly drawn to discussions of Newtonian physics. During a visit to London, Benjamin Franklin encouraged Paine to sail for America, which he did in October of 1774. Talk of revolution was heard everywhere in the Colonies in the 1770s, and Paine began to write pamphlets that eventually made him one of the independence movement's principal proponents. His wildly popular pamphlet *Common Sense* played a decisive role in

convincing many colonists that separation from England was inevitable.

"The Age of Reason." Paine had long believed that Christianity prevented people from thinking about the injustices of government, and was convinced that a free and just government could not exist simultaneously with Christianity. For Paine, the Deists' veneration of Reason was the only true religion, and it could not exist side by side with Christianity. "Tyranny in religion" is the worst of all tyrannies. Always a popularizer, Paine provided Americans in the 1790s what Deists of the 1730s provided England—a clear and accessible argument for rejecting the Revealed Word in favor of a "religion of Reason."

Voltaire vowed to show the world that, if it took only twelve men to establish Christianity, it would take only one to destroy it. Similarly, Paine boasted that he would "march through the Christian forest with an axe." *The Age of Reason* was to be that axe. So extreme were the views expressed in this book that Samuel Adams and Benjamin Rush refused to associate with Paine after its publication. The publisher of the book's first edition was actually tried for blasphemy and imprisoned. Paine's deep hatred of Christianity rang clear in the book's pages. "Whenever we read the obscene stories, the voluptuous debaucheries, the cruel and torturous executions, the unrelenting vindictiveness, with which more than half of the Bible is filled," he wrote, "it would be more consistent to say that it was the word of a demon than the word of God. It is a history of wickedness that has served to corrupt and brutalize mankind; and, for my part, I sincerely detest it as I detest everything that is cruel."[10]

While *The Age of Reason* is infamous for such antireligious sentiments, Paine's argument for a religious hope in science is seldom recognized. Nevertheless, he incorporated into this caustic and provocative work a groundbreaking view of science as spiritual solace, as the source of a new religion suited to the modern world. *The Age of Reason* is his manifesto on a new era in human consciousness, his plea for taking leave of all of the errors of the past and embarking on a new scientific path in religion. Paine spent many pages in *The Age of Reason* rehearsing the Bible's errors and other offenses to reason, making the case that Reason, not the Bible, leads us to God. "It is only by the exercise of reason that man can discover God," he wrote.[11]

Paine was above all a highly capable rhetorical tactician, and two strategic goals regarding religion are evident in *The Age of Reason*. The first is to undermine the Revealed Word perspective through corrosive biblical criticism of the type pioneered by the Deists and with which Paine was intimately familiar. The second is to advance an alternative religious perspective based on Science, one that prefigures

components of the New Religious Synthesis. Paine sets about accomplishing these goals by writing as an angry opponent of all superstition and rational tyranny. Tyranny in the spiritual realm was even more objectionable than tyranny in the political realm, and Paine knew better than anyone how to rouse public ire over tyranny.

But Paine's tone changes in the second book of *The Age of Reason*. Here he writes as the reader's friend and guide into the mysteries of an incomparably complex and wonderful universe. Book Two presents Paine as the diligent student of nature and nature's God, a thinker and observer ready to share discoveries that might actually form the basis of a new perspective on religion.

A glimpse of this new religious perspective is afforded in Paine's discussion of the Bible's two worthy passages. The book of Job and the nineteenth psalm garner Paine's approval because they "take the book of creation as the Word of God, they refer to no other books, and all the inferences they make are drawn from that volume [of creation]."[12] The physical world—Paine's "book of creation"—is elevated in these two portions of Scripture in a commendable, scientific way. More to the point, Paine is particularly interested in what careful study of the sky reveals about the original human theology.

Paine argued that Psalm 19 and the book of Job "are theological orations comformable to the original system of theology."[13] That is, all theology can be, and originally was, derived from observing nature, especially "the structure of the universe."[14] Like the magical scientists of the Renaissance, Paine sought to understand the underlying principles of the cosmos—for this is all he can mean by "theology"—through a study of the stars. As Hugh Kearney writes, these early scientists sought "to recognize the fundamental structure of reality."[15] It was thought that such a science placed its practitioner in virtual control of the cosmos.

Science, understood as grasping the mathematical structure of the universe through study of the planets and stars, has always been, according to Paine, Christianity's mortal enemy. Indeed, he alleges that early Christian leaders tried to prevent science's development. They "could not but foresee that the continually progressive knowledge that man would gain, by the aid of science, of the power and wisdom of God, manifested in the structure of the universe and in all the works of creation, would . . . call into question the truth of their system of faith." Thus, these first Christian leaders actively opposed the development of science. They "cut learning down to a size less dangerous" to faith, and so "restrict[ed] the idea of learning to the dead study of dead languages."[16]

Christian myth versus scientific pantheism. If Christianity cannot be supported by science, how should we understand the faith? For Paine the Deist, faith is simply "another species of mythology" and a corruption of "an ancient system of theism."[17] To reclaim this pre-Christian system of rational belief, one must turn to science, especially astronomy. In fact, Paine traces the rise of theism itself to the worship of the planet Saturn. "The supposed reign of Saturn was prior to that which is called the heathen mythology, and was so far a system of theism that it admitted the belief of only one god." He adds, "All the corruptions that have taken place in theology and in religion have been produced by admitting of what man calls *revealed religion*," that is, the Revealed Word tradition and all of its offshoots.[18] Rational religion, on the other hand, derives from the scientific examination of nature, especially the careful study of celestial bodies.

In a section entitled "Comparing Christianism with Pantheism," Paine recommends a scientific alternative to Christianity. He labels this faith Deism, but it is a brand of pantheism that locates God in creation. "How different is [Christianity] to the pure and simple profession of Deism! The true Deist has but one Deity," he announces, "and his religion consists in contemplating the power, wisdom and benignity of the Deity in His works," that is, in nature.[19] For Paine, the Judeo-Christian tradition is a corruption of an ancient pantheism that can be reclaimed through science—the study of God "in His works." Nature does not so much point to a God outside of itself as it suggests that there is something divine in nature.

Astronomy, extraterrestrial life and scientific religion. Paine compared Science as the study of "the structure of the heavens," with the various "systems of religion."[20] Science, "the progression of knowledge," was the one true source of religion. Early Christians had recognized this fact, and thus tried to stop Science. Had Christianity not stifled Science, human knowledge of the cosmos would have developed indefinitely. This limitless scientific knowledge would have become the foundation of a scientific religion based on the mathematical structures of the universe and resulting in the limitless "progress of the human mind."[21] Christians had, then, prevented the advent of heaven on earth by their vision of a heaven beyond life.

Paine began developing his theology of Science at an early age. Even as a youth he "doubted the truth of the Christian system or thought it to be a strange affair."[22] From early childhood the "natural bent" of his mind "was to science." Thus, as soon as he was able he "purchased a pair of globes and attended the philosophical lectures of Martin and Ferguson" and became acquainted with other eminent as-

tronomers.[23] He made himself master of the use of globes and of the orrery," a term referring to a "machinery of clock-work representing the universe [solar system] in miniature." Paine eventually became convinced of "the infinity of space, and the eternal divisibility of matter."[24]

In a section entitled "Advantages of Life in a Plurality of Worlds," Paine explains that this idea of an infinite space filled with divine life led him, as it had earlier led Giordano Bruno, to speculate that there are other intelligent species in the universe. "Since, then, no part of our earth is left unoccupied, why is it to be supposed that the immensity of space is naked void, lying in eternal waste?"[25] Rather, as we contemplate its vastness, "the immensity of space will appear to us filled with systems of worlds."[26] Recognizing that the universe contains "a *plurality* of worlds" should elicit "the gratitude of man as well as his admiration." Paine is confident that these other worlds are inhabited, and that "the inhabitants of each of the worlds of which our system is composed enjoy the same opportunities of knowledge as we do."[27] Though he claims to be following Science alone, Paine ends in speculation about inhabited planets in other parts of the universe as a source of religious awe and spiritual comfort.[28]

"The cheerful idea of a society of worlds" ought to function as an antidote to Revealed Word's puny vision of a single inhabited planet. "In the midst of those reflections, what are we to think of the Christian system of faith that forms itself upon the idea of only one world, and that of no greater extent, as is before shown, than twenty-five thousand miles? . . . Alas, what is this to the mighty ocean of space, and the almighty power of the Creator?" Christianity is wrong, for when one reflects on the skies "every evidence the heavens afford to man either directly contradicts it or renders it absurd."[29] Nature clearly teaches a religion, but that religion is not the Revealed Word.

Morality and transcendence. The perennial religious contest, then, pits the Revealed Word and its God against Science and Nature. Rather than trusting "that which is called *the Word of God,* as shown to us in a printed book that any man might make," Paine commends "the real word of God existing in the universe."[30] However, Paine faced two problems in advocating a scientific religion that venerated the natural order.

The first problem was finding moral content for a new religion inspired by merely contemplating the vastness of space and the numerous inhabited planets swimming in that vastness. Paine discovered a solution to this problem that has

been employed many times since—morality in the new scientific faith derives from "contributing to the happiness of the living creation that God has made." This is the chief moral duty of scientific religion.[31] "Living creation" is an important phrase for Paine. Despite his references to a creator God, his strong implication in the second book of *The Age of Reason* is that the creation is, in fact, a living thing generating other living things.[32] Thus, actions that increase the happiness of the living natural order are moral, while those that work against its happiness are not.

Second, Paine needed a source of transcendence to replace the worship of the Revealed Word's personal God. Again, he invents a source of reverent awe often repeated since his day. Transcendence is discovered in contemplating the intricate order of the cosmos, an act of worship for Paine. Religious feelings "become enlarged in proportion as we contemplate the extent and structure of the universe."[33] Thus, Science can provide a sense of wonder that expands our spiritual consciousness and deepens our religious feeling.[34]

For Thomas Paine, Science was the basis for a new spiritual hope. Pantheism coupled with a close study of the structures of the universe—"the real word of God"—generates a rational, unifying religion as an alternative to the old, irrational tradition of the Revealed Word. Paine's argument hearkens back to the magical scientists of the sixteenth and seventeenth centuries who "looked forward to a Golden Age of universal wisdom (pansophia)" that would follow our deciphering of the secrets of the cosmos.[35] As the Enlightenment closed, Thomas Paine became an ardent advocate of this universal and scientific religion. His vision was pursued in the next century by a great American orator whose admiration for Paine was well known.

ROBERT GREEN INGERSOLL: SCIENCE AND DELIVERANCE

The public lecture was a popular form of entertainment in nineteenth-century America, and an important means of disseminating ideas. In the absence of radio, television and national newspapers, the public lecture performed some of the functions of modern mass media. Well-known political, religious and academic figures held large audiences in thrall with their eloquence and erudition. Even in small towns large crowds gathered on Main Street to hear Abraham Lincoln and Stephen Douglas debate, or congregated in a lecture hall to contemplate the philosophy of Ralph Waldo Emerson or the political ideas of Susan B. Anthony. Particularly famous speakers made regular appearances on the Chautauqua, Lyceum

or other prominent lecture circuits. The Lyceum Movement, established in 1834, at one time had more than three thousand local branches.

Among the most famous and successful of these traveling speakers was a former army officer and Attorney General of the state of Illinois, Robert Green Ingersoll (1833-1899), known to his Christian opponents as Mr. Injure-soul. Born in Dresden, New York, the son of a Congregational minister, Ingersoll had little opportunity for formal education as a child but diligently educated himself. After studying law, Ingersoll was admitted to the Illinois bar in 1854, eventually developing a legal practice that brought him considerable income. He served as a Union cavalry colonel during the Civil War, and following the war became involved in politics as a persuasive Republican spokesman during presidential campaigns.

Ingersoll's interest in arguments against Christianity, coupled with his legal training and oratorical skill, led him to write volumes in opposition to traditional faith. He eventually became a highly sought-after speaker with a national reputation for eloquence and wit. At the peak of his fame in the 1870s and 1880s Ingersoll commanded the astonishing sum of $3,500 for a single evening of speaking. A prolific writer and lecturer, he published numerous books, articles and lectures on a variety of subjects, but was most famous for his brash attacks on Christianity and the Bible. The personal cost of his passionate assault on the Revealed Word was substantial, as Republican leaders refused to appoint Ingersoll to prestigious cabinet and diplomatic posts.

Ingersoll more than any other figure in late nineteenth-century America popularized a virtually religious faith in scientific progress. His lectures were intelligent, provocative, bombastic and superficially scientific. Ingersoll presented himself as a freethinking citizen asking tough questions and looking for honest answers. He was an ordinary person of common sense too clever to be duped by biblical myths and legends. Ingersoll invited his audiences to join the ranks of forward-looking, scientifically minded thinkers liberating themselves from outdated and unexamined religious notions. His most famous and influential speech, "The Mistakes of Moses," dismantles key narratives in the Pentateuch using scathing satire and biting wit. The speech places science in the dual role of critic of the old superstitions and source of a new spirituality. Ingersoll thus reflected a view of science now characteristic of the New Religious Synthesis.

According to Ingersoll, "all religious systems enslave the mind."[36] No existing religion is founded on "the facts of nature" as revealed by science. The goal of Sci-

ence is "to go into partnership with these forces of nature" in order to benefit humankind.[37] No longer would modern thinking people need the Revealed Word's superstitions to explain either their existence or their destiny. Religious ideas bear no relationship to scientific knowledge. "What does religion have to do with facts? Nothing. Is there any such thing as Methodist mathematics, Presbyterian botany, Catholic astronomy, or Baptist biology?"[38] Liberating the popular mind from the dictates of the Revealed Word became Ingersoll's great public work. To light the way out of the dungeon of unscientific religious belief he held aloft "the torch of reason." And Science was reason's purest flame.[39]

The scientific attack in "The Mistakes of Moses." Ingersoll's goal in "The Mistakes of Moses" was to challenge on scientific grounds certain claims in Genesis and Exodus. He lived his entire life during the nineteenth century, a century of astonishing advances in the various sciences. Scientific discoveries in biology and geology seemed to render miracles incredible and the earth incalculably ancient. Ingersoll cast his critical gaze on famous biblical passages such as the creation of Eve from Adam's rib, the miraculous crossing of the Red Sea and the Israelite's subsisting on manna in the desert, subjecting them to scornful examination. Ingersoll attacked the Genesis notion that the sky is a "firmament" over the earth. "The man who wrote that believed the firmament to be solid. He knew nothing of the laws of evaporation."[40] He ridiculed the Noahic flood in Genesis. "How deep were these waters? About five and a half miles. How long did it rain? Forty days. How much did it have to rain a day? About 800 feet. How is that for dampness?"[41] Concerning the rainbow that appeared after the flood, Ingersoll asked his audiences the scientific question, "Now, can anybody believe that that is the origin of the rainbow? Are you not all familiar with the natural causes which bring about those beautiful arches before our eyes?"[42] In these and many similar examples Ingersoll hoped to demonstrate that Science employed by common sense overturns a literal reading of the Bible. And Science would also provide the Revealed Word's replacement.

The creed of Science: a new salvation. Ingersoll repudiated the Christian notion of salvation by faith. "Are we to get to Heaven by creed or by deed?" he asked. "Shall we reason, or shall we simply believe?" Christ's substitutionary atonement was an "infamy" that taught "that one man can be good for another, or that one man can sin for another." According to Ingersoll, "you have to be good for yourself; you have to sin for yourself." Thus, "the trouble about the atonement is, that it saves the wrong man." His alternative to such unscientific religion is summarized in three

words: "Liberty, love, and law." With minds unencumbered by worries of an after-life, our goal becomes to make ourselves and others happy. "One world at a time is my doctrine," Ingersoll told his audiences. "Let us make some one happy here. Let every man try to make his wife happy, his children happy . . . and God cannot afford to damn such a man."

Ingersoll's gospel was that "humanity is the only real religion." Guided by Science, a new humanity will reject destructive ideas such as hell, sin, guilt and judgment and will "grasp each other's hands in genuine friendship."[43] A new spirituality elevates the title "human" above labels such as Baptist or Methodist. "Forget that [you] are Baptists or Methodists, and remember that [you] are men and women. These are the biggest titles humanity can bear—man and woman; and every title you add belittles them. Man is the highest; woman is the highest."[44] Recognizing our common humanity is spiritual fulfillment enough for the dawning age. "Instead of loving God, we love each other." In this way "real religion" is to "live for each other." A scientific society will emerge when we "build the fabric of civilization on the foundation of demonstrated truth."

To hasten the advent of this new spiritual order, scientifically minded people must "destroy the guide-boards that point in the wrong direction," a reference to the old spirituality of the Revealed Word. Like the futurist prophet that he understood himself to be, Ingersoll called his audiences to "dispel the darkness of ignorance" by turning toward "the sun of science."[45] And what is the creed suggested by the rising sun of Science?

In an important speech entitled "The Foundations of Faith," Ingersoll set out his moral code for the new religious age. He entitled it "The Creed of Science," though it makes no direct reference to science. Like the Deists' Reason, Ingersoll's Science teaches an ethic evident in the natural order of things. In fact, Ingersoll referred to this natural and universal morality as "the religion of reason." I will present the creed in its entirety, as it is the clearest and most complete statement of the scientific moral perspective Ingersoll hoped would replace the Revealed Word:

To love justice, to long for the right, to love mercy, to pity the suffering, to assist the weak, to forget wrongs and to remember benefits—to love the truth, to be sincere, to utter honest words, to love liberty, to wage relentless war against slavery in all its forms, to love wife and child and friend, to make a happy home, to love the beautiful; in art, in nature, to cultivate the mind, to be familiar with the mighty thoughts that

genius has expressed, the noble deeds of all the world, to cultivate courage and cheer-fulness, to make others happy, to fill life with the splendor of generous acts, the warmth of loving words, to discard error, to destroy prejudice, to receive new truths with gladness, to cultivate hope, to see the calm beyond the storm, the dawn beyond the night, to do the best that can be done and then to be resigned—this is the religion of reason, the creed of science. This satisfies the brain and heart.[46]

For Robert Green Ingersoll, then, Science had a clear spiritual dimension. It sought not simply facts about the physical universe, but a universal moral order. Only "the sun of science" could provide religious insight. Despite his experiences in the Civil War—a vicious conflict ignited by a loathsome practice—Ingersoll remained confident that natural human goodness, informed by Science, would provide the foundation of a new spiritual awareness destined to replace the Revealed Word. Science was the engine of religious progress, the source of a new religion that would carry us to a bright future.

CARL SAGAN: FROM *THE DEMON-HAUNTED WORLD* TO ALIEN *CONTACT*

No writer of the late twentieth century did more to popularize science than Carl Sagan. Prior to his death from cancer in 1996, Sagan was the David Duncan Professor of Astronomy and Space Sciences and Director of the Laboratory for Planetary Studies at Cornell University. He had also held such prestigious positions as the Distinguished Visiting Scientist at the Jet Propulsion Laboratory, California Institute of Technology. Sagan was cofounder and President of the Planetary Society, the world's largest space interest group. A prolific writer and television commentator on scientific issues, Sagan was a Pulitzer Prize recipient as well as the recipient of the Public Welfare Medal, the highest award offered by the National Academy of Sciences. Sagan was also involved in the American space program for many years. He received twenty-two honorary doctorates and the Oersted Medal from the American Association of Physics Teachers.

Sagan's public fame resulted from books such as *Cosmos* (which became an Emmy and Peabody Award-winning television documentary), *Billions and Billions* and the science fiction novel *Contact*, which was made into a popular movie starring Jodie Foster. *Cosmos* was the most widely read science book ever written. Carl Sagan wrote these extraordinarily popular scientific and fictional works as a bona fide scientific scholar, an expert with few peers. To unquestioned expertise he added

charm, wit and transparency. Sagan brought science out of the laboratory and into the living room. Science was now for everyone's enjoyment, and it had wonderful and unexpected things to teach us. For his vast and attentive audience, Carl Sagan spoke as an unquestioned authority.

However, despite his impeccable credentials, numerous awards and unprecedented fame, Sagan was a controversial figure in the scientific community. This controversy had one source—Sagan's life-long interest in discovering intelligent beings on other planets. An enthusiastic backer of SETI, the Search for Extraterrestrial Intelligence, his passion for this project led to his rejection by many scientists who considered his quest to be pseudo-science.[47] Undaunted, the charismatic Sagan placed all of his considerable influence and personal charisma behind the project. He lived to see Harvard University establish the 8 million channel META/Sentinel survey, and an even more powerful NASA program begun as part of the ongoing search for intelligent life in the cosmos.

"The Demon-Haunted World." The Demon-Haunted World: Science as a Candle in the Dark was Carl Sagan's last book. The metaphor in the subtitle is revealing: in the twentieth-century's gathering darkness of rampant superstition and religious fundamentalism, science is a saving presence, a lone light in a dark place. In short, science offers humanity's only real *spiritual* solace. The book is a historical exploration of how scientists and other critically minded individuals have fought to expose spiritual charlatans, overturn groundless superstitions, and still the voices of religious enthusiasts. *The Demon-Haunted World* also elevates science as a source of wonder and transcendence, and argues that science and democratic values will provide the foundation for a progressively improving and increasingly peaceful human future.

According to its title, Sagan's lengthy statement on "science as social hope" is written against a religious idea—that demonic or other hidden spiritual forces exist and that they influence the daily lives of human beings. This benighted notion of a "demon-haunted world" becomes Sagan's metaphor for all that science seeks to dispel—occult causes, esoteric knowledge, dark superstitions, religious fundamentalism, barbaric persecutions and inhumane inquisitions. Though one would expect that the late twentieth century would no longer be witness to such irrational excesses, they are, in fact, on the increase. Moreover, this new dark night of the mind threatens to engulf the most scientifically advanced culture ever produced on planet earth. The world is again on the verge of submitting to the demons of our darker imagination, and in the process losing all that science has achieved. The

light of science can alone rescue us from the new Dark Age. The fight is on.

Throughout his book Sagan contrasts fruitless religious practices with productive scientific ones. For example, he draws attention to science's enormous progress in overcoming human diseases. What hope does religion provide in such cases? Sagan poses the dilemma between science and faith: "We can pray over the cholera victim, or we can give her 500 milligrams of tetracycline every 12 hours."[48] And yet, Sagan can employ essentially religious phrasing to describe science. Of medicine's progress he writes, "This is a precious offering from science to humanity—nothing less than the gift of life."[49] Science is a magnificent edifice of demonstrable facts, while faith is an illusory house of imaginary cards. Thus he writes, "For me, it is far better to grasp the Universe as it really is than to persist in delusion, however satisfying and reassuring."[50]

Like Ingersoll and Paine, Sagan confidently affirmed that science would displace all spiritual explanations, and thus all false hopes. We have already embarked on the path of trading one worldview for another. "Plainly there is no way back. Like it or not, we are stuck with science. We had better make the best of it."[51] Nevertheless, some of us stubbornly try to make the return trip. Because of our discomfort with the power and sobriety of science we reach out to "pseudo-science," such things as creationism and alternative medical practices. These function as "a kind of halfway house between old religion and new science, mistrusted by both."[52] *The Demon-Haunted World* is as much an assault on pseudo-science as it is a rejection of religious explanations. And though Sagan is willing to concede that "science is far from a perfect instrument of knowledge," it nevertheless remains for him "the best we have."[53]

Responding spiritually to the cosmos. Sagan was a staunch opponent of what he took to be the excesses of religion. However, he was no enemy of "spirituality," by which he meant the human quest for the transcendent. Like many scientists writing for the trade book market today, he argues in *The Demon-Haunted World* that "science is not only compatible with spirituality; it is a profound source of spirituality." But, what does this surprising statement mean? By way of example, Sagan writes that "when we recognize our place in an immensity of light-years and in the passage of ages, when we grasp the intricacy, beauty, and subtlety of life, then that soaring feeling, that sense of elation and humility combined, is surely spiritual."[54] Scientific spirituality, then, means having an appropriate emotional response to the vastness and complexity of the cosmos science reveals. Sagan was not bothered that he lacked a scientific basis for calling such feelings spiritual. He simply chose

to label them as such, apparently assuming his readers would find the label apt.

Sagan willingly blurred the line between what science can provide—explanations of physical events—and what it cannot—transcendence, moral guidance and a sense of the spiritual. *The Demon-Haunted World* is salted with such unscientific terms and phrases as "our place," "beauty," "subtlety," "soaring feeling," "elation" and "humility." Such ideas as these, however, have no empirical verification; no study provides their proof. On the other hand, terms such as "immensity," "light years," "ages" and "intricacy" may be scientific because they imply units of measure, or comparisons of physical phenomena. But Sagan freely mixed such terms and notions in his effort to find a transcendent science to satisfy the human soul, itself an entity incapable of scientific verification. Sagan the *scientist* held that only those objects and events that are physically present and empirically verifiable are "real" in any meaningful sense. As he said, "it is far better to grasp the Universe as it really is than to persist in delusion, however satisfying and reassuring."[55]

New objects of worship for a New Religion. For Sagan, science makes determinations about existence, and thus about worth. That is, science reveals what actually exists, and what actually exists is all that is worthy of our attention. In this discovery of true worth through science—the term *worship* literally meaning "to attribute worth"—Sagan replaced Revealed Word theology with what might be called Scientific Cosmology. By spiritualizing the cosmos, physical objects of worship replace spiritual ones in Sagan's new scheme. Similarly, Paine's worship of "God in his works" or Ingersoll's worship of "humanity" replaced Revealed Word worship of the God who created both the cosmos and humanity. Nevertheless, Sagan denied that his goal was to make science a matter of faith and worship. "Is this worshipping at the altar of science? Is this replacing one faith with another, equally arbitrary? In my view, not at all."[56]

However, Carl Sagan repeatedly opposed the Revealed Word to science, thus suggesting a contest between two *religious* views. Each claims a source of transcendence—God on the one hand, the cosmos on the other—and each recommends appropriate human emotional response to that transcendence. After all, Sagan urged that the appropriate response to the immensity of the cosmos is "a soaring feeling" and a "sense of elation and humility combined." A feeling of absolute, suicidal despair at the emptiness of space apparently is not an appropriate emotional response. Truth about the physical universe provides, for Sagan, the doctrine of a new scientific religion. Accordingly, scientists like Sagan function as a new order of

priests assisting us to respond with the correct emotions to these truths.

In fact, Sagan argued that science is a better religion than the Revealed Word because science tests its doctrines empirically. Sagan asks, "What sermons even-handedly examine the God hypothesis?"[57] Forcing a face-off between the Revealed Word and science for the role of the one true religion, Sagan taunts: "Despite all the talk of humility, show me something comparable [to testing hypotheses] in religion." Divine inspiration and miracles are two ideas central to the Word, and neither idea can be tested empirically. Thus, each is rationally suspect. "Scripture is said to be divinely inspired—a phrase with many meanings. But what if it's simply made up by fallible humans? Miracles are attested, but what if they're instead some mix of charlatanry, unfamiliar states of consciousness, misapprehensions of natural phenomena, and mental illness?" Traditional religion is simply less reasonable than science when scientific standards are applied to it. "The fact that so little of the findings of modern science is prefigured in Scripture to my mind casts further doubt on its divine inspiration."[58]

Science thus becomes the only legitimate source of transcendence for Sagan. Even modern religions, those established after the rise of science, fail to "take sufficient account of the grandeur, magnificence, subtlety and intricacy of the Universe revealed by science."[59] Sagan's commitment to exploring the intersection of science and transcendence is even more pronounced in his science fiction work *Contact*.

"Contact." In Sagan's 1985 novel *Contact*, the brilliant maverick astronomer Ellie Arroway fights against great odds to convince a hidebound scientific establishment that a search for extraterrestrial life is a good use of scientific research funds. She succeeds, but only to have her funding yanked by self-interested scientific bureaucrats who are too narrow minded and ambitious to see the brilliant possibilities in her search.

Ellie Arroway is, then, a thinly veiled representation of Carl Sagan himself. On a shoestring budget she manages to set up a listening station with radio telescopes pointed heavenward. The climactic day finally arrives when a clear signal from outside our solar system reaches Ellie's listening station—beams of prime numbers, repeatedly transmitted. The heavenly signals, called suggestively "the Message," come from the Vega star system, and are followed by an enormous amount of numerical data which, it turns out, is a long series of instructions for building some sort of space craft. In Sagan's prophetic vision the stars have finally yielded up their numerical secrets.

Eventually Ellie Arroway secures funding from an eccentric and secretive billionaire who makes it possible to actually build the craft. Ellie and four others are allowed to enter the craft—referred to in the novel as "the Machine"—and are whisked away through a series of black holes and wormholes until they reach Vega thirty-three light years away from earth. The trip takes little more than an hour.

On Vega, Ellie carries on a long conversation with a Vegan who has assumed the exact appearance of her deceased father in order to alleviate her fears of the first contact. Sagan writes in a strikingly religious way of this strange encounter: "It was as if her father had these many years ago died and gone to Heaven, and finally—by this unorthodox route—she had managed to rejoin him. She sobbed and embraced him again." Ellie concludes, "this was their way of calming her fears. If so, they were very . . . thoughtful."[60] As it turns out, the aliens had entered her dream life the one night she slept on the new planet and taken memories of her father as the plans for this model. Apparently alien thoughtfulness does not extend to respect for the privacy of one's memories.

The Vegan who has assumed her father's form reassures Ellie that her science fiction notions of the work of intergalactic empires are passé. The Vegans are not space warriors, but cosmic bureaucrats.

VEGAN: "Don't think of us as some interstellar sheriff gunning down outlaw civilizations. Think of us more as the Office of Galactic Census. We collect information. I know you think nobody could learn anything from you because you're technologically so backward. But there are other merits to a civilization."

ELLIE: "What merits?"

VEGAN: "Oh, music. Lovingkindness. (I like that word)."[61]

Presumably, the Vegans are died-in-the-wool scientists like Sagan himself. And yet they, like Sagan himself, exhibit peculiarly unscientific moral preferences. The alien tells Ellie, "last night we looked inside you. All five of you. There's a lot in there: feelings, memories, instincts, learned behavior, madness, dreams, loves. Love is very important."[62] Love may be very important to Sagan, but is this a concept that can find validation through science, Sagan's candle in the dark?

Alien creators. As the dialogue between Ellie and the Vegan alien progresses, more facts come to light. It turns out that the Vegans are producing galaxies by redirecting energy that is being sucked into two black holes at the very center of the Milky Way. The galaxy currently under construction, Cygnus A, is one with

which Ellie is familiar. Not surprisingly, she is surprised. "You're *making* Cygnus A?" The alien answers nonchalantly, "Oh, it's not just us. This is a . . . cooperative effort of many galaxies. That's what we mainly do—engineering." Civilizations abound in Sagan's universe as they did in Paine's. "You mustn't think of the Universe as a wilderness. It hasn't been that for billions of years," he said. "Think of it more as . . . cultivated."[63]

The reason for alien interest in galaxy creation is simple—the universe is slowly winding down. The Vegan explains:

> The basic problem is easily stated. . . . The universe is expanding, and there's not enough matter to stop the expansion. After a while, no new galaxies, no new stars, no new planets, no newly arisen lifeforms—just the same old crowd. Everything's getting run-down. It'll be boring. So in Cygnus A we're testing out the technology to make something new. . . . It's good honest work.[64]

The Vegans and their allies are working to create new matter in a universe that will eventually disappear without their efforts. That is to say, these superevolved, godlike beings are controlling the destiny of the universe itself. In fact, the Vegans already were involved in "galactogenesis"—the creation of galaxies—before life on earth had even gotten a good evolutionary start.

Scientific religion: pi in the sky. Ellie says at one point in her conversation with the alien: "I want to know about your myths, your religions." She then asks, "What fills you with awe? Or are those who make the numinous unable to feel it?" Here is the big question: What do virtual gods think about God? What is their understanding of ultimate reality, of "the numinous"? Sagan created the ultimate authority to answer our ultimate questions, presumably from a scientific point of view. The alien's answer is both intriguing and instructive. "I'll give you a flavor of our numinous. It concerns pi, the ratio of the circumference of a circle to its diameter." He continues, "After calculating pi out to ten billion places, the randomly varying digits disappear, and for an unbelievably long time there's nothing but ones and zeros." Ellie replies, "And the number of zeros and ones? Is it a product of prime numbers?" "Yes," he says, "eleven of them." "You're telling me there's a message in eleven dimensions hiding deep inside the number pi? Someone in the universe communicates by . . . mathematics?"[65]

This sequence of numbers, the virtually infinite calculation of pi, is referred to in *Contact* as "the Message," and the entire visible universe is created to reveal this hidden message to those knowledgeable enough to read and understand it. Ancient

mathematicians such as Pythagoras, Renaissance astronomers like Brahe, even the great eighteenth-century physicist Sir Isaac Newton: all sought such a numerical key to the cosmos. Sagan reveals what he thought this key might be, thus aligning himself with an earlier scientific tradition. Is this the mystery of the universe unveiled, the final answer to humankind's religious longings?

Sagan the scientist, a determined materialist, suggested a source of transcendence in superevolved extraterrestrials, a means of conquering death through complete re-creation of individuals, the possible origins of some galaxies by the engineering feats of intelligent beings, and the notion that the universe is constructed around a numerically coded message. Carl Sagan wished that the world might find in science what he found there—hope, a sense of transcendence, and an antidote to religious superstition. Carl Sagan propagated the hope in science of the New Religious Synthesis as a source of numinous awe. As we shall see in the next section, the distinction between new and old religions is breaking down under pressure from a new breed of scientists who, like Paine, Ingersoll and Sagan, find in science a spiritual hope to rival the Revealed Word.

THE NEW PHYSICS: SCIENCE AND ANCIENT WISDOM

In his book *From Atom to Kosmos: Journey Without End,* Gordon Plummer demonstrates how the insights of astronomy reestablish "ancient wisdom."[66] Plummer is not alone in his assertion that what has been called the New Science confirms an old spirituality. Gary Zukav provided an early indication of the trajectory of much New Science writing in his bestselling book *The Dancing Wu Li Masters: An Overview of the New Physics,* published in 1979. After examining some of the findings of quantum physics, Zukav determined that the greatest insights of modern science were actually ancient theological insights capable of transforming Western spirituality. "The development of physics in the twentieth century," he writes, "already has transformed the consciousness of those involved with it."[67]

The specific religious insights of the New Science often contradict those of the Revealed Word, while simultaneously confirming Eastern religious thought. Zukav writes, "the study of complementarity, the uncertainty principle, quantum field theory, and the Copenhagen Interpretation of Quantum Mechanics produces insights into the nature of reality very similar to those produced by the study of eastern philosophy." He adds, "We need not make a pilgrimage to India or Tibet. There is much to learn there, but here at home, in the most inconceivable of places,

amidst the particle accelerators and computers, our own Path without Form is emerging."[68] Ancient wisdom and the New Science are so similar, teach so many of the same truths, that the terms *experiment* and *pilgrimage* become synonymous.

Science in the New Religious Synthesis is a means of discovering spiritual knowledge. But for many of its advocates, science also confirms ancient wisdom. Thus, Marilyn Ferguson writes in *The Aquarian Conspiracy,* "Science is only confirming paradoxes and intuitions humankind has come across many times but stubbornly disregarded."[69] This ancient wisdom—of consciousness in stars and planets, of spiritual energy in objects, of magical properties in numbers, of mystical forces in nature, of fundamental spiritual unity in the human race, of a spiritual world just beyond our sensory experience—anticipates many discoveries of the New Science. "The new science," writes Ferguson, "goes beyond cool, clinical observations to a realm of shimmering paradox where our very reason seems endangered."[70]

Advocates of the New Science present these paradoxes as scientific discoveries. For example, physicist Amit Goswami suggests that science now shows that "consciousness is fundamental" to all that exists. Moreover, "science proves the potency of monistic philosophy over dualism—over spirit separated from matter."[71] That is to say, science proves that God and the physical universe cannot be two different things, as the Revealed Word suggests they are. This scientific discovery is, Goswami admits, essentially a religious tenet. "This philosophy accommodates many of the interpretations of human spiritual experience that have sparked the various world religions."[72] Still, Goswami and other New Scientists treat it as a scientific discovery.

Another physicist writing about the New Science, Fred Alan Wolf, also finds ancient wisdom to be proven by modern scientific investigations. Hindu philosophy posits that present experience is *maya,* a self-generated illusion. Wolf maintains that science proves that "the universe is being created in a dream of a single spiritual entity" and that our own consciousness and our own dreams are but reflections of that one great cosmic soul. "Reality," writes Wolf, "is not made of stuff, but is made of possibilities that can be coherent so that possibility forms into matter."[73] Again modern science confirms the ancient Eastern religious idea that we create our own personal realities.

Fritjof Capra is quite explicit that such spiritual insights came to humankind originally through religious channels, not through science. In his groundbreaking 1974 publication *The Tao of Physics,* Capra announced that even though the "changes brought about by modern physics have been widely discussed by physicists and philosophers over the past decades, very seldom has it been realized that they all seem to lead

in the same direction, toward a view of the world which is very similar to the views held in Eastern Mysticism."[74] He writes, "In modern physics, the universe is always experienced as a dynamic, inseparable whole which always includes the observer in an essential way." Capra adds that this experience "is very similar to that of the Eastern Mystics. The similarity becomes apparent in quantum and relativity theory, and becomes even stronger in the 'quantum-relativistic' model of subatomic physics where both theories combine to produce the most striking parallels to Eastern Mysticism."[75]

More recently, Capra has again asked readers to reject "the concepts of an outdated worldview"—apparently the Revealed Word—and called on them to embrace a new spirituality supported by the insights of a new physics. Science now provides us with "spiritual or religious awareness." He adds, "It is . . . not surprising that the emerging new vision of reality is consistent with the so-called perennial philosophy of spiritual traditions, whether we talk about the spirituality of Christian mystics, that of Buddhists, or the philosophy and cosmology of the Native American traditions."[76] Thus, not only is science the source of fundamental spiritual insights, but it is also the source of a new pluralism that unites various religious traditions.

The Revealed Word tradition, however, insists upon the reality and persistence of individual identity. That is, individuals possess an identity or "self" that continues to exist even after the end of physical life. But, Capra argues, science proves that such a view is unfounded. "The Buddhist doctrine of impermanence includes the notion that there is no self—no persistent subject of our varying experiences. It holds that the idea of a separate individual self is an illusion, just another form of maya, an intellectual concept that has no reality." Science, then, proves Buddhism correct in its assumption that our experience of a fixed reality and a separate identity are more apparent than real. Buddhism teaches that "to cling to this idea of a separate self leads to the same pain and suffering (dukha) as the adherence to any other fixed category of thought." Interestingly, "science has arrived at exactly the same position."[77] The Revealed Word repudiates such a view, and must now do so in the face of scientific objection.

The old distinction between religion and science, then, has all but disappeared. Goswami writes that "today, modern science is venturing into realms that for more than four millennia have been the fiefdoms of religion and philosophy." Under the guidance of science, we are evolving to a higher level of spiritual understanding that confirms the ancient wisdom. "We are privileged to be a part of this evolutionary and transcendent process by which science is changing not only itself but also our perspective on reality."[78]

CONCLUSION

Canadian anthropologist Jeremy Narby has written recently that while "shamanism, as classically defined is reaching its end, . . . bringing scientists and shamans together seems more like a beginning."[79] Narby's suggestion would have been unthinkable to any self-respecting member of the scientific community forty years ago, but something dramatic occurred in the sciences during the second half of the twentieth century. The wall between the scientific and the spiritual was breached, and spiritual insight became a matter of scientific interest as it was for the medieval alchemists and Renaissance magical scientists. Zukav has written that we should "not be surprised if physics curricula of the twenty-first century include classes in meditation."[80] What are these popularizers of science as spirituality telling us about the impending spiritual future?

They may be telling us that the Revealed Word's role in that future will be limited, for its assumptions impede the progress of scientific spirituality. First, Revealed Word theology is dualistic, separating God and the physical universe, but science now proves that all things are a single thing or essence. Second, a writer like Carl Sagan would likely say that the very idea of a Creator impedes scientific advancement by filling the world with unobservable "demons." Third, the Revealed Word renders nature a mere artifact of such a Creator, thus obscuring its inherent divinity.

Writers in the New Science are also telling us that science's role as a source of spiritual insight and guidance will only increase, and for good reason. More than a century ago, Ingersoll argued that science promotes harmonious human relationships and conquers humanity's perennial ills such as war, hunger and disease. Two centuries ago Paine was already contending that science provided a sense of transcendence as we contemplate the vast inhabited spaces of the cosmos. Today, a host of writers urge that science confirms the perennial philosophy, that ancient wisdom of primitive human spirituality lost under the disastrous dominion of the Revealed Word. In fact, among the New Science's two principal goals today is to establish on empirical grounds this ancient wisdom, the early and foundational spiritual outlook of the human race before we were encumbered by Revealed Word theology. Its other great goal is explored in the next chapter—infusing modern religious thought with the hope of humanity's inevitable and complete spiritual transformation through evolutionary change.

6

EVOLUTION AND
ADVANCEMENT

The Darwins' Spiritual Legacy

❧

As I lay in the tub thinking, I wondered how long it would be before scientists would find ways to verify the evolution of the soul in the same way that they had verified the evolution of the body.

SHIRLEY MACLAINE, Dancing in the Light

The soul has come to the body, and the body to life, for the purpose of evolution. You are evolving, you are becoming.

NEALE DONALD WALSCH, Conversations with God

Evolution is a continuous breaking and forming to make new, richer wholes. Even our genetic material is in flux. If we try to live as closed systems, we are doomed to regress. If we enlarge our awareness, admit new information, and take advantage of the brain's infinite capacity to integrate and reconcile, we can leap forward.

MARILYN FERGUSON, The Aquarian Conspiracy

Where do advanced human souls go? There are many forms of Life that exist as advancements of this one. There are literally millions of options. There is life in numerous galaxies.

GARY ZUKAV, The Seat of the Soul

❧

The young prophet spoke confidently, his words an unquestioned revelation to his rapt listeners. The death of a friend that year, 1844, had prompted a discourse on the human soul, the nature of God and the relationship between the two: "There are very few beings in the world who understand rightly the character of God," he announced, and some clarity on this question was needed. "I will go back to the beginning, before the world was, to show what kind of being God is." The prophet promised to reveal "the designs of God in relation to the human race, and why he interferes with the affairs of men."[1]

His next statement, which the prophet termed "the great secret," clearly demarcated his theology from the Revealed Word and its preexistent divinity: "God himself was once as we are now, and is an exalted man, and sits enthroned in yonder heavens. That is the great secret." Were a human being able to see God, "you would see him like a man in form—like yourselves, in all the person, image, and very forms as a man." The traditional idea that "God was God from all eternity" was erroneous, for "God himself the Father of us all, dwelt on earth." Of perhaps even greater import to the listeners gathered that April day in the frontier town of Nauvoo, Illinois, was the admonition, "you have to learn how to be Gods yourselves ... by going from one degree to another, and from a small capacity to a great one."[2]

Employing an apt analogy for gradual spiritual ascent, the Prophet continued his exposition on the advancing soul. "When you climb a ladder, you must begin at the bottom, and ascend step by step until you arrive at the top; and so it is with the principles of the Gospel: you must begin with the first, and go on until you learn all the principles of exaltation." Their own minds and spirits could develop endlessly, with divinity itself within their grasp. "All the minds and spirits that God ever sent into the world are susceptible of enlargement."[3] This truth of the enlarging mind, the expanding soul, the ever-evolving, divinity-destined human spirit was central to the new gospel of Jesus Christ, as it had been delivered to the prophet Joseph Smith.

Bestselling research psychologist Robert Ornstein has written extensively on the topic of the evolution of human consciousness, and is today perhaps the leading expert on the subject. His books include *New World, New Mind: Moving Toward Conscious Evolution* and *The Evolution of Consciousness: The Origins of the Way We Think.* Ornstein thinks the time has come for human beings to seize control of the evolution of the mind. The human mind possesses "an endless supply of possible capabilities, waiting to be called on in response to the new necessities of the new world we've created." Thus, we must undertake "conscious evolution," a process that "may be easier, closer at hand, and more liberating than we might normally think."[4] "Conscious selection," as opposed to natural selection, is the means by which we "take our evolution in our own hands by developing the ability to select parts of the mind."[5] In *New World, New Mind* Ornstein and coauthor Paul Ehrlich call for a "solution" to our inability to adapt to a rapidly changing world. They write, "the 'solution' is not simple—to generate the social and political will to move a program of conscious evolution to the top of the human agenda."[6]

Ornstein's vision of evolving consciousness is neither new nor unique. It also

occurred to many readers of Darwin's *On the Origin of the Species* in 1859 and is today a foundational component of the New Religious Synthesis. Even prior to Darwin, progressivist thinking had suggested continual evolution of the body and the spirit. Joseph Smith's progressive theology was fully developed by 1844, while Herbert Spencer had postulated in 1855 that "mind had evolved out of life as a form of adaptation."[7]

This chapter considers several early proponents of continuing human evolution, including Charles Darwin's brilliant grandfather Erasmus Darwin. But not until Charles Darwin provided evolution with a credible scientific foundation was it possible for writers such as T. H. Huxley in England and Ernst Haeckel in Germany to make a convincing public case for continuing evolution as human destiny, one resting on more than speculation or prophetic utterance. After Darwin's *Origin of the Species*, proponents made continuing human evolution seem inevitable, indeed morally essential. The scientific vision of a spiritually evolving human race set the stage for writers of fiction to furnish us with vivid images of an exalted future for the human race.

ERASMUS DARWIN

Charles Darwin's brilliant and eccentric grandfather Erasmus (1731-1803) was England's most famous physician and perhaps its most knowledgeable scientist at the end of the eighteenth century. His advanced studies began at St. John's College, Cambridge, and his medical degree was completed in 1756 at Edinburgh University. The elder Darwin was also a tireless inventor, a talented poet and an ardent opponent of Christianity. He helped to start the Industrial Revolution in England along with other members of the famous Lunar Society of industrialists and inventors, including Josiah Wedgwood and Richard Edgeworth. Erasmus Darwin was also a theorist of education, basing many of his ideas on the work of Rousseau, with whom he corresponded.[8]

Despite his reputation as an original thinker and talented writer, admirers of his famous grandson at one time suppressed Erasmus Darwin's works. This tactical historical censorship was an effort to save Charles Darwin from the charge that his grandfather's strange theories—Erasmus believed that plants possessed a soul—had any influence on his own. Moreover, Erasmus Darwin, for all his brilliance, was an eccentric who delighted in writing erotic poetry and whose romantic escapades were legendary. Any link between Erasmus and Charles Darwin might compromise the latter's status as an original and respectable scientific thinker.

Fluid materialism. Erasmus Darwin's greatest influence came through his own theory of evolution. His famous book, *Zoonomia, or the Laws of Organic Life* (1794-1796), is a massive medical treatise arguing a straightforward evolutionary hypothesis.[9] In *The Temple of Nature*, a popular poem setting out his evolutionary views for the public, he "traced the progress of life from microscopic specks in primeval seas to its present culmination in man."[10] These works advance a concept dubbed "fluid materialism." As Edward Reed explains, "For [Erasmus] Darwin all of animate nature was possessed of sensibility and feeling, even plants." Thus, Darwin "sought the material basis for this sensibility in a subtle fluid or ether in the body and nerves, basing his ideas on the influential fluid theory of electricity developed by his friend Benjamin Franklin."[11] Darwin subjected many of his medical patients to electrical shocks in hopes of understanding the universal life force he was so certain existed. His theories and experiments gave Mary Shelley the idea for her book *Frankenstein*.

Erasmus Darwin believed that life evolves toward higher levels of complexity and happiness, a commitment that became for him a virtual religion. As one biographer notes, Darwin "weaves his evolutionary ideas into the wider philosophy of organic happiness."[12] Thus, "evolution was no casual speculation" for Erasmus Darwin, "but a belief he lived with for thirty years and one which moulded his whole philosophy of life."[13] As we shall see, Erasmus's grandson Charles shared much of his grandfather's faith.

Finding a cure for religion. According to Erasmus Darwin, the human mind or soul has a physical basis. In both *Zoonomia* and *The Temple of Nature*, Darwin speculated that "objects of thought" were merely "the movements of the relevant neural fibers" and that these movements were vibrations, an idea found earlier in the work of David Hartley.[14] The upshot of Darwin's speculation was to put human mental or spiritual life on a biological and evolutionary plane, making all aspects of our conscious existence products of natural processes. Thus, human religious feelings and beliefs—including those expressed in the Revealed Word—also were material in nature, simple movements of "relevant neural fibers."

In fact, the staunchly anti-Christian Darwin found conventional religious beliefs pathological and prescribed appropriate psychological cures in *Zoonomia*. To cure the mental illness of belief in hell, for instance, Darwin prescribed the remedy of ridicule. "Those who suffer under this insanity are generally the most innocent and harmless people," he conceded. And though "the voice of reason is ineffectual . . . that of ridicule may save many."[15] Religious beliefs result from environmental

factors such as early training, which cause "intellectual cowardice" to be "instilled into the minds of the people from their infancy." This cowardice "prevents inquiry" into religious beliefs. The medical cure in such cases "is to increase knowledge of the laws of nature." In this way we are able to "emancipate ourselves from the false impressions we have imbibed in our infancy, and to set the faculty of reason above that of imagination."[16] That is, science is the proper cure for religious belief. Similarly, so-called sins were simply the result of nerve vibrations, and could also be cured by proper therapy. Wrong action was merely a matter of doing what one's nerves told one to do; right action could be engendered by sound nerve therapy. Moral guidelines would be derived from what Darwin termed "universal love."[17]

Darwin, Frankenstein and the Romantics. Though his name and ideas are not widely known today, Erasmus Darwin's influence on writers and thinkers of his own day was enormous. Considered by some contemporaries to be the greatest intellectual figure of the day, his idea of fluid materialism was particularly influential in the early development of Romantic thought. Around the time of Darwin's greatest popularity, the poet William Blake in his *Marriage of Heaven and Hell* has the devil repeat a distinctly Darwinian idea: "Energy is the only life and . . . Reason is the bound or outward circumference of Energy."[18] Edward Reed writes that his "relative obscurity nowadays should not lead us to ignore the impact of Darwin's fluid materialism, which was, at the very least, one of the major physiological and psychological theories propounded between 1798 and 1815."[19] Among those falling under the Darwinian spell was the great English surgeon William Lawrence and, through Lawrence, his patient Percy Shelley. Shelley's wife, Mary, was the author of the famous novel *Frankenstein*, a work she acknowledged to have written while pondering Erasmus Darwin's ideas. She and her husband "talked of the experiments of Dr. Darwin," concluding that "perhaps a corpse would be re-animated" through electrical shock treatment if "the component parts of a creature" could be "brought together, and endued with vital warmth."[20] Darwin had suggested to the great writer that life—physical, mental and moral—might arise out of matter alone without divine intervention.

Erasmus Darwin's influence on a generation of English thinkers and artists was extraordinary. Coleridge, Wordsworth, Percy Shelley and Keats all took Darwin's ideas seriously. Desmond King-Hele writes that "Darwin was the most important single influence on the English Romantic poets."[21] For Wordsworth and Coleridge, Darwin's *Botanic Garden* "had a longer and stronger effect"

on their thinking than did the French Revolution.[22] Wordsworth "came to adopt a religious creed very similar to Darwin's, including the idea of a vague Power lying behind the processes of Nature, and as much concerned with Nature as with Man." In addition, Shelley's great poem *Prometheus Unbound* advocates "regeneration of the world through Universal Love" on the model of Darwin's *The Temple of Nature*. Blake, Byron and Crabbe are among the other English Romantics who looked to Darwin for inspiration.[23]

Erasmus Darwin was a skilled public advocate, one remarkably successful in propagating his ideas about evolution, nature and the progress of life. He wrote with the intellectual confidence of a noted medical expert, but also with the grace and force of a poet. His ideas were both popular and controversial from the moment they appeared in *Zoonomia* and *The Temple of Nature*. Many contemporaries considered the elder Darwin the greatest and most original thinker of the age. Others understood that this eccentric scientist's ideas were revolutionary and intentionally anti-Christian. Within two years of its first publication, Thomas Brown answered *Zoonomia* in his 560-page *Observations on the Zoonomia of Erasmus Darwin*.

LAMARCK AND SPENCER

Herbert Spencer (1820-1903) is an important transitional figure in the development of ideas about human evolutionary progress. Before Charles Darwin had published *On the Origin of the Species*, Spencer had already formulated and advocated a theory of human social progress based on the early evolutionary theories of French naturalist Jean Baptiste Lamarck (1744-1829). Lamarck's theory emphasized progress and improvement, and "Spencer must have delighted in the notion, easily extractable from Lamarck," that both nature and society were on "an exciting, buoyant, optimistic course, bouncing onwards and upwards."[24] Spencer, armed with his Lamarckian view of an ever-progressing cosmos, exerted tremendous influence over nineteenth-century thought. John Passmore writes that Spencer's "agnostic-evolutionary philosophy" literally "swept the world."[25]

Lamarck rejected the traditional notion that animal species were unchanging. His *Philosophie zoologique* (1809) argues the descent of current species from earlier ones, but his ideas about *how* evolution occurred were not convincing. Lamarck imagined organisms adapting to actual physical constraints more or less on the spot, and then passing these changes on to their offspring. In his most famous example, early and greedy giraffes slowly stretched their necks to reach leaves at the

tops of trees. As these giraffes were more successful at getting food, they also had a greater chance of reproducing. Though eventually overturned, Lamarck's theories were nevertheless employed to justify various theories of human progress. Spencer never abandoned Lamarck's theory.[26] However, when Darwin's more plausible theories were made public, Spencer recognized their greater persuasive potential for supporting his theory of human social and moral progress.

An evolving society, an evolving race. Spencer argued in *Social Statics* (1850) that human progress was inevitable, the increasing complexity of organisms over time being his chief evidence. Spencer, not Darwin, coined the phrase "survival of the fittest," and he argued for a ruthless social system of free enterprise that paid no heed to the needs of the "unfit" poor. Some human beings are more advanced than are others, and they demonstrate this fact by their capacity to acquire knowledge, wealth and power.

Racism seemed always to emerge from evolutionary thinking at this time. According to Spencer, the European race was the most highly evolved. In *First Principles,* Spencer wrote of the residents of Papua New Guinea, "Though often possessing well-developed body and arms, the Papuan has very small legs; thus reminding us of the man-apes, in which there is no great contrast in size between the hind and fore limbs." However, "in the European, the greater length and massiveness of the leg has become marked." Similarly, facial features proved the higher evolutionary status of Europeans. Spencer argued that "the higher forms" of human race are "distinguished by the relatively larger size of the bones which cover the brain, and the relatively smaller size of those which cover the jaws." Moreover, "this trait, which is stronger in Man than in any other creature, is stronger in the European than in the savage."[27] And, we might add, even more pronounced in the celluloid alien than in the European, a notion to which we will return toward the end of this chapter.

Spencer's melding of the metaphysics of progress and the biology of evolution would have many imitators, and he remained a major figure in the development of the doctrine of progressive evolution. A. N. Wilson has written that Spencer "bolstered up two . . . key superstitions: the idea of life as perpetual progress— the life of the universe as well as the life of societies and individuals; and, secondly, the idea that Science would provide the key instrument of progress."[28] These "key superstitions" of the Victorian age have now been incorporated into the New Religious Synthesis.

CHARLES DARWIN: NATURALIST PROPHET

The period from 1840 to 1900 was one of profound and extensive intellectual change in the Western world. In the wake of the Enlightenment's caustic criticism of the Revealed Word, powerful new explanations of the human condition emerged to challenge the traditional account of creation, fall and redemption. The most influential intellectual figure of this period was Charles Darwin (1809-1882), whose *Origin of the Species* (1859) changed forever how life's origins and development on earth were understood.

It goes without saying that Darwin's evolutionary hypothesis has affected assumptions about biological life's development. Most educated people today accept that biological advancement takes place by degrees over a long period in response to external pressures. This basic biological hypothesis has also greatly influenced thinking in a range of disciplines including religion. Darwin's life is important to understanding his most famous idea and its considerable influence on contemporary religious thought.

Charles Robert Darwin was born into a prominent and prosperous British family in 1809. His mother was the daughter of the wealthy potter and industrialist Josiah Wedgwood—friend of Erasmus Darwin—and his father was the successful doctor Robert Waring Darwin. Darwin's early life was one of unusual social privilege and stimulating intellectual contact. Robert Darwin, son of Erasmus, adopted his father's beliefs about both evolution (he accepted it) and Christianity (he rejected it). Thus, though Charles Darwin was born six years after his brilliant grandfather's death, Robert Darwin became a conduit to his son of much of Erasmus Darwin's thought.

Charles Darwin received a good early education, and in 1825, at his father's direction, he went on to study medicine in the family tradition at Edinburgh University. A sensitive boy, Darwin was repulsed by macabre scenes in the dissection theatres. Consequently he turned most of his attention to naturalism. In Edinburgh Darwin came under the influence of the famous marine biologist Charles Gray, an evolutionary theorist in his own right. But Charles was not seriously committed to his studies and spent much of his time hunting and collecting natural specimens.

In 1828 his father directed him to enter Cambridge University to study for the ministry. Darwin had no real interest in the ministry, but a clerical position would allow him leisure to pursue his real passions—hunting and naturalism. Darwin spent much of his time in Cambridge collecting and categorizing species of beetles.

In December 1831, at the recommendation of his beloved botany professor, Reverend John Stevens Henslow, Darwin was made naturalist on the *H.M.S. Beagle*, which was sailing to the South American coast. This famous voyage lasted nearly five years, Darwin returning to England October 1836. During the *Beagle's* long Pacific adventure, Darwin became an expert on the plants and animals of several regions.

Between 1836 and 1846, Charles Darwin's reputation as a naturalist grew due to his many publications on topics ranging from volcanic islands to the anatomy of tropical birds. He had become one of England's leading naturalists. In 1844—fourteen years prior to publication of the *Origin*—Darwin developed a theory of the means by which one species gradually changes into a distinct and separate species. That year he wrote to his friend, the botanist James Hooker, "I think I have found out . . . the simple way by which species become exquisitely adapted to various ends."[29] He termed the mechanism of evolutionary change "natural selection."

Though he arrived at his fully developed theory of evolution by natural selection in the early 1840s, Darwin waited to announce his speculations in a scientific paper read in 1858. His theory of transmutation from one species to another resulted from long and serious study of natural phenomena, including painstaking collection and dissection of many species of animals, barnacles being his special interest. Darwin finally published his theory of evolution in book form in 1859, largely due to concern that another naturalist would get credit for it. This other naturalist, Alfred Russel Wallace (1823-1913), had not only developed a theory of evolution strikingly similar to Darwin's, but had also arrived at the mechanism Darwin called natural selection. Wallace sent a manuscript describing his own evolutionary theory to Darwin for review in 1858, an act that finally persuaded Darwin to publish *On the Origin of the Species*.

Darwin's famous book first appeared November 1859 and went rapidly through six editions. Though the initial print runs were small, *On the Origin of the Species* was soon selling as many volumes in England and America as were the novels of Dickens.[30] The *Origin* created enormous controversy and is one of the few works whose publication can be said to have changed all subsequent intellectual life.

Darwin's diminishing religion. Darwin's famous theory has created as much controversy in the realm of religion as it has in the life sciences, and for understandable reasons. His hypothesis challenges the Revealed Word view of special creation by providing a scientific justification for believing that life on earth progressed from

single-celled organisms to human beings without divine intervention in the process. Darwin's religious views apparently influenced his interest in evolution and may have shaped both his basic theory and the arguments he employed publicly to defend that theory. But what were Darwin's religious views, and what relationship do they bear to his ideas about evolution? The answer to this question has been the subject of much speculation and controversy.[31] The following facts seem matters of general agreement.

Raised in a family of Unitarian women and skeptical men, Darwin was not much exposed to traditional Christian thought in his home. As his views on evolution developed, his faith in God diminished further. The apparent cruelty and randomness of nature eroded his trust in Paley's argument from design. Darwin found nature a ruthless, barbaric battleground in which the random variations of survivors accounted for the physiological features of all species. Paley's argument from design had once drawn Darwin toward theism, but his own theory of evolution by natural selection tended to "banish design from the universe."[32] Darwin eventually saw no need for God or design "to explain the beautifully effective hinge of a bivalve shell or even more perfect adaptations."[33] The power behind nature was not a personal and creative God but impersonal natural forces producing design through evolution. For Darwin, brute biological facts argued against a benevolent God and for the heartless "deity" of natural selection.

The Unitarianism with which he grew up also affected Darwin's thinking about spiritual matters. Theology is insignificant in Unitarianism because God is an inexpressible enigma. The universe operates according to natural laws that preclude miracles, and these laws render God's activity in nature unnecessary. Darwin came to embrace a completely materialist view—nothing exists but physical matter. As his biographers Adrian Desmond and James Moore write, Darwin concluded that "wild animals are not the product of God's whim any more than planets are held up by his will."[34] Frank Brown adds, "Considerably after Darwin's rejection of Christianity, theism itself began to seem to him difficult to establish."[35]

Once Darwin's case against Revealed Word assumptions was fully developed in his own thinking, the great naturalist became an ardent foe of the faith. "Disbelief crept over me at a very slow rate, but was at last complete," he wrote. "The rate was so slow that I felt no distress and have never since doubted even for a single second that my conclusion was correct."[36] The strident nature of Darwin's opposition to Christianity is not well known in part because relatives excised from his papers an-

grier comments about the faith so as to save the family embarrassment and to protect Darwin's public image. These hostile comments have now been restored to the text of his autobiography.

"The mystery of the beginning of all things is insoluble by us," he wrote, "and I for one must be content to remain an Agnostic."[37] But this bland statement hardly captures the real tenor of Darwin's thought on the issue. His position regarding Christianity resembles the adamant Deism of his grandfather Erasmus. "I can hardly see how anyone ought to wish Christianity to be true, for if so the plain language of the text seems to show that the men who do not believe, and this would include my Father, Brother and almost all my best friends, will be everlastingly punished. And this is a damnable doctrine!"[38]

Darwin had other reasons for rejecting traditional Christian teachings. An intensely sensitive man prone to various illnesses, Darwin found it difficult even to be present in public settings. Throughout his long life he was deeply bothered by the suffering that he knew to be an inherent part of natural existence. The suffering of animals was for Darwin a powerful argument against God's care for living things. Like Voltaire, Darwin reasoned that God, if he exists, must be omnipotent. And yet, if God is omnipotent he has chosen not to prevent the suffering of animals. Darwin concluded that the idea of a benevolent and omnipotent God "revolts the understanding, for what advantage can there be in the suffering of millions of the lower animals throughout almost endless time?"[39] The loss of a beloved daughter to a painful disease at the age of ten cemented Darwin's conviction that the Christian idea of a loving God was a charade.

Charles Darwin, then, made public his argument for evolution for a variety of personal and professional reasons. He sought to advance science by presenting a plausible mechanism for the development of different species. Darwin also wanted recognition for an important scientific discovery, fearing credit might go to Wallace if he did not publish his views. But Darwin was also interested in arguing from biological science against the Christian doctrine of an omnipotent and benevolent deity.

Darwin the rhetorical strategist. Darwin did not disseminate his ideas in public lectures nor in the classroom; his patrician social status ensured that he never actually had to teach or lecture to earn a living. Rather, his advocacy of evolution was done through his many publications. As Edward S. Reed writes, "The most famous scientist of the [nineteenth] century never once gave a public presentation of his revolutionary theory, not even in the form of a classroom lecture!"[40] But the suc-

cess of Darwin's ideas was not hindered by the absence of their author from the public lecture stage, for Charles Darwin was a skilled rhetorical strategist and an accomplished writer of persuasive prose.

Though readers assume that Darwin wrote as a scientist for other scientists, he is clearly also seeking to persuade the general reading public in *On the Origin of the Species*. He certainly sought fame beyond the halls of the academy, and his great work was intended for the common reader as much as it was for the scientist. One measure of his rhetorical success is the fact that the *Origin*'s impact has always been felt as dramatically in popular thinking about science, society and religion as it has been in the realm of professional biology. Darwin's rhetorical maneuvering deserves closer examination.

Darwin scholar John Campbell has focused attention on Darwin's efforts to make his ideas persuasive to a dubious public.[41] Both the scientific world and the public were disinclined to accept that species of plants and animals emerged gradually through evolutionary change, and were thus not the products of special divine creation. Even Darwin's term "natural selection" was selected more for its persuasive potential than for its actual descriptive accuracy.

In positing natural selection, Darwin was applying to biology the theories of controversial English economist Thomas Robert Malthus (1766-1834). Malthus observed that "food supply increases arithmetically while population increases geometrically." The result is that "not as many organisms live as are born." Darwin added this "thoroughly negative" economic doctrine to the biological notions of variation and inheritance. Campbell notes that "when one combines variation, inheritance, and the struggle for existence" the result is "differential reproduction"—the idea that some members of a species have a reproductive advantage over others. "Allow differential reproduction to continue over virtually unlimited time in an unlimited variety of changing environments and the result is organic change or evolution."[42]

This, in a nutshell, is Darwin's theory of evolution, and it owes much to Malthus's ruthless reasoning. As Franklin Baumer states the point, Darwin pictured nature as "a great battleground, not unlike the world of contemporary economics." In the economic world of mid-nineteenth-century England, "individuals competed for an insufficient food supply, and . . . victory went to luck rather than to cunning."[43] Many readers then and now import the notion of progress to Darwin's basic theory, the idea that evolution involves not merely change, but improvement. However,

progressivism is not actually present in Darwinism as advanced in *On the Origin of the Species*. Evolution under the Darwin theory is random, unintentional and undirected. His carefully chosen metaphor of "selection," with its implied analogy to domestic animal breeding, suggests something the theory does not deliver. Biological life in a Darwinian world is not headed anywhere in particular—it just happens.

Darwin on progress: nature imperfectly solving problems. Darwin was himself largely responsible for the interpretation that evolution is progressive, for his carefully chosen language was intended to implant the idea in his readers' minds. Darwin writes in the *Origin*, "natural selection tends only to make each organic being as perfect as, or slightly more perfect than, the other inhabitants of the same country with which it has to struggle for existence. And we see that this is the degree of perfection attained under nature."[44] Within the limits of his theory, however, Darwin's term "perfection" can only mean "reproductively advantageous change." In the same section in which he mentions "perfection," Darwin also draws attention to the limits of that perfection. The stinger of a honeybee, for instance, functions in such a way that the bee dies after stinging an intruder. This, clearly, is not a perfect design, though the bee's actions benefit the colony.[45]

Darwin's strategic reason for placing the notion of "perfection" next to examples of "imperfection" is to argue a specific point: natural selection, not a divine hand, solves practical problems in the natural order. Improvements do occur in the evolutionary process, but they are not the perfect solutions one would expect of God. A divine designer would not create the stinger that kills the bee. This contrivance came about because at one time the stinger was a tool for boring—thus, barbed or serrated—that later was "adapted" to use as a weapon of defense. God would never have set out to design the bee's stinger in this clearly imperfect way, creating in the very process of design a fatal disadvantage to the individual creature. However, the bee's adaptation is still perfect in a limited sense, that is, reflecting the "degree of perfection attained under nature." Darwin's argument from an "imperfect perfection" is tactical, allowing him to argue *for* adaptation by natural selection while at the same time arguing *against* divine design.[46]

Darwin also sought to make *ultimate* progress by means of natural selection appear benevolent compared to certain temporary natural states which, if the result of divine design, rendered God cruel. Darwin thus strategically presented these biologically momentary states as mere steps along the way to something more advanced, that is, as stages in a progressive succession toward "higher" or more complex forms

of life. As Campbell points out, "Darwin takes several of nature's ingenious adaptations and underscores the embarrassment they cause to the customary belief in divine goodness." Campbell quotes a relevant passage from Darwin's works:

> Finally, it may not be a logical deduction, but to my imagination it is far more satisfactory to look at such instincts as the young cuckoo ejecting its foster-brothers—ants making slaves—the larvae of the ichneumonidae feeding within the live bodies of caterpillars—not as especially endowed or created instincts, but as small consequences of one general law, leading to the advancement of all organic beings.[47]

Darwin's argument is couched in such a way as to make evolution *compatible with* theism, a view Darwin had himself already relinquished. It appears that he wished to maintain the public appearance of faith in God, while arguing the opposite thesis throughout the *Origin*. Darwin argued that if evolution moves toward improved species or "higher animals," then God is saved from the charge of cruelty. But, as we shall see, saving the dignity of God clearly was not Darwin's motive in advancing this argument and thus his theory.

Natural and artificial selection. The master strategy behind Darwin's eventual persuasive success was his metaphor of "natural selection" itself, an implied comparison of the undirected and wholly physical processes of evolution to the highly intentional, goal-directed work of the animal breeder. In deploying this metaphor, Darwin walked a very fine line between rhetorical stratagem and outright deception. Darwin compares nature to a breeder, both of whom "eliminate certain individuals from their breeding stocks." But, Campbell adds, "nature is not like the breeder in that nature does not consciously choose certain animals or plants to achieve a foreseen end."[48] Campbell notes that Darwin's particular use of the term "selection" in the *Origin* "is unusual and technically false," "misleading" and "inaccurate." And, we should add, enormously successful, for Darwin was able to not only win a hearing for his views, but to convince many readers who, frankly, did not understand his argument while being convinced that they did.

Charles Darwin eliminated the need for divine involvement in the biological world. In fact, he seemed to have eliminated the need for purpose in nature altogether. There was no Designer behind the design of nature, and even the apparent design, if one looked closely, was flawed in just such a way as to suggest that all living things were the survivors—albeit improved survivors—of a great battle rather than the products of a divine craftsman. A playwright behind nature's scenery was unnecessary to explain the

drama of life; it was all about a fight over food among the players on stage. "If Darwin's hypothesis was correct, then mind was indeed 'pitchforked' out of the universe, as Samuel Butler put it."[49]

Darwin the progressivist: a new divinity. Nevertheless, another component must be added to the story of Charles Darwin and his theory before considering its later applications. Apparently Darwin *did* believe in evolutionary progress, and himself held out the hope of a physically and morally perfected human race. In spite of the fact that his famous theory clearly is not progressive, Darwin both believed in ultimate human progress and thought his theory supported such a belief.

The leading expert on the question of Darwin's views on progress is Robert Richards of the University of Chicago. In his book *The Meaning of Evolution* Richards points out that "Darwin expressed his belief in a progressive, natural selection dynamic" in his notebooks as early as 1839, twenty years before the publication of the *Origin.*[50] In fact, Richards argues that Darwin's "notion of an innate tendency to change gradually faded in his theory" and was replaced by "the supposition of environmental forces producing the kind of variation that could be transmuted into progressive forms during the development of species."[51]

What is Richards saying? Just this—that Charles Darwin increasingly attributed to the completely undirected process of natural selection a virtually willful concern for progress. As Richards writes, "In the *Origin,* Darwin augmented the power of this progressive dynamic by attributing to natural selection the beneficent concern for the good of creatures, a concern that had been formerly expressed by the recently departed Deity." For Darwin, "natural selection altruistically looked to the welfare of the creatures selected."[52] Thus, the theory of evolution, with its central mechanism of natural selection, was specifically intended by Darwin to take the place of God in a scheme of natural relationships that tended inherently toward progress. Richards adds that progressivism had been incorporated into every theory of evolution that had influenced Darwin's thinking, including those of his teacher Grant, his grandfather Erasmus Darwin, the great French scientist Lamarck and several others.[53]

Darwin's theory "banished God from the universe" and introduced in his place the possibility of scientifically justified "progress." Of course, the Darwin theory does not posit a mechanism for continuing improvement or progress through evolutionary change. Rather, Darwinian change within members of a species is random and does not tend toward any particular culmination point or eventual

destiny. It may be said to suggest improvement only when that term is defined as "improved capacity to reproduce," or perhaps as "greater biological complexity." Thus, though Darwinism is popularly taken to imply gradual progression toward "higher forms of life" and perhaps eventually toward biological perfection, his theory of evolution does not support such an interpretation. When Darwin spoke of progress, he was not speaking as a biologist

Some Darwin defenders have argued that progressivism was a misinterpretation of evolution by those wishing to use the theory to support political and social concepts. However, according to Richards, progressivism was close to Darwin's heart, and Darwin himself was largely responsible for this erroneous interpretation of his theory. Hopeful of a meaningful natural world tending in some discernable direction, Darwin sometimes spoke as a believer in progressivism. For instance, he wrote in his autobiography: "Believing as I do that man in the future will be a far more perfect creature than he now is, it is an intolerable thought that he and all other sentient beings are doomed to complete annihilation after such long-continued slow progress."[54] Thus, the Revealed Word notion that the human race would one day be annihilated with an ensuing judgment was an intolerable doctrine to Darwin. His rival hope, now a mainstay of the New Religious Synthesis, was for ultimate human perfection by means of evolution.

Edward Reed writes, "The mid-nineteenth century was a time when most serious thinkers in Europe were eager to hear progressivist accounts of both natural and civil history."[55] In the nineteenth and early twentieth centuries, however, progressivism could not be separated from racism, and for most European believers in progressivism, the future of the human race was a white future. "Humans were the most highly developed creatures on earth, were they not? And certain humans (European, male, well heeled) were the best of the best—who could doubt it?"[56] It is not clear whether Charles Darwin himself accepted the racist implications of evolutionary progressivism, but he also did not attempt to overturn the use of his theory to prop up such speculations by others. After all, belief in racial progress helped to promote his theory, something Darwin never obstructed.

Many Victorian intellectuals found Darwin's dismissal of God from the universe spiritually liberating, in large measure because it seemed to open the way for unlimited human progress. God's dismissal put humanity squarely in the cosmic spotlight and placed human destiny in human hands. George Bernard Shaw, always on the lookout for an exotic theory to prop up his humanistic egoism, wrote

that Darwin's friends "actually regarded the banishment of mind as 'a glorious enlightenment and emancipation' from a moribund theology and Biblicism. 'We were intellectually intoxicated with the idea that the world could make itself without design, purpose, skill or intelligence: in short, without life.'"[57]

Frederick Pollock recalled the reaction of Cambridge students after steeping themselves in the basics of Darwinian antitheology: "We seemed to ride triumphant on an ocean of new life and boundless possibilities. Natural Selection was to be the master-key of the universe; we expected it to solve all riddles and reconcile contradictions. Among other things, it was to give us a new system of ethics." W. K. Clifford, a friend of Pollock's at Cambridge, developed a system of ethics based on natural selection.[58] As we shall see, the tendency to appropriate the progressive aspects of Darwin's theory have persisted, and they have been propagated in various arenas including popular religious thought.

THE SPIRITUAL VISION OF DARWIN'S EARLY DEFENDERS

The notion of perfecting the human race was a potent idea well before Darwin published his *Origin* in 1859. For example, the lapsed American Congregational minister John Humphrey Noyes (1811-1886) advocated controlled breeding to achieve human progress in the 1840s. Procreation was strictly forbidden in his Oneida Community (est. 1848) without Noyes's approval. He called his approach to eugenics "stirpiculture," and considered it a logical outgrowth of progressive thinking. Noyes determined which men and women would be allowed to reproduce in order to propagate certain physical, mental and spiritual characteristics.

Noyes wrote before such thinking about human progress had any real scientific grounding, however. Following the publication of *The Origin of the Species*, a host of English and Continental intellectuals speculated about the moral and spiritual possibilities inherent in Darwin's solidly scientific theory. These thinkers often authored works for the general public that provided a highly credible, scientifically grounded case for a new view of human advancement.

Prominent British scientist, physician, lecturer and close Darwin family friend T. H. Huxley (1825-1895) was known as "Darwin's bulldog" for his tenacious defense of Darwin's theory of evolution. Huxley, perhaps the leading naturalist of his day, did what the reticent Darwin could not—mount an energetic, even flamboyant public defense of evolution through natural selection. A charis-

matic speaker and gifted debater, Huxley relished the opportunity to address large crowds of working class men—the "cloth hats"—about the new scientific discoveries that were challenging the settled convictions of the church. Huxley sought nothing less than to foment a revolution in religious thought predicated on his friend Darwin's discovery.

T. H. Huxley recognized the many implications of Darwin's evolutionary ideas for an emerging Western culture that would be governed by a scientific rather than a Christian worldview. What principle would provide the moral foundation of a world without traditional "revealed" religion? Perhaps evolution itself suggested the contours of a new morality. Huxley often speculated about the possibilities of human moral evolution, a progression from survival of the fittest to survival of the morally soundest. In his book *Evolution and Ethics* (1893), for instance, he wrote that "social progress" for human beings meant "checking the evolutionary process at every step" and substituting for biological evolution the process of moral evolution, "which may be called the ethical process." The result of this process is the survival of the morally fittest. Though Huxley detested the spiritualism and occultism that had captivated the Victorian mind, he did view life's emergence through biological evolution as a springboard into an even more astounding possibility—the process of human evolution from one level of moral attainment to another. That is, Huxley recognized that Darwin had discovered the spiritual future of the human race, a future free of the constraints of religion.

Another British scientist directly influenced by Charles Darwin on the point of human advancement was Darwin's own cousin, Francis Galton (1822-1911). Galton, with Darwin's approval, advanced the first fully developed theory of eugenics in books such as his *Hereditary Genius* (1869). His ideas took Darwin's strategic analogy of evolution to animal husbandry and applied it to the breeding of humans. J. W. Burrow writes, "One decided whom one wanted to breed and rear offspring and then tried to arrange the environment accordingly. It was akin to what Darwin in *The Origin* had called 'artificial selection.'" Such selective breeding of humans was to be overseen by "a rational elite."[59]

Many of Darwin's ideas were also adopted and developed by the phenomenally popular German evolutionary theorist, Ernst Haeckel (1834-1919). The first important advocate of Darwinism in Germany, Haeckel popularized the idea of human evolutionary progress in Europe through his many books and lectures. His ideas provided a foundation for eugenic theories and experiments in the late nineteenth and

early twentieth centuries. Just one of Haeckel's books, *The Riddle of the Universe*, sold 100,000 copies in one month soon after its publication in 1899. The tone of his writing was ferociously anti-Christian, and he argued strenuously for a new religion founded on evolutionary theory. The details and surprising success of Haeckel's effort to found an evolutionary religion will be discussed in the next chapter.

As noted above, the hope of scientifically improving the human race intoxicated a wide range of European intellectuals in the late nineteenth and early twentieth centuries. Eugenics was often viewed as a vehicle to achieve a physically and morally perfected human race. The examples of intellectual figures who promoted the practice are too numerous to list, Haeckel being one of the more prominent and credible. Another important figure in the eugenics movement was the French psychiatrist August Forel (1848-1931). Forel wrote, "We hope that the eugenics of the future, if well applied, will even be able to improve by small degrees the quality of our higher races," by which he meant Europeans.[60]

Forel, like Haeckel, was enamored of the evolutionary possibilities for human advancement and envisioned a future in which science supplanted religion. He advocated a "scientific religion of man's well-being" that would be "the religion of the future." Sounding much like Robert Green Ingersoll, Forel wrote that this religion "must be free from doctrine and metaphysics, uniting all that is truly good and purely human in the ancient religions."[61] The doctrine-bound Revealed Word tradition would have to be set aside in favor of a modern, scientific religion capable of encouraging evolutionary advances.

The works of Huxley, Haeckel, Galton, Forel and many other leading European intellectuals at the end of the nineteenth century show some tenets of the New Religious Synthesis already solidly in place. Clearly, any notion of a sovereign God directing human destiny had been rejected, and reason was given the task of shaping humanity's destiny following the principles of evolution. Science replaced the Revealed Word as a source of religious hope by providing the techniques necessary to bring about humanity's perfection. The spiritual future of the human race would derive from humanly directed, evolutionary moral advancement.

JULIAN HUXLEY: TRANSHUMANISM AND THE MORAL ELITE

T. H. Huxley's grandson Sir Julian Sorell Huxley (1887-1975), brother of the famous essayist and novelist Aldous Huxley, has been called the greatest Humanist of

the twentieth century. An accomplished scientist and graduate of Balliol College, Oxford, Huxley was appointed the first director of the United Nations Educational, Scientific and Cultural Organization (UNESCO) in 1947. In the mid-twentieth century Huxley was a famous news broadcaster and a frequent lecturer in America and England. His many books include *Religion Without Revelation* (1927), *Evolution: The Modern Synthesis* (1942) and *New Bottles for New Wine* (1958). Huxley was a leading figure in evolutionary biology and a highly successful popularizer of both scientific findings and his own metaphysical speculations based on those findings.

Julian Huxley presented his message of freethinking, human evolutionary destiny and moral advancement to hundreds of thousands in the Western world. His "transhumanism" was a doctrine of evolutionary progress toward a morally or spiritually perfected human race. The religion of the new human race would consist in the reverent contemplation of its own evolutionary destiny. A fundamental change in the universe occurred when evolution finally produced human consciousness. "As a result of a thousand million years of evolution, the universe is becoming conscious of itself, able to understand something of its past history and possible future."[62]

The conscious life of a human being is the ultimate goal that biological life has been seeking from the very beginning. The next stage in human evolution is cosmic self-awareness—a conscious awareness of the direction and purpose of human evolution. This stage of development is "being realized in . . . a few of us human beings." Though it offends liberal notions of democracy, the idea that only an elite will take the next evolutionary step seems in keeping with the basic mechanics of evolution. So only a few human beings are destined to take remarkable evolutionary bounds. "Do not let us forget that the human species is as radically different from any of the microscopic single-celled animals that lived a thousand million years ago as they were from a fragment of stone or metal."[63]

Evolution, metaphysics and human destiny. In his hugely successful and frequently reprinted work *Evolution: The Modern Synthesis,* Julian Huxley described the current state of evolutionary science for English and American readers between 1942 and 1974.[64] For Huxley, as for his brother Aldous, evolution was undeniably progressive, a fact the public readily accepted. "The confusion appears to be greater among professional biologists than among laymen," Huxley writes.[65] Evolutionary progress was crucial to Huxley's metaphysical system, and he drives the point hard against those who reject the idea as unscientific.

For Huxley, "dominant types" branch out and take over territory inhabited by

other species. Such biological conquest demonstrates, not just change, but progress. It is clear that these dominant types reveal "efficiency in such matters as speed and the application of force to overcome physical limitations."[66] The "final results" of progress appear in "the historical fact of a succession of dominant groups" occupying ever more territory.[67] Thus, "evolutionary progress" means "increased control over and independence of the environment," and by this criterion humans are the current evolutionary leaders.[68]

Though he was a scientist, Huxley's interest in evolution was ultimately metaphysical, focusing on a human race whose evolutionary destiny had to be recognized in order to be realized. In the climactic section of *Evolution*, entitled "Progress in the Evolutionary Future," Huxley argued that "conscious and conceptual thought is the latest step in life's progress." There will not be a proliferation of new species from the human stock, but rather one new species resulting from the "crossing and recombination" of human genetic material. Human beings will "set limits" on this process based on the environment available for the new species to inhabit.[69]

In keeping with New Synthesis thinking, science will direct the creation of this new human species. Scientists must insist on "greater disinterestedness and fuller control of the emotional impulse," an idea Sir Julian attributed to his brother, Aldous. Old-fashioned moral restraint of the type suggested by the Revealed Word, as well as irrational limits on scientific research rooted in concerns over "playing God," must be dispensed with. The "brain's level of performance could be genetically raised" in various ways. "Castes" could be created with special capacities needed by the society.[70] The very best among us—"the best endowed ten-thousandth"—would be the model and goal of such experimentation with human genetic engineering. "Nor is there any reason to suppose that such quantitative increase could not be pushed beyond its present upper limits."[71]

Progress, mysticism and the religious impediment. Capacities such as "telepathy and other extra-sensory activities of the mind" would be goals of genetically guided evolution in humans. Of course, inherited traits that hinder advancement may have to be eliminated from a more evolved humanity, just as our earlier ancestors got rid of scales and grew hair. Human "values" themselves must be examined and determinations made about which ones to keep and which ones to jettison. "Control and independence," the twin criteria of progress, would guide such decisions.[72]

Huxley muses that "true human progress consists in increases in aesthetic, intellectual, and spiritual experience and satisfaction." His foundational concern ap-

pears to be spiritual, with a particular spiritual tendency viewed as the most desirable—the mystical experience. "Control" rests with the human being when he achieves "independence of inessential stimuli and ideas." The result is "the satisfaction of mystic detachment and inner ecstasy."[73] His brother's well-known experiments with hallucinogens may have suggested such a view.

Rejecting as "wholly false" the idea that human destiny is directed by "some external power"—the view of Darwin's rival, Alfred Russel Wallace—Huxley argues for *human* directedness in future evolution. "It is we who have read purpose into evolution," he writes. "If we wish to work towards a purpose for the future of man, we must formulate that purpose ourselves. Purposes in life are made, not found."[74] And finding such purpose is our destiny. "The future of progressive evolution is the future of man," he writes. "The future of man, if it is to be progress and not merely a standstill or a degeneration, must be guided by a deliberate purpose."[75] That "deliberate purpose" ought to be the ultimate driving force of science.

A great conflict of fundamental human values will occur between those who can envision the human evolutionary future and those who cannot, those who have moved beyond the traditional religious values of the Revealed Word, and those who remain rooted in the past. Repeating Darwin's own complaint against Christianity, Huxley writes, "another struggle still in progress is between the idea of a purpose directed to a future life in a supernatural world," that is, in heaven, "and one directed to progress in this world." However, "until such major conflicts are resolved, humanity can have no single major purpose, and progress can be but fitful and slow."[76] The Revealed Word's dominance in the Western world, where science is the most advanced, has been the principal impediment to human evolutionary advancement. "Man must work and plan if he is to achieve further progress for himself and so for life."[77] This "work" might reasonably involve propagating a new spiritual view more amenable to such progress.

PIERRE TEILHARD DE CHARDIN: REACHING THE OMEGA POINT

French Jesuit priest, geologist and paleontologist Pierre Teilhard de Chardin (1881-1955) was perhaps the twentieth century's greatest advocate of spiritual evolution. "During his formative years, Teilhard was greatly influenced by both of his parents: his father was an avid naturalist while his mother was a devout mystic." As a result, from an early age "Teilhard became interested in both science and reli-

gion."[78] One commentator writes that Teilhard offered "a new framework for those believers who take science seriously and concern themselves about the future of humankind."[79] The Catholic Church withheld publication of many of his works until after his death, fearing that his ideas were unorthodox. His books are now foundational works of progressive spiritual thought.

Henri Bergson's book *Creative Evolution* (1907) "convinced Teilhard of the truth of evolution." He thus "devoted the rest of his life to a personal attempt at reconciling science and theology within an evolutionary interpretation of this dynamic universe."[80] Evolution was the fundamental principle of the cosmos, and Teilhard afforded humans a central place in the "evolving universe." The evolution of the cosmos was "both progressive and directional."[81] Teilhard dubbed the terminus of human evolution the Omega Point, a state of "mystical unity" and "spiritual love."[82]

Writing in *The Future of Man* (1959), Teilhard praised the efforts of Aldous Huxley "to formulate and crystallize . . . the basis of a common philosophy on which all men of goodwill can agree in order that the world may continue to progress." Teilhard believed such an effort would hasten the day when, "in religious thought as in the sciences, a core of universal truth will form and slowly grow to be accepted by everyone." He asked, "Can there be any true spiritual evolution without it?" In Teilhard's vision, "mankind is to achieve a breakthrough straight ahead by forcing its way over the threshold of some higher level of consciousness."[83]

One commentator writes, "Teilhard always maintained that the whole universe is evolving spirit (since matter is energy and, for him, all energy is ultimately spirit)."[84] Humanity as part of this evolving universe is destined to evolve with it. Teilhard referred to the elite group destined to achieve a spiritual evolutionary breakthrough as the "Sacred Union" and "the active minority" of the human race. These spiritually gifted individuals constitute the "solid core around which the unanimity of tomorrow must harden."[85]

The final step in spiritual evolution results in "all the separate consciousnesses of the world converging" into one great consciousness centered on love. When this breakthrough occurs, humanity will have created out of itself a new divinity. This is the Omega Point, the messianic moment when an evolving, converging human consciousness issues in "the rise of God."[86]

Teilhard de Chardin joined the scientific and the religious ideas of a new age, making the evolutionary notion of constant, incremental improvement the foundation of a new spirituality. Recently a number of popular writers have developed this

idea to the point that it has become the centerpiece of the New Religious Synthesis. One of those authors is the focus of the next section.

JAMES H. AUSTIN: EVOLVING BRAIN, EVOLVING SPIRIT

James H. Austin is emeritus professor of neurology at the University of Colorado. His recently published *Zen and the Brain: Toward an Understanding of Meditation and Consciousness* is an encyclopedic 840-page synthesis of brain research and Zen philosophy. His book serves as a bridge between the biological progressivism of Darwin and the more spiritually oriented evolutionary thinking explored in the next chapter.

Austin, writing as a recognized expert in brain science, argues that Zen Buddhism's emphasis on meditative techniques holds the key to understanding the brain's continuing evolution. He contends that Westerners, accustomed to understanding God as the Creator, are not immediately open to Eastern explanations of human consciousness. However, "as we learn more about Zen's subtler mechanisms, we shall discover . . . [that] its messages are not really that alien to the West after all." In fact, Austin suggests that "human brains everywhere gravitate toward the same kinds of natural messages."[87] And these natural messages are more closely aligned with Eastern than with Western spiritual systems.

Following his exhaustive overview of the literature on the brain's development, Austin offers his readers a musing on the future of the brain and, indeed, of the human soul. He accepts the notion of continuing human evolution, one of the most persistent consequences of the Darwinian worldview and a mainstay of the New Religious Synthesis. Austin asks his readers to consider whether "still other forces" in addition to biological ones might have been at work in our continuing evolution. "The Jesuit Teilhard de Chardin thought so," he notes. "He perceived that humankind was also progressing through sequences of *spiritual* development" as a "natural consequence of the fact that the human species was still evolving biologically."[88]

Evolution and human destiny. Where will this continuing process of human spiritual evolution end? Teilhard apparently believed that at some distant moment that he termed the Omega Point all human beings would achieve the equivalent of the Buddha's enlightenment. Austin is less sanguine. When looking at the history of the human race, the idea of "universal enlightenment" sounds to Austin "like too grandiose a Utopia."[89] Nevertheless, Austin finds various kinds of evidence pointing to the spiritual progress of at least a portion of the human race.

For instance, he argues that early Buddhist philosophers "were especially far-sighted" about our evolutionary destiny. "In the old city of Nara, there exists today a sublime statue which depicts their long-range faith" in our spiritual evolutionary progress. This seventh-century statue is of "*Miroku* (Maitrea), the Buddha of the future" and this statue bears "remarkably 'modern' facial features." Moreover, "a closer look discloses another curious feature about this Buddha of the future." The statue, as it turns out, "has *two* protrusions, one on either side of the top of the head *next* to the midline" when other Buddha heads "are limited to only one *ushnisha* in the midline." Austin asks, "Was the remote sculptor sending us some kind of message? Will evolved brains of the future be twice as enlightened?"[90]

Austin explores the crucial assumption of the New Religious Synthesis that human spiritual evolution follows directly from the notion of biological evolution, though he lacks Teilhard's confidence that such evolution is in store for everyone. "So, how realistic is an expectation that fallible human beings will evolve" to a point where they are "*all* Buddha-like in their degree of enlightenment?"[91] Still, some of us are already spiritually well on our way. Those capable of experiencing "advanced alternate states of consciousness" demonstrate that at least some human brains possess great capacity for change. Thus it seems likely that "some of our adaptable descendants," in particular "those whose education has gentled them and made them more flexible," are certain to "build on their experiences" and thus "become increasingly free to adapt creatively to survive future crises."[92] Some future humans with the right genetic equipment and access to the right kind of education will evolve to the next plane of spiritual achievement.

New Age stirpiculture? For Austin, the key Darwinian mechanism of natural selection may carry us onward to our spiritual destiny. "Let a few more persons multiply who had survived because they had greater capacities for such adaptability, and the resulting series of events might go on slowly to change the ethical and religious climate of the far distant future."[93] But why wait for the spiritual future to arrive by the slow conveyance of natural selection when we can speed up the process of change? "One can at least imagine," Austin writes, "a new era when some religious group within a culture might decide that it needed to raise and train a new leader." In the distant future "the ancient custom of searching all over for the right baby" would have disappeared. Moreover, "'reincarnation' would finally be appreciated as something determined solely by the laws which govern the human genome."

Lining up these possibilities, Austin concludes that "in this far-distant future it

might be realized that the desired child could best be conceived in a test tube and nurtured in a surrogate mother." Sounding a bit like John Humphrey Noyes, Austin writes, "entering into the ever-braver union would be the ovum donated perhaps by a virginal nun, plus the sperm from an exemplary monk, both of whom had been screened and selected on the basis of their outstanding lineage and capacity." And what ought our response be to such hopeful spiritual eugenics? Austin replies, "Our task is to take a deep breath and to accept that such a blessed event is now *technically* possible. And not to scoff too quickly."[94]

For Austin, the progression from biological to spiritual evolution is a natural one that suggests the trajectory of ultimate human destiny. "Infinitesimal steps" akin to those of biological evolution slowly reveal "the human potential to evolve toward illumination at more advanced levels. For ours is still a species on an endless journey into an unimaginable future."[95] In addition, Austin seems confident that this future may be hastened by scientific research into the mechanisms of the brain, under the direction of the insights of Zen and other meditative traditions. Such research might suggest how to direct the process of evolution toward enlightenment. "As one of the byproducts of such research, it would be of interest to develop ways of identifying at a young age, *prospectively*, those persons who do have the potential to mature into our classic ideal of the saintly sage: a next Dalai Lama, a future Mother Theresa, or a Krishnamurti in the making, so to speak."[96] Austin's speculations bring us to the brink of an intentional union between spirituality and reproductive science in the search for our spiritual future.

JAMES REDFIELD: THE CELESTINE PROPHET

Spiritual evolution is now a potent spiritual idea reflected in a wide range of both popular nonfiction and fiction. James Redfield's bestselling adventure story *The Celestine Prophecy* (1993) reflects the concept's centrality to a new genre of spiritual fiction. For Redfield, spiritual advancement is a direct outgrowth of biological evolution, and his story presents the idea in a winsome and persuasive fashion as a matter of modern common sense. *The Celestine Prophecy*'s protagonist searches a Latin American country for a mysterious manuscript bearing spiritual secrets. In an instant of cosmic insight after reading the manuscript, he realizes that he is on an evolutionary journey that began with the first helium atoms beginning to "vibrate." Vibration is the fundamental principle of life itself in *The Celestine Prophecy* and has been a common theme in evolutionary writing since the days of Erasmus Darwin and "vitalism."

According to Redfield, evolutionary progress is tied directly to an individual's insights into the evolutionary process itself, a view not far removed from Julian Huxley's thinking on the matter. "I perceived everything to be somehow a part of me," Redfield's unnamed narrator tells us, this insight triggering a personal recollection of the evolutionary hypothesis in an almost mystical vision. "The science of evolution had always bored me, but now, as my mind continued to race backward in time, all the things I had read on the subject began to come back to me . . . [and] the recollection allowed me to look at evolution in a new way."[97]

Matter, he realizes, is not solid, but rather is vibrating energy operating under a "ruling principle" that causes it to continuously organize itself into more and more complex forms. Basic matter—hydrogen—organized itself into helium, helium into stars, and hydrogen and helium into lithium. "The stage was now set," he understands in an instant of illumination, "for the next step of evolution."[98] To make a long evolutionary story short, matter continues to organize itself into progressively more complex systems until "great lightning storms" on earth cause matter in "shallow pools and basins" finally to "leap past the vibratory level of carbon" to become amino acids. Inevitably life appears, and then more complex life. At the end of it all, "the progression ended. There at the pinnacle stood humankind."[99]

As Redfield tells the grand story, evolutionary progress came about through increasingly higher pitched "vibration." The progressive evolution of matter, guided by a "ruling principle," produces "humankind" as its final outcome. But, as with Julian Huxley and Teilhard de Chardin, humanity is not a finished work.

The spiritually sensitive Father Sanchez patiently explains the mechanics of spiritual evolution in *The Celestine Prophecy*. "We fill up, grow, fill up and grow again. That is how we as humans continue the evolution of the universe to a higher and higher vibration." In this way, "evolution has been going on unconsciously throughout human history." This fact "explains why civilization has progressed and why humans have grown larger, lived longer, and so forth. Now however," Sanchez adds, "we are making the whole process conscious. That is what the Manuscript is telling us. That is what this movement toward a world-wide spiritual consciousness is all about."[100] The emerging "world-wide spiritual consciousness" will involve the elimination of all distinctions among the world's various religions as realization dawns that each in its own way is assisting human spiritual evolution. The new consciousness also means the elimination of unhelpful concepts such as a fall from grace, sin and evil as inherent components of human nature.

SCIENCE FICTION AND HUMAN EVOLUTIONARY DESTINY

Inevitable human progress through evolutionary processes is a theme in some of the most imaginative and persuasive science fiction. It is particularly important to the works of three pillars of British science fiction: H. G. Wells (1866-1946), Olaf Stapledon (1886-1950) and Arthur C. Clarke (b. 1917). That Wells would have devoted attention to human evolutionary advancement is not surprising considering that he was a student at Huxley's London School of Science.

Bulwer-Lytton's "The Coming Race." The idea of human evolutionary progress appears in some of the very earliest works in the science fiction genre. Sir George Edward Bulwer-Lytton (1798-1871) was a popular English fiction writer of the nineteenth century who produced an extraordinary number of novels and short stories between about 1835 and his death in 1871. Among his last works was the strange novella about a journey beneath the surface of the earth entitled *Vrilya: The Power of the Coming Race*, better known simply as *The Coming Race*. The book "created a sensation" when it first appeared in 1871.[101] A skilled storyteller, Bulwer-Lytton combined current scientific theories, racialist dogma, speculation about the ancient Egyptians and a love story to create a captivating but troubling early work of science fiction.

The Coming Race bears a haunting message about the possible racial and cultural implications of evolutionary theory. Bulwer-Lytton, a Rosicrucian and occultist with an interest in languages, presents the Vrilya people as descendants of the original Aryan race that once inhabited the earth's surface. Following a great deluge early in human history the Vrilya were forced to develop their civilization below ground and largely in isolation from other races. Adolf Hitler is known to have been influenced by Bulwer-Lytton's works, and may even have absorbed this Victorian writer's theories about a master race descended from the Aryans.[102] Madame Blavatsky, herself a racial theorist and proponent of Aryan superiority, was also known to have been a fan of *The Coming Race*.

In *The Coming Race* a young American explorer falls through a chasm in the lower reaches of an abandoned mine shaft. The protagonist finds himself in a new world inhabited by advanced human beings—the Vrilya—who are physically perfect, extraordinarily intelligent, godlike creatures capable of flight with artificial wings. Seeing a member of this superrace "reminded me of symbolical images of Genius or Demon that are seen on Etruscan vases or limned on the walls of Eastern

sepulchres—images that borrow the outlines of man, and are yet of another race."[103] This creature had "the face of man, but yet of a type of man distinct from our known extant races." As if encountering a god, the narrator's initial "terror" gives way to "a sense of contentment, of joy, of confidence in myself and in the being before me."[104] Appearing like "sculptured gods," these new people constitute "a race akin to man's, but infinitely stronger of form and grander of aspect, and inspiring [an] unutterable feeling of dread."[105]

The Vrilya have mastered a mysterious force known as Vril. By means of Vril—a kind of psychic or spiritual energy providing enormous power—the subterranean humans illuminate their dark world. Vril also powers their air ships and land vehicles. The Vrilya are vegetarians, and practice a benign form of fascism, having dispensed with democracy as a "crude experiment." In every way, including spiritually, the Vrilya have evolved beyond their surface-dwelling cousins. And like Julian Huxley's "dominant types," the Vril intend one day to return to the earth's surface and annihilate the inferior human species living there.

The inexplicable force known as Vril is used to perform virtual miracles. It provides a limitless source of light and can be employed to control the thoughts and actions of others. Vril is the Life Force itself, the key to godlike control over all that exists and the key to extending life indefinitely. "These people," says the protagonist, "consider that in Vril they have arrived at the unity in natural energic agencies, which has been conjectured by many philosophers above ground."[106]

The Vrilya discovered Vril because they perceived by scientific means that "the various forms under which the forces of matter are made manifest have one common origin."[107] That is, science led the Vrilya to monism, and monism led them to Vril, the power that propels life forward toward ever more perfect states. The highest point so far attained in the evolutionary progress of life is the Vrilya themselves. The protagonist is calmly informed by a leader of the master race that they will one day return to the surface of the earth and subjugate or destroy the other races. This is their destiny and the destiny of life itself as it moves toward ultimate perfection. That which is inferior must be set aside to make room for that which is progressing toward perfection—this is the rule of life.

George Edward Bulwer-Lytton used The Coming Race as a forum in which to advance his theory of a spiritually evolved master race destined to rule or destroy all other races.[108] And his theories proved quite popular with his Victorian reading audience. Vril societies formed in England and on the European Continent, lasting

well into the twentieth century. The Vril Society of Munich attracted several members who would later become prominent figures in Hitler's National Socialist Party.

"Close Encounters." In closing this chapter, I would like to look briefly at two other examples of science fiction as a messenger of continuing human evolution. Steven Spielberg's classic 1977 UFO movie, *Close Encounters of the Third Kind*—the title a reference to direct human contact with aliens— was among the first of many highly successful big-budget science fiction blockbusters. In the film a small number of humans are subconsciously instructed to await a visit by aliens at a mountain location in Wyoming. There, the process of instructing human beings in their further progress will begin. As one character says in the opening moments of the actual visit, "This is the first day of school."

In the climactic scene of Spielberg's *Close Encounters,* alien beings emerge bathed in light from an enormous spacecraft to make contact with humans. Suggestively, these aliens look vaguely like some members of the gathered humans waiting breathlessly for this moment of contact with a more advanced species. The camera focuses on the now familiar face of a celluloid alien—narrow chin, large eyes, high forehead, pale skin. Then, the camera pans the human audience, focusing at last on a similar human face—narrow chin, large eyes, high forehead, pale skin. Through the juxtaposition of cinematic images, Spielberg seems to be making a point—the aliens reflect what the human race is destined to look like somewhere in the distant evolutionary future. In addition, some of us have already taken important genetic steps in this direction.[109]

One is reminded of Herbert Spencer's speculation that among the various human races "the higher forms [are] distinguished by the relatively larger size of the bones which cover the brain, and the relatively smaller size of those which cover the jaws, etc. Now this trait, which is stronger in Man than in any other creature, is stronger in the European than in the savage."[110] And, apparently, stronger yet in the extraterrestrial than in the European. Spielberg and Spencer seem to be reading from the same script. As *Close Encounters* closes, a minister reads the biblical passage "He will give his angels charge over you," as actor Richard Dreyfuss is awarded the unimaginable privilege of entering the alien craft and departing on a grand cultural adventure. Alien culture, it is suggested, will become for us a source of innumerable insights, certainly scientific, perhaps also spiritual.

"Star Trek." Another example of science fiction exploring the evolutionary hypothesis is important if for no other reason than its massive cultural impact. *Star*

Trek is perhaps the most popular and long lasting and influential media phenomenon of all time. So vast has been its cultural influence that a number of terms and phrases have entered the English language through the show.

In a groundbreaking study of the hidden messages of *Star Trek* from the first appearance of the television program through the latest movie manifestation of the saga, Daniel Bernardi has examined, among other issues, how the writers and producers of *Star Trek* treat the topic of evolution. Under the doctrine of "parallel evolution"—the notion that humanoid beings would have evolved at a rate approximately that of humans on earth—*Star Trek's* creator Gene Rodenberry and subsequent writers have often speculated about where humanity is headed, both physically and spiritually.[111] According to Bernardi, "the pinnacle of evolution in Trek is a creature who looks white and becomes god-like." A virtually divine race of beings known as the Organians choose "to take humanoid form, thus representing our divine destiny." Mr. Spock comments regarding these minor divinities: "I should say the Organians are as far above us on the evolutionary scale as we are above the amoeba."

According to the Trek myth, human evolution began when aliens seeded the earth's oceans with their DNA. In a *Next Generation* episode entitled "The Chase," a holographic image of an early galactic humanoid states, "the seed codes directed your evolution toward a physical form resembling ours."[112] Thus, the human race is created—not in the Revealed Word's image of God—but in the image of a dying race of aliens anxious to perpetuate itself throughout the galaxy.

If this is where we started, the nearly divine character Q may be where we finally will arrive on our evolutionary march. The first episode of the television series *Star Trek: The Next Generation* featured Q, an "omniscient being who can manipulate the space-time continuum with the snap of a finger."[113] Played by actor John de Lancie, Q is an arrogant and sarcastic demi-god who represents the evolutionary terminus of a species that apparently started its cosmic climb in a fashion similar to human beings. In several episodes featuring immortal, omnipotent and omniscient Q, the point is made that human beings also are embarked on an evolutionary journey and will one day resemble Q and the members of a guild of gods known as The Continuum. In this way, *Star Trek*, like much science fiction, incorporates evolutionary spirituality and its vision of a divine future for the human race.

CONCLUSION

Aldous Huxley, Sir Julian's brother, wrote in 1947, "Human progress in happiness,

virtue, and creativeness is valuable in the last analysis, as a condition of spiritual advance toward man's Final End." For Aldous Huxley, "If happiness, morals and creativeness are treated as ends in themselves instead of means to a further End, they can become obstacles to spiritual advance no less serious, in their way, than wretchedness, vice, and conventionality."[114] That is, all of the aspiration, attainment and virtue of our present lives are simply preparing the way for something grander and more consequential—the ultimate spiritual End of human evolution. The idea that human beings are embarked on an inevitably successful and increasingly self-directed journey toward spiritual perfection via the mechanisms of evolution is now a crucial and taken-for-granted component in much religious thought. This idea exerts a powerful grip on contemporary religious thinking.

Under the New Religious Synthesis, evolution is the principle animating the cosmos. Human beings, evolution's conscious products, can now achieve ever-higher levels of consciousness by directing their own evolution. The goal is spiritual fulfillment, absolute consciousness, blissful experience. Most advocates of spiritual evolution agree that humans can and should hasten the process. Marilyn Ferguson wrote in *The Aquarian Conspiracy* of a "new paradigm" that now "attributes evolution to periodic leaps by small groups." The efficient operation of this new paradigm will require "a mechanism for biological change more powerful than chance mutation," which will open "the possibility of rapid evolution in our time."[115] For some theorists of the "next step," assistance is available to us from entities further along the evolutionary path. Gary Zukav, for example, refers to such helpers as Angels. "An Angel," he writes, "might be thought of as a force of consciousness that has evolved into an appropriate teaching modality for the planetary village called earth."[116]

Charles Darwin saw evolutionary perfection as a rival to the Revealed Word's hope of heaven, and he certainly was not alone in looking forward to an era of a fully evolved human race. Similarly, Darwin's grandfather Erasmus found in evolution a mechanism for moral as well as biological progress, provided we cured the plague of conventional religious thinking. Herbert Spencer did much to popularize the notion of human evolutionary progress. Spencer also recognized that evolution could assist the invention of a powerful moral philosophy, indeed, a new religious view, provided traditional religion could be jettisoned. This idea is still powerfully with us. A. N. Wilson asks, "Do we not share with Spencer a generalized belief that the scientific outlook, however that may be defined, compels the religious outlook to be modified, if not actually abandoned?" Wilson adds that "the existence on this planet

of two generations of Europeans who believed Herbert Spencer to be the greatest thinker of their time might have something to do with our own outlook."[117]

Franklin Baumer writes that evolution "persuaded people to think of everything in nature as the fruit of a gradual growth rather than an original creation." Such gradualist thinking means that it is "now difficult if not impossible for an educated man to conceive of a primitive revelation such as traditional Christianity taught, or even of an original natural religion from which men had declined." This difficulty arises because "in an evolving world, perfection obviously lay, not in the past, but in the future."[118] Evolutionary, progressivist thinking has reversed the direction of Western spirituality—we did not fall from perfection, we are gradually heading toward it. Moreover, the idea of "conscious evolution" has shifted the locus of spiritual agency: we do not need to turn to God for salvation; we shall do that work ourselves as we learn to control evolution.

Darwin's idea is now taken as final proof that the universe is governed, not by a divine will that created humans out of dust, but by a virtually divine force Darwin called natural selection. Having produced human consciousness, evolution may now, according to its prophets, be brought directly under the control of its own product. Humanity, the accomplishment of natural selection, is on the threshold of mastering Darwin's divinity. The hope of the New Religious Synthesis is that the mechanisms of evolution can be taken by force and consciously employed to guide human progress toward the next level of existence, Aldous Huxley's "Final End."

7

PANTHEISM IN THE MODERN WORLD

Nature or God

"What is that mysterious force?" I asked.
"It's a force that is present throughout everything that is," he said.

CARLOS CASTANEDA, The Fire from Within

Science proves the potency of monistic philosophy over dualism—over spirit separated from matter.

AMIT GOSWAMI, The Self-Aware Universe

Pantheists usually believe that God, so to speak, animates the universe as you animate your body: that the universe almost is God, so that if it did not exist He would not exist either, and anything you find in the universe is part of God. The Christian idea is quite different.

C. S. LEWIS, Mere Christianity

Teilhard de Chardin saw in the rising religious awareness of humankind "the progressive Spiritualization of Matter." The destiny of the cosmos is for spirit and matter to be revealed as "the same cosmic stuff."[1] The universe is "falling . . . in the direction of spirit," which is its "stable form."[2] The matter of which the universe is made up is not inanimate, but carries within itself "an extraordinary capacity" for "complexification."[3] That is, matter continually organizes itself into more and more complex forms, with consciousness being the end of the process. Human consciousness is finally awakening to the reality and inevitability of the universe's evolutionary process, while at the same time recognizing that it—human consciousness, that is—represents the very pinnacle of the universe's spiritual evolution.

Teilhard claims that even as a child he recognized in himself the operation of "Cosmic" and "Christic" forces, which led him into a virtually worshipful relation-

ship first with a piece of iron and later with quartz. He writes that these substances "opened my groping mind into the vast structures of the Planet and Nature."[4] And what did he see when viewing these "vast structures"? He saw that the earth is enveloped, not just in an atmosphere, but also in a "noosphere," a thinking layer of spirit that is, in fact, the sum of all human minds. The noosphere is, in his words, "totalized Mankind," all human minds as one great Mind.[5] Moreover, this noosphere drives forward the evolution of the universal spirit. The noosphere is not static, but is currently experiencing an "accelerated drift toward ultra-human states, under the influence of psycho-physical convergence (or Planetization)."[6] We are, that is, becoming something other than, something higher than human. We are gradually but inexorably becoming one with the divine consciousness that is in everything that exists.

The idea that nature or the cosmos is divine is an ancient and persistent one that stands in direct contradiction to the Revealed Word's personal and transcendent God. The notion appears throughout history in a variety of guises. Ancient writers such as Plotinus imagined a universe in which "soul" animated all physical objects. "It is the soul that lends all things movement," he wrote.[7] In the seventeenth century, the Dutch philosopher Benedict de Spinoza advocated pantheism. Shortly afterward the idea was popularized in the controversial writings of the Irish religious radical John Toland. A form of pantheism was at the root of the vast nature-worshiping movements in Europe during the nineteenth century. Richard Noll has written that "the 1890s in Central Europe were marked by the rise of volkish utopianism" based on the rejection of Christianity "and emphasis on the worship of nature." Noll takes this movement to have been rooted in the pantheistic monism of the enormously influential German naturalist Ernst Haeckel.[8] Haeckel wrote that it was "quite certain that the Christian system must give way to the monistic," that is, to an understanding of all things as one divine entity.[9]

Writers in the New Science genre now routinely describe a universe charged with divine energy or consciousness. For example, physicist Fred Alan Wolf writes of "our present modern vision of an abstract God and mysterious eternal soul" present in all material things.[10] Wolf believes that pantheism returns us to an earlier, more fundamental human spiritual view. The "early modern vision of raw and to-be-conquered nature" he finds to be "vastly different from that of the pre-Greeks." Moreover, "this pre-Greek vision of the soul, life and death" that incorporated the notion that "everything in nature, including rocks, mountains, the sky,

animals, and plants, was alive, bristling with sacred energy" is a worldview Wolf sees "returning to our time."[11]

This basic idea is found in many contemporary spiritual works as well. For instance, in Helen Schucman's *A Course in Miracles,* students are instructed to repeat the "lesson" that "God is in everything I see." Schucman instructs, "Begin with repeating the idea to yourself, and then apply it to randomly chosen objects about you, naming each one specifically, . . . 'God is in this coat hanger. God is in this magazine. God is in this finger. God is in this lamp.'"[12] Pantheism has become an essential component in the New Religious Synthesis. God is no longer outside of creation, no longer either "wholly other" or personal. Rather, the new god is in all things as a divine energy, animating force or cosmic consciousness.

This chapter considers the reemergence of pantheism as a popular religious idea and building block of the Other Spirituality. John Toland coined the term *pantheism* in the early eighteenth century, and Toland's influence on religious ideas in England and later in France, Germany and America was great. Indeed, this early pantheist was the first truly successful and popular religious radical in the modern period. This chapter also explores pantheism's development as a popular religious idea in America under the influence of Ralph Waldo Emerson. Emerson exerted extensive influence over religious thought in the rapidly expanding American republic of the 1800s.[13]

From Emerson we will shift our focus to the pantheistic monism of Ernst Haeckel, a late-nineteenth-century scientist, evolutionist and popular writer who for years held Europe in thrall on a wide range of scientific and metaphysical topics. So successful was Haeckel's case for seeing all that exists as one entity that monistic churches began to spring up on the Continent. Moving from the sciences to the arts, we will consider the pantheism inherent in an important play by the English playwright George Bernard Shaw. The chapter concludes with a consideration of the fundamental pantheism inherent in much of the New Science.

SPINOZA AND TOLAND

Baruch or Benedict de Spinoza (1632-1677) was a member of the Jewish Diaspora in the Netherlands. For his unorthodox writings he was expelled from the Synagogue of Amsterdam in 1656. The reclusive Spinoza made his living grinding lenses for telescopes and other optical instruments, and once refused a prestigious chair in philosophy in order that he might continue to live a tranquil life as a lens

grinder. Spinoza is famous for his attacks on the Bible in *Tractatus theologico-politicus*. The *Ethics* sets out his pantheistic view that the natural realm is God, and God is all of nature. Spinoza's view is captured in a famous Latin phrase, *Deus sive natura* (God or nature). The two terms are, for Spinoza, interchangeable. This god/nature is infinite, one substance extended indefinitely in such a way as to preclude the possibility of any other entity in the cosmos. That is, Spinoza literally leaves no room in the cosmos for God. There is no mind behind the physical matter of Spinoza's universe, and thus no divine purpose in the cosmic order of things. Matter in motion is the only principle at work in the universe. The material/divine universe is all of one essence. Human beings and all other physical objects share this common essence. This makes human beings a part—albeit a uniquely rational part—of the vast cosmic order.

In his own day, Spinoza's rendering God equivalent to the physical world was taken as simple atheism. But Spinoza insisted he had a theology and that it was in keeping with an ancient Jewish tradition. That tradition, however, was the kabbalistic mysticism of writers such as Rabbi Moses Cordovero, the author of the famous mystical work *A Garden of Pomegranates*. Cordovero argued that "God the knower" and the objects that God knows are one and the same thing, partaking of the same essence. Thus, Spinoza may have seen himself as providing philosophical grounding for a theological view that had been alive in Judaism for centuries. To identify God with nature is to make science and theology the same discipline. As Daniel C. Dennett writes, "Benedict Spinoza, in the seventeenth century, *identified* God and Nature, arguing that scientific research was the true path of theology."[14]

Spinoza influenced a number of late seventeenth and early eighteenth-century religious radicals. One famous skeptical work that circulated in this period, *The Treatise of the Three Impostors*, provided curious readers a sensational and popularized version of many of Spinoza's skeptical arguments. The Irishman John Toland (1670-1722) was among the most colorful and controversial of the public religious advocates directly influenced by the great Dutch philosopher. He is, in fact, credited with having coined the term *pantheism* in a 1705 publication, the word coming into general use among English speakers by the time of Toland's death in 1722. His most important work was *Christianity Not Mysterious* (1696), in which he attacked the Bible on the argument that the true religion of humanity was established well before Christianity.

In works such as *Pantheisticon* (1720) Toland advocated a pantheistic theology

that popularized the ideas of both Spinoza and the earlier Dominican writer Bruno, who had championed the infinity and "divinity of the universe" as well as the plurality of habitable worlds.[15] If Bruno was correct that the universe was infinite, Toland reasoned, this left no room for a God who exists externally to it. Thus, if there is a God he must be indistinguishable from the physical universe. Moreover, in an infinite universe shot through with a life force, intelligent life might be expected to arise and flourish in many places.

Such views were dangerous to express in the early eighteenth century, and so Toland adopted a strategy of advocating pantheism without appearing to be committed to the idea. Thus, historian Robert Sullivan notes that "insinuation" of pantheism into the minds of the British reading public became Toland's "ultimate literary purpose."[16] Avoiding direct statement of his religious views was in keeping with Toland's approach to religion generally. A believer in esoteric theology, he found secrecy a necessary means of guarding spiritual truths against the corrupting influence of the public.

John Toland was committed to the pantheistic principle that "everything was full of God, who was in everything."[17] In *Pantheisticon* he wrote of "the Force and Energy of the Whole, the Creator and Ruler of All, and always tending to the best End is GOD, whom you may call the Mind, if you please, and the Soul of the Universe."[18] Sullivan writes that "Toland's aim was to eliminate both the separation of God from the universe and the distinction between a supreme intellect (or soul) and the natural activity of matter." That is, Toland sought to usher out of the Western mind the Revealed Word's conception of God. However, Toland's new deity was incapable of providing either "divine guidance of individuals" or "loving care, and intervention."[19]

Toland studied the texts of a wide range of ancient and modern religions, often in the original languages. He was particularly fascinated with the ancient British Druids, reading their works in Celtic. His interest in the Druids was driven largely by his desire to discover the most primitive human religious beliefs and practices. Druid nature worship, Toland argued, suggested that the primitive religion of humanity was pantheism, not theism. Early humans did not worship a transcendent and personal God, but nature itself as god. In *Pantheisticon*, Toland developed his fullest argument to the effect that pantheism was the natural religion of the human race. It was also, he claimed, the spiritual view expressed by "all wise men" at all times.[20] Among the groups that he believed to have been pantheistic in their theology were the Pythagoreans of Greece and the Brahmans of India.

Many others also held to this view of a unity between God and the physical universe. These included "most ancient Egyptians, Persians, and Romans, [and] the first Patriarchs of the Hebrews," all of whom understood "the simplicity of the Divine Nature."[21] In *Letters to Serena*, Toland remarks that "a great many eminent Persons in Europe and Asia, both understood themselves the Origins of the Religions commonly received . . . and thus asserted the Unity of the Deity."[22] Thus, Toland viewed his project as "laboring to restore forgotten truths" by reintroducing pantheism to human religious thinking.[23] After all, pantheism was the natural religion of the human race. Sullivan remarks that Toland's account of human spirituality's devolution from pantheism into belief in various personal gods "dominated European writing on the subject for almost two generations after his death."[24] This view—that all religious faiths share a common ancestry in primitive pantheistic and mystical spirituality—is now an important component of the New Religious Synthesis.

RALPH WALDO EMERSON

Ralph Waldo Emerson (1803-1882) was the son of a Unitarian minister, William Emerson, who died in 1811 when Ralph Waldo was eight. Born in Boston at the opening of the nineteenth century, Emerson grew up in the context of a religiously saturated and spiritually jaded New England. Emerson's father was fond of both Paine and Priestley, and so a strong deistic influence is evident in the elder Emerson's thinking. One of Ralph Waldo Emerson's biographers calls the religion of the great essayist's father "calm deism." In this way, the religious atmosphere in which Emerson grew up was remarkably similar to that in which Charles Darwin, born only six years after Emerson and dying the same year, was reared. Emerson's mother is described as "deeply religious," but was drawn to works of "spiritual self-help" rather than to theology.[25]

However, the greatest early spiritual influence on Ralph Waldo Emerson was his aunt Mary Moody Emerson, a self-styled mystic, visionary and prophet compared by one writer to the German mystical writer Jakob Böhme.[26] This strange woman wrote and traveled a great deal, wore a burial shroud when she traveled, and slept in a bed fashioned in the shape of a coffin. Mary Emerson's "effect on [Ralph Waldo Emerson] was permanent."[27] She was drawn to authors with pantheistic, mystical and deistic leanings—Plotinus, Spinoza, Goethe, Law, Coleridge—and Emerson himself owed a great debt to these same authors.

It is no mere coincidence that Mary Baker Eddy, Joseph Smith, Henry David

Thoreau and Emerson all were born around the same time and in the same region of the United States. Each threw off the dominant Protestantism of New England and suggested an exotic spiritual alternative that drew adherents into a variety of closely related teachings. The New England of the first half of the nineteenth century has been called the "burned over region" because of the extensive evangelizing that had taken place there and the resultant spiritual weariness of the residents.

Emerson entered Harvard at the age of fourteen, where he studied John Locke's empiricism, Dugald Stewart's commonsense philosophy and William Paley's ethics. Graduating in 1821, he was drawn increasingly toward the ministry and became a Unitarian minister in 1829. Emerson married Ellen Tucker in 1829, a woman for whom he had a deep and passionate love. She died only eighteen months later, dealing a severe blow to Emerson's beliefs about the immortality of the individual soul. At this time, around 1831, he began to formulate his distinctive religious ideas.

Swedenborg, Schleiermacher and Reed. To understand Emerson it is important to recognize the writers he read, admired and emulated. Emerson owed a considerable debt to Emanuel Swedenborg (1688-1772), the enormously influential Swedish mystic who claimed numerous conversations with spirits over a period of several years. Swedenborg repudiated Christianity's historical orientation, stressing instead the inner search for divine consciousness. Biographers have difficulty reconciling Emerson's apparent genius with his profound interest in Swedenborg's strange theology.

Another writer who profoundly influenced Emerson was Friedrich Schleiermacher (1768-1834), the prominent German theologian who also stressed the importance of interiority, emotion or feeling (*Gefühl*), and individual reflection in the religious life. Critics labeled Schleiermacher a pantheist, perhaps because he advocated a central mystical core common to all religious faiths. Jesus was unique only in the degree of his God-consciousness, that is, his awareness of the divinity at work in the world. Sin, for Schleiermacher, was a matter of wrong belief, rather than evil, and could be overcome by increasing one's God-consciousness. In both Swedenborg and Schleiermacher, Emerson found a religion of interior experience and god as a diffuse spiritual essence in nature.

Emerson was also drawn to the mental evolutionist Sampson Reed, for whom humanity was in the midst of a "revolutionary change."[28] In Reed's major work, *Observations on the Growth of the Mind*, he wrote, "all the changes which are taking place in the world originate in the mind."[29] Another of Emerson's mentors was the mys-

tical and gnostic writer Guillaume Oegger, especially through his work *The True Messiah*.[30] The seventeenth-century mystic and gnostic Jakob Böhme (1575-1624) was another strong influence on Emerson. Böhme, who claimed direct divine illumination in 1600 and again in 1610, believed the external, physical world was a projection of an inner spiritual power. His theology is set out in the book *Aurora*.

Finally, Emerson was influenced by eastern religious works, and he himself eventually popularized in America a fundamentally Hindu religious view for the first time. Philip Jenkins writes that "Emerson was influenced by the Upanishads, and in 1883 his widow hosted a lecture by a visiting Hindu teacher."[31] Emerson apparently also read magical works and advanced a theory of correspondence like the one undergirding occult thinking. The view is summarized in the adage, "As above, so below." That is, there is a correspondence between the physical world of events and objects in the spiritual world; thus, the former is an analogy or map for the latter.

Emerson's career. Emerson was one of those rare intellectual figures who both ably translate their ideas into the language of ordinary citizens and relish the opportunity to write for that audience. Moreover, Emerson was unusually successful in this enterprise of popular persuasion. As far as the public was concerned, he was the most compelling thinker of his age—and his age lasted a very long time indeed. Because Emerson had such extensive influence on religious ideas as both a lecturer and author of popular essays, it will be helpful to understand the course of his public career.

Ralph Waldo Emerson assumed the pulpit of the Second Unitarian Church of Boston in 1831. As his theological views drifted ever further from even liberal Christian thought, he resigned from the church and traveled to Europe where he met both Wordsworth and Coleridge. But it was his visit with Thomas Carlyle that moved him most. The two carried on a famous correspondence for the next thirty-eight years. In 1834 Emerson received an inheritance from Ellen Tucker's estate, the money being sufficient to ensure that he did not have to hold a steady job ever again. Eager to disseminate his developing theological views, Emerson became involved in the growing Lyceum movement of public lectures. Part education, part entertainment, the Lyceum circuit gave Emerson the opportunity both to promote and to hone his ideas.

As his fame increased, newspapers often reprinted his lectures. Emerson's many public addresses over several decades popularized an unorthodox spiritual view that has come to be known as Transcendentalism. His short book *Nature* (1836) and his lecture "Address Before the Divinity Class" (1838) are perhaps his

best-known explications of his now well-developed theology. The basic argument in these addresses is that individual consciousness is the one crucial component in religion, not doctrine, creed or ceremony. This subjective religious consciousness is triumphant over all historical and cultural constraints, including the teachings of all religions.

Emerson held that "the religious spirit does not reside in external forms, words, ceremonies, or institutions," affirming that "the one thing of value in the universe is the active soul." Thus, "subjective consciousness" is the essence of religion.[32] But Emerson also insisted on the general similarity of religious consciousness in all people. Holding to the idea of "one mind and common humanity," he argued that individualism was wrong because it tended to isolate us from those of other religious persuasions.[33] This unifying view of human religious experience was joined in Emerson's thought to a pantheistic understanding of divinity itself. When the term *god* carried any meaning at all for Emerson, it described a spirit present in all things. His radically subjective spirituality created controversy when he first expounded it. But by the end of the 1830s Emerson was beginning to be accepted as America's heterodox prophet of pantheism, the divine self and reverence for Nature.

By 1840 Emerson was directing most of his writing and speaking to the general public, and his influence was considerable. This "confident American prophet" traveled and lectured extensively in the Northeast and along the Atlantic seaboard.[34] He felt, as one biographer records, "that the nation needed him."[35] His fame continued to grow throughout the 1840s and 1850s, and his lecturing now took him to the Midwest. Emerson was a "magnificent rhetorician," according to one biographer, a speaker with "the power to communicate feelings even better than ideas."[36]

Emerson was the forefather of today's motivational speakers, and in this role served as spiritual counselor to thousands of Americans. Audiences found him inspiring even when they did not adopt or perhaps even fully understand his philosophy. Still, some ideas stuck, becoming part of the American religious consciousness: place your trust only in self, it is a cosmic law that good deeds are rewarded and bad deeds punished, God is present in all nature.

Emerson's religious thinking. It has been said that Emerson set about to invent a religion, doing so at a time when inventing religions was an American growth industry. Most of Emerson's writing is theological, whether implicitly or explicitly, and he has been accused of attempting to force all of his thinking into each essay, book and speech. Moreover, he aggressively sought converts to his point of view

and was quite successful in this effort. From 1835 through 1870 he was the most respected and influential American religious teacher. What religion, then, did Emerson teach?

It is clear that Emerson's personal and public theology was a reaction *against* Christian theology. Though never an orthodox Christian, Emerson moved further and further from Christianity throughout his life. Influenced by Romantics, mystics and naturalists, his "skepticism toward Christianity" was also bolstered by German biblical criticism.[37] Emerson developed his spiritual system as a tool for overturning Christianity and replacing it with something he thought better—an American version of monistic pantheism. God was not a divine judge or father, but rather a spirit present in all physical objects. He appears, Emerson wrote, "with all his parts in every moss and cobweb."[38]

On this "divinity in nature" view, Emerson erected an anthrotheology common to other nineteenth-century theological speculators: Humanity is the embodiment of the divine spirit moving through the universe, and thus each individual person is, in this sense, god. It followed that trust could be placed only in the self. In his essay "Self-Reliance," he writes about the individual as akin to a deity. For instance, spiritual peace must be discovered in the resources of the individual and not in an external deity. "Nothing can bring you peace but yourself," he writes.[39] Moreover, the individual explores the unmapped inner regions of consciousness in the search for religious truth. Only the self can explore the "undiscovered regions of thought."[40] The individual is embarked on an internal spiritual quest to discover the divinity residing within the human soul.

"I am part or particle of God." The similarity between the human mind and nature was so thoroughgoing for Emerson that he could write, "The whole of nature is a metaphor for the human mind."[41] And if nature is a *metaphor* for the human mind, nature was *identical* with the divine mind. In *Nature* Emerson affirms two essences in the universe, "Nature and the Soul," with Soul being his name for the divine spirit in all things and in each individual.[42] Because the human mind is analogous to the divine mind infusing nature, Emerson's theology led him to the view all pantheists eventually arrive at—the individual is divine. In Emerson's radically subjective theology, the observing, experiencing, intuiting self displaces a transcendent creator God. Moreover, the divine self takes on qualities traditionally attributed to God, such as omniscience and omnipresence. In *Nature* Emerson writes: "I see all. The currents of the Universal Being circulate through me; I am part or particle of God."[43]

For Emerson, truth comes not from a Revealed Word but rather from within the divine self. Malcolm Cowley notes that for Emerson, "each of us can find the laws of the universe by searching his own heart."[44] Similarly, the search for God also takes one on an inward path. Thus, in his "Divinity School Address" Emerson affirms that "if a man is at heart just, then in so far is he God; the safety of God, the immortality of God, the majesty of God do enter into that man with justice."[45] His "sub lime creed" was that "the world is not the product of manifold power" as taught by the Revealed Word. Rather, the world is the product of what Emerson terms "one will" and "one mind." That "one mind," he writes, "is everywhere, in each ray of the star, in each wavelet of the pool."[46] All things emerge "out of the same spirit, and all things conspire with it."[47] For reasons not clearly articulated, this spirit in all things is a moral spirit, which encourages right action and discourages wrong.

For Emerson, a cosmic "law of laws" awakened "the religious sentiment" which is the source of "our highest happiness." All of the world's religions are expressions of this sentiment because it called each of them into existence. This "sentiment lies at the foundation of society, and successively creates all forms of worship," Emerson assured the Divinity School students.[48] The same elemental religious spirit also teaches human beings that they are divine, suggesting that the concept of human divinity resides at the heart of all religious systems. "This thought dwelled always deepest in the minds of men in the devout and contemplative East; not alone in Palestine, where it reached its purest expression, but in Egypt, in Persia, in India, in China."[49]

Life is a great mystery that the individual unravels, resulting in spiritual self-reliance. Mind, not the Revealed Word's God, rules in Emerson's cosmos. Emerson grew ever more suspicious of the physical nature of human beings, and thus ever more inclined to spiritualize human existence. This spiritualizing tendency eventually led him to reject the central emblem of human physicality—the act of procreation itself. In *The Conduct of Life* (1860), his last important book, he urged his readers to invest themselves "in spiritual creation and not in begetting animals."[50]

In his own day, Emerson's more astute critics understood his views to be derived from Swedenborgian mysticism, Romanticism and ancient pantheism. As Hershel Parker writes, "all the reviewers understood *Nature* was not a Christian book but one influenced by a range of idealistic philosophies, ancient and very modern, Transcendentalism being merely the latest name for an old way of thinking."[51] Emerson's influence on American thinking in his own day was considerable; his was the most

important hand shaping the nation's religious views in the mid-nineteenth century. Emerson's influence was always felt more keenly by searching individuals than by the society as a whole. Richardson writes, "Transcendentalism did not transform American life, but it did change—and continues to change—individual American lives."[52]

ERNST HAECKEL AND *THE RIDDLE OF THE UNIVERSE*

Ernst Haeckel (1834-1919), professor of zoology at the University of Jena, was one of the leading scientific voices on the European continent at the end of the nineteenth century. An ardent proponent of Darwinism in Europe, the first in Germany, this daring explorer and gifted writer and artist exercised extraordinary influence on popular thought. Haeckel sought a religious view rooted in scientific study of the natural realm, a religion he dubbed "monism." On Haeckel's view, the old religious system was "dualistic" in that it posited both nature and a God outside of nature, with worship properly directed to the latter. Monism, on the other hand, affirmed a single essence in all things. In this way the cosmos itself became the only possible god.

Haeckel envisioned nothing less than a new model of culture built on the foundation of a new scientific religion. Richard Noll writes that Haeckel "designed secular paths of cultural renewal or regeneration that were greatly influenced by evolutionary biological training."[53] Haeckel's new way in religion, his monistic religion, was explicitly "anti-Christian."[54] The utopian Volkish movement that swept central Europe in the 1890s rejected Christianity and emphasized "the worship of nature (particularly the sun)." Haeckel's bestselling *The Riddle of the Universe* (1899)—an early version of the popularized science genre—openly promoted pantheism as the basis of a new order of civilization. Noll adds, "Haeckel himself exhibited a messianic zeal in promoting his logical, new pantheistic 'nature religion'" to a public ready to be persuaded that science provides solid answers to ancient metaphysical puzzles.[55]

Under Haeckel's monistic-pantheistic religious revolution, nature alone demands our adoration. Modern people should not repeat the ancient mistake of placing a Revealed Word above reason, thus derailing religious thought. Haeckel's *The Riddle of the Universe* presents "our godlike reason" and its clear superiority to revelation. "We must at once dispose of this dangerous error" of thinking that revelation ought to rule reason.[56] Reason employing "triumphant" science would lead humankind out of the darkness of revealed dualism and into a bright new monistic day.

Science as the foundation of monistic religion. For Haeckel, science was a metaphysical as well as a physical enterprise. "The greatest triumphs of modern science—the cellular theory, the dynamic theory of heat, the theory of evolution, and the law of substance—are *philosophic achievements*," he writes in *The Riddle*.[57] Moreover, the philosophy revealed by science is pantheistic monism, the same view advocated by the great German Romantic writer Goethe, who stood for Haeckel as a modern prophet. "At the end of the nineteenth century we have returned to that monistic attitude which our greatest realistic poet, Goethe, had recognized from its very commencement to be alone correct and fruitful."[58]

And what distinguishes this monistic religion that both science and the Romantics have taught us? "Monism," writes Haeckel, "recognizes one sole substance in the universe, which is at once 'God and nature'; body and spirit (or matter and energy) it holds to be inseparable." Monism thus stands opposed to "the extra-mundane God of dualism," belief in whom "leads necessarily to theism." However, "the intra-mundane God of the monist leads to pantheism," the one true religion for a scientific age.[59] Haeckel explains that "matter cannot exist and be operative without spirit, nor spirit without matter." He referred to "spirit" and "energy" as simply "sensitive and thinking substance." Spirit and energy are then the "attributes or principal properties of the all-embracing divine essence of the world, the universal substance."[60] Thus Haeckel the scientist rejects Revealed Word dualism in favor of a universe comprised of a divine energy defined as "sensitive or thinking substance."

The soul's evolution. One of Haeckel's principal interests in *The Riddle of the Universe* was to develop a case for the evolution of the human soul based on two principles: pantheism and the evolutionary theory of Charles Darwin. "It becomes one of the main tasks of modern monistic psychology," he writes, "to trace the stages of the historical development of the soul of man from the soul of the brute."[61] Haeckel grounds his argument in a theory of a "soul substance" capable of creating consciousness. Within us resides a "protoplasm which seems to be the indispensable substratum of psychic life." Haeckel dubbed this substance *psychoplasm*, which he defined as "the 'soul-substance,' in the monistic sense."[62]

The cells exhibiting the greatest capacity for a soul life are the "sexual cells," all cells in any way connected with the human sexual response. "Each of these sexual cells," he writes, "has its own 'cell-soul'—that is, each is distinguished by a peculiar form of sensation and movement." In such cells are found "potential energies" that

are "inseparable from the matter of the protoplasm."[63] That is, there is no need to posit a soul *in addition to* the biological functions of cells within the human body. The soul—a name for our capacity to think, feel and move—evolved in a cellular fashion as did all other human functions.

In this way Haeckel's spiritual version of materialism renders dualism unnecessary. Of course, a key strategic purpose of *The Riddle* is to refute a major component in the Revealed Word worldview—that the human soul is a special creation of God. Haeckel believed that his argument about the souls of cells sufficed "for the destruction of the still prevalent superstition that man owes his personal existence to the favor of God." On the contrary, the soul's origin "is rather to be attributed solely to the 'eros,'" or sexual life of some human cells.[64] Thus, in the evolution of sexuality and the erotic impulse is found "the evolution of the soul."[65]

The highly specialized sex cells "not only conduct the commerce between the muscles and the organs of sense, but they also affect the highest performances of the animal soul, the formation of ideas and thoughts, and especially consciousness."[66] The "soul" function of these cells leads eventually "to that marvellous structure of the human brain which seems to entitle the highest primate form to quite an exceptional position in nature."[67] Thus, Haeckel believed that his sexual/cellular evolutionary theory of the soul demonstrated that "consciousness is simply a natural phenomenon like any other psychic quality, and that it is subject to the law of substance like all other natural phenomena."[68] Where does all this leave us with regard to rational religion? In a rather unexpected place, as it turns out.

Sun-worship as scientific religion. Haeckel recognized that directing his readers to reverent contemplation of nature might fail to arouse the sense of transcendence found in traditional religion. He thus sought a brilliant divinity worthy of the new pantheistic/monistic faith he had invented. Haeckel found his new god in the sky. The nature-worshiping Volkish movement sweeping central and Eastern Europe as the nineteenth century waned revered the sun as nature's true god. For Haeckel as well, the sun became the perfect emblem of the constant cycle of evolutionary advancement that characterizes the cosmos. "This universal movement of substance in space takes the form of an eternal cycle or of a periodical process of evolution," he wrote, and the sun perfectly represents this cyclical, universal and eternal process.[69]

Evolution was the very basis of the cosmos, its foundation and organizing principle. And, in keeping with this conviction, Haeckel understood human beings as but a point along an evolutionary trajectory toward something grander. "Human-

ity is but a transitory phase of the evolution of an eternal substance, a particular phenomenal form of matter and energy," he affirmed.[70] The sun best manifested this eternal progression of cosmic energy, leading Haeckel the scientist to a remarkably unscientific conclusion: "Sun-worship (solarism, or heliotheism) seems to the modern scientist to be the best of all forms of theism."[71]

Interestingly, Haeckel found sun-worship a more scientific faith than worship of a triune God. In a striking passage he wrote, "in the light of pure reason, sun-worship, as a form of naturalistic monotheism, seems to have a much better foundation than the anthropistic worship of Christians."[72] For support, Haeckel turned to the leading lights of science and philosophy. "Many distinguished scientists and philosophers of the day, who share our monistic views, consider that religion is generally played out," he claimed. In short, the Revealed Word tradition was dead; monism had taken its place as the faith of thinking people, and was thus the basis of a new religion. "Clear insight into the evolution of the world which the scientific progress of the nineteenth century has afforded us will satisfy, not only the causal feelings of our reason, but even our highest emotional cravings."[73]

Science reveals evolution as the foundational principle of the cosmos, and evolution in turn instructs us that our new religion is pantheistic monism—everything is one thing, and that one thing is divine. Haeckel is now "convinced" that "truth unadulterated is only to be found in the temple of the study of nature," a conclusion Thomas Paine had arrived at a century earlier in his *The Age of Reason*.[74] And thus, with prophetic confidence Haeckel affirms that "the modern man who 'has science and art'—and, therefore, 'religion'—needs no special church, no narrow, enclosed portion of space."[75]

Monistic morals, self-love and a world religion. Of course, any religion worthy of the name must instruct us about how we ought to live. And, according to Haeckel, any adequate ethic "must be rationally connected with the unified conception of the cosmos which we have formed by our advanced knowledge of the laws of nature."[76] What, then, is the unified moral system taught by Haeckel's new monistic religion? Clearly it must not simply replicate the moral view of the Revealed Word, the perspective Haeckel set out to destroy.

Sounding like his contemporary and fellow countryman, the anti-Christian philosopher Friedrich Nietzsche—and Nietzsche's twentieth-century disciple Ayn Rand—Haeckel takes Christianity to task for overemphasizing love of others. He writes, "The supreme mistake of Christian ethics . . . is its exaggeration of love of

one's neighbor at the expense of self-love." Haeckel is offended that "Christianity attacks and despises egoism on principle." And yet, the natural selfishness we call egoism "is absolutely indispensable in view of self-preservation," while love of others—"a very ideal precept"—is "as useless in practice as it is unnatural."[77] Darwinian science and its spiritual offspring, pantheism, direct us down another moral pathway—self-preservation through self-love.

Haeckel realized, of course, that the Revealed Word tradition and his scientific monism were diametrically opposed spiritual forces. Christianity denounced "all that invaluable progress of science, especially the study of nature, of which the nineteenth century is justly proud." Christians find "worthless" the scientific advances that enjoy "so high a value in the eye of the monist," or so Haeckel argued.[78] For Haeckel, science and Christianity are sworn enemies locked in a "culture war" to determine control of the Western mind. "Christianity is to be found an enemy to civilization, and the struggle which modern thought and science are compelled to conduct with it is . . . a 'cultur-kampf.'"[79] Haeckel was nevertheless confident that "the older view" was "breaking up with all its mystic and anthropistic dogmas." A new religion—scientific monism— was already rising out of the ashes of Christianity. In a heroic flourish Haeckel asserted that "upon the vast field of ruins rises, majestic and brilliant, the new sun of our realistic monism, which reveals to us the wonderful temple of nature in all its beauty. In the sincere cult of 'the true, the good, and the beautiful,' which is the heart of our new monistic religion, we find ample compensation for the anthropistic ideals of 'God, freedom and immortality' which we have lost."[80]

Haeckel proposed that a single unified religious view—monism—be adopted throughout the world in the coming twentieth century. "We may, therefore, express a hope that the approaching twentieth century will complete the . . . construction of pure monism" and thus "spread far and wide the desired unity of world-conception."[81] The spread of Haeckelian monism was, in fact, surprising. "By 1904, groups all over Central Europe had formed and were known as *Monistenbund* (the Monistic Alliance), with some trying out rituals based on this new scientific religion."[82] Haeckel actually organized the various cells of the *Monistenbund* under "a single administrative umbrella." Moreover, the new religion of "the Monistenbund attracted prominent cultural, occultist, and scientific celebrities as members."[83] The movement spawned various other organizations devoted to the worship of a "'life-principle' in all matter."[84]

BERGSON AND SHAW

Belief in a pantheistic "Life Principle" or "Vital Impulse" was widespread among intellectuals in the early twentieth century, and its foremost advocate was the French philosopher Henri Bergson (1859-1941). As Bergson influenced many twentieth-century advocates of a divine principle at work in the evolving cosmos, it will be helpful to survey his thought on this point. Bergson, like many writers of his day, affirmed that the Vital Impulse worked through the mechanism of evolution, and that its principal activity was evident in the evolutionary ascent of the human race. Physical matter was being organized by the Impulse into organisms of greater and greater complexity, and thus higher and higher levels of consciousness. The Vital Impulse was "an inward impulse that passes from germ to germ through individuals, that carries life in a given direction, toward ever higher complexity."[85]

In human beings this impulse expresses itself in various forms of higher order intelligence, each form a step along the way to divinity. "The creative effect progressed successfully only along that line of evolution which ended in man. In its passage through matter, consciousness assumed in that case, as it were from a mould, the shape of tool-making intelligence."[86] Such high-order intelligence was also the source of what Bergson called "the myth-making function that contrives the patterns of religion."[87] In other words, religion—including the Revealed Word variety—is an expression of the myth-making quality found only in highly evolved human intelligence. Thus, our myth-making ability binds us together as producers of religions, the ability to create religion being itself simply a stage in our evolutionary development.

However, human evolutionary progress does not manifest itself in all places equally for Bergson. Some races clearly lead the pack in the race toward human spiritual destiny. Bergson spoke freely of "the inferior races" who did not show the signs of advancement, brackish evolutionary backwaters cut off from "a great current of creative energy" that is the main stream of the Vital Impulse's flow toward the larger evolutionary sea. He also spoke of "static religions" that kept people from recognizing their destiny, spiritual systems that insisted on a fixed dogma, an unchanging orthodoxy unresponsive to developments in human evolution.

Shaw's Supermen. George Bernard Shaw (1856-1950) was one of the twentieth century's most prolific and influential writers and is considered by many the most important English playwright since Shakespeare. Shaw was also a strident political polemicist and a speculative religious advocate. A member of the socialist Fabian

Society, Shaw tirelessly promoted radical social change as well as revolutionary ideas in religion. Not the least of these ideas was the spiritual evolution of the human race under the direction of a pantheistic presence Shaw referred to as the Life Force, a variation on Bergson's Vital Impulse.

Shaw's Life Force continually organizes itself into higher and higher forms of life. Such is the basis of life in the cosmos most clearly present in Shaw's play *Man and Superman* (1903). A principal character in the play speaks of "the working within me of Life's incessant aspiration to higher organization, wider, deeper intenser self-consciousness, and clearer self-understanding."[88] This continually advancing Force directs the cosmos toward a specific goal. In Shaw's vision, Revealed Word religion was "a mere excuse for laziness, since it had set up a God who looked at the world and saw that it was good." The alternative was better: "The instinct in me that looked through my eyes at the world and saw that it could be improved."[89]

Shaw advocated "evolving a mind's eye that shall see, not the physical world, but the purpose of Life."[90] Developing such a perspective will "thereby enable the individual to work for that purpose." Shaw thus praises the person who seeks "to discover the inner will of the world," and who, on the basis of that discovery, takes "action to do that will." In other words, the person of great intellect and great will works in consort with the moving spirit in nature to shape the evolutionary future of the human race. Thus, the wise or strong individual "chooses the line of greatest advantage," becoming nothing less than "Nature's pilot."[91]

The Life Force's goal is to ensure that intelligence in the universe evolves to the point of divinity. In *Man and Superman* Shaw states the point this way: "Life is a force which has made innumerable experiments to organize itself... [and] to build up that raw force into higher and higher individuals, the ideal individual being omnipotent, omniscient, infallible, and withal completely self-conscious: in short, a god."[92] The fully evolved divine human race will rule the cosmos. Our guide to this glorious future is not the Revealed Word's suffering servant, but rather Shaw's "Man of Philosophy," a determined and talented student of the Life Force who masters its power.

"The Revolutionist's Handbook." Though Shaw was a proponent of human advancement, he utterly rejected the Victorian notion of inevitable social progress. In an essay attached to *Man and Superman*, entitled "The Revolutionist's Handbook and Pocket Companion," Shaw argues that unless we take evolution into our own hands and provide the Life Force some assistance in perfecting us—an idea borrowed from T. H. Huxley—we humans will never see significant progress. As

Shaw urges, without evolution "we must frankly give up the notion that Man as he exists is capable of net progress."[93] All apparent evidence of progress is "an illusion." Thus, he concludes, nothing will become of the human race "unless we are replaced by a more highly evolved animal—in short, by the Superman." Without these highly evolved Supermen, "the world must remain a den of dangerous animals among whom our few accidental supermen, our Shakespeares, Goethes, Shelleys, and the like, must live as precariously as lion tamers do."[94]

In order to hasten the advent of this new breed, Shaw advocated "the selective breeding of Man," thus providing assistance to "human evolution." Progress by means of "political, scientific, educational, religious or artistic" developments—so far as we remain in our present evolutionary state—is simply meaningless. "Our only hope, then, is in evolution. We must replace the man by the superman."[95] And as we seek superman, "we must eliminate the Yahoo" as well, lest he ruin the eugenic project.[96] Government could assist the Life Force by establishing a "State Department of Evolution." Such a bureau might develop a "private society or a chartered company for the improvement of human live stock."[97]

It goes without saying that Shaw's proposal for directing human evolution toward the goal of a new race of supermen assumed the rejection of Revealed Word theology and ethics. The "men and women" who would give themselves to Shaw's exalted plan of directed human advancement are individuals who "no longer believe that they can live forever." Having rejected the Revealed Word's notion of spiritual transformation through repentance and salvation, citizens of a new world "seek for some immortal work into which they can build the best of themselves before their refuse is thrown into that arch dust collector, the cremation furnace."[98] Shaw's new hope—a highly evolved race of superhuman beings transforming life on earth— replaces the antiquated Revealed Word hope of eternal spiritual existence with God. His Darwinian vision was joined to a pantheistic faith in a universal Life Force that drove the cosmic evolutionary project ever forward. With human assistance, the terminus of this project would be superman.

At the end of the twentieth century and beginning of the twenty-first, a pantheism akin to that of Toland, Emerson, Haeckel, Bergson and Shaw found support among members of the scientific community. The following section overviews recent efforts in popular scientific writing to provide empirical grounding for a self-organizing Life Force driving the life of the universe. New Physics writers claim to have irrefutable scientific proof for the foundational pantheism of the Other Spirituality.

A NEW PANTHEISTIC PHYSICS

German physicist Max Planck revolutionized the study of physical phenomena in 1900 when he announced a theory that light acted like it was comprised of particles. As Catherine Albanese writes, "Planck described energy 'packets' in which, he said, light was emitted and absorbed. He called these packets '*quanta*,' and in his work quantum mechanics, the 'new physics' of the twentieth century, had its early beginnings." Quantum theory opened not only a new era in physics, but a new era in metaphysical speculation as well. The cosmos, once apparently made of solid matter and bound by inflexible laws, now seemed composed of energy operating according to indecipherable rules. "At the subatomic level, many scientists were saying, matter was not the solid entity that appeared to commonplace observation [and so] the line between matter and energy was fluid, the boundary not so fixed as it seemed."[99] Furthermore, if this boundary was flexible, perhaps so was the boundary between the material and the spiritual. In fact, perhaps the physical *was* the spiritual. In this way the new physics gave birth to a new pantheism.

In *The Quantum Society*, science writers Danah Zohar and Ian Marshall advocate a new pantheistic psychology and sociology grounded in quantum theory. Sounding much like Emerson positing his famous analogy between the human mind and nature, they assert that "there is an uncanny analogy between the structures and processes underlying quantum reality, and the structures and processes underlying the conscious mind."[100] This section explores the new pantheism as presented in Zohar and Marshall's fascinating and engaging *The Quantum Society*.

Emerson once referred to himself as an invisible eye observing nature, but at the same time participating in the formation of what he observed. More recently, Zohar and Marshall have affirmed what they term "the mutually creative relationship between the observer and the observed in the quantum domain." They explain that "the quantum observer does not stand outside his observations. He does not see nature as an object. Rather he *participates* in nature's unfolding" because "the observer is *part of* what he observes." No longer is the human agent distinct from the natural order, with a creator God standing above both. Rather, humans reside within that order, while at the same time participating in its creation through their observations of it.

Zohar and Marshall discover a breathtaking range of practical implications in the "fundamental physics that underlies all else that is in the universe." A common physics of existence suggests a new view of the self, of society and of personal and social ethics. But such is only to be expected, for "the nature of the mind, the nature

of society, and the nature of nature are all one and the same thing," for all three are "linked by a common physics."[101] But the ultimate discovery of the New Physics is a final scientific proof of the basic correctness of Benedict Spinoza's pantheistic theology—nature *is* god. The components of that proof are worth setting out in some detail, and they focus on a particle called the *boson*.

Bosons: particles of relationship. Zohar and Marshall describe bosons as "one of only two *basic* sorts of 'particles' that make up the whole universe. The other sort are called *fermions*." Fermions, they explain, "are particles that make up things." Thus, fermions include "protons, neutrons and electrons, the basic constituents of the atom." In other words, "all of the matter of the universe is made of fermions."[102] Thus, there are two kinds of things in the universe, and all of one kind of thing is what we call matter or the physical universe. What does this leave? The inescapable answer appears to be that bosons must be *spiritual* or *mental* particles, though our authors prefer "particles of relationship." They explain that "all the fundamental forces that bind the universe together—the electromagnetic, the gravitational, the strong and weak nuclear—are made of bosons." Bosons actually exhibit "social" qualities. For instance, they appear to "like clustering together" in various experiments. In fact, Zohar and Marshall posit that "consciousness itself" may be a "boson phenomenon."[103]

Sounding at times more like philosophers than physicists, Zohar and Marshall contend that "there is a whole new 'metaphysic' of the human in this history of boson evolution." They contend that the boson is implicated in basic evolutionary process, thus taking on metaphysical implications. "If the same tendency of two bosons to bunch together at the most basic level of early physical processes can be traced in unbroken sequence to the principles underlying the physical basis for conscious mind," they write, then "we have traced the origins of the human mind back to primordial physical reality." That is to say, in the social tendencies of bosons we have discovered the evolutionary origins of the human soul itself. The boson provides a critical link between the previously immaterial human soul and the entire evolutionary process of both biological life on earth and of the universe itself. "The self carries within itself the whole history of the physical universe," they write.[104]

Of course, if this is the case then the Revealed Word idea that the human soul makes us distinct from the rest of creation is erroneous. "There is no basis, then, in the quantum worldview for any ontological distinction between the human and the natural." Zohar and Marshall recognize that this conclusion represents "a radical shift away from the whole earlier Western worldview." They also find, how-

ever, a new source of ethical insight to be derived from this new metaphysical view. When we move to a "deeper level" we discover a "quantum source of empowerment to act as personal and moral agents" rooted in "the nature and function of what physicists call the 'quantum vacuum.'" Emerging understanding of this vacuum "and our relationship to it" is causing a "revolution in our understanding of human reality."[105] What, then, is the nature of the quantum vacuum that may prove the foundation of a new reality and a new religion?

Confronting the void: Buddhist Sunyata and modern science. When physicists and astronomers probe the deep recesses of the universe, they find an indefinite and apparently infinite field of energy. As Zohar and Marshall put it, "We are confronted by a 'void,' a background without features and that therefore *seems* empty." Of course, the particles and waves of physicists must be made of something, but what? The answer to this question tells us where all physical objects originate. "All the waves and particles that we can see and measure, literally, as in the Greek, *ex*-ist or 'stand out from' an underlying sea of potential that physicists have named the vacuum . . . just as waves undulate on the sea."[106] This "sea" of proto-physicality is "an all-pervasive, underlying field of potential—the vacuum." On this view, all physical objects are surfaces on the underlying cosmic vacuum. "It is as though all surface existing things are in constant interaction with a tenuous background of evanescent reality."[107]

This view is strikingly similar to some Hindu and Buddhist accounts of the origins of physical objects as emanations from the One. In fact, Zohar and Marshall do not dispute this similarity. "The vacuum spoken of by quantum physicists, like the Buddhist concept of *Sunyata,* or the Void, to which it is so similar, is replete with all potentiality." The ineffable vacuum or void is, moreover, the ground of all true religious experience. The Buddhists say that "it is the basis of all . . . the absolute, the truth, that cannot be preached in words." The void, then, is that ultimate and divine ground of being experienced by mystics. As the beginning and ending of all reality, the vacuum is "the vast sea of all else that is." Moreover, "*We* are excited states of the vacuum."[108] The vacuum is, then, ultimate reality. "In more religious language, the vacuum is *the* All of everything."[109]

Perhaps Zohar and Marshall's most striking conclusion is that "the vacuum has the same physical structure as human consciousness." If this is the case, then the soul of the universe and the human soul are one and the same *substance.* "There is, then, quite possibly a common physics linking human consciousness to the ground state of 'everything that ever existed or can exist' in the universe," write Zohar and Mar-

shall. They add, "This is a very exciting idea, filled with wide implications."[110] Thus, one of religion's perennial questions receives a scientific answer—we now know with certainty who we are. "We are *part* of it. Each one of us as an individual *is* an excitation of the vacuum, an individual being on the sea of Being." That we are part of the vacuum, that the structure of consciousness is the structure of the universe "is a straightforward conclusion of orthodox physics. It is, if you like, proven."[111]

Mysticism and modern physics. For Zohar and Marshall, recent physical discoveries provide us "a whole new sense of finding human beings at the center of things." But perhaps these findings are new only to science, for this essentially religious insight has been understood in other arenas for ages. That the universe is consciousness and that we are part of that consciousness "is a vision more common to the great wisdom traditions of native peoples or to the ancient Greeks, but here it is derived from the latest insights of science." Science has discovered the divinity of the great mythic and mystical traditions, the god of the New Religious Synthesis. "If we are looking for God in physics, the vacuum would be the most appropriate place to look," they write. "As the underlying ground state of all that is, the vacuum has all the characteristics of the immanent [all-pervading] God, or of the Godhead, spoken of by mystics, the God within, the God who creates and discovers Himself through the unfolding existence of His creation."[112]

The vacuum is posited as a new and scientifically proven god, though certainly not the personal and wholly other God of the Revealed Word. The New Physics has birthed a new myth with the power to inform and unify an array of religious traditions. "In this new 'myth' of the vacuum, all things that are, are expressions of the immanent God's being. All are precious and awe-inspiring, all 'filled with spark of the divine.'" Science proves that our consciousness participates in cosmic consciousness. Thus, "there is no real sense in which we are 'created in God's image.'"[113] It would be more accurate to say that we are becoming godlike.

Zohar and Marshall embrace a version of spiritual evolutionism built upon a new *gnosis*—the knowledge of quantum physics. "Because we may be possessed of *the most complex version of physics in the universe,* we may, in a strict physical sense, actually be at the vanguard of evolution." This new *gnosis* of physics, then, provides the key to our spiritual ascent. That is, because we are aware of our own thoughts, there is "a real, physical importance to the constructs of human reason." Could it be that our minds are evolving toward godhood? "This is the true, the awesome, significance of 'being created in God's image.'" That is, we are directing our own

evolution, and thus the very evolution of god.[114] This notion is common to various ancient and modern gnostic and mystical systems, a fact that Zohar and Marshall acknowledge. "Indeed," they write, "there is a similarly uncanny link between many older, mystical visions and recent scientific insight."[115]

CONCLUSION

Pantheism has a long history in Western religious thought and has now, as we have seen, taken up residence in Western science. The English Deist John Toland reintroduced the ancient notion into popular religious discourse in the early eighteenth century, and since that time it has found many advocates. In America, a species of pantheism found a powerful advocate in Ralph Waldo Emerson, while in Europe the philosopher Henri Bergson provided the concept with intellectual credibility. Pantheism continued to appear in a number of popular authors in Europe and America in the early twentieth century, George Bernard Shaw being an important example. Other literary figures exploring pantheism included the German novelist and 1946 Nobel laureate Herman Hesse, who achieved extraordinary popularity in Europe in the 1920s and 1930s, and in America of the 1950s and 1960s, and who affirmed the fundamental unity and divinity of the cosmos. In his Buddhist novel *Siddhartha,* the principal character affirms, "This stone is a stone. It is also animal, God and Buddha." This fundamental insight gained through arduous effort and self-discipline leads Siddhartha to a worship of the god in nature. "This is what pleases me," he states, "and seems wonderful and worthy of worship."[116]

More recently, as we have seen, scientists and popularizers of science have found in quantum physics a new foundation for pantheistic thinking. Under the banner of pantheism, science and theology become virtually indistinguishable in some writers. Consequently, mystical spirituality is increasingly advocated by writers in the genre of the New Science, often presented as a rediscovery of an ancient spiritual truth. Clearly the appeal of pantheism and its "older, mystical visions" extends to scientists other than Danah Zohar and Ian Marshall. Daniel C. Dennett, Director of the Center for Cognitive Studies at Tufts University, also finds in pantheism a religion for a new era. This expert on the evolution of consciousness writes in his book *Darwin's Dangerous Idea* that "Darwin has shown us how, in fact, *everything* of importance is just such a product" of what Dennett terms "mindless, purposeless forces." He adds, somewhat incongruously, "Spinoza called his highest being God or Nature (*Deus sive Natura*), expressing a sort of pantheism."

So why does Dennett's book on Darwinian evolution end with a discussion of Spinozan pantheism? Apparently because Dennett finds in Darwin "a convincing *explanation* of just how God is distributed in the whole of nature." Darwin's convincing account of what can only be called pantheism draws support from "the distribution of Design throughout nature." This fact alone suggests "an utterly unique and irreplaceable creation, an actual pattern in the immeasurable reaches of Design Space that could never be exactly duplicated in its many details."[117] In other words, the design of nature is itself a kind of divinity for Dennett that does not require positing the Revealed Word's personal and wholly other deity in the cosmos. The cosmos *is* deity because the cosmos is design. Dennett asks, "What miracle caused it? None. It just happened to happen in the fullness of time." But this amazing product of happenstance does not lead Dennett to reject the idea of a spiritual reality behind the physical universe. Rather, it issues in a pantheistic faith in a divinity that *is* the universe. "The Tree of Life," Dennett's shorthand for the exquisitely designed cosmos, "created itself . . . slowly over billions of years." Does this make the cosmos "a God one could worship? Pray to? Fear? Probably not." Nevertheless, the universe "is surely a being that is greater than anything any of us will ever conceive of in any detail worthy of its detail." So what should be our response to this sort of "being"? Dennett's response recognizes it as sacred. "Is something sacred? Yes, say I with Nietzsche. I could not pray to it, but I can stand in affirmation of its magnificence. The world is sacred."[118]

Similarly, physicist Fred Alan Wolf hearkens back to an earlier time in our religious history when human spiritual vision was clearer, revealing a universe more in keeping with the findings of modern science. "According to many historians," he writes, "our ancient forebears saw God everywhere, in all nature and in all the universe. . . . Gods were seen as nature itself and observed everywhere."[119] These early spiritual explorers—Wolf dates the insight at three to four thousand years B.C.—found God to be indistinguishable from the physical objects making up their world. "Our ancient forbears envisioned a universe forming from a great void sometimes imagined to be primordial waters." Our ancestors "discovered the Creator of the universe . . . was in all nature and in all of the universe, constantly becoming."[120]

This "creator" was "contained by the creation He created" according to Wolf. This "creator," however, so common in New Synthesis writing, is certainly not of the kind envisioned in the Revealed Word, a God who willfully creates a universe that exists as something other, something distinct from its creator. Rather, Wolf's

creator is the "world soul" of the pantheists, a divine essence within all things. And our own souls are simply a part of this world soul. Perhaps, he writes, "the soul inside you and the soul inside me are simply reflections of one soul living . . . in the universe at large." If this is the case, "then my soul is your soul is the only soul that ever was or ever will be."[121]

Certain implications follow from this insight. For instance, Wolf argues that suffering results from believing that I am an independent entity with lasting personal identity, a concept at the heart of the Revealed Word tradition. However, "when we realize that at another level, perhaps at a mythic one, we are God—the Universe—our children—our mothers—the apes in the trees—the rocks on the ground—when we see that we are all that there *is*, all suffering appears to melt away just as the boundaries separating our visions of ourselves vanish."[122] Can this be right? Does pantheism eliminate the problem of suffering? We will be pursuing this and other spiritual implications of New Synthesis pantheism in subsequent chapters, as pantheism has ushered in a number of ancient spiritual practices now dressed in modern garb.

8

THE REBIRTH OF GNOSTICISM

The Secret Path to Self-Salvation

His study fits a mercenary drudge,
Who aims at nothing but external trash
Too servile and illiberal for me
When all is done, divinity is best.
CHRISTOPHER MARLOWE, Dr. Faustus

The fallen angels are in prison, that is, embodied, so that Man is an apostate Angel and a Body.
JACOB ILIVE, The Oration Spoke at Joyner's Hall

You have got to learn how to become gods yourselves; to become Kings and Priests to God, the
same as all gods have done, by going from a small degree to another.
JOSEPH SMITH, King Follett Discourse

Now open your eyes and look at all the gods in hiding.
JEAN HOUSTON, A Passion for the Possible

The scene in the mansion at 18241 Colina Norte Drive in Rancho Santa Fe shocked the world. Thirty-nine bodies of men and women of various ages, identically clad in black, lay within the estate, the victims of mass suicide ordered by Marshall Applewhite, leader of the Heaven's Gate UFO cult. Among them were a thirty-nine-year-old mother of five from Cincinnati, a seventy-two-year-old grandmother from Iowa, and the fifty-nine-year-old brother of an actress from the original *Star Trek* television series. The Hale-Bopp comet, according to Applewhite, announced the arrival of a vehicle from another dimension that would usher "a select group" of followers to their destiny in the stars.[1] All they had to do was "shed

their containers," the bodies containing their preexistent spirits, and move to the "Next Level."

Applewhite had been preaching his message of celibacy, secret knowledge and cosmic ascent for more than twenty years. Recruits were told that they were "highly evolved" and thus were among the "chosen ones." According to a report in *U.S. News & World Report,* "Applewhite believed that he and his followers were aliens who had been planted [on earth] years ago."[2] Descending from "a level above human in distant space," they sought to return to "their world," or the place of their cosmic origin, by following secret teachings and, eventually, destroying the material containers—their bodies—that were not part of their true nature.

THE FUNDAMENTALS OF GNOSTICISM

Marshall Applewhite's message was derived from gnosticism, a spiritual view reasserting itself today and an important component in the New Religious Synthesis. The term *gnosticism* may conjure up images of second- and third-century Christian heretics practicing secret rites, disseminating occult knowledge and challenging the stability of Christian theology.[3] For some scholars, the term *gnosticism* has itself become a contested category.[4] While *gnosticism* itself may be difficult to define with precision, a spiritual inclination I will term the gnostic impulse has been both powerful and persistent in Western religious thought.[5] This impulse manifests itself in the veneration of secret spiritual knowledge, the elevation of spiritual elites in possession of such knowledge, a denigration of time and history, a tendency to view the physical realm as evil and a corresponding tendency to view human embodiment with suspicion. The elements of the gnostic impulse are increasingly important to contemporary spiritual thought, often being joined to the notion of spiritual evolution. As will be shown in the following chapter, shamanism—the idea that secret spiritual knowledge comes by way of spirit guides—also plays a part in the gnostic impulse. Some voices for a new gnosticism will occupy our attention in the present chapter. But first it will be helpful to gain a fuller historical view of gnosticism itself.

Gnosticism is often traced back to Simon Magus (fl. A.D. 40-55), whom Peter opposed in Acts 8, and his student Menander (fl. A.D. 90-100). Valentinus, a second century teacher condemned as a heretic, was also a major figure in the establishment of Gnosticism in Europe, as was Marcion of Pontus (fl. A.D. 135-145), who actually established a series of Gnostic churches in the Roman Empire. Other early sources of Western Gnosticism include Mani (216-275), whom Augustine followed before

his conversation to Christianity, and the various Neo-Platonic philosophers such as Plotinus (205-270) and Proclus (d. 466). Much of the available information about the teachings of such early Gnostics, however, comes from Christian sources who opposed them. Mystical speculation of the type that later Gnostics drew upon in developing their views can also be found in Greek philosophers, including Plato and Pythagoras, and even earlier in the works of Zoroastrian writers.

As already noted, gnosticism was a persistent and highly influential force in the development of the Western religious tradition, one constantly in tension with the Revealed Word. I will be arguing in this chapter that gnostic thought has powerfully reasserted itself over the past three centuries. However, because gnosticism is itself a contested term, it will be important to clarify what I take to be the defining marks of the gnostic impulse in contemporary spiritual systems. So, what makes a religious view gnostic?

Rising above it all: transcending time and the physical. In its most elemental form, gnosticism is the systematic spiritual effort to escape the confines of history and physical embodiment through secret knowledge (*gnosis*) and technique (magic). Gnostics seek to rise above the crowd of ordinary mortals who lack the will to break the chains of time and earthly existence. Thus, Henri-Charles Puech has called gnosticism "a 'revolt' against all myths and belief systems which purport to give time some indwelling meaning."[6] Time, history and the earthly realm are the gnostic's enemies. Conventional religious "myths" that give history legitimacy and that make the physical world a significant place—Christianity with its emphasis on both history and incarnation being the singular example—must be demolished. Yuri Stoyanov, an expert on medieval gnosticism, notes that gnostics advanced "allegorical interpretations of the gospels and parts of the Old Testament" because of their aversion to history and historically based faith.[7] One is reminded here of both Woolston and Strauss.

Gnostic spirituality, then, exhibits a deep suspicion of history and any attendant notions such as God's redemptive work in history. The gnostic dispenses with the historical Christ of Christianity, choosing instead to pursue self-salvation through secrets that come from beyond the earthly and historical scheme of things. Sin—a historical category associated with the Fall as well as with particular actions in time—is not humanity's captor, as the Revealed Word would have it. Rather, ignorance is—particularly ignorance of liberating spiritual secrets or *gnosis*. Thus, *gnosis*, not the Revealed Word's divinely initiated redemption, is the solution to our

collective predicament. Gnosticism also typically involves demeaning the creator God of the Old Testament, the God of history and of the entire physical realm that he created in time and out of matter. True divinity—known to gnostics as the *pleroma* or fullness—is inaccessible and unknowable in our present limited state.

Secrecy and the spiritual elite. The central component in gnosticism is *gnosis* itself, esoteric knowledge unavailable to and, importantly, unattainable by the general run of humanity. Such secret knowledge usually developed around a myth about a titanic struggle between the highest divine being along with his cohort, and a lower creator God over the creation of the human race itself. In short, humanity resulted from a misdirected effort to combine pristine spiritual consciousness with fallen physical matter. To apprehend this myth, this *gnosis,* was to take the first step toward spiritual self-liberation. Other steps followed as additional secrets were learned. Thus, gnostics "purported to offer knowledge of the otherwise hidden truth of total reality as the indispensable key to man's salvation," writes Hans Jonas.[8] Gnosticism taught "salvation by enlightenment," and enlightenment always came in the same way—by mastering hidden knowledge. *Gnosis* allowed the soul's ascent into the higher reaches of spiritual experience, divinity itself being the ultimate tantalizing possibility.

In all gnostic systems, ancient or modern, spiritual awareness comes to and through a small minority of the spiritually capable. The members of this spiritual elite go by many names: seers, ascended masters, prophets, pneumatics, *perfecti,* shamans, illuminati, mystics, magi and adepts. Typically these individuals alone determine which other mortals will enter the inner sanctum of *gnosis.* As Carl Raschke writes, gnosticism always depends on "esoteric wisdom accessible only to the privileged or initiated few."[9]

Spiritual elitism, then, is an essential aspect of the gnostic impulse. Moreover, the enlightened ones loath the unenlightened as spiritually inferior beings incapable of spiritual ascent. The initiated or *pneumatikoi* are the "truly 'spiritual' people, despising the uninitiated as *psuchikoi,* doomed to an animal life on earth."[10] As a result of their exalted spiritual perspective, spiritual masters often reject conventional morality as belonging to a lower order of things, and thus consider themselves to be living lives above morality. The gnostic master, writes Hans Jonas, is "free from the yoke of the moral law, and all things are permitted to him."[11]

The power promised to initiates by gnostic masters of the ancient world was truly mind-boggling. Divinity itself loomed as a seductive possibility. Disciples

were taught to envision themselves as one with the universe. Jack Lindsay, a leading expert on the spiritual beliefs of the classical world, quotes an ancient source of gnostic lore known as the *Asclepius*. A man possessing the appropriate secret knowledge is promised dominion over a world, or "as the Greeks say more correctly, an order [cosmos]."[12] The initiate literally takes on the qualities of a God. "Grasp . . . in your mind that nothing is impossible for you," he is taught. "Consider yourself immortal and capable of understanding everything. . . . Gather into yourself the sensations of creation, fire and of water, of dryness and of humidity, imaging that you are at one and the same moment everywhere, on earth, in the sea, in the heaven, that you have not yet been born, that you are beyond death."[13]

JACOB ILIVE: ENLIGHTENMENT GNOSTIC

Carl Raschke has written that a "wistful recollection of a marvelous prehistory" animates the gnostic mind, a yearning for a time before historical forces corrupted human religious belief.[14] The spiritual view of the earliest human beings has often been seen as a key to discovering an authentic spirituality that would provide the basis for a new religion to replace the Revealed Word. In pristine prehistory, it is assumed, human beings enjoyed uninhibited access to spiritual truth. For instance, Enlightenment Deists affirmed a primitive and universal religion of Reason, a faith uncorrupted by a devious priestly caste and literal notions of history. According to the Deist Jacob Ilive, Adam and Eve practiced a pure religion of Reason. But modern religions have departed "so far from their origin" that they have "lost their primitive intention."[15] Ilive and many others set about to reclaim that early religion or to invent a new religion that would capture its content. His work in this regard is intriguing and has proven surprisingly influential.

Jacob Ilive (1705-1763) was a prominent member of the London printers' guild. As early as the 1730s he began delivering lectures in London guildhalls. He affirmed that the human soul was not created, but preexistent and eternal.[16] Ilive identified this eternal human soul with the key Deist term *reason*. More startling was his additional claim that each human soul was a fallen angel imprisoned in a human body.[17] Over a period of twenty years Ilive reinvented and popularized a brand of gnosticism in which his unusual theory of human origins and spiritual progress played a prominent role.

Fallen angels on their own planet. Like most other ancient people, early gnostics found the stars crucial to shaping human destiny. The force of such "astral fatal-

ism" in the ancient world is difficult for modern people to apprehend, but even educated and powerful people feared to make a major decision or begin a journey
without consulting the stars. Moreover, the stars were thought to reflect the actual
presence of spiritual beings—sometimes referred to as elemental spirits—who
held the keys to human spiritual advancement. Some of these star-dwelling beings
had at one time been humans who employed spiritual secrets to achieve their divine
ascent. Ilive brought such ancient notions to life again between 1730 and 1750.

In a 1733 lecture presented at the London Joyner's Hall, Ilive envisioned a massive and ancient struggle for control of heaven. A lower divinity named Jesus de-
feated Lucifer, who was subsequently expelled from the celestial realm.[18] Lucifer and
his host of fallen angels were imprisoned on earth where human bodies were fashioned as "certain little Places of Confinement for the reception of [these] apostate
Angels."[19] However, the highest God was intent on "bringing back again the rebellious and apostate angels" by putting them through a series of purgatorial exercises
on the prison-planet earth.[20] Thus, in keeping with the dominant gnostic myth, the
human race was created as the consequence of a spiritual struggle, and represents
the imperfect combination of deposed angelic spirits and physical bodies.

Ilive also imagined numerous other inhabited planets, founding his speculations
on Jesus' statement, "In my Father's house are many mansions." These other planets are "Celestial Mansions" that humans may eventually inhabit and govern provided sufficient progress toward their spiritual redemption is achieved. Greater
advancement will be rewarded with assignment to more prominent planets. But
for now the purgatorial period must be endured. Earth, "that Globe we now inhabit," is hell, which is not so much a place of torment as it is a correctional facility
created specifically "for the reception of the Rebellious Angels." Thus, "no new Order of Beings was created on Purpose to people [the earth]" as the Revealed Word
tradition affirms.[21] Far from being the special creations of God, humans are "fallen
Angels . . . in Prison," each of us being "an apostate Angel and a Body."[22] Repeatedly
Ilive affirmed the myth at the center of his new *gnosis*: "the very fallen Angels [are]
cloathed in Flesh, and . . . the Place we now inhabit, is Hell, and no other place."[23]
This account closely parallels second- and third-century Gnostic accounts of a
"world dominated by the evil angels."[24] But Gnostics held out the hope that these
fallen spirits might "return to the heights of knowledge" provided they gained access to the appropriate mythic secrets, or *gnosis*.[25]

Other Enlightenment writers were familiar with gnostic thinking, and some

hinted at its merits. Charles Gildon commended the view of "the *Pythagoreans* and *Chaldeans*," who believed human souls "were created in Heaven, and thence transmitted to the Bodies for punishment." As a result, "we are Devils."[26] Charles Blount in *Anima mundi* (1678) elevated the gnostic myth that "the fall of those evil Angels" who assisted Lucifer in his rebellion "occasioned our Corporeal Creation." Human bodies are places for "those wicked Spirits" to be imprisoned, the spirits being now human "souls." These fallen angels were placed in human bodies "for expiating their guilt," and thus "our Sublunary Orb," or earth, became "the only Hell."[27]

"Astro-Theology." Ilive found support for his gnostic theology in an earlier eighteenth-century work, William Derham's *Astro-Theology* (1715).[28] Derham had argued, based on astronomical observations, that the universe contained innumerable planets. These other planets "consist in all probability of Land and Water, Hills and valleys, having atmosphere about them, and being enlightened, warmed and influenced by the Sun, whose yearly visits they receive as Seasons, and frequent Returns for days and nights."[29] Some of Derham's planets, comets and stars are, like Ilive's earth, hells.[30] There is much more going on in the universe than we can know from our puny planet, which, Derham points out, is insignificant on a cosmic scale.[31]

Derham claimed that the Dutch astronomer Huygens had observed planets orbiting other stars. "The usual Question is," Derham writes, "what is the use of so many Planets as we see about the Sun, and so many as are imagined to be about the Fix'd Stars? To which the answer is, that they are *Worlds*, or places of *Habitation*, which is concluded from their being *habitable*, and well provided for habitation."[32] Some astronomers, according to Derham, had actually seen human-like beings moving about on these planets. Thus, extraterrestrials make an Enlightenment appearance, and in direct connection with a new theological view—Ilive's gnosticism. As we saw at the beginning of this chapter in the description of the Heaven's Gate UFO cult, the connection between extraterrestrials and new gnostic theologies is an active one on the contemporary spiritual scene.

Moses the magician. Scholars have often wondered about the "fierce anti-Jewish polemics of ancient Gnosticism."[33] Gnostics rejected anything to do with the Jews or the Old Testament, treating Yahweh the Creator-God as a bungler or worse. Anti-Semitism, hating this inferior God's chosen people, followed logically. A similar anti-Semitic thrust is clear in Ilive's writings. Moses in particular comes in for harsh treatment. The great and deadly plagues that struck Egypt were "wrought by Moses's Knowledge in the Magick Art."[34] Moses and his general Caleb plotted

and personally helped to carry out the murder of all of the first-born children of the Egyptians. He and his henchmen were guilty of "killing the harmless babies while they sleep."[35] Moses also masterminded the theft of Egyptian property. Thus, Ilive concludes that "by Murder and Theft [Moses] procured their Freedom" from Egypt. Far from being the chosen people of God, the Jews are portrayed as a murderous band of renegades under the leadership of the vicious general Caleb and the cunning sorcerer Moses. For Ilive the biblical history of the Jews is a lie, and "the *Jewish* Religion . . . a grievious Yoke."[36]

The Book of Jasher. In 1751 Ilive published a transparent forgery entitled *The Book of Jasher*, a lost book mentioned twice in the Old Testament, once in Joshua 10:13, and again in 2 Samuel 1:18. This unusual and controversial work—which is still published by the Rosicrucians—is moral fiction intended to register a series of theological points or, more accurately, corrections. That is, *The Book of Jasher* is a myth based on stories from Genesis and advances several speculative theological ideas that support Ilive's gnostic views. The book's wide readership for two centuries and its lasting influence suggest it is worthy of our attention.

As noted above, Deists speculated that early human beings practiced a pure religion of reason, an idea central to Ilive's theology. Early gnostics often taught a similar concept—that early and universal knowledge of *gnosis* had been lost to humanity over long eons of time. Gnostic interpretations of the Garden of Eden narrative cast the serpent in a hero's role as the bringer of liberating knowledge, an idea also reflected in the Deist Peter Annet's theology. The Fall was thus a "fall up," as humans gained knowledge that set them on a path toward divinity. In similar fashion, Ilive's recounting of the Eden incident in *Jasher* involves no human fall into sin. Ilive affirms in *Jasher* that Adam practiced a pure religion, later corrupted by the first priest, Enos, who invented something Ilive terms "the worship of the body."[37] Enos and his ilk wrongly directed humanity's religious thinking away from the unsullied realm of reason and spirit, and toward the physical and the temporal.

Moreover, the concept of sin—a time-bound notion rejected by gnostics—developed out of early religious stories corrupted during centuries of transmission. Ilive is at pains to remove the stain of human sin from the Genesis stories through strategic retellings in *Jasher*. For example, Cain never actually murdered his brother Abel; he merely slew Abel's beast, and the story was related with the crucial error that one brother had killed the other. "From this act of Cain slaying the beast of Abel, it seemeth, arose that story recorded in the book of Moses, that Cain slew

Abel." Nor did God employ a flood to punish human sin. Rather, Noah simply invented "a floating cave, a vehicle, a house to remain upon the surface of the waters."[38] Other biblical stories were similarly corrupted over time. For instance, Abraham was not instructed to sacrifice Isaac, but misunderstood the angel's instructions.[39]

In *The Book of Jasher* Ilive also sought to provide natural explanations for miraculous events. Miracles were offensive to the Deist mind as violations of the rule of reason by which the cosmos operated, and which even God was bound to follow. Gnostics rejected the notion of miracle as well, for the transcendent God—always distinguished from the lower Creator God—does not meddle in the evil material world. Thus, the miracle of Isaac's birth to Sarah and Abraham after Sarah had grown too old to conceive is creatively refashioned. In Ilive's telling, Isaac is born to the aging patriarch and his wife after Sarah instructs her husband to circumcise himself, thus allowing a stronger flow of semen. In one stroke, so to speak, what appeared to be a miraculous pregnancy is explained away.[40]

In sum, by his strategic rewriting of Genesis accounts, Ilive suggested to his readers—many of whom would have believed they were reading a translation of a lost Hebrew text—that the Bible they usually read was not a Revealed Word but a priestly deception. Moreover, his approach to history in *Jasher* as an invented narrative to be shaped and adapted according to theological need reflects the gnostic's disdain for history. Another author drawn to imaginative historical reconstruction began shaping the American religious mind early in the nineteenth century. As with Ilive, gnosticism likewise informs the religious invention of Joseph Smith.

JOSEPH SMITH'S YANKEE GNOSTICISM

Americans are so familiar with the Mormon Church, a common name for the Church of Jesus Christ of the Latter Day Saints, that they have difficulty imagining that its theology is only vaguely Christian. And yet the teachings of Mormonism's founder, Joseph Smith, are much closer to those of ancient gnostics than they are to New Testament Christianity. Smith (1805-1844) helped to popularize a gnostic cosmology in mid-nineteenth-century America.[41] Harold Bloom correctly observed in 1992 that "the Gnostic components in Mormonism are overt, but called by different terms," and it is to these components that I wish to drawn attention in this section.[42] As one of the fastest growing religious groups in the world, and one of the most aggressively evangelistic, Mormonism wields tremendous influence and demands attention.

Spirit guides and secret revelations. Joseph Smith insisted that the revelations on which he based Mormonism were private, coded and delivered to him by spirit guides, each element in this set suggesting his gnostic orientation. Spirit or angel visitation was a feature of Smith's young adulthood. He claimed to have been visited in 1820, at the age of fourteen, by two spiritual beings now referred to as angels by the Mormon Church. In 1823, another spiritual entity identifying himself by the name Moroni appeared to Smith. The Moroni visitations continued yearly between 1823 and 1827. D. Michael Quinn notes in his well-researched book *Early Mormonism and the Magic World View* that these visitations always occurred on the autumnal equinox, September 22, in keeping with Smith's deeply rooted astrological convictions regarding auspicious days for such contact.[43]

Moroni directed Joseph Smith to a number of golden plates buried in a hill near Palmyra, New York. The plates contained the narrative history of North America's ancient inhabitants, one among them being Moroni himself during his physical life on earth. Smith had to visit the specified site near Palmyra regularly over a period of three years before he was allowed to actually take possession of the plates.[44]

Smith alleged that the golden plates were inscribed with characters from a hitherto unknown version of Egyptian hieroglyphic. Moroni, the spirit guardian of this golden textual treasure, gave Smith permission to translate the plates into English with the help of the Urim and Thummim, stones in a breastplate that Smith found with the inscribed plates. Witnesses familiar with Smith's magical inclinations claim that the stones were actually "peepstones" of the type Joseph and his father had used to seek treasure. We will take a closer look at the Smiths and their alleged treasure hunting shortly.

From Smith's private translation of these plates—knowledge of this unusual Egyptian symbol system was limited to Joseph himself—came *The Book of Mormon*, a historical work cast in prose reminiscent of the King James Version of the Bible. *The Book of Mormon* describes several ancient immigrations to North America by Semitic peoples, some of whom are the lost tribes of Israel. Great battles on the North American continent between the Israelites, or Nephites, and other Semitic tribes called the Lamanites, resulted in the complete destruction of the former. This history is of vital importance to Mormonism, and yet its authenticity has always been a matter of great doubt. Jan Shipps, a leading student of Mormonism, comments that "in Mormonism, history has always been at one and the same time unusually significant and very problematic."[45]

Shipps is certainly right if Smith's historical accounts were intended as ordinary textbook history. But another reading is possible. *The Book of Mormon*, like Ilive's *Book of Jasher*, may reflect a disregard for ordinary history, presenting instead Smith's own mythic history or *gnosis*. Before considering Smith's unorthodox approach to history and history's relationship to his gnostic leanings, it is crucial to understand something of the singular social setting in which he was reared.

Magic and hidden treasures: the Smiths of Palmyra. Michael Quinn writes that the family in which Joseph Smith grew up was deeply immersed in legends and folk magic common on the American frontier of the early nineteenth century. Quinn notes that Smith's mother practiced divination of various kinds, "including palm reading."[46] Moreover, Smith's father, like many American men of his day, was "preoccupied with treasure-digging."[47] The Smith family owned "implements of ritual magic," which included a "magic dagger" and three ritual parchments "inscribed with signs and names of ceremonial magic."[48] It is perhaps not surprising, then, that as a young man Joseph Smith was associated with Luman Walter, a "conjurer and Smith's mentor."[49] Throughout his life, Smith was an ardent believer in astrology.[50]

Joseph Smith and his father and brother were well known for their treasure seeking activities.[51] According to a contemporary witness, Martin Harris, Joseph and his father "dug for money in Palmyra, Manchester, also in Pennsylvania, and other places."[52] Treasure seeking was a common activity among the rural residents of upstate New York in the early nineteenth century, fueled by legends about buried pirate loot and deposits of Spanish gold. The hills of some districts were pockmarked with the shallow mines of men desperate to find forgotten gold, silver and jewels. Treasure seeking typically involved the use of magical devices such as divining stones and rods, as well as astrological charts, talismans and other paraphernalia owned by the Smith family.

The idea that secret knowledge led one to personal advancement pervaded the atmosphere Joseph Smith breathed as a young man. Moreover, such notions were intertwined with spiritistic supernaturalism and magical practices. In such a setting, the youthful Joseph Smith claimed he had discovered a pearl of great price: ancient and mysterious golden plates buried in a hillside. It is also understandable why Smith would give the discovery a religious meaning, why spirit beings directed him to the plates, why they were written in a code and why magical stones were required to decode them.

The Book of Mormon: sources. Smith's story of his angelic visitations and subse-

quent translation of the golden plates has been contested from the beginning. However, the polemical nature of virtually everything written by or about the Mormons during the first decades of the organization makes it difficult to know which accounts to believe. It is thus perhaps more productive to focus on the one point of objective agreement between Mormons and their critics—that *The Book of Mormon* with its epic stories of North America's early residents is crucial to Mormon history and theology. What, then, are the most likely sources of Smith's mythic histories if one does not accept the story of angelically revealed ancient golden plates written in an unknown and unknowable hieroglyphic? Again, social milieu is important.

The origin of Native Americans was a topic of great controversy virtually from the moment Europeans set foot on North American soil. Speculation often focused on the ten mysterious lost northern tribes of Israel. Perhaps, somehow, members of these tribes had traversed the Mediterranean Sea and Atlantic Ocean and established a new life in the New World. As early as the 1650s published versions of this theory appeared in the English colonies. By the early nineteenth century, then, such speculation had known almost two centuries of development. It mattered little to a fascinated American public that legitimate historians dismissed such accounts, and it mattered not at all to the young backwoodsman Joseph Smith Jr.

In 1823, Ethan Smith—not related to Joseph—published a book entitled *View of the Hebrews*. Harry L. Ropp notes that Ethan Smith's *View of the Hebrews* presents a detailed theory that the American Indians are descended from the Israelites, suggests that a book of their early history in America is buried somewhere on the American continent, and discusses early Egyptian documents. In other ways as well *View of the Hebrews* is similar to Joseph Smith's *The Book of Mormon*.[53] *View of the Hebrews* was republished in 1825, both the first and second printings occurring in Poultney, Vermont. Poultney was the place of residence of one of Joseph Smith's early partners, Oliver Cowdery. In 1825 Cowdery moved to New York and met Joseph Smith.

Other possible sources for *The Book of Mormon* include an epic tale of ancient North American tribes in conflict by Reverend Solomon Spaulding. Spaulding's manuscript, never published, also developed the theory that Native Americans were descendants of the Israelites. Spaulding wrote his fictional work in 1809 while living in Conneaut, Ohio. Ropp writes:

In 1812, Spaulding and his family moved to Amity, Pennsylvania, near Pittsburgh,

and there he turned his manuscript over to Robert Patterson, a local printer, to be published. Patterson had an employee, J. H. Harrison, who was a friend of Sidney Rigdon. Rigdon frequently lounged around the printing office, and when the manuscript came up missing, Rigdon was suspected of the theft.[54]

Rigdon was critically important to Mormonism's founding. In fact, some scholars speculate that Mormon theology owes more to Rigdon than to Smith.[55] According to this theory, "Rigdon reworked the [Spaulding] manuscript with the aid of Smith and Cowdery, and this we have as the *Book of Mormon.*"[56] However, Harry Ropp entertains the possibility that Smith used several sources—the Bible, the Spaulding manuscript, Ethan Smith's *View of the Hebrews*—to prepare *The Book of Mormon.* The controversy surrounding Smith and Rigdon's sources will likely never be resolved to the satisfaction of all interested parties. That there are parallels between Smith's *Book of Mormon* and the ideas of both Ethan Smith and Solomon Spaulding is strongly suggestive but not conclusive. Both his cosmology and the fact that it was founded on a mythic *gnosis,* a secret spiritual history, places Joseph Smith in the tradition of ancient gnosticism. That remarkable cosmology has had enormous impact on the American religious mind.

Smith's cosmology. Like early Gnostic mythologies, *The Book of Mormon* represents a rhetorical revolt against the whole Revealed Word tradition. Smith's encoded golden plates and spirit visitations provided him private access to *gnosis* or liberating spiritual secrets.[57] The spiritual truths derived by these magical means were held as personal secrets, the full contents of which were shared only with a small inner circle.[58] Several components in Mormon cosmology reflect gnostic influences.

Mormonism finds humans to be embodied preexisting souls, with earthly life being an important step on a journey toward divinity that is directed by the teachings and rituals of the church, some of which remain secret to outsiders. The end of the process of one's progressive escape from mundane restraints is elevation to divinity itself. "You have got to learn how to become gods yourselves; to become Kings and Priests to God, the same as all gods have done, by going from a small degree to another," Smith taught his followers. Harold Bloom has written, "though many Mormons now are uncomfortable with their very human God, their prophet was emphatic in his insistence that God had begun as a man upon our common earth, and had earned godhood through his own efforts."[59]

According to Smith, God the father and his wife are continually engaged in the

propagation of spirit children who in turn await birth into human bodies in order to begin their ascent toward divinity. Adam of the Garden of Eden is also understood as a god who had been assigned to earth by a higher deity. Jesus, like Adam, resides in a lower echelon of gods. Anthony Hoekema sums up some of the gnostic principles of Mormon theology in a fashion strikingly reminiscent of Ilive's accounts in the Joyner's Hall address. Hoekema writes, "all gods first existed as spirits, came to an earth to receive bodies, and then, after having passed through a period of probation on the aforesaid earth, were advanced to the exalted position they now enjoy in the heavenly realm."[60] The Revealed Word's sharp distinction between the Creator and the creature is lost in Smith's cosmic progressivism that renders God an evolved human being, and all human beings potential gods. The idea that humans evolve or progress toward divinity is central to Mormon cosmology. Reflecting the gnostic astrological interest in stars and planets as residences of ascended human beings, Smith also promised faithful followers lordship over celestial bodies. Harold Bloom has correctly noted that "Mormons have a Gnostic freedom from the world of nature, a necessary liberty for men who aspire to become gods, each with his own planet, a world altogether his own."[61]

Such astral speculation, like spiritual evolution, was crucial to Smith's worldview.[62] Smith was taken with the stars, finding them critical to human spiritual progress. As noted above, Quinn argues that Smith's visits with Moroni occurred at astrologically propitious times. Moreover, a great star called Kolob was the site, according to Smith, where a council of divine beings initiated the vast spiritual plan in which humans still participate. Earth is a planet created jointly by Jesus (called Jehovah) and his father (Elohim) for carrying out the plan. Also involved in earth's creation were Michael (Adam in preexistent form), maybe Noah and Enoch, and perhaps even Joseph Smith before he was born. "The creation of this earth," writes Hoekema, "was thus a kind of cooperative venture between the gods and the spirits of certain preexistent men."[63]

All of these elements in the Smithian cosmology are at odds with central commitments of the Revealed Word tradition, which teaches the earth's creation *ex nihilo*—out of nothing—by the one true God. Smith taught, on the other hand, the gnostic idea that the "creation" of earth was merely a reorganization of existing matter. Bruce McKonkie, a Mormon writer, argues that "to create is to organize." Thus, "it is an utterly false and uninspired notion to believe that the world or any other thing was created out of nothing." Another Mormon authority concurs,

writing that God "cannot conceivably originate matter."[64] Thus, on Smith's interpretation the creative activity of the various gods was limited to reorganizing matter into various physical forms, one of which was the human body.

Joseph Smith embraced and taught a cosmology that more closely resembles gnostic thinking than the theology expressed in the Revealed Word. Smith affirmed spiritual ascent toward divinity through the combination of disciplined effort and *gnosis* or spiritual secrets. Joseph Smith conceived of himself as the human conduit of these secrets from the spirit world. Moreover, he viewed physical embodiment as a probationary condition temporarily endured for the sake of human spiritual advancement to higher realms of existence—from telestial through terrestrial to celestial. For all of these reasons, Smith can be understood as a potent advocate of gnostic spirituality in nineteenth-century America. In the last century and a half millions have embraced Smith's message, and many others who have not become Mormons have been influenced by his basic cosmology.

CARL JUNG AND THE GNOSTIC IMPULSE

Few writers or thinkers have had a greater shaping influence on contemporary thought than the Swiss-born psychoanalyst Carl Jung (1875-1961). Joseph Campbell refers to Jung as "a scholar in the grand style, whose researches, particularly in comparative mythology, alchemy and the psychology of religion, have inspired and augmented the findings of an astonishing number of the leading scholars of our time."[65] Major shaping influences in the development of Jung's own thoughts about religion include, among others, Nietzsche, Eastern religious thought and ancient gnostic writers.

Jung's principal role in the twentieth century may not have been the propagation of psychoanalytic theories. Rather, he has been a highly successful proponent of a closely related set of religious ideas, some of which are at the center of the New Religious Synthesis. He retrieved for modern Western readers many ancient Eastern, gnostic and occult ideas such as the divinity of the individual, the existence of spiritual *gnosis*, the reality of a spiritual elite and the legitimacy of parapsychological phenomena. He is famous for affirming that humanity's various divinities are generated from deep within the human psyche and that individual human minds are connected by a vast psychic force he termed "the collective unconscious." Moreover, Jung found the individual to be "the maker of history."[66] Jung disseminated these ideas in his many books and essays on psychoanalysis, religious psychology

and mythology. A leading expert on Jung's spiritual ideas, Richard Noll, writes, "Such ancient ideas, ironically, are what Jung is best known for introducing as modern innovations." Indeed, Noll comments, these ideas "are so widely spread in our culture through their connections to psychotherapeutic practice, New Age spirituality, and neopaganism that they continue to be the subject of innumerable workshops, television shows, bestselling books, and video cassettes, and they form the basis of a brand of psychotherapy with its own trade name: Jungian analysis."[67]

A return to gnosticism. Jung grew up as part of a social elite in late nineteenth-century Switzerland. Consequently, "Nietzschean ideals of a new nobility were . . . grounded in Jung's personal and practical experience."[68] But from the time he was a young man, Jung also had a strong interest in spiritistic phenomena, also probably derived from his family situation. Whereas Jung's father was a Protestant pastor, his mother maintained a decided interest in the occult. Jung recalls his mother's involvement with a spiritual medium, and he was known to take notes at seances. His mother also "introduced him as a child to Hindu gods, for which he maintained a lifetime fascination."[69] He eventually rejected the Christian theology of his father, cultivating in its place an intense fascination with ancient mystery cults, especially the Roman cult of Mithra.[70] One commentator writes, "Jung's works abound in selections from Gnostics, mystics, and alchemists, all of whom pointed to the God within."[71]

Indeed, Jung came to affirm "mankind's native divinity" and called for "a return to the Gnostic sense of God as an inner, directing presence."[72] This required turning away from the external forces of both history and the wholly other God of the Bible, and toward the interior life of the soul. His vehement rejection of Christianity and the entire Revealed Word tradition was focused specifically on this point—that it had "emptied the soul of a native divine presence" and made God external.[73] Jung also held, in keeping with gnostic theories, that the soul experienced "imprisonment in the body" from which it could be led into unity with the divine through techniques of psychic magic.[74] Jung's effort to found a new religion based on gnostic thought was fueled by moral outrage against Revealed Word thinking and its enfeebling effect on the human psyche. A return to gnosticism was the true path to spiritual liberation for the Western world.

The Volk and the East. Perhaps because of his strong interest in gnostic and occult thought, Jung was drawn to the Volkish movement that Nietzsche helped to foment. Jung "undoubtedly felt himself to be part of the community of Germanic

Volk united by its faith in a field of life-energy, with all of its accompanying transcendent spirituality and pantheistic beliefs."[75] With its foundational concept of an Aryan spiritual elite, the Volkish movement created some of the preconditions for the rise of Nazism in Germany. Jung became an important proponent of Volkish thinking, and many in Europe and America were influenced by his views. Historians have often obscured the connection between the widely admired Jung and a movement with decidedly racialist tendencies. According to Jung biographer Richard Noll, Jungians "seem to place more value on preserving an image of Jung as a divinely inspired human vessel for dispensing the eternal truths of the spirit."[76]

Jung was also a devoted student of Eastern religious thought, finding it superior in many ways to the Western theology expressed in the Revealed Word. In his essay "The Difference Between Eastern and Western Thinking" Jung wrote that "the East" possessed "a superior psychic proficiency [which] is throwing our spiritual world into confusion."[77] This was a spiritual confusion of which Jung most decidedly approved. The West was destined to jettison the outmoded spirituality of the Revealed Word tradition in favor of a blend of ancient wisdom and modern psychological insight. Only in this way could it save itself from the destructive tendencies of monotheism. In fact, Jung held that all religious traditions would be transcended by "a religious consciousness much richer and more encompassing than any that had yet been manifested."[78] This new and universal religion of humanity would arise from within the human psyche itself.

Jung foresaw the advent of an Eastern inspired Religious Synthesis in the West, albeit an advent largely hidden from direct view. "We have not yet hit upon the thought," he wrote, "that while we are overpowering the Orient from without, it may be fastening its hold on us from within."[79] Jung's vast study of religious systems convinced him that "the East is at the bottom of every spiritual change we are passing through today."[80]

A new spiritual path for the West. Jung believed that the West was "at the threshold of a new spiritual epoch." He was himself a major force pushing Europe and American toward that threshold. Noll writes that "Freud may still be the genius of choice for the learned elite of the late twentieth century, but it is clear that, in sheer numbers alone, it is Jung who has won the cultural war and whose works are more widely read and discussed in the popular culture of our age."[81] While "practitioners and theoreticians" advocate Jungian psychoanalysis, "far greater numbers" of Westerners are drawn to Jungian "spirituality."[82] Jung is more important today as

a spiritual guide than as a clinical theorist, and the spiritual guidance he offers is fundamentally gnostic and esoteric in outlook. Jungian groups "sponsor programs and workshops related to New Age spirituality and neopaganism." Noll adds that "most Jungian analytic-training institutes" also provide "practical classes or programs on astrology, the I Ching, palmistry, and other practices associated with the occult sciences."[83]

At least one leading Jungian analyst, Edward Edinger, "openly acknowledges Jung's role as a prophet in the twentieth century," a voice ushering in a new religious age. Edinger terms Jung's *Collected Works* "a divinely inspired 'new dispensation' to succeed the Jewish and Christian dispensations of the Old and New Testaments." Jung's works are "read as part of the services of a New Age 'Gnostic Church' in San Francisco, as they are alongside the works of Emerson at some Unitarian services." Noll openly wonders if with the "Jungian movement and its merger with the New Age spirituality of the late twentieth century we are witnessing the incipient stages of a faith based on the apotheosis of Jung as a God-man." He concludes, "Only history will tell if Jung's Nietzschean religion will finally win its Kulturkampf and replace Christianity with its own personal religion of the future."[84] In the enormously influential works of Carl Jung, the confrontation between the New Religious Synthesis and the Revealed Word could not be more pronounced.

JEAN HOUSTON: GNOSTICISM AND THE NEW AGE

Bestselling author and sought-after speaker Jean Houston (b. 1941) is one of the leading proponents of the idea that new scientific discoveries are assisting a revolutionary understanding of human spirituality. Some of Houston's many books include *The Possible Human, Mind Games, The Search for the Beloved, A Mythic Life* and *The Hero and the Goddess.* Among the greatest influences on Houston's thought and writing are Carl Jung and Joseph Campbell. Houston focuses attention on mythology, spiritual evolution, and techniques for exploring the realm of the psyche including meditation and guided experiences. She offers courses in developing personal spiritual potential through her Mystery School in Oregon and Institute for Mind Research in New York.

Jean Houston affirms that the modern residents of the industrialized West stand at the threshold of a new religious era. In *A Passion for the Possible,* a popular book that resulted in a PBS television series, she sets out both the Darwinism and monism that underlie her own theories of unlimited spiritual evolution. "Our

cells," she writes, "contain the memories of all things past—the birth of stars, the coming of life, the experience of being fish and amphibian, reptile and early mammal, monkey and human, and the lure now calling us from beyond the horizon to enter the next stage of our becoming."[85] Within each one of us lies latent an unlimited spiritual potential awaiting an awakening. Indeed, Houston contends that within each of us there exists deity itself.

Exploring of the inner realm of myth and mind will characterize the new spiritual age, much as exploring outer space characterized the scientific era of the late twentieth century. At the very core of the emerging religious paradigm shift is the monistic recognition that all things are one thing. "Eventually the worlds within and without," writes Houston, "are recognized as inseparable parts of the One Reality in which we live and move and have our being."[86] Houston urges her readers to follow her on a quest for the truths that this basic insight provides when taken to its logical, or spiritual, conclusion. Thus, she issues an exciting and winsome call to the new religious seeker to "whet your appetite for inner adventure."[87] This inner journey toward enlightenment is distinctly gnostic, with spiritual secrets important to one's progress being revealed during an interior passage through the psyche.

Going inside to find activating intelligence. Houston presents herself as a friendly, supportive and knowledgeable guide to the realm of the soul. The "inner adventure" begins with readers imagining that they are "climbing a spiral path up a small mountain."[88] On the ascent, various thresholds must be crossed, doorways entered and spirit beings confronted. Light plays a prominent role on this upward and interior journey. "Suddenly you see a light. Another doorway is before you. Its shiny surface is a mirror." This is the entrance "to the realm of the Psyche."[89] Once inside this new realm we realize that we are not alone, for within us reside many selves, in fact, "a vast crew."[90] Houston affirms that the members of this crew are simply expressions of the varieties of the self—a thinker, an artist, a psychologist.

This crew, however, is under the direction of its own Guide, an entity Houston draws attention to throughout this and other of her books. This being is "a presence that all the other selves regard with awe and respect." Houston identifies this dominant presence as the evolved self, the "you who has evolved into all that you could be." Houston acknowledges that "the presence is sometimes called the Daimon— the activating intelligence that guides your life."[91] This notion of a guiding daemon is central to much ancient gnosticism. She adds that when you "enter consciously into close relationship with this presence, your life takes on purpose and energy."[92]

This internal presence plays an enormously important role in one's spiritual evolution, the next step in which process is death.

Death, power and the Self. For all of her spiritual optimism in A Passion for the Possible, motifs of death play a major role in Houston's spirituality, as do exotic locations associated with death such as the Egyptian pyramids and coffins. The reader is encouraged to "walk on until you come to a pyramid." Opening a door, we "follow a long upward path into a chamber where there is an empty sarcophagus—the King's coffin." At this point, "something beckons you to lie down in it." The tomb becomes a place "from which you will be birthed to a richer, more complex life. Your gestation complete, you rise and continue your journey."[93] Thus, the reader is encouraged to embrace death in order to move on spiritually.

Following one's death experience, the spiritual guide is reintroduced as "the Beloved of your Soul—your angel, your divine other half, your life's spiritual partner." Once in "the Beloved's embrace," we find that "all yearnings are fulfilled" and experience "the wonder of unconditional love." At this point "you and your allies"—the Beloved and the crew— return across the threshold of amplified power." Though departing, they assure you that "they live forever within you to give you protection and guidance."[94] Various techniques have assisted some in reaching out to the inner crew, understanding spiritual advancement, and continuing the psychic journey, including "hypnosis, meditation, inward focusing and even electrical stimulation of the brain."[95]

Some readers may be reluctant to yield themselves to a spiritual friend accompanied by an "inner crew." Houston assures us, however, that this is nothing to worry about, that our fears reflect the remnants of Western thinking, specifically the notion of a persistent, unified self. "If the idea of having so many 'beings' within yourself seems strange, it's because our culture puts so much emphasis on each person having a single, consistent personality or role."[96] The Beloved is merely a manifestation of what each of us may become, provided we have the right guidance and the necessary courage to evolve spiritually. This daimon or activating intelligence is a trustworthy friend who "holds the totality of your life and memories" while at the same time offering you the opportunity to "contribute to the design of your life."[97]

Houston's role as a contemporary gnostic master emerges gradually in A Passion for the Possible. First, she is familiar with the spiritual realm and with the spiritual keepers of secrets residing there. Second, Houston has an acquired understanding of how one navigates the spiritual world, a knowledge or *gnosis* without which the

wandering reader would be lost and perhaps even in danger. Finally, she possesses personal knowledge of the interior transactions with spirit entities that lead to spiritual release and development. For example, she knows how one ought to proceed through the pyramid scenario. Finally, as will become clear in a moment, Houston holds that human beings possess a divine spark waiting to be reunited with the larger divinity of the cosmos.

Myth and evolution. Gnostic systems always involve a myth of human origins, the *gnosis* itself. Jean Houston, like her mentor Joseph Campbell, is a devotee of mythology and its place in spiritual evolution. Myth as the carrier of the stages of ascent is crucial to individual spiritual progress, according to Houston and our spirit guides. The Inner Friend himself reveals that "most of the world's great myths" express that "imbedded in the human psyche" are the various "stages of our evolution."[98] The use of the qualifier "most" in this sentence is suggestive, perhaps implying that the Revealed Word tradition—which has resisted the idea of a purely interior spirituality—may not carry the knowledge necessary for one to "wake up to a higher destiny."[99]

A crucial role of myth in Houston's system, as in ancient gnostic theories, is to provide the knowledge important to overcoming the guardians who would prevent our spiritual advancement. "The Threshold Guardian," for example, "is a monster who guards the gateway to the larger reality we seek." Consequently, "one is required to prove oneself faster, wiser, and more ingenious than the Guardian in order to make safe passage."[100] And there are many such guardians in Houston's cosmos, just as there were in the cosmos of ancient gnostic masters. "As you feel the power of this Guardian fade, cross the threshold. Then return to confront another of the Guardians."[101] Once having conquered the various guardians, we "become aware of a Force within ourselves that links our life to Great Life."[102]

Commitment to the Inner Friend. A surprising passage occurs near the end of *A Passion for the Possible.* Here Houston leads her readers through what can only be described as a spiritual wedding ceremony. Readers are urged to "be acknowledged by the one who is known as the Beloved or Heavenly Partner." While insisting that "this glorious being" is actually "your other half," Houston adds that the Friend "dwells in the depth world" and is rightly referred to as "the Divine Other." The appropriate response to this Divine Other is, apparently, nothing less than total commitment and submission. "Go out in the evening or early morning," she writes, "when Venus is bright in the sky, and using the planet of love as the symbol of the

Beloved, say words such as these: 'From this moment forth I am with you always. From this moment forward, I am your partner in the human realm. From this moment forward, I will bring you, my Beloved, and your ways into time. I know you will ignite the fire in my mind.'"[103]

At this point, the last great barrier having been traversed, one finally achieves the gnostic realization that "each person is really 'God in Hiding.'"[104] The divinity of the individual human is the final great spiritual insight toward which all this inner journeying has been leading. This insight is only possible because of Houston's guidance into the realm of spirit and out of the imprisonment of "the habits of consciousness that sustain the brain's cataracts."[105] As ancient myths related repeatedly, "each person holds a Godseed, a divine essence that can be nurtured through spiritual practice into a fully matured expression of the Godstuff within."[106] Houston helps her readers to recognize this fact about themselves and to engineer their inner divinity's escape from time and ordinary existence.

In *A Passion for the Possible* the reader's spiritual advancement is achieved with the help of a person specially qualified to direct our path through her familiarity with the secrets of the spiritual realm. This process of spiritual evolution is accomplished with the assistance of one who knows well the guiding spirits. Houston thus plays the role of gnostic master, a knowledgeable pathfinder through the spirit realm and a guide to the secrets of spiritual growth and escape.

SCIENCE FICTION: THE FINAL GNOSTIC FRONTIER

Science fiction, among the most popular of literary and cinematic genres, has long been a carrier of religious ideas. This genre is particularly influential in shaping the thinking of its legions of young devotees, but always maintains a sizeable adult following as well. From the genre's inception, science fiction has embraced evolutionary thinking. Several prominent science fiction writers added to the basic Darwinian plot the idea that a small elite of the human race possess the special capacities required to master the secrets and techniques that enable the next step in mental or spiritual advancement. Adding a third factor to evolution and elites—namely, that the secrets of human ascent were delivered by entities from other planets or dimensions—launched hundreds of science fiction stories.

Gnostic thinking and space stories have often enjoyed a natural union. In fact, the two ideas have been almost inseparable in the modern period. Jacob Ilive imagined creatures thrown out of heaven (space) and falling to earth where they were

given human bodies. While on earth they were to regain the knowledge that would allow their reentry into the cosmic realms. Other inhabited planets played a role in Ilive's cosmology as well, each performing a specific function in a vast scheme of cosmic ascent. It is also interesting to reflect that Joseph Smith's account of human origins involves an extraterrestrial being (Adam) from a distant star (Kolob) coming to earth to help the human race—embodied spirit entities from another realm—to begin the process of achieving its cosmic destiny of reattaining the celestial realm.

By the middle of the twentieth century—particularly following a series of well-publicized UFO sightings in 1947—many spiritual masters with gnostic leanings began to portray their spirit guides, not as Blavatskian Tibetan ascended masters, but as "space commanders" and "aliens."[107] Catherine Albanese reports that "from 1954 Englishman George King—a yoga adept long familiar with theosophical tradition—began, according to his own report, to have a series of unusual experiences." Specifically, King reported that "he had been designated by Venusian Master Aetherius as the 'Primary Terrestrial Mental Channel.'" By 1956, King's followers became "the Aetherius Society in London, and in 1959 he moved to Los Angeles, where his movement grew."[108]

With King we have a direct link between the fundamental building blocks of much science fiction and religious invention in the world of actual human affairs. Others have followed his lead. Marshall Applewhite's suicidal Heaven's Gate UFO cult, briefly described in the introduction to this chapter, is just one recent example of the phenomenon of fitting gnostic spirituality to a science fiction narrative. Another example of the apparently natural connection between science fiction and gnostic thought is the fiction of writer and religionist L. Ron Hubbard (1911-1986). Hubbard authored a series of pulp science fiction books in the 1940s. In 1950 he turned his attention toward religion, writing his now famous *Dianetics: The Modern Science of Mental Health*, the foundational work of a new faith.

Hubbard's gnostic leanings are evident in his account of human origins. According to Hubbard, humans are embodied alien beings called Thetans who were banished to earth 75 million years ago by a cosmic tyrant known as Xenu. Once this hidden truth about our nature is recognized, a process known as "auditing" can begin to undo the damage done by the Thetans within. In Hubbard, ideas first expressed in science fiction are seamlessly transformed into a worldwide religion with affinities to gnosticism.

"Star Wars" and "The Matrix." Several of the most popular science fiction mov-

ies in recent years have woven a gnostic cosmology into their narrative fabric. Two examples will suffice to illustrate the point. George Lucas's wildly popular *Star Wars* movie series introduced American audiences to Yoda, a diminutive master of spiritual secrets that allowed one to control and benefit from a vague spiritual force known as, well, The Force. Protagonist Luke Skywalker studies under Yoda's direction until he is able to control The Force and communicate with deceased individuals and spirit beings. In learning Yoda's secrets, Luke has taken an important step toward spiritual enlightenment. Another suggestion of the movie series is that Luke's special pedigree—he is the descendant of a select group known as Jedi Knights—enables him to master the secrets of The Force. Presumably an ordinary human might not have what it takes to control this potent spiritual force akin to Bulwer-Lytton's Vril.

More explicitly gnostic than *Star Wars, The Matrix* was one of the most popular films among America's teenage audience in 1999. Its protagonist, Neo, is selected by an ascended master named Morpheus to learn the grand secret—a mythic *gnosis*—behind all apparent reality. Morpheus reveals that the entire human scene is, in fact, an elaborate illusion. Embodiment is a trick played on the human mind by computers, the consequence of a cosmic struggle between evil intelligences and human beings that the humans lost. By learning the *gnosis* that unlocks the secret of human existence—something within the reach of only a select elite—Neo enters a special order of ascended spiritual adepts. Within this small community, life is monastically simple. All fleshly appetites are denied, rejected as elements of the deception of embodiment. The struggle with the evil intelligences—called Agents—for the souls of humanity is the central purpose of the small community of futuristic *pneumatikoi*.

In a detailed analysis of the film's gnostic message published in *Envoy* magazine, Steve Kellmeyer identifies a number of parallels between the movie's plot and ancient gnostic doctrine. *The Matrix* affirms that "we live in an illusion, creation is an evil prison in which we serve its creator, and we must be freed."[109] He adds, "Once we're acquainted with this worldview, we can see how *The Matrix* clearly unfolds as a modern retelling of the Gnostic version of salvation history."[110]

CONCLUSION

In his now classic 1969 work *The Teachings of Don Juan*, Carlos Castaneda relates his apprenticeship to a Sonoran Indian medicine man. Don Juan teaches Castaneda to become "a man of knowledge." But not just anyone can master the secret

knowledge necessary to achieving such status. Moreover, the master himself must specially select the student of such secrets, albeit guided by spiritual entities. "Don Juan as a teacher," writes Castaneda, "selected [as] his apprentices" individuals possessing "a certain disposition of character, which [he] called 'unbending intent.'" Castaneda adds regarding the selection process, however, that "the final decision in matters of who could learn to become a man of knowledge was left to an impersonal power that was known to don Juan, but was outside his sphere of volition."[111] Like a true gnostic master, don Juan recognizes that spiritual insight and liberation are not attainable by all people. Unlocking the secrets of the spirit realm demands an arduous effort to acquire secret knowledge and great discipline to employ that knowledge correctly once acquired.

The gnostic impulse is at work in a variety of contemporary religious and spiritual movements. This impulse elevates a spiritual elite who, through secret spiritual knowledge, are enabled to transcend time, the body and conventional morality. Gnostic thinking seeks to shake off the restraints of Revealed Word thinking with its restrictive personal morality, its sovereign deity, its regard for time and history and its veneration of the physical as part of the good creation of God. Carl Raschke writes, "Through private, internal excursions into the spirit realm the Gnostic learns the secrets that bring mastery over the great mysteries of death and eternity." He concludes that gnosticism is thus a "'religion of revolt' against conventional religion, its symbols, and its terminology."[112]

For the gnostic, the human mind or soul possesses virtually unlimited capacity for expansion provided it apprehends *gnosis*. Knowledge of *gnosis* may come in the form of a myth about the human predicament—we are fallen angels or eternal souls trapped in bodies—as techniques of spiritual ascent or perhaps simply as a revelation about the power of one's own mind. However, modern gnostics remind us, as did their predecessors, that ordinary human beings limit their spiritual potential through adhering to various cultural constraints on thought and action. They thus can never achieve the breakthrough to spiritual self-liberation.

This chapter has considered several important religious, philosophical and literary works that have served to reintroduce the Western religious mind to gnosticism. The Enlightenment Deist Jacob Ilive had somehow absorbed and then replicated a pure strain of ancient gnosticism, advocating it in a series of public lectures in eighteenth-century London. Biblical history was for Ilive the product of a priestly caste, and he set about to rewrite Genesis history to comport with gnostic

ideas. The surprising demonology of his Joyner's Hall address is inexplicable except when read as a return to an earlier gnostic tradition. In a similar fashion, Joseph Smith advocated that human beings were temporarily embodied preexistent souls working their way back to a more elevated cosmic realm and eventually to divinity. His own mythic *gnosis* was revealed by spirit beings and encrypted, rendering it inaccessible to anyone but Smith and an inner circle.

The early twentieth-century European intellectual Carl Jung also revived ideas at the heart of the gnostic impulse, including the reign of the powerful individual, the crucial role played by spiritual elites and the place of magic in unlocking spiritual secrets important to unlimited self-expansion. More recently the cluster of ideas that animates gnostic thought has shown up in writers in the spiritual self-help genre, including Jean Houston, and in the extraordinarily popular narratives of science fiction. Secrets are taught by knowledgeable adepts to those specially equipped to receive them, and spiritual elevation results from mastering techniques and apprehending *gnosis*.

The contrast between gnostic and Revealed Word spirituality could not be starker. The Revealed Word has always been radically public in nature. It is a proclaiming perspective, a disclosing faith view devoid of secrets. Moreover, the Revealed Word affirms history as ardently as gnosticism denies it, and elevates the physical as determinedly as gnosticism demotes it. The creating God of Genesis creates both humanity and history, treating the former as good and the latter as a serious fact. Finally, the Revealed Word eschews the notion of an inner circle of adepts learning spiritual secrets from an ascended master, repudiating the very idea that salvation comes by way of apprehending secrets of spiritual ascent.

As the following chapter reveals more clearly, gnosticism is often closely aligned with occultism—the pursuit of spiritual power through ritual magic and spirit communication. Theodore Adorno writes, "the tendency to occultism is a symptom of regression in consciousness" toward a "metaphysics of dunces."[113] Nevertheless, the gnostic affirms that the liberating use of *gnosis* depends on the work of a few rationally gifted and spiritually advanced individuals. Under the influence of the gnostic impulse "the rescue of society and culture" is brought about by "great, gifted, powerful and autonomous individuals" under the direction of a leader "whose vision traverses and transcends time and space, and who sings of the return of a golden age."[114] So, which assessment of the gnostic master—metaphysical dunce or spiritual genius—is correct?

The New Religious Synthesis has revived the ancient gnostic tradition, so long opposed by the Revealed Word. *Gnosis* is on the rise, and spirituality is again being construed as a matter of mastering secrets that make self-deliverance possible. The path back to *gnosis* from grace was opened by writers like Ilive, explored by Smith, celebrated by Jung, popularized by Houston and rendered in winsome narratives by the writers of science fiction. Gnosticism is now a crucial building block in the New Religious Synthesis, a foundational complement to components such as spiritual evolution and pantheism in the formation of a contemporary Western religious mind. The Revealed Word with its images of redemption, faith and universally available grace has been displaced in that mind by a vision of the spiritual struggle of an ever-ascending elite in possession of secret knowledge. The following chapter explores the alleged source of some of these spiritual secrets, and it examines the private conversations of several leading spiritual masters with voices from beyond the physical realm.

9

MODERN SHAMANISM
Spirit Contact and Spiritual Progress

Since I wished to know what the people of Mercury were like in face and body . . . a woman was displayed to my gaze, who was very much like the women on earth. She had a comely face, but one smaller than women on earth have.

EMANUEL SWEDENBORG, The Worlds in Space

It was absolutely astonishing. I saw the form of a very tall, overpoweringly confident, almost androgynous human being. A graceful, cream-colored garment flowed over a figure seven feet tall, with long arms resting calmly at its side.

SHIRLEY MACLAINE, Dancing in the Light

As we approached the door we encountered two taller, thin men with gigantic, black, almond shaped eyes. . . . It was hard to be in their presence. One of them said, "He isn't ready yet."

WHITLEY STREIBER, Transformation: The Breakthrough

This experiment seemed to show that scientists can learn a good deal by working with Amazonian shamans. Some observers have suggested that shamanism, as classically defined, is reaching its end. But bringing scientists and shamans together seems more like a beginning.

JEREMY NARBY, Shamans Through Time

The term *shaman* originated among the Tungus-speaking people of Siberia, and it described an individual who professed to have healing powers and the ability to see the future and to summon demons.[1] Sixteenth- and seventeenth-century European explorers in South America also observed local healers who claimed to communicate with spirits, often with the aid of tobacco, hallucinogenic drugs and self-inflicted wounds. Exorcised by Catholic monks and debunked by Enlightenment philosophers, shamans eventually became a curiosity that Westerners associated with new worlds and exotic lands.

However, if the essence of shamanism is to gain hidden knowledge through contact with spirits, demons, the dead or beings from other worlds, then the practice of shamanism has its own long and vigorous tradition in the Western world as well. Magicians, witches, mediums and alchemists have claimed for centuries to receive information or direction from spirits. Moreover, in recent times shamanism has experienced a surprising resurgence of public interest and is today complementary to the spiritual outlook I have termed the New Religious Synthesis, particularly as a source of the secrets that assist spiritual evolution. How, in an allegedly scientific and rationally enlightened age, has shamanism managed to reassert itself? As with other components in the Other Spirituality, persuasive public texts have played an important role.

Philip Jenkins underlines the importance of the 1932 publication *Black Elk Speaks,* which "introduced a White audience to the riches of Native American spirituality and shamanism," adding that "Black Elk's words proved a major inspiration to many hopeful White imitators in the 1960s and beyond."[2] Jeremy Narby and Francis Huxley write that in the 1950s "western observers began participating in shamanistic sessions involving hallucinogenic plants, [and] found, to their astonishment, that they could have experiences similar to those described by shamans." A major story in *Life* magazine in 1957 popularized the idea of shamanism for many American readers. "In Mexico, American banker Gordon Wasson ate psilocybin mushrooms in a session conducted by Mazatec shaman Maria Sabina." Wasson described to *Life*'s readers "flying out of his body." Narby and Huxley report that "hundreds of thousands of people read Wasson's account, and many followed his example."[3]

In the 1960s Carlos Castaneda described his apprenticeship with a Yaqui Indian shaman named don Juan in an enormously popular series of books that were read by hundreds of thousands of university students. *The Teachings of Don Juan: A Yaqui Way of Knowledge* and its sequels "became worldwide bestsellers."[4] Castaneda's training involved in part the use of the hallucinogen peyote and techniques for conjuring spirits. "In the wake of Castaneda's books, millions of people became interested in shamans in a hands-on way," write Narby and Huxley. "There was a great flowering of neo-shamanism in the New Age movement, concentrated in the United States, but increasingly spreading around the world."[5] The 1980s and 1990s saw the publication of dozens of New Age accounts of messages channeled from spirit beings and direct contact with a host of otherworldly entities.

This chapter explores the reemergence of shamanism in the modern Western

world and its place in the New Religious Synthesis. That members of a spiritual elite can garner important information from beings in another realm or on another planet is now a widely accepted component of religious thought. Spirit contact, once limited to occult works, surfaces today in popular fiction, the personal accounts of New Age aficionados, the literature of the UFO movement, spiritual biographies, the literature of angelic visitation, countless movies and in a variety of other genres.

This chapter examines several important documents that have assisted in again popularizing the ancient practice of communication between human and intelligent nonhuman entities. We shall begin by considering an early modern proponent of human-spirit contact, the famous religious writer Emanuel Swedenborg, who claimed to have been instructed by beings on other planets as well as by angels. We will then take note of the explosion of occult interest that occurred in Victorian England and America, a social phenomenon that radically altered public attitudes about spirituality while at the same time undermining Revealed Word prohibitions on the practice of mediumship or shamanism. Twentieth-century advocates of shamanism and related practices to be considered include the Harvard psychiatrist John Mack and his surprising accounts of sessions with UFO abductees, as well as spiritual counselor Paul Ferrini and his conversations with Jesus.

EMANUEL SWEDENBORG

Eighteenth-century Swedish scientist, engineer, artisan and mystic Emanuel Swedenborg (1688-1772) had an important influence on a variety of nineteenth-century writers and thinkers including Ralph Waldo Emerson and Joseph Smith. Swedenborg's theology is complex and difficult to apprehend due to his tendency to mask heterodox ideas with Christian terminology. What is particularly striking about Swedenborg's theology is his claim about its ultimate source. He insisted that virtually everything he wrote on spiritual matters after 1744 was revealed to him directly by spirits in almost daily episodes of direct spirit contact.

The corpus of Swedenborg's work is massive, and I have chosen here to focus on one particularly unusual and popular short book in which he claims to have traveled among various planets and learned from their inhabitants a variety of spiritual secrets. The original Latin title of this book was *Telluribus in universo,* and it was first published in 1758. The first English translation, *The Worlds in Space,* appeared in London in 1787. The book has maintained a readership for more than two hundred years and is still published by the Swedenborg Society.

Though others had speculated about the possibility of life on other planets prior to the 1750s—Bernard Bouvier de Fontenelle wrote *Conversations on the Plurality of Inhabited Worlds* in 1686—Swedenborg likely invented the genre of the first-hand account of alien contact. This rhetorical invention, an early version of science fiction, proved irresistible to many readers then as now, and the space alien narrative remains a highly persuasive carrier of religious ideas.

Talking with alien spirits: questing for knowledge. Swedenborg opens *The Worlds in Space* by claiming, "I have been enabled to talk with spirits and angels, not only those in the vicinity of our earth, but also those near other worlds."[6] These other worlds include Mars, Venus, Saturn, Mercury and Jupiter, planets well known to eighteenth-century astronomers. Swedenborg's "space" travel is, however, a strictly interior, spiritual journey in which he encounters beings he terms "spirits" who belong to the planets of our solar system. He writes, "as I have said several times before, a spirit is taken from place to place by nothing but changes in his inner state."[7] Swedenborg journeyed in a similar fashion, entering an altered mental state in order to achieve the spirit contact he alleged was a daily experience for him for more than twelve years.

Many of the planetary spirits whom Swedenborg encountered desire human contact because of their great thirst for knowledge, which is the key to their own spiritual attainment. When happening upon a knowledgeable human being, "they review everything in his memory, calling up from it whatever suits them," a technique reminiscent of the aliens in Sagan's *Contact* as discussed at the end of chapter five.[8]

The point of Swedenborg's quest for alien contact is to increase his own knowledge of the true spiritual nature of the universe. In fact, much of *The Worlds in Space* is taken up with passages in which planetary spirits correct the false teachings of Christian orthodoxy on such issues as the Trinity and the incarnation and resurrection of Christ. One of the principal lessons conveyed in this unusual book is that the literal sense of the Revealed Word is insignificant when compared to the true or spiritual meaning of the Christian Scriptures. "Everything in the literal sense of the Word corresponds to Divine things in heaven," and it is these things in heaven, or space, that are preeminent.[9] Just as the Deist Thomas Woolston claimed that only the spiritual sense of Scripture mattered—an idea he occasionally attributed to spirit contact as well—so Swedenborg is at pains to instruct his readers that planetary spirits have conveyed to him undiluted spiritual truth.

"Correspondence" is a key component in Swedenborg's cosmology in *The*

Worlds in Space, an idea he borrows from Hermeticism and the occult tradition. The familiar phrase from the world of magic states "as above, so below." That is, the microcosm of the visible world and nearby worlds is a miniature representation of the macrocosm that is the vast system of an invisible spiritual universe. For Swedenborg, each planet and its spirits correspond to a particular part of something he calls "The Grand Man," a gigantic cosmic entity that is the sum of the many parts of a vast, invisible world. "The whole of heaven corresponds in every part to a human being," he writes.[10] This notion was also common to earlier works on alchemy and the occult: the elements of the zodiac were thought to correspond to parts of the human body, and the cosmos itself was understood as fashioned on the model of an enormous man.

For Swedenborg, to understand the spirits and planets and their various places in the cosmic scheme of things is to achieve potentially great spiritual power. As Swedenborg admits, however, there are certain risks associated with the work of acquiring cosmic knowledge through direct spirit contact.

Alien abuse. Swedenborg as modern shaman is a conduit to humans of secret spiritual knowledge. Yet he is also at the mercy of alien beings who themselves wish knowledge from him. Oddly, though in keeping with contemporary alien contact literature, Swedenborg frequently mentions the physical abuse these planetary spirits are more than ready to inflict on uncooperative hosts. For instance, when Swedenborg fails to comply with an alien request for information, he reports: "So as to show their annoyance they brought a kind of painful contraction of the right side of my head as far as the ear."[11]

Similar incidents are frequently reported in *The Worlds in Space*. Some of his alien acquaintances from Jupiter reveal to Swedenborg how they "draw out from a person's memory all he has done and thought." If they "find fault with his actions or thoughts," their response is to "chastise him by means of pains in the joints, the feet or the hands, or around the epigastric region."[12] Another punishment for bad thinking was "spells of choking until the victim was very distressed . . . and finally a death sentence."[13]

More than once Swedenborg mentions that the abuse aliens inflict on humans or on their own kind extends to the sentence of death. Bad theology—such as accepting the historical accounts of Jesus' life—might bring such a harsh penalty. Swedenborg suggests that planetary spirits often inflict the penalty of death on anyone or any family on their planet holding to false theological ideas. It is the aliens' practice

"to get rid of any family so infected . . . by spirits suppressing their breathing and so taking their lives, after they had passed sentence of death on them."[14] It is an inescapable feature of Swedenborg's account that alien entities are inclined toward violence, a characteristic that attends shamanistic practices both ancient and modern.

Alien advances: the body and science. Many of the alien spirits Swedenborg encounters resemble humans, but are smaller and of slighter build. In keeping with racialist notions of physical and spiritual evolution, the aliens' faces "resembled the faces of people of our world, white and handsome, with a look of sincerity and modesty shining from them."[15] Imperfections are not allowed among these advanced races from space. Faces with "warts and spots, or otherwise disfigured . . . were never to be seen among them." However, "they did approve of some faces, the ones that were cheerful and smiling, and had slightly pouting lips."[16] Of a later alien encounter, Swedenborg writes, "their faces were not unlike those of people in our world, except that the eyes are smaller, and so were the noses."[17] Implicit, then, in alien encounter is the notion of physical perfection—including white skin, beautiful faces and delicate facial features—as characteristic of more advanced humanoids.[18]

The advances enjoyed by aliens—physical and otherwise—are the result of scientific researches. Among some of the alien spirits with whom Swedenborg communicates, the "sciences" are treated as "spiritual riches" that may be used to open the "path to the light of heaven."[19] In a later episode, he proudly explains "various achievements of our world" to some planetary spirits, "especially about our possession of sciences unknown elsewhere, such as astronomy, geometry, mechanics, physics, chemistry, medicine, optics, and philosophy." Through science and technical advances such as printing, "there was a revelation permanently operating in our world."[20] Science, then, had important spiritual significance for Swedenborg, who began his circuitous public career as a highly regarded scientist. Of all human achievements it is science that he is most eager to explain to the spirits, and in which they take the most interest.

History, on the other hand, does not fare so well. When informed about the earthly and historical life of Jesus Christ, the spirits reply that this is "of no interest to them," though Jesus' spiritual nature and authority were deemed important.[21] Other historical details of Jesus' life such as "that he was born as a baby, lived as a man, looked like any other man, was crucified and so forth" were considered among enlightened spirits to be "scandalous ideas."[22]

The qualities of a shaman. To be a shaman, to communicate with spirits, one

must possess special qualities. "Only those whose interiors are open," writes Swedenborg, "can hear those speaking from heaven." Special faith and a great capacity for love are important to this capacity for contact. "No one is allowed to talk with spirits and angels . . . unless he is, as regards faith and love, capable of associating with angels." Because so few meet these criteria "there are few today allowed to talk and converse with angels."

Of course, crucial to this process is "belief in spirits and angels" as well as the belief that "these put a person in touch with heaven."[23] Being in touch with heaven means "travelling . . . in spirit" as one is "guided through varying states of inner life, which appear . . . like travels through space." Both "the outward and return journeys" require "continuous guidance" from spirits.[24]

This is the essence of shamanism—to be found qualified to speak with spirits and to be guided by them on an inner journey that involves risks, pain, ecstatic experience and vast personal knowledge. Swedenborg helped to reintroduce this ancient spiritual practice to the Western world. Through his influence and that of a host of other public advocates, the notion of spirit contact has made its way into the New Religious Synthesis. The following section explores shamanism's tremendous appeal in England a century after Swedenborg's death.

VICTORIAN SHAMANS: OCCULTISM, THEOSOPHY AND SPIRITUALISM

The late nineteenth-century occult movement was vast, complex and somewhat surprising in a nation engaged at that time in creating the modern Christian missionary movement. Through books and especially cheap periodicals, the mysteries of the occult, witchcraft, magic and Satanism became matters of public curiosity and even devotion in the British Isles. Shamanism was at the center of this wildly popular spiritual phenomenon. I want to take note of a few of the major characters and characteristics of Victorian occultism and shamanism, as this movement played a major role in shaping the public religious mind in the direction of the New Religious Synthesis.

Bulwer-Lytton and Crowley. In the 1830s and 1840s a series of popular novels by authors such as the Rosicrucian and occultist George Edward Bulwer-Lytton popularized occult practices and familiarized the European and American reading public with the idea of contacting spirits, demons and ascended masters using secret techniques. Bulwer-Lytton, a nineteenth-century Stephen King, churned out

spine-tingling page-turners at an astonishing rate, each one finding a waiting audience. His novels incorporating occult themes include *Godolphin* (1833), *Asmodeus at Large* (1833), *Pilgrims of the Rhine* (1834) and *The Last Days of Pompei* (1834).[25] Bradford Verter calls Bulwer-Lytton "a fictive popularizer of esoteric philosophy" who published almost without a break from 1828 through 1873. "Through collected editions and cheap reprints," writes Verter, "his work would continue to find an audience into the early twentieth century."[26]

But Bulwer-Lytton's most famous and influential occult novel was without doubt the 1842 bestseller *Zanoni*, the story of a five thousand year old alchemist and his student, set during the French Revolution. Such was the demand for *Zanoni* in America that "readers could buy pirated editions for as little as six cents."[27] Philip Jenkins writes that "characters like Zanoni . . . exercised a powerful spell on the esoteric subculture on both sides of the Atlantic."[28] Reading *Zanoni* amounted to taking an introductory course in magic and spiritism. The most riveting element in the novel, however, was the young hero's encounter with spirits from another realm who imparted to him esoteric knowledge. The book attracted the attention of occultists, religious opponents, social reformers and the simply curious. One effect of the novel, however, was to assist in popularizing the traditional practices of shamanism, a fact that did not escape the notice of the subject of the next section, Madame H. P. Blavatsky.

Bulwer-Lytton's works were among the required reading for students of the greatest English occultist of the first part of the twentieth century, Aleister Crowley.[29] It would be impossible to exaggerate the scandal, controversy and general social alarm that attended the man who called himself The Beast, or to overstate his influence. Crowley more than any other figure popularized ritual magic for Westerners. He was instrumental in developing the highly influential occult organization known as the Order of the Golden Dawn. Crowley authored dozens of books and pamphlets between 1911 and 1940, and he managed to keep himself almost continuously before the public eye. He saw himself as "the prophet of a New Aeon that would supplant the Christian Era" and the developer of "nothing less than a full-fledged successor religion" in which humans would "become the gods" we had previously "merely worshipped."[30] A self-professed occultist, Satanist and magician, Crowley created intense pubic interest in the occult with books such as *Magick* (1911), *The Book of Lies* (1913), *Confessions of a Drug Fiend* (1922) and *The Confessions of Aleister Crowley* (1929). Biographer Lawrence Sutin writes that Crowley "anticipated the spread of Eastern spirituality in the West."[31]

A master rhetorician, Crowley recognized the persuasive power of a sensational novel as well as did Bulwer-Lytton. "The publication of *Confessions of a Drug Fiend*," his most popular novel, "garnered Aleister Crowley more press coverage than his mystical texts ever received."[32] Occult novels, according to Verter, "proved to be an effective means of expanding the readership base for occultist literature, and thus served as a method of propaganda and recruitment."[33] The shamanistic elements in these novels—their instruction in conjuring spirits, seeking secret knowledge from departed individuals or lashing out at enemies with demonic assistance—provided their greatest intrigue. Public thirst for stories of the occult knew no bounds from the late eighteenth century through the early twentieth.[34] Throughout this period, popular fiction and nonfiction advocating contact with spirits, ghosts and demons helped lay the groundwork for a new religious outlook that would compete with the Revealed Word perspective.

Nineteenth- and twentieth-century occult shamanism combined several elements associated with the New Religious Synthesis—rejection of biblical theology, the elevation of reason and science, and a pantheistic belief in a divine energy permeating the cosmos. Particularly prominent was the notion of spiritual evolution, for "great mystics or prophets might represent souls in a very advanced state of spiritual progress, who should be regarded as the rightful teachers of humanity, Masters or Secret Chiefs."[35] Among the most influential of these "advanced souls" was the great Victorian occult leader Madame Blavatsky.

Madame Blavatsky. Evolutionary progression was a central component in Theosophy, founded in America by Madame Helena Blavatsky and others in the last third of the nineteenth century. Her spiritual system is eclectic in its sources, but fundamentally occult and shamanistic in orientation. She, like Joseph Smith, saw herself as a human conduit of secret spiritual truths from another realm. In several lengthy books Blavatsky argued strenuously that mystical, astrological, gnostic, Hermetic and magical teachers of old understood the cosmos correctly. She rejected the Revealed Word tradition out of hand. No less a student of spiritual culture than Carl Jung noted in the 1930s that Madame Blavatsky and Theosophy were the harbingers of a completely new spiritual orientation for the Western world.[36]

Madame Blavatsky traveled extensively in search of hidden spiritual knowledge. She claimed that much of her knowledge had been obtained in the lamaseries of Tibet and other exotic sites. Her 1877 publication, *Isis Unveiled*, denounces conventional Western science—though not true Science—and argues for spiritual

insight through mysticism and occultism. "Science finds herself in a very disagreeable dilemma," Blavatsky wrote in 1877: "She must either confess that the ancient physicists were superior in their knowledge to her modern representatives, or that there exists something in nature beyond physical science, and that *spirit* possesses powers of which our philosophers never dreamed."[37]

Despite such criticism of empirical science, Blavatsky fancied herself a determined advocate of true Science—the systematic study of a cosmos charged with occult energy. A friend and associate, Colonel Henry Steele Olcott, wrote at the time of her death that she "desired that science should be brought back to the true ground where life and intelligence are admitted to be within and acting upon and through every atom in the universe. Hence her object was to make religion scientific and science religious."[38]

Helena Petrovna Blavatsky (1831-1891) was born in Russia on August 12.[39] At the age of seventeen she was married to a Russian nobleman named General Nicephore Blavatsky. After a year she fled from her husband, disappearing "from an English ship bound for Constantinople."[40] This episode began nearly twenty years of travel, the numerous contradictory allegations about this lost period of her life becoming part of the extensive Blavatsky legend. During her travels she claims to have carefully studied firsthand the religious, spiritualist and magical traditions of Europe and the East.

The period of her life from 1850 to 1875 was a closely guarded secret, and Blavatsky forbade friends and biographers alike from inquiring about it.[41] She did intimate late in life that during an 1851 visit to London with her father (which contradicts the claim that she traveled alone) she was directed by a mysterious "tall Hindu" to form the Theosophical Society, "and shortly afterwards left London for India."[42] Rumors of numerous illicit love affairs and equally numerous illegitimate children, egregious deceptions of her many followers, and a host of other scandals haunted Blavatsky throughout her life.

Theosophy. Along with Colonel Olcott (1832-1907) and William Q. Judge, Blavatsky founded The Theosophical Society in New York in 1875. In 1878, Olcott and Blavatsky traveled to India, where they settled. Eventually the headquarters of The Theosophical Society was established in Madras where local Christian missionaries feverishly opposed its work. In December of 1878 Blavatsky made a visit to England where she was welcomed by a number of spiritual explorers. From 1879 through 1888, Blavatsky edited *The Theosophist*. She wrote incessantly on

magic, the occult and spiritualism, her collected works running to fourteen volumes. Blavatsky was involved in an extensive and widely publicized scandal in 1884 when the British press accused her of faking dramatic spiritual phenomena. She was forced to go into seclusion and wrote her most famous work, *The Secret Doctrine* (1888), shortly before her death.

Theosophy did not develop a significant following until Blavatsky and Olcott moved to India, where the native population was quite receptive to a system that incorporated many Hindu teachings, including reincarnation. At the height of its influence, "the Theosophical movement directly involved hundreds of thousands, if not perhaps millions, of individuals."[43] Eventually, Blavatsky's influence was felt strongly in the West. Some adherents of Blavatsky's gnostic shamanism were famous and influential: "Prominent among these were poets Lord Tennyson and W. B. Yeats; the young Mahatma Gandhi; the Goethe scholar, spiritualist medium, and founder (in 1913) of the rival occultist tradition Anthroposophy, Rudolf Steiner; and Thomas Edison, who was busy in the 1890s trying to invent a phonograph-like device to speak to the spirit world."[44] The rapid rise and surprising influence of Theosophy further illustrates how occult spirituality achieved great popularity in nineteenth-century America and Europe.

Ascended masters, secret doctrines and lost races. Blavatsky built Theosophy out of various elements including occultism, spiritism, mysticism, her peculiar understanding of world religions and what she accepted as advances in science. A committed spiritualist, Blavatsky "chose the name *theosophy* ('knowledge of God' or 'divine wisdom') for her doctrine, which was based on the idea that all of the world's religions and spiritual traditions down through history were derived from a long-lost 'secret doctrine' that had been revealed to her by . . . divine beings." Blavatsky referred to these divine beings as the brothers, the Mahatmas or the Masters, and alleged that they resided in Tibet and communicated with her telepathically and in visions.[45]

The knowledge Blavatsky claimed came to her by shamanic means was of ancient origin and had been carefully preserved to be revealed at the appropriate time and to carefully selected individuals. At various times Blavatsky allegedly received secret information from a host of spirits, masters and departed spiritual leaders. Philip Jenkins writes that she "relied on material channeled from great spiritual Masters, members of the Great White Brotherhood, a select club that included Jesus, the Buddha, Confucius, Mesmer, and Cagliostro, as well as real-life occultists she had consulted over the years."[46]

"Isis Unveiled" and the sources of Theosophy. Blavatsky's first major work was her massive polemical survey of ancient magical and occult sources entitled *Isis Unveiled.* Originally published in 1877, *Isis Unveiled* provided the philosophical groundwork for Theosophy, and is still published by the Theosophical University Press in Pasadena, California. Encyclopedic in its coverage of the magical tradition, this two-volume, 1,200-page work reflects throughout Blavatsky's preoccupation with Indian thought. She embraced the pantheism advocated by European writers from Pythagoras to Spinoza, a perspective consistent with Hindu cosmology. "The universe is itself Brahman," she wrote. "This is the philosophy of Spinoza which is derived from that of Pythagoras; and it is the same for which Bruno died a martyr."[47]

Like many public advocates of the New Religious Synthesis from the late seventeenth century onward, Blavatsky labeled Christianity and the Revealed Word tradition a spiritual aberration that deviated from its ancient mystical and pantheistic sources. Blavatsky adhered to the idea, advocated by the Deist Woolston and recently resurrected by several prominent scholars including Marcus Borg, that Jesus was a mystic and a magician who practiced the *"divina sapientia."*[48]

Theosophical thought draws heavily on standard gnostic sources such as Simon Magus and Valentinus, the medieval mystic Meister Eckhart, Renaissance writers in the school of Bruno, the German mystic Jacob Böhme and some Romantic philosophers. However, with Indian cosmology being so important to Blavatsky, Olcott and Annie Besant, the Hindu Vedas, Upanishads and Bhagavad-Gita are perhaps the richest source of theosophical ideas. The tributary of Buddhism also flowed into the stream of theosophical speculation. Olcott himself authored the highly successful *Buddhist Catechism* in 1881, a book translated into several languages.

Spiritual evolution and racial superiority. Blavatsky contended that modern science supported her spiritual system. She was especially intrigued with Darwinian evolution, so powerfully present in late nineteenth-century religious speculation. According to Blavatsky, human evolution would eventuate in a *spiritually* perfected human race, a theme repeated by numerous Victorian writers. She maintained that a lost continent, which she dubbed Lemuria, was once home to a master race. "Historical accounts of this lost society," according the Philip Jenkins, "were mainly derived from mediumship and channeling."[49] From this now lost race, a variety of races have descended. Blavatsky and the other developers of Theosophy used Darwin's evolutionary theory as the basis for a racialist scheme featuring seven "root" races. The fifth of these root races included the Aryans.

Linguistic analysis featured among the various approaches Blavatsky employed to determine which current races were intellectually and spiritually the most advanced. Highly evolved races, it was argued, spoke highly evolved languages. She employed the analytic work of linguists such as August Schleicher (1821-1868) to support her case that Europeans represented the human spiritual vanguard. Richard Noll writes that Schleicher's diagrams were "widely adapted by Blavatsky and the Theosophists to give the appearance of seriousness and scholarly legitimacy" to their racial theories. On such linguistic grounds, Blavatsky argued that the Aryan race "contained the highest spirituality of all mankind."[50] Philip Jenkins notes that occult groups often "drew on the scientific findings of the era, at least as far as they understood them, and this apparent ultramodernity was part of their appeal."[51]

In true shamanic fashion, however, Blavatsky augmented her scientific argument for racial superiority with messages from two of the Mahatmas—Koot Hoomi and Morya—who conveyed their views by means of "spiritual communication from beyond" to Blavatsky's associate A. P. Sinnett.[52] In addition, she posited that Maitreya Buddha, "the Buddha of the final age" would inaugurate "a new stage in the human evolutionary cycle."[53] This "evolutionary cycle" was something Blavatsky found taught in many of the world's magical traditions. The Hermetic writers, for instance, maintained that the human race must "inevitably and collectively . . . in accordance with the law of evolution . . . be finally *physically* spiritualized."[54] This eventuality—physical spiritualization—represents the final stage in human evolution. But, despite her apparently inclusive language—"inevitably and *collectively*"—this apogee of human evolution is not to be achieved by all members of the human race.

Blavatsky endorsed spiritual racism, for some races were simply spiritually superior to others. Blavatsky had imbibed this view from the eminent scientist Alfred Russel Wallace, who arrived at the theory of natural selection at the same time as did Darwin. Blavatsky writes, "In his lecture on *The Action of Natural Selection on Man*, Mr. Alfred R. Wallace concludes his demonstration as to the development of human races under that law of selection by saying that, if his conclusions are just, 'It must inevitably follow that the higher—the more intelligent and moral—must displace the lower and more degraded races.'"[55] Wallace, like Blavatsky, was a spiritist who held that the course of the human race was being directed by "higher intelligences." Eventually, Wallace set about "revamping evolution to take account of unseen spirits."[56]

Blavatsky held, along with many Victorian intellectual figures, that the evolutionary juggernaut leaves behind the "lower and degraded" human races, while a homogenous, perfected race gradually but inexorably emerges. The perfected humans' "mental constitution may continue to advance and improve, till the world is again inhabited by a single, *nearly homogenous race, no individual of which will be inferior to the noblest specimens of existing humanity.*"[57] Blavatsky, the notorious spiritual charlatan of Victorian London, apparently included herself among these "noblest specimens." Moreover, Blavatsky noted that such a racist and evolutionary view was fully consistent with the magical tradition generally. She writes, "What he [Wallace] says" about evolution and the rise of a superior race "clashes in no way with our kabalistic assertions."[58]

Interestingly, Blavatsky had read with approval the work of Bulwer-Lytton, especially *Zanoni* and *The Coming Race*. She apparently derived her idea of ascended masters "from the novels of Bulwer Lytton, which were enormously influential in the English-speaking world as well as in Europe."[59] *Isis Unveiled* was published in 1877, just six years after the appearance of Bulwer-Lytton's *The Coming Race*, and at the height of Vril excitement in Europe. When "ever-progressing nature" follows "the great law of 'survival of the fittest,'" she wrote, then we will see in the "future the possibility—nay, the assurance of a race, which, like the Vril-ya of Bulwer-Lytton's *Coming Race*, [and] will be but one remove from the primitive 'Sons of God.'"[60] Similar racialist-evolutionist ideology is one of the most disturbing aspects of a large number of new religious groups as well.[61]

JOHN MACK AND UFO ABDUCTION

John Mack is a professor of psychiatry at Harvard Medical School. Thus, he is perhaps an unexpected expert on the experiences of individuals who claim to have been abducted by aliens. Nevertheless, Mack's bestselling book *Abduction: Human Encounters with Aliens,* reports his interviews with several persons who allege that beings from another dimension or another planet have contacted and even kidnapped them.[62] Other books in this genre by Mack include *Secret Life: Firsthand, Documented Accounts of UFO Abductions* (with David M. Jacobs, 1993) and *Passport to the Cosmos: Human Transformation and Alien Encounters* (1997).[63] Mack's unusual clinical work finds a place in this chapter because of his suggestion that abductees are themselves modern shamans with important spiritual messages from beyond.

Mack addresses his readers from the perspective of a medical expert in search of the facts behind his clients' curious reports and the explanations for their bizarre

experiences. As a trained psychiatrist and member of the Harvard faculty, he carries unusual credibility. Mack's book recounts clinical sessions in which clients are encouraged to remember the details of their abductions, often after being placed into a hypnotic trance to assist their recall. But he is quick to point out that he may be dealing with something other than actual memory in his interviews with the abducted. To think of memory "as 'true' or 'false,'" he writes, "may restrict what we can learn about human consciousness" from abductees.[64] Mack's curious qualification—that thinking of memory as true or false is restricting—makes sense if one considers his clients not victims of abductions but mouthpieces for guiding spirits, that is, shamans.

A cosmos filled with intelligences. Mack's extensive experience with UFO abductees has convinced him that the cosmos, like Swedenborg's planets and Houston's realm of the psyche, is filled with "intelligences." He writes, "What the abduction phenomenon has led me (I would now say inevitably) to see is that we participate in a universe or universes that are filled with intelligences from which we have cut ourselves off, having lost the senses by which we might know them."[65] Surrounded by intelligences with whom we no longer know how to communicate, the need for shamanic intermediaries between humanity and these higher minds is clear. The alien intelligences can guide us into truths unknown to us, Mack contends, teaching us to stop war, ecological disaster and racial conflict.[66]

Apparently we have been in contact with such beings for a very long time indeed. Mack writes of the "long story of humankind's relationship to vehicles and creatures appearing from the heavens that goes back to antiquity."[67] Moreover, mythology traditionally has provided a language for communicating the essence of these encounters. This "connection between humans and beings from other dimensions has been illustrated in myths and stories from various cultures for millennia."[68] Thus, myth is as central to Mack's explanation of the alien abduction phenomenon as it is to Houston's understanding of the encounters of inner journeying.

But the West's understanding of consciousness has prevented Western people from recognizing the true nature of contacts with the other side. "Throughout history, many societies have acknowledged consciousness as something more potent than we have in the west—as a sieve or receiver and transmitter of communication with forces, not always visible, other than ourselves."[69] Thus, Mack concludes, "It would seem that today's UFO abductees are continuing an amply documented tradition of ascent and extraterrestrial communication." The meaning of "extraterrestrial

communication" is relatively clear, but what does Mack mean by "ascent"? Apparently a spiritual issue comes into play here, with abductees taking a step up spiritually through their experiences with alien beings.

As support for the view that abductees are on a spiritual journey, Mack cites folklorist Peter Rojcewicz, who "has compared the experience of today's abductees" with "aerial and abduction phenomena" in earlier times and other cultures. Rojcewicz finds "the possibility of the existence of an intelligence, a spirit, an energy, a consciousness behind UFO experiences and extraordinary encounters of all types, that adapts its form and appearance to fit the environment of the times."[70] Thus, Mack believes that, in addition to UFO abductees, "contemporary examples of such entities in the West might be the spirit guides that are reported by many individuals."[71]

The shamanic connection. In *Abduction*, John Mack entertains the idea that consciousnesses from another dimension are actively seeking to contact and influence the human race. But in order to receive the benefits of such contact, one's worldview must include openness to these cosmic conversations. Religions and worldviews that allow for such a possibility are commended. Those that limit the view of consciousness or that demonize contact with spirits are to be censured, for we are on the verge of a new, shamanic religious consciousness.

"What function," he asks, "do events like UFO abductions and various mystical experiences play in our psyches and in the rest of the cosmos?"[72] His answer to this question appears to be a religious one: "The UFO abduction experience, while unique in many respects, bears resemblance to other dramatic, transformative experiences undergone by shamans, mystics, and ordinary citizens who have had encounters with the paranormal."[73] The abductee takes on the crucial role of providing a bridge between mundane experience and the spirit world beyond, and she does this in much the same way as the mystic or shaman of lore. "The mystic or shaman, like the abductee, makes a pilgrimage, usually with ardor, to receive a new dimension of experience or knowledge."[74]

Mack even finds that abductees often perceive their alien visitors as animals—"owls, eagles, raccoons, and deer"—which he quickly points out is remarkably similar to the reports of tribal shamans regarding their encounters with beings from the spirit world. "The connection with animal spirits is very powerful for many abductees." Mack believes that "this shamanistic dimension needs further study" because such events "cannot be understood within the framework of the laws of Western science," even though "they are fully consistent with beliefs developed

thousands of years ago by other non-Western cultures."[75] Joseph Campbell also noted that the Hindu term *marga* "means 'path or track, trail of an animal, to be followed,' and this is precisely what is implied by C. G. Jung's term 'the archetypes of the unconscious.'" Following these animal guides "we are led—if we can follow—beyond maps, according to the Indian view, to the seat from which all the gods have sprung, which is the revelation of the deepest source and being of ourselves."[76]

Mack notes that abductees, like all shamans, possess a peculiar openness to diverse spiritual experiences. "I have the impression that the abductees as a group are unusually open and intuitive individuals, less tolerant than usual of societal authoritarianism, and more flexible in accepting diversity and the unusual experiences of other people."[77] Abductees may, in fact, be of an entirely different species than the rest of us. Mack writes about some abductees "being told by an alien female that she was their true mother." The abductees felt that "in some vague but deep way that this is actually true, i.e., that they are not 'from here' and that the Earth mother and father are not their true parents."[78] Mack suggests in *Abduction* that such accounts of alien parentage, as well as of strange sexual experiments reported on some abductees, are related to alien efforts to prepare the human race for the next stage in its physical and spiritual evolution.

The abductee is for Mack, then, a uniquely spiritual being, a religious seer, a shaman bearing messages from another realm and the harbinger of a new human race. Many other modern day shamans have claimed that beings from other planets were trying to contact and educate the human race, usually on the rationale that our spiritual and social progress would thus be enhanced. Sometimes the initial contact is more spiritual than physical. Thus, Wilfred Kellogg claimed that his massive *The Urantia Book*, a "history of the galaxy and the solar system," came to him through channeling messages from aliens.[79]

Mack's work with UFO abduction claimants is remarkable, both in the fact that his own status lends credence to the reports of abductees and in his tendency to view the abductees as contemporary shamans. In a fashion typical of New Religious Synthesis efforts to appropriate science to spirituality, Mack argues that Western science is currently undergoing "spectacular advances in physics, biology, neuroscience, and psychology," which may "shed light on" abduction experiences and other mystical or shamanistic phenomena.[80]

In a similar vein, Whitley Streiber has written about his experiences with aliens in enormously popular books such as *Communion* and *Transformation: The Break-*

through. He has also collected various evidences for alien contact in *Confirmation: The Hard Evidence for Aliens Among Us.*[81] As the titles of these books imply, Streiber finds a virtually religious significance in human encounters with aliens, which he terms the "visitor experience." He writes, "The 'visitor experience' is old. Two hundred years ago a farmer might have come in from plowing and said, 'I just saw fairies dancing in the glen.' A thousand years ago he might have seen angels flying." Though the experience is ancient, it now has a new dimension. "That we could ever conceive of being in relationship with this force is what is new about the visitor experience in modern times." This is possible because, "thankfully, the very way we think and perceive our universe may be changing."[82]

As we shall see in the next section, sources of spiritual wisdom from nonhuman entities are not limited to UFO abductees. In fact, Jesus himself has recently been transformed into a spirit guide.

PAUL FERRINI AND THE JESUS PHENOMENON

Paul Ferrini, a "spiritual counselor" from Massachusetts, has written a number of books advocating a new approach to religion, one with shamanic overtones. In one of his most influential books, *Love Without Conditions: Reflections of the Christ Mind*, Ferrini claims to bring a message directly from Jesus Christ.[83] He urges his readers to cultivate their own capacity to make direct contact with a consciousness existing beyond ordinary experience. Moreover, the Jesus to whom Ferrini introduces his readers shares similarities with the "Inner Friend" described by Jean Houston—an interior guide to spiritual truth, perhaps another name for the self. "To think of Jesus as being outside of and independent of your mind," Ferrini writes, "is to miss the point. For it is in your mind that Jesus addresses you." Ferrini even describes his Jesus as "your most intimate friend speaking to you, sometimes in words, often beyond words."

Ferrini's Jesus makes no unique claims to divinity or spiritual authority and, in fact, advocates religious pluralism. Jesus is merely the mouthpiece of something called "the Christ Mind," a universal consciousness expressed in varying ways in many religious traditions. Thus, Jesus is not unique; he is simply one among many spirit voices of universal truth. "Let us be clear," writes Ferrini in his role as shaman, "that Jesus has no exclusive place or position in the Christ Mind." Rather, "Krishna, Buddha, Moses, Muhammad, Lao Tze, and many others are consciously joined with him there, or perhaps I should more accurately say 'here.'" Thus, we

may address Jesus by any number of names. "If you feel more comfortable addressing yourself to Buddha or Krishna, please do so. Jesus will not be offended. Indeed he will be pleased because you are following his teaching of non-separation."[84] All people "commune and communicate with the Christ Mind (you can say Buddha Mind or Brahman or Holy Spirit if you prefer)." This is because "we are all joined with the mind of God."[85]

Ferrini advocates an essentially gnostic spirituality in which this One Mind shows up as a divine spark in all people. "Each of us has a tiny spark of light that illuminates the darkness of our unconsciousness." This "divine spark of awareness" keeps our "connection to God alive."[86] With these framing considerations in mind, what does Jesus have to say to us through Ferrini?

Jesus speaks: lessons from the Christ mind. Ferrini insists in *Love Without Conditions* that he is not "channeling" Jesus. He does claim, however, shaman-like contact with a being he labels Jesus, and this spiritual contact becomes a source of authority for a wide range of teachings. One of the first lessons we learn through Ferrini's Jesus is that religious division is wrong, that "divisions into religions are relics of this world." Jesus informs Ferrini that "such boundaries do not exist in the Christ Mind, where all beings join in a single goal."[87] Thus, the foundational Revealed Word notion that Christianity is uniquely true is categorically false; Jesus himself says so. Ferrini assures us that "Jesus does not ask us to convert to Christianity, for there is no such thing." For the Jesus with whom Ferrini communicates, "Christianity is a myth of separation. It divides the Christian from the Jew or the Muslim or the Buddhist." Ferrini asks rhetorically, "Do you think that Jesus would advocate such an idea? Of course not."[88]

There is more to learn from Jesus than the message of religious pluralism. Among other things, Jesus is *not* concerned about sin, in fact, he does not even believe in the concept. "My teaching is a simple one: I teach the forgiveness of sins. I teach that sin itself is not real."[89] It follows that human evil is also an illusion. Moreover, the body is not important, for the true individual is a spirit that experiences neither birth nor death. "You are not the body, for the body is born and dies, and you are not born, nor do you die."[90] The Revealed Word teaching that the body *is* significant is an unhelpful thought, and "unhelpful thoughts must be eliminated. This is the essence of mind training."[91]

Ferrini demotes the Jesus of history—whose teachings have been twisted by Christians—and elevates the *spirit* Jesus who can inform us directly and accurately.

The latter states through Ferrini that "my teaching has been and will continue to be distorted because it threatens every thought which is false."[92] At the heart of Jesus' true spiritual teaching is a central tenet of the New Religious Synthesis— that we are embodied for a time, only to be released eventually through a process of spiritual evolution. Feelings of guilt are themselves just part of an evolutionary process taking place while we remain in our embodied stage. In this way "unresolved issues of self-worth" are being worked out as we progress spiritually. Oddly, Jesus teaches that each of us "selected" our parents in order, he tells us, to "exacerbate your guilt so that you can become conscious of it."[93] Once conscious of guilt, it can be eliminated as a false concept. Conversely, feelings of guilt are not the result of any actual wrongdoing on the reader's part.

Paul Ferrini's performs a shamanic function in *Love Without Conditions*, making contact with a spiritual entity named Jesus who speaks truth derived from a diffuse divinity called the Christ Mind. Ferrini's Jesus has much to say that assists the reader in making spiritual progress, much of it in direct contradiction to the Revealed Word tradition as expressed in the New Testament. Ferrini's message of a unity at the heart of all faiths will be taken up in the next chapter when we consider how, in the New Religious Synthesis, the shaman's experience of a direct encounter with the realm of the spirit has now become a crucial argument for religious pluralism.

CONCLUSION

In his bestselling book *The Seat of the Soul* (1989), frequent Oprah Winfrey Show guest Gary Zukav takes for granted the existence of "nonphysical Teachers" who come to us from "levels of Light" that are beyond our immediate perception.[94] These "impersonal consciousnesses" are often involved in instructing human beings in the higher spiritual truths, such as the evolutive nature of the cosmos and the fundamental unity of all things. In other words, these spirit beings accept some of the basic tenets of the New Religious Synthesis and are here to teach them to us. "This is not their home, so to speak. They are teachers to our plane. They are free to teach in our plane without being of our plane." That these Teachers can come to us in our plane without becoming one with our plane is a result of their having transcended duality altogether. They live in the plane of the ultimate unity of all things, and this "is simply the natural dynamic of evolution." Zukav assures his readers that "as you evolve beyond [duality], and also when you leave your physical body and journey home to your nonphysical plane of reality, you will not exist in dualism."[95]

Zukav takes for granted several foundational elements of the New Religious Synthesis: the fundamentally evolutive nature of the universe, the spiritual evolution of human beings and the essential unity and divinity of all things. Compatible with these is the presence of spirit teachers to guide us on in our evolutionary progress. Moreover, these entities and "advanced human souls" go on to inhabit "millions, indeed, billions of life-filled planets."[96] In fact, he asserts that "there is not one planet that lacks a level of active consciousness, some of it akin to our human form, and some of which does not come close to our form." These members of "the Angelic kingdom" are here to "guide and interact with us" in order to assist our evolution. Moreover, they have assisted with "the evolution of other galaxies and Life forms there."[97]

Zukav's fundamental thesis is compatible with the position outlined by Emanuel Swedenborg more than two hundred years ago and has been reiterated in innumerable popular religious texts in the modern period. It is present not only in Madame Blavatsky's treatises, but also in John Mack's alien abductee accounts. Other examples of this position appear in contemporary popular religious writing. For example, Neale Donald Walsch affirms in his *Conversations with God* that there is life on other planets, that human beings have been visited by aliens and that we currently are being observed.[98]

In the cosmos of the New Religious Synthesis there is no sovereign deity, though minor deities abound. They may be identified as spirits or aliens, inner guides or higher selves, ascended masters or highly evolved intelligences. Whatever the name they are called, they have something of profound spiritual significance to tell humanity. Often they seek to instruct us through their human mouthpieces in proper theology, or at the very least to correct theological misconceptions.

The theological perspective articulated by spirit guides contradicts that of the Revealed Word. Swedenborg's planetary spirits repudiate the historical details of the Christian gospel, while Blavatsky's ascended masters reveal ancient spiritual secrets that prove Christianity to be a spiritual aberration. And so it goes right down to the present—Paul Ferrini's Christ proclaims a distinctly unchristian religious pluralism.

Lacking a sovereign deity, the Other Spirituality's evolutive universe yields up its secrets by two means—scientific enquiry and spirit contact. And, as it turns out, both sources say complementary things. Similarly, Jeremy Narby reports experiments in which shamans help research scientists resolve difficult experimental

issues. Of one such collaborative effort he writes, "This experiment seemed to show that scientists can learn a good deal by working with Amazonian shamans." Thus, he concludes, "Bringing scientists and shamans together seems more like a beginning."[99] In the Other Spirituality, shamanism and science embrace. The next chapter explores in detail the case for religious pluralism embedded in the shaman's mystical experience.

10

THE MYSTICAL PATH
TO PLURALISM

Discovering That All Is One in Religion

⟳✕⟲

It is striking how similar the analysis of human "interior life" reads among mystics of all the great religions, be the individual Jewish, Zen-Buddhist, Sufi, or Christian.

RICHARD ROHR, The Enneagram

There is a unity at the heart of all religions. More than moral it is theological, but more than theological it is metaphysical in the precise sense of the word. The fact that it is thus transcendent, however, means that it can be univocally described by none and concretely apprehended by few.

HUSTON SMITH, *introduction to*
The Transcendent Unity of Religions

Evidence suggests that the deepest origins of religion are based in mystical experience.

ANDREW NEWBERG AND EUGENE D'AQUILI,
Why God Won't Go Away

Is Jesus Christ the unique mediator of salvation? I was one of five panelists assigned to address this question at a recent meeting of Catholic theologians. I was the first to speak and, as it turned out, the only panelist prepared to advance an unqualified affirmative response to this question.

J. A. DI NOIA, *in* First Things

⟳✕⟲

In his recent book *The Mystic Heart*, Catholic lay brother Wayne Teasdale has written that mystics and "some enlightened philosophers" have long "known and proclaimed the essential interconnectedness of all things," which is "consciousness itself!"[1] Human consciousness is, for Teasdale, simply our participation in "*a community of consciousness*" that is present everywhere.[2] Science, for Teasdale, supports this spiritual insight. He invokes Amit Goswami, "one of the most eloquent voices

in physics today," to confirm "a familiar new paradigm: that consciousness is the basis of reality."[3] That is, science proves that consciousness, not the Revealed Word's personal God, is "the basis of reality."

According to Teasdale, "the real religion of humankind can be said to be spirituality itself, because mystical spirituality is the origin of all the world's religions." He predicts that "the religion of the third millennium" will be pluralistic in nature—"the sharing of ultimate experiences across traditions."[4] Mystical experience, then, is the common core of all religious traditions, and as such the basis of a new spiritual paradigm to replace the Revealed Word. Mysticism "points to the realization that although there are many spiritual paths, a universal commonality underlies them all."[5]

Teasdale acknowledges that some mystics are seeking contact with a personal God. However, these "mystics" are in the minority and misunderstand the nature of the mystical experience. The "mystery and reality known for tens of thousands of years by mystic sages" includes the truth that "we are all already divine, and we simply have to wake up and realize it."[6] Despite theological differences that tend to divide people of different faith traditions, mysticism unites the various faiths through a common experience of Ultimate Reality. Through mystical experience, the human race will learn to transcend the restraints of differing theologies.

Teasdale also acknowledges that in Buddhism and Christianity one finds an apparently irreconcilable contradiction between atheism and theism. As he articulates the point, "the basic contradiction lies between the Buddhist concept of no god, and the Christian commitment to God."[7] Nevertheless, he writes that "Buddhism and Christianity have a historic mission to create, together, a new vision for the world." These two historic faiths will lead the way to religious unity by making "a precious contribution toward the evolution and communication of a new consciousness all around the world."[8] Such a "breakthrough" will take us to "a higher level of awareness."[9] For Teasdale, the awareness that transcends theological contradictions will come not through theology but through "mystical practice and a new spirituality." He adds, "The resulting spirituality or mystical practice will embrace the totality available from the vast deposit of humankind's inner experience."[10]

Pluralism has come to dominate the Western religious scene in the past thirty or so years. The pluralistic perspective affirms that all religions provide unique insights into the transcendent and reflect a similar human longing for the divine. In addition, pluralism insists that no single faith can make an exclusive claim to

truth and that there is no superior spiritual perspective from which other perspectives can be assessed.

The presence of a strong and apparently inextinguishable human religious impulse has itself been advanced to support pluralism, and the goal of much scholarship over the past two centuries has been to discover the common origin of all religions. The project of discovering what Mircea Eliade has called "the *fundamental unity* of all religious phenomena," then, has been at the center of religious research and speculation in the modern period.[11] Though this is a long and complex chapter in Western intellectual history, an overview of some important developments provides us with a sense of the project's history.

English Deists of the seventeenth and eighteenth centuries believed that Reason was the source of an early and universal religion. In *De religioni laici* (1645), Lord Herbert of Cherbury (1583-1648) observed that each faith shares many points in common with the others.[12] In *Of Truth* (1624), he argued that the universal practice of worship and sense of repentance indicated that human reason apprehended a common spiritual truth in the cosmos. In 1794, a French writer by the name of Dupuis published a three-volume treatise entitled *On the Origin of all Forms of Worship*, in which he maintained that all human religions could be traced back to astrology and the worship of the stars.[13]

In the early nineteenth century, the great theologian Friedrich Daniel Ernst Schleiermacher (1768-1834) contended that Jesus Christ represented a starting point in a new phase of human spiritual progress. Just as biological life progressed, so spiritual progress followed a similar path. Jesus Christ represented this "first point" in an ongoing spiritual process, a man "entirely unique in that he was dominated by the consciousness of God as no man had been before and no man has since been."[14] Christ reflected "absolute dependence upon God," an experience noted in all faiths, each expressing the concept in differing but legitimate fashions.

By the middle of the nineteenth century, psychological theories emerged that placed the origin of religion within the human mind. In *The Essence of Christianity* (1841), Ludwig Feuerbach (1804-1872) argued that human beings possess an innate desire to create an ideal humanity, really an ideal self. This overwhelming desire for personal perfection leads us to create gods who embody the virtues we would like for ourselves. Thus, Feuerbach "reduced religion to unconscious self-projection."[15]

The twentieth century produced additional explanations of religion's universality. Rudolf Otto's book *The Idea of the Holy* (1917) found a human encounter with

"the numinous"—something divine and awe inspiring—to be at the heart of all authentic religious experience. Religious feeling arises from "that strange and profound mental reaction to the numinous," which Otto referred to as "'creature feeling' or creature consciousness." This awareness of a divine reality, even of a divine person, beyond our sensate comprehension leads to "the diminution of the self into nothingness."[16] Even the early "Religion of Primitive Man" reflects such a "numinous dread" that later matures into "more highly developed forms of numinous emotion."[17] Otto saw Christianity as the highest and most fully developed expression of what he took to be an authentic human encounter with the divine. In Christianity, the primitive dread of the numinous "invades the mind mightily . . . with the words: 'Holy, holy, holy.'"[18]

Not all twentieth-century explanations were so complimentary of the religious believer, however. Sigmund Freud (1856-1939), in his 1927 work *The Future of an Illusion*, advanced the now famous hypothesis that early human beings personified nature in order to gain a sense of control over its forces.[19] Thus were created gods responsible for rain, fire, sun and wind. These gods helped to ameliorate human fear in the face of the extraordinarily powerful forces at work in the natural world. Nature gods eventually became supernatural parents who were at once feared, appeased, petitioned and worshiped. The Jews invented the notion of a single parent-God.[20]

Freud's associate and disciple Carl Jung developed a theory of his own as to the origins of human religions. Jung had an abiding interest in religion and was particularly taken with gnosticism. Like Freud, he maintained that all religious ideas, including the idea of God's existence, are generated within the human mind. Unlike Freud, he affirmed the existence of a source of religious ideas common to all human minds, which he dubbed the "collective unconscious." The collective unconscious is a kind of deep and common memory that binds human beings to one another and to their ancestors. Thus, religions are the products of "a deity-engendering faculty within the human psyche."[21]

Other explanations of religion have turned upon a society's need for a mutually binding moral code, the search for meaning in human experience, the structure of the human mind, the devious efforts of a priestly caste to gain social dominance, and human wonder in the presence of great power such as that of the sun. The famous primatologist Jane Goodall suggested in 1970 that the exuberant reaction of apes watching a waterfall revealed the evolutionary origins of the sublime feelings in humans that were the source of the first religions.[22] Recent

speculation about the evolution of the brain, however, has turned increasingly to a hypothesis close to the center of New Religious Synthesis thinking. In *The Mystical Mind: Probing the Biology of Religious Experience,* psychiatrist Eugene G. D'Aquili and physician Andrew B. Newberg argue that the brain's evolution has equipped it specifically for the mystical experience.[23] Moreover, this universal mystical encounter with a realm beyond the physical accounts for the variety of human religions. Thus, at least some scientific research is moving in the direction of a particular argument for religious pluralism.

This chapter explores one of the "common source" arguments for religious pluralism that advocates of the New Religious Synthesis have endorsed with remarkable consistency. This approach finds mystical experience or the experience of spiritually sensitive individuals to be the source and center of human spirituality throughout the ages. Historian Roland Bainton has noted that "mysticism is actually found in all religions, and can very readily conceive of Christianity as simply one among many valid approaches to God."[24] This effort to bring the Revealed Word under the mystical umbrella runs contrary to its two most foundational and controversial claims about itself—that it is directly revealed by a personal and wholly other God and that it is uniquely true among the world's religious traditions. This chapter considers several important efforts to render mysticism the essence of human religious experience, and in this way to make it the basis of a powerful argument for religious pluralism emerging out of the New Religious Synthesis.

The chapter begins by considering some important early efforts to discover a common source of the human religious experience. We will then turn our attention to the specific effort to ground an argument for pluralism in mysticism. One major proponent of this view is the nineteenth-century Canadian physician R. M. Bucke, who argued that mysticism was an essential stage in the evolution of the human spirit. Frithjof Schuon is another prominent voice in the effort to place mystical or "esoteric" experience at the center of human spiritual life, and we will consider both his argument in *The Transcendent Unity of Religion,* as well as comparative religions scholar Huston Smith's endorsement of Schuon's ideas. One of the more persuasive voices for religious pluralism in the last fifty years has been Joseph Campbell. We will consider how mysticism plays an important role in his arguments for a new approach to accommodating religious diversity. The chapter concludes by exploring Marcus Borg's argument that Jesus himself should be understood as a mystic whose experience of the realm of the spirit has been shared by many founders of religions.

AN ORIGINAL RELIGION

As noted in chapter two, several prominent European scholars of the Renaissance period advocated an undifferentiated view of religion. Bainton notes that Renaissance mystics in particular "sought to discover the same set of truths beneath the symbols of many systems: in the lore of Zoroaster, the mysteries of Hermes Trismegistus, in the alluring number speculations of the Jewish cabala." Some sought to establish a World Parliament of Religions based on mystical insights.[25] Fifteenth-century scholar Nicholas of Cusa argued in 1453 for "a fundamental harmony linking all faiths to the worship of a common hidden God," not the self-revealing God of the Revealed Word. Bradford Verter notes that in Nicholas and other similar thinkers we find "seeds of both esoteric mysticism and theological unitarianism."[26] The important Renaissance writer Pico della Mirandola blended Neo-Platonism, Hermeticism, Christianity and the kabbalah as part of his search for a mystically based religious unity.[27]

European colonial expansion provided additional impetus for pluralistic theories. Religious documents from the Eastern world in particular contributed to the sense that a single, unifying source lies at the foundation of all religions. Some European scholars concluded that "all of Eastern religion must have been reducible to a single pattern," which might be considered "a gentile approximation of Christianity," albeit with an important difference.[28] Eastern faiths tended to posit a diffuse divine essence rather than the personal God of the Revealed Word, an essence best understood through mystical experience rather than rational apprehension.

Not until the seventeenth century did pluralistic arguments begin to achieve genuinely popular acceptance. Charles Blount (1654-1693) was the first successful proponent of a religious pluralism based on comparing various faiths. Blount collected the views of ancient religions on an afterlife in his work *Anima mundi (World Spirit)* (1678).[29] This work introduced British readers to several religions of the Near and Far East, advocating in the process their underlying pantheism and direct experience of the divine. Blount systematically compared a number of religions in order to demonstrate that there exists in each an irreducible pantheistic core, the fundamental element, he argued, of a natural human religion. Personal experience of a divine essence and a corresponding religious pluralism rooted in such experience were already being advocated in tandem as components in a new religious understanding.

In *Oracles of Reason* (1693), Blount compared various ancient religious sources

and examined the foundational doctrines of Islam, Hinduism and Zoroastrianism.[30] In his search for an argument supporting pantheism and condemning Revealed Word exclusivity, Blount scoured classical and contemporary religious texts including works by early Christian heretics such as Philostratus, Porphyry and Celsus. He also examined classical writers such as Lucian, Seneca and Cicero, the Arabian philosopher Averroes and European Humanists and skeptics such as Erasmus, Montaigne, Bacon, Spinoza, Hobbes and Locke.[31] The result was a catalog of religions and religious philosophy, initially intended as a sourcebook for skeptics.[32] Blount's efforts to discover a common basis for human religions, however, inspired a generation of writers seeking an argument for religious pluralism as an antidote to Revealed Word exclusivity.

True religion that recognized the divine in nature was universal. So how did the misleading Revealed Word tradition arise? The notion of a personal God who demanded a particular kind of belief for salvation, it was argued, grew out of the efforts of a priestly caste to overturn natural religion. The Deists' name for this error was "Priestcraft." Blount argued that the conspiracy against direct experience of the natural divinity started when a priestly class began exploiting the fear of death. The original priest was a "crafty discerning person, who having observed what is most dear to Mankind" pretended that he was "able to assist in the preservation of life." This proto-priest's goal was purely self-serving; he sought "esteem and credit in the world."[33] From such common ancestors the whole class of priestly types descended, seizing spiritual power by exploiting primal fears.[34] Freethinkers throughout history, however, employed reason to cut through the thick fog of fear and priestly deception, keeping alive the native human religion.

An intriguing eight-page pamphlet appearing on the streets of London in 1753 advanced anthropological evidence for an original and natural human religion. Its title, *A Speech Delivered by an Indian Chief in Reply to a Sermon Preached by a Swedish Missionary*, did not suggest the pamphlet's true intent—to affirm a universal religion still known to primitive people. Presented with the Christian gospel, a Native American tribal chief asserts that "every Man is possessed with sufficient Knowledge for his own salvation," and that this saving knowledge comes through "natural religion." Moreover, the chief was adamant that the missionary's Bible "can't add to natural religion."[35]

The argument for a universal religion of humanity received a boost in eighteenth-century Europe with the diligent work of the French scholar Anquetil du

Perron (1731-1805) to introduce Westerners first to Zoroastrianism and then to Hinduism. In 1754, when only twenty-three, du Perron visited India, where he became acquainted with the members of the Parsee sect, descendants of ancient Zoroastrians. A scholar named Dastur Darab introduced du Perron to the teachings of Zarathustra. In 1771, du Perron presented his French translation of the Avesta, the sacred book of Zoroastrianism that had shaped the religious thinking of the entire Eastern world. The book created an immediate and heated controversy when Christian missionaries and scholars challenged it, a controversy that only contributed to its readership.

Throughout his life du Perron published papers and books for a Western audience on the religions of the East. In the opening years of the nineteenth century du Perron returned from India with "a translation of the *Oupnek'hat*—a collection of fifty *Upanishads*—which gave the Western world its first deep insight into the baffling mind of the East." Carl Jung wrote that du Perron "brought the Eastern mind to the West, and its influence upon us we cannot as yet measure." Jung, ever the student of mystical experience, held that du Perron's work introduced to the West "the secret, spiritual influence of the East," and thus threw the Western spiritual mind into "confusion."[36] Mystical experience and the interior psychic life were now elevated in a fashion that permanently changed how Europeans and Americans thought about both the spiritual world and the origins of religion. The Revealed Word perspective with its external and personal God could no longer claim unchallenged dominance of Western religious thought. Moreover, the foundation of a new religious pluralism was in the making.

R. M. BUCKE

At the end of the nineteenth century, a Canadian physician advanced a surprisingly durable theory regarding the biological and religious evolution of the human race. Richard Maurice Bucke (1837-1902), in *Cosmic Consciousness: A Study in the Evolution of the Human Mind*, argued from historical evidence that certain individuals in the human family had already taken the next step in spiritual evolution and that this step involved mystical awareness or what he termed "Cosmic Consciousness." Bucke wrote that "this consciousness shows the cosmos to consist not of dead matter governed by unconscious, rigid, and unintending law; it shows it, on the contrary as entirely immaterial, entirely spiritual and entirely alive." Thus, Cosmic Consciousness opens one to the fact of pantheism, revealing that "the universe is

God and that God is the universe, and that no evil ever did or ever will enter into it."[37] The experience of Cosmic Consciousness also "shows that death is an absurdity, that everyone and everything has eternal life." The experience of Cosmic Consciousness is "called in the East the 'Brahmic Splendour,'" while in "Dante's phrase," the experience is "capable of transhumanizing a man into a god."[38]

Cosmic Consciousness is, for Bucke, the third stage in the evolution of human consciousness. It follows simple consciousness or awareness of one's basic existence, and self-consciousness or awareness that one exists as a self distinct from others. In keeping with the New Religious Synthesis emphasis on science as a source of spiritual insight, Cosmic Consciousness will lead humankind into a scientific study of the divine that will enhance the human capacity to continue its spiritual evolution toward even greater consciousness. Developing an adequate science of God will take a great deal of time, according to Bucke, but is an important component in the spiritual destiny of the human race. Bucke writes, "If it has taken the race several hundred thousand years to learn a smattering of the science of humanity since its acquisition of self-consciousness, so it may take it millions of years to acquire a smattering of the science of God after its acquisition of Cosmic Consciousness."[39] Bucke, then, turns science in the direction of an ultimate theology, much like contemporary authors in the New Science genre.

Cosmic Consciousness is already known in some religions, though certainly not in all. It is the foundation of "the higher religions and the higher philosophies and what comes from them, and on it will be based, when it becomes more general, a new world of which it would be idle to try and speak today."[40] This next evolutionary step comes when our present minds are "overcrowded" with increasingly "larger, more numerous and more and more complex" concepts. Eventually, "the chemical union of several [such concepts] and of certain moral elements takes place," resulting in "cosmic consciousness."[41] That is, chemical pressures in the advanced human minds cause an eruption into the next level of consciousness. Thus we continue our "beginningless and endless ascent" toward a "higher life than any heretofore experienced or even conceived."[42]

Evolving consciousness, the moral nature and lunacy. In Bucke's late nineteenth-century theorizing, the "savage" represented an early stage in human mental development, as did the human child. Thus he could write that "as the individual physical man begins at the very bottom of the scale as a unicellular monad, so does the physical man begin on the bottom rung of the ladder of mind." For Bucke, the

"lower minds" of savage races lack important spiritual qualities such as "faith, courage, personal force, sympathy, and affection."[43] Only higher minds would be capable of advancing to Cosmic Consciousness, while lower human minds represent an evolutionary dead-end.

Something Bucke called "the moral nature" guides the evolution of higher minds. This "moral nature" determines "for the race at large" and "from age to age" what sort of place we experience the cosmos to be.[44] The general direction of the "moral nature" is to create a cosmos that is increasingly friendly and accepting. Already the whole world is better than it once was. "The whole human race and all living things have put on," writes Bucke, "a charm and sacredness which in the old times they were far from possessing." Our view of the divine is more sanguine under evolutionary pressures as well. "The governing powers of the universe (obedient to the same beneficent influence) have been gradually converted from demons into beings and forces less and less inimical, more and more friendly to man."[45] All of this is proof of our spiritual evolution, which "is a simple matter of growth strictly analogous to the unfolding of the branch from the bud, or the plant from its seed."[46]

Some races are evolving rapidly toward Cosmic Consciousness; others are moving more slowly. But there is hope, for spiritual evolution begins in individuals and spreads to larger groups. "When a new faculty appears in a race, it will be found, in the very beginning, in one individual of that race; later it will be found in a few individuals."[47] Still, evolved faculties appear only in those members of a race *who have reached full maturity*," for the spiritually immature "cannot over-pass or go beyond a mature individual of the same race."[48] Such spiritual maturity is often found in those we call mystics, and mystics may appear to us at first as lunatics.

For Bucke, a psychiatrist, "the large number of mental breakdowns, commonly called insanity, are due to the rapid and recent evolution of those [new] faculties" in the human race.[49] Some true mystics are taken to be insane only because they demonstrate abilities the rest of us do not yet have. However, "cases of cosmic consciousness should become more and more numerous" as well as "more perfect, more pronounced." Bucke was even willing to assert that "at least thirteen cases are so great that they can never fade from human memory—namely Gautama, Jesus, Paul, Plotinus, Muhammad, Dante, Las Casas, John Yepes, Francis Bacon, Jacob Behmen, William Blake, Balzac, Walt Whitman."[50]

Evolution toward pluralism. Cosmic Consciousness occurs with increasing frequency as history progresses. Bucke counts "five cases" in the eighteen-hundred-year

period from Gautama the Buddha to Dante, or "one case to every three hundred and sixty years." However, "from Dante to the present day" there have been more than six hundred cases. This means that "cosmic consciousness has been 4.8 times more frequent during the latter period than it was during the former."[51] Eventually, it will be a common experience, and finally, one spread throughout the human race. Thus, in the distant future distinctions among religions will disappear because every human being will share Cosmic Consciousness. For now, however, the rest of us must look for religious guidance to "the few who have been illumined."[52]

Cosmic Consciousness produces harmony among religious teachers, even ones whose followers mistakenly think they are at odds with the adherents of other faiths. Bucke states categorically that "there is no instance of a person who has been illumined denying or disputing the teaching of another who has passed through the same experience."[53] Thus, if Jesus' followers took him to be claiming that he was unique in some way, they misunderstood his message. According to Bucke, Jesus was "a Specialist—that is, he had Cosmic Consciousness."[54] But he was not the Son of God in the sense that the Revealed Word tradition means that term to be understood. He did, however, "have the earnest temperament" from which "the Cosmic Sense springs."[55]

Despite the coming religious egalitarianism, the Cosmically Conscious currently constitute a spiritual, emotional and physical elite. Bucke affirms that "in order for a man to enter into Cosmic Consciousness he must belong . . . to the top layer of the world of Self-Consciousness." The candidate for Cosmic Consciousness "must have a good physique, good health, but above all he must have an exalted moral nature, strong sympathies, a warm heart, courage, strong and earnest religious feelings."[56] Bucke's opinion as to whether a woman could take this next evolutionary step is uncertain.

The experience. Bucke gathered from the works of various mystics and visionaries their accounts of the initial leap into Cosmic Consciousness. The experience itself involved the sense of "suddenly, without warning . . . being immersed in a flame, or rose coloured cloud, or perhaps rather a sense that the mind is itself filled with such a cloud or haze."[57] At the very same time the Cosmically Conscious person is "bathed in an emotion of joy, assurance, triumph, 'salvation.'"[58] Following this "like a flash there is presented to his consciousness a clear conception (a vision) in outline of the meaning and drift of the universe."[59]

Insights arising from this mystical experience are almost doctrinal in nature, and

often contrary to the Revealed Word. They include the sense that "all life is eternal," that the universe is "a living presence" and an "infinite ocean of life," that "the soul of man is as eternal as God is" and that "the happiness of every individual is in the long run absolutely certain."[60] On the difficult issue of sin, which clearly and irreconcilably separates the Revealed Word from Cosmic Consciousness, Bucke is unyielding—the concept is false and misleading. "It is not that the person escapes from sin; but he no longer sees that there is any sin in the world from which to escape."[61] The work of drawing the human race out of error and toward Cosmic Consciousness "has been going on within us since the dawn of life on this planet."[62]

FRITHJOF SCHUON AND TRANSCENDENT RELIGIOUS UNITY

Perhaps the foundational text for all subsequent discussions of mysticism as the essence of pluralism is Frithjof Schuon's (1907-1998) classic *The Transcendent Unity of Religions*. In this dense polemical work, first published in 1957, the Swiss comparative religions scholar sets out his now famous distinction between exoteric and esoteric approaches to faith. Schuon argues that the latter takes a more open approach to religion, emphasizing experience over the exoteric's doctrine. Esoterics, for Schuon, represent a more advanced stage of religious attainment, as well as a path to religious enlightenment.

Born in Basel, Switzerland, on June 18, 1907, Schuon eventually immigrated with his family to France. From an early age he was drawn to the texts of Indian religion, especially the Upanishads and the Bhagavad-Gita. An avid student of Arabic, Schuon traveled in North Africa in the 1930s, becoming familiar with Islam. In 1939 he visited India, returning to Switzerland where he lived for forty years following World War II. On visits to America in the late 1950s, he lived with members of the Sioux and Crow tribes and studied their religious practices. The author of more than twenty books, Schuon was a world-renowned scholar in religion. In 1980 he took up residence in the United States, where he continued to write until his death in 1998.

Schuon's distinction between the exoteric and the esoteric religious believer has been widely adopted.[63] The exoteric believer demands literal understandings of external and accessible religious symbols, thus insisting, for example, that the Bible is to be read literally and historically rather than symbolically or allegorically. This leads to conclusions such as that Jesus actually *is* God in some literal sense, rather than recognizing that a phrase such as "Son of God" is to be taken as a symbolic ex-

pression of a spiritual reality. The esoteric seeker, on the other hand, recognizes that religious symbols are just that—representations of something incapable of linguistic description or of historical manifestation. The esoteric thus possesses a more sophisticated and flexible understanding of spiritual matters than does the exoteric.

For Schuon, a single divine reality lay behind various religious experiences and expressions. As renowned religions scholar Huston Smith explains, "Intimations and realizations of this supreme identity appear in varying degrees of explicitness in all revealed religions and constitute the point at which they are one."[64] Schuon found that the exoteric was "anchored" to a particular spiritual spot, believing in a single, uniquely true revelation. The esoteric, on the other hand can accept that "revelation has multiple and equal instances" and thus that "no single instance can be absolute." Smith notes that for Schuon, religious unity can only be realized "on the esoteric plane," even though esoterics constitute a "minority" of religious believers "who realize that they have their roots in the Absolute."[65] Exoterics are "less supple in their capacity for 'spiritual abstraction'" and are thus unlikely to realize commonality with members of other faiths.[66] The esoteric would be, in R. M. Bucke's terms, ready to take the next step toward Cosmic Consciousness.

Schuon sought to liberate religion from the Revealed Word notion of personal salvation rooted in exoteric doctrines such as the uniqueness of Jesus Christ and his atoning death.[67] Schuon found the exoteric's self-interested emphasis on personal salvation to deflect attention from Ultimate Reality, the true source of spiritual experience. "Exoteric ideology," he writes in *The Transcendent Unity of Religions*, is "limited to a relative point of view, that of individual salvation" which constitutes "an interested point of view."[68] "The exoteric point of view," he writes, "cannot comprehend the transcendence of the supreme Divine Impersonality. . . . Such truths are of too high an order, and therefore too subtle and too complex . . . to be accessible by the majority or formulated in a dogmatic manner."[69]

Schuon thus rejected the uniqueness of Jesus Christ as a manifestation of the divine Logos, albeit on a rather strange argument. "If Christ had been the only manifestation of the Word . . . the effect of His birth would have been the instantaneous reduction of the universe to ashes."[70] This is because "a universal Reality cannot have only one manifestation to the exclusion of others, for in that case it would not be universal."[71] In other words, Jesus Christ cannot be the one manifestation of the Divine, for then the Divine would not be universal.

Schuon finds "the Divine Authority" to be "inherent in every Revelation."[72] He

posited an early, unified and unsullied religion, which he termed "the Primordial Tradition" and which is "the only unique religion possible."[73] Under this Tradition, humankind experienced "thousands of years of sane and balanced existence," but then went astray. But the idea that God would save humanity through "a means so materially and psychologically ineffective as a new religion" like Christianity would render the Divine "monstrous."[74] The "ideology of 'the believers'" in a single, unique revelation is "nothing but an intentional and interested confusion between the formal and the universal."[75]

"Indispensable" religious ideas are not owned by one faith. "Indeed, the more important and indispensable any particular means of grace may be, the more certain it is that it will be found in all the orthodox forms in a mode appropriate to the environment in question."[76] In a famous formulation he affirmed that "the Divinity manifests Its Personal aspect through each particular Revelation and its supreme Impersonality through the diversity of the forms of Its Word."[77] Consequently, perceptive thinkers will recognize that Christ was one among many "God-men," individuals specially gifted both to experience and to express the inexpressible ultimate reality behind all religious symbols.[78] These are the most advanced esoterics, humanity's spiritual guides along the path to religious unity.

Prophets, inner reality and esoteric elites. Esoterism is not the religious view of most people, nor does it seek to explain the religious experience of the majority. In fact, Schuon held that "esoterism is reserved, by definition and because of its very nature, for an intellectual elite necessarily restricted in numbers."[79] Certain specially endowed individuals throughout human history—including both Christ and Muhammad—reflect an "inner reality" in which they are "identified with the Word," Schuon's term for an ultimate divine reality.[80] Indeed, "every being who has achieved metaphysical reality" is identified with Ultimate Reality or the Word.[81] Thus, Jesus of the Revealed Word represents but one among many expressions of the divine Word.

These spiritually attuned individuals are the God-men among us, and "without the idea of the 'God-man' esoterism would be deprived of an aspect of its very existence."[82] The fact that God-men experience Ultimate Reality in an extraordinary way undergirds statements such as Jesus' famous remark, "I and the Father are one." Such a man will join "his essential identity with the divine principle that alone is real."[83] On the other hand, those not so equipped for special spiritual experience are relegated to the status of "the collective average" who become "passive and un-

conscious transmitters of the symbols."[84] Thus, though Schuon's theory accommodates religious pluralism by finding the special experience of the esoteric at the heart of all legitimate spiritual expression, it may, like Bucke's account, result in a kind of spiritual elitism.

JOSEPH CAMPBELL: THE PERENNIAL PHILOSOPHY AS PLURALISTIC HOPE

Joseph Campbell (1904-1987) was one of the most famous intellectual figures of the twentieth century. His public fame was due to his many publications that clearly presented the history, geography and theory of myth. Campbell was the author of such widely read works as *The Hero with a Thousand Faces* (1949), the four-volume work *The Masks of God*, the five-volume *The Historical Atlas of World Mythology*, and innumerable book chapters, published lectures and essays. But Campbell was perhaps best known and remembered for his enormously popular television specials, *The Power of Myth*, with Bill Moyers on Public Broadcasting System, and *Transformations of Myth Through Time*, a televised series of lectures produced by Stuart Brown and William Free. The lectures from *Transformations* were published in book form in 1990, three years after Professor Campbell's death. Campbell contributed significantly to public acceptance of a religious pluralism rooted in myth and mystical experience.

Campbell popularized the idea that myths reflect recurring themes in human experience of the transcendent. He writes, "Throughout the mythologies and religious systems of the world, the same images, the same themes are constantly recurring." These he referred to as "elementary ideas," following the work of Adolf Bastian.[85] Campbell was a devoted student of Bastian's work and cites it frequently. Bastian's concept of *Elementargedanken* or elementary ideas is of particular importance to Campbell's theory of myth. Elementary ideas "characterize the recurrent themes and motifs that [Bastian] was everywhere encountering." Bastian also recognized that "wherever and whenever they appeared it would be in costumes local to that region."[86] Thus, basic religious ideas recur throughout the world, albeit dressed in native mythic costume.

Myths, power and pluralism. Campbell emphasized those myths conveying what he, like Aldous Huxley, liked to call the Perennial Philosophy, particularly "the mythologies and the interpretations of the myths in India."[87] The Perennial Philosophy posits an undifferentiated Ultimate Reality of consciousness in the universe, elevates

mystical experience as contact with this Ultimate Reality, and venerates the special spiritual knowledge of mystics. Campbell took the Indian Vedas, for example, as records of this experience of Ultimate Reality, literally as what has been *heard* by those who experience the Reality. He writes, "the word *veda* is from a Sanskrit root, *vid*, which means 'knowledge.'" Thus, "the Vedas are the manifestation of a specific kind of knowledge. It's called *sruti*, which means 'heard.'" In the Indian tradition, "the Rhishis, or saints, were people who did not invent the poems, the hymns of the Vedas. They heard them, just as anyone who listens to the muse will hear." The special knowledge of the Vedas can be employed to summon the gods. "Those who have heard deeply the rhythms and hymns and words of the gods can recite those hymns in such a way that the gods will be attracted." The Vedas, then, convey spiritual power to those who know them well. "The Vedas form the substance of the rituals by which the powers of nature, personified as gods, are invoked to support the intentions of Aryan society. You invoke the gods to do your will."[88] Those who control such power are "stronger than the gods." Thus, "an illuminated man is stronger than any deity. This is the great thing in the universe, and this is what the Brahman is."[89]

A component in the Perennial Philosophy, then, is that divine power is present in anyone who learns how to "turn in" and discover the deity within himself or herself. "All those gods that you are invited to worship through public sacrifice are projections of the fire of your own energy." This belief supports a kind of religious pluralism, for regardless of the god one says one is worshiping, one is worshiping oneself. "There's a wonderful passage in the Chandogya," writes Campbell. "Worship this god, worship that god, one god after another; those who follow this law do not know. The source of the gods is in your own heart. Follow the footsteps to that center and know that you are that of which the gods are born."[90] This idea, writes Campbell, is "the basic idea of the Perennial Philosophy. Deities are the symbolic personifications of the very energies that are yourself."[91]

The deep well of the human psyche. Campbell supported his case for the Perennial Philosophy, and for the religious pluralism that is its byproduct, with passages from the Tibetan Book of the Dead, a manual of instructions to help the spirits of the recently deceased find heaven. Though the full content of Campbell's description of this book need not detain us, one of its instructions is particularly relevant to the question of pluralism. The lama guiding a departed soul by the Book of the Dead tells it the following: "Try to bring into your consciousness the image of the lord that has been of your worship throughout your lifetime." Campbell adds, "this may be

any god, so long as that god has been understood as the supreme image of the powers of the energizing energies of the universe as they have operated in your lifetime. . . . Any deity that's been your top deity, this is the place to contemplate it."[92]

But even this deity must be released as the soul attempts union with Ultimate Reality by letting go of itself. The departed soul seeks "absolute Brahma, undifferentiated consciousness; that's what we're intending all the way here. You may speak of it as the Void, you may speak of it as the abyss, you may speak of it as mother light."[93] Undifferentiated consciousness is the ground of all genuine religious experience and thus a unifying factor in the case for religious pluralism. It is also the source of the universal myths arising from the "bottomless, deep and dark" well of "the human psyche itself."[94] These myths give voice to the unspeakable experience of direct contact with the unknowable, the "sphere of the intelligible," Ultimate Reality, or god. But Ultimate Reality clearly is not the personal and transcendent God of the Revealed Word whose consciousness is differentiated from that of human beings.

Funerals and hallucinogens. Ancient funerary rituals are, for Campbell, an important source of human mythology and thus of the Perennial Philosophy. These rituals often were efforts to make contact with Ultimate Reality in which hallucinogenic drugs played an important role. Campbell writes that "at one important site, at Shanidar in northern Iraq, there has recently been discovered a cave containing a number of burials, in one of which the body had been laid to rest on a bier of evergreen boughs overspread with flowers, the pollens of which could still be traced, and all of which have turned out to be plants with hallucinogenic properties. Some sort of belief in a life beyond death is here indicated, inspired perhaps by visions."[95] At least some early human mystical experiences implanting the idea of an Ultimate Reality, then, were drug-induced.

Huston Smith has recently made a similar observation about early human religious experiences and hallucinogenic drugs. In his most recent book, *Cleansing the Doors of Perception,* Smith writes that shamans, the "Native American Church" and some mystics employed "virtually nonaddictive mind-altering substances that are approached seriously and reverently," and suggests the word "entheogens" as a substitute for psychedelic in this regard.[96] For Smith "a connection exists" between entheogens and some human encounters with "God and the Infinite," a connection that he finds too often underestimated and insufficiently appreciated.[97]

In addition to the visions inspired by sacred drug use, traditions once vibrant in the West reflected the Perennial Philosophy, in Campbell's estimation. How-

ever, the West endured "a gradual attack on the mythological ideas," which separated its religious thought from "the elementary ideas." Nevertheless, Campbell notes that the elementary ideas endured in fringe traditions such as "Gnosticism, alchemy, and many of the discredited manners of thought that carry on this interest in what might be called the perennial philosophy."[98] Primitive people did not approach religion in an analytic fashion, and thus maintained a purer contact with the Perennial Philosophy. Campbell repeats Smith's point that the loss of primal religion is due to confusing concrete religious symbols with their abstract referents such as Ultimate Reality. "One of the great dangers to be avoided in the interpretation of *all* symbolic systems is that of mistaking the symbol for its reference—which, curiously, seems to be a mistake more likely to be made by teachers and students of our own symbolic heritage than even by illiterate hunters."[99] Thus, to make particular historical claims central to a religious system—as the Revealed Word does—is a mistake of this type.

Tribal hope. According to Campbell, the best hope for Westerners to retrieve the Perennial Philosophy is to return to tribal wisdom. Campbell finds such wisdom to parallel the aforementioned European traditions that were eventually abandoned. For instance, a twelfth-century translation of the Hermetic work *The Book of the Twenty-Four Philosophers* includes a statement "very much like his [Sioux medicine man Black Elk], which has been quoted, through the centuries, by a number of significant Western thinkers . . . and which is a wonderfully apt epitomization of the mystery that speaks to us everywhere through mystic vehicles: 'God is an intelligible sphere, whose center is everywhere and circumference nowhere.'" Campbell adds that "that is the elementary idea, and the function of all ethnic ideas is to link, as by a flexible tethering, all the acts, thoughts, and experiences of our daily lives—individual and social—to this realization."[100]

The true and central religious idea at the core of myth, mystical experience and the Perennial Philosophy, then, is the mystic's insights that God is "an intelligible sphere, whose center is everywhere and circumference nowhere." Religious systems adhering to this assertion are true and unifying, while those not recognizing such a theology are false and divisive. It follows that shamans and mystics are right to teach that God is a consciousness to be experienced, and that Revealed Word advocates are wrong to insist that God is a divine person to be worshiped. Clearly the latter perspective does not square with Campbell's notion that the individual is divine, the "source of all gods."

MARCUS BORG AND JESUS THE SPIRIT PERSON

Founding director Robert W. Funk of the University of Montana first convened the Jesus Seminar in 1985 under the auspices of the Westar Institute. The stated purpose of the Seminar is to investigate the figure of the "historical Jesus"—a term the group's website also puts in quotes—using the best scholarship and sources available. The Jesus Seminar has published a large number of books and other materials through Polebridge Press and has achieved a level of fame and generated a degree of controversy unusual for academic study groups. The Seminar's participants have not limited their public comments to biblical criticism, but also have advocated positions on a variety of religious issues including religious pluralism.

Marcus J. Borg is perhaps the most widely read member of the Jesus Seminar. Borg, a graduate of Oxford University, teaches in the Department of Religion and Culture at Oregon State University. The author of nine books, Borg has been both a provocative and persuasive voice in the recent Western religious conversation. In one of his bestselling books, *Meeting Jesus Again for the First Time*, Borg writes, "I agree with those who speak of each religious tradition as a 'cultural linguistic world.'" Though the religions of the world are "clearly not all the same," Borg is convinced that "the impetus for creating these cultural-linguistic worlds" of the different religions "comes out of certain kinds of extraordinary experiences that are cross cultural."[101] In *Meeting Jesus*, Borg seeks to redefine the historical character of Jesus as a mystic, a person in touch with the spirit world, a conduit of truth from another realm. As a mystic, Jesus becomes for Borg part of an argument for religious pluralism that complements the New Religious Synthesis.

Reconceptualizing God as "holy mystery." Borg's personal quest for a path to religious pluralism started with the realization that "God does not refer to a supernatural being 'out there' (which is where I had put God ever since my childhood musings about God 'up in heaven')." Rather, he writes, "I began to see, the word *God* refers to the sacred at the center of existence, the holy mystery that is all around us and within us."[102] God, for Borg, is transformed from the Revealed Word's wholly other and personal being—a view Borg associates with childhood—to a "holy mystery" that is everywhere and even in each one of us. "God, was no longer a concept or an article of belief, but had become an element of experience."[103]

Borg argues that traditional Revealed Word conceptions of a historical Jesus and a personal God reflect a "precritical naivete," which one grows beyond in the "critical thinking of adolescence and adulthood" when it is no longer necessary to demand

that the Bible's accounts be "literally true."[104] An evolution of theological thought occurs as the believer leaves literalism behind and moves on to find truth in the "extraordinary experience" of the God that is "all around us and within us." That is, mature theology is more clearly represented in the mystic's direct experiences of the spiritual realm than in the church's historical creeds and biblical literalism.

Jesus, spirit people and the mystic experience. Borg's research into the life of Jesus of Nazareth and the origins of religion leads him to classify Jesus as a "spirit person" rather than as the Revealed Word's Messiah or God incarnate. Indeed, Jesus the spirit person is difficult to distinguish from a mystic. Borg argues that the insight that Jesus was a spirit person is "foundational to everything else Jesus was." He continues, "the most crucial fact about Jesus was that he was a 'spirit person,' a mediator of the sacred, one of those persons in human history to whom the Spirit was an experiential reality."[105]

Borg indicates that it took him "a long time" to come to this realization about Jesus' true mystic nature. "The process began," he relates, "with the realization that there really are such phenomena as experiences of Spirit and spirit persons." Religions that recognize mysticism as the foundational human spiritual experience were the source of this insight for Borg. "The realization came to me initially not from the study of the Bible of the Christian tradition, but from the study of non-Western religions and cultural anthropology." When Jesus' mystic role is recognized, a new vista is opened on his life and ministry. "This illuminating category helps us see much about Jesus that we otherwise might miss," writes Borg.[106]

Borg explains that "spirit persons are known cross-culturally." They "have vivid and frequent experiences of another level or dimension of reality," experiences that "involve momentarily entering into nonordinary states of consciousness and take a number of different forms." These different forms include "visionary experiences" and "journeying into another dimension of reality" which is, to quote Borg, "the classic experience of the shaman."[107] This "other dimension of reality" that the spirit person, mystic or shaman enters is known by many names, such as "Yahweh, Brahman, Atman, Allah, the Tao, the Great Spirit, God."[108] Thus, making Jesus a shaman becomes for Borg both a source of great insight about Jesus and a step toward religious pluralism.

Borg renders mystic experience a defining quality of religious leaders; then he brings Jesus into the category of spirit person or mystic. The implication of such a maneuver is clear—all spiritual pioneers experience mystical entrances into the spirit world, a world parallel to our own, which is incapable of any genuine descrip-

tion in language and which must be experienced by the mystic directly. Thus, John Mack's comparison of his clients' ordeals with the experience of the mystic fits with Borg's understanding of the spirit person. "The mystic or the shaman," writes Mack, "like the abductee, makes a pilgrimage usually with ardor, to receive a new dimension of experience or knowledge."[109] Western science may eventually help us to understand these experiences, if it can accept dramatic changes in its presuppositions about the universe.

The spirit world of the mystic, the other reality that the spirit person experiences, is directly adjacent to our own. "This other reality it is important to emphasize," he argues, "is not 'somewhere else.' Rather, it is all around us, and we are in it."[110] Borg insists that Jesus was just another person capable of making the short passage to the Other Reality and then telling us about it. "Jesus was clearly a spirit person," he writes. Specifically, Jesus was a Jewish mystic: "The more we realize that there was a form of Jewish mysticism in first-century Palestine, the more likely it seems that Jesus stood in that experiential tradition."[111]

Moreover, Jesus is not unusual in this regard, for prophets, seers, mystics and shamans have always grounded religion on experience. Thus, the Revealed Word understanding of Jesus as unique mediator of human salvation, as revealer of the character of God himself, must be set aside in favor of a new perspective. "The image I have sketched views Jesus differently: rather than being the exclusive revelation of God, he is one of many mediators of the sacred." Borg adds, "Even as this view subtracts from the uniqueness of Jesus and the Christian tradition, it also in my judgment adds to the credibility of both."[112] Thus, he reasons that capitulating to the Other Spirituality actually strengthens the Revealed Word tradition.

Promoting Christianity by demoting Jesus. As I have indicated, embedded in Borg's account of Jesus as spirit person is an argument for religious pluralism. A single communication of divine truth in human history is highly unlikely. "What are the chances that God would speak only through this particular groups of people [the Jews]?"[113] Borg does not answer his rhetorical question, but clearly he is bothered by the logic of theological exclusivism. Mysticism thus becomes an important argument for religious pluralism—each tradition advances individuals who have experienced the "other reality," and Jesus is but one of these. Jesus had an "enlightenment experience similar to such experiences reported of other great sages."[114]

Jesus as spirit person is no longer understood as Son of God in the unique Revealed Word sense of the phrase. He is, rather, one among many sons and daugh-

ters of god, mystics who have traveled from this dimension to another and returned with a life-giving message. Borg writes, "This recognition subverts the common impression that Christian faith involves believing that Jesus was *literally* 'the Son of God.'" But this "is a helpful subversion," because "the literalist reading of 'Son of God' narrows the scope of Christology by giving primacy to one image."[115]

Borg overturns traditional understandings of the life and ministry of Jesus Christ, moving him outside of the frame of history and redefining him as a 'spirit person' in the mystic tradition. As a witness in support of this position, Borg brings Jesus himself. "His own self-understanding," Borg writes of Jesus, "did not include thinking of himself and speaking of himself as the Son of God whose historical intention or purpose was to die for the sins of the world, and his message was not about believing in him." Instead, Jesus cast himself in the role of "a spirit person, a subversive sage, social prophet, and movement founder who invited his followers and hearers into a transforming relationship with the same Spirit that he himself knew."[116]

The New Testament as myth. Consistent with New Synthesis constructions of the Bible, Borg's view of Jesus and his consequent reduction of Christianity to a mystic faith founded by a spirit person depend upon reading the Gospel accounts as narrative or myth. "The centrality of narrative in the Bible is also pointed to by the fact that it contains literally hundreds of individual stories." Moreover, "at the center of Scripture are a small number of 'macro-stories'—the primary stories that shaped the religious imagination and life of ancient Israel and the early Christian movement."[117]

Borg's point is reminiscent of David Strauss's search for mythi, recurrent mythical themes in the New Testament. Again the biblical account of Jesus is read, not as history, but rather as myth, as a narrative about the journeys of a spirit person to another reality. In this way, Jesus the spirit person is to be understood as similar in kind to many hundreds of such mystics and shamans throughout human history.

CONCLUSION

Religious pluralism rooted in the twin concepts of the divine as an Ultimate Reality and mystical experience as an encounter with that Reality is an important component of the New Religious Synthesis. Closely connected to spiritual evolution, mystical pluralism sees belief in concrete religious images and fixed revelations as an early stage in religious development, and thus as an impediment to the coming age of religious unity. An obstacle in the road toward that new day is the historically grounded Revealed Word tradition. In the Other Spirituality, all human reli-

gions are inadequate human attempts to express the inexpressible truth of a divine essence or consciousness beyond ordinary human experience.

Renaissance scholars in the Hermetic tradition hoped to discover the common core of all religious experience. The goal of their researches into the occult traditions of the ancients was a single world religion centered on mystical experience, guided by secret teaching and led by a priesthood of *magi* or enlightened spiritual masters. As John G. Burke, a leading expert on Renaissance Hermetism, has written of the notorious Dominican monk Giordano Bruno, "Bruno shared the feelings of his contemporary Hermetists that there should be one universal religion, but it was not a reformed Christendom that he desired. Instead, it was a return to the worship of ancient Egypt as described in the Hermetic literature."[118]

In the modern period, the ancient hope of a single world religion has had numerous advocates. At the end of the seventeenth century, Charles Blount affirmed an original, natural faith that began with the human race itself.[119] More recently, advocates of a new approach to religion have focused much attention on mystical experience as the likely source of that primordial human religious sense. We have noted how R. M. Bucke found mysticism to be a step along the path to spiritual maturity for the human race. More recently, Frithjof Schuon and Huston Smith have claimed the presence of an esoteric and mystical core at the heart of all faiths. Joseph Campbell, in apparent agreement, calls us to affirm the centrality of a direct experience of the spiritual realm to the world's great faiths. Finally, Marcus Borg makes Jesus a "spirit person," an individual with a peculiar capacity for encountering that realm. In this way, Jesus resembles the founders of other world faiths. These writers affirm a potent source of religious unity in the experiences of these spiritually gifted individuals. Similarly, Wayne Teasdale writes that "the real religion of humankind can be said to be spirituality itself, because mystical spirituality is the origin of all the world's religions."[120] He adds that "the religion of the third millennium" will be "the sharing of ultimate experiences across traditions."[121]

Mystical experience is the common core of all religious traditions, and as such the basis of a new spiritual paradigm, another spirituality to replace the Revealed Word. Mysticism "points to the realization that although there are many spiritual paths, a universal commonality underlies them all."[122] Similarly, Gary Zukav suggests that the special spiritual experiences of evolving human masters, "such as those after whom religions have been named on earth," accounts for the multiplicity of religions.[123] However, the argument for a new pluralism via mysticism runs

dramatically at cross-purposes to the internal logic of the Revealed Word. That logic states that God entered human history one time in the person of Jesus Christ, that Christ's atoning death occurred at a particular historical moment, and occurred but once, and that personal knowledge of God is available through faith rather than through mystical experience.

11

CONCLUSION

A New Spirituality for a New Age

In the beginning God created the heavens and the earth.
GENESIS 1:1 NIV

I have invented the world I see.
HELEN SCHUCMAN, A Course in Miracles

If a kingdom of heaven is desired, it must be synthesized from the available stuff.
JOSEPH CHILTON PEARCE, The Crack in the Cosmic Egg

We do not realize that while we are turning upside down the material world of the East with our technical proficiency, the East with its psychic proficiency is throwing our spiritual world into confusion.
CARL JUNG,
"The Difference Between Eastern and Western Thinking"

A dramatic shift in popular Western religious assumptions has occurred during the modern period, starting around 1700, and public religious advocates have played a central role in bringing about this fundamental alteration in spiritual outlook. We have surveyed the component parts of what I have called the New Religious Synthesis, a comprehensive religious view now successfully contesting the dominance of the Judeo-Christian tradition, or Revealed Word. The Revealed Word had affirmed a sovereign and personal God intervening continuously in human history, a single uniquely true revelation, a fallen humanity incapable of correcting its spiritual predicament, a central and historical act of atonement and the open proclamation of a message of forgiveness grounded in that divine act of redemption.

The New Synthesis reverses each major tenet of the Revealed Word. The Word's insistence on history as faith's foundation gives way to myth as the universal mode of spiritual expression. Salvation through faith in God's grace yields to the mystical episode as the elemental religious experience. An evolving universe infused with divine consciousness supplants a wholly other God, while human beings evolving toward a divinity of their own are no longer created in the image of such a God. Our rational self-awareness—Reason, Mind, Consciousness, Intellect—is the first inkling of our own latent divinity.

Science, Reason's instrument, provides theological insight to guide our quest for spiritual awareness and attainment. Among science's greatest revelations—second only to its confirmation of evolution as the operative principle of the cosmos—is that monism and pantheism are proven by deep inspection of physical matter. This massively significant discovery confirms ancient ideas about universal unity originally delivered through shamans and mystics and still reflected in tribal spirituality.

The New Synthesis affirms a new *gnosis* consisting of spiritual and scientific secrets. These keys to our spiritual advancement are available first and most clearly to a knowing elite of shamans and scientists—the new gnostics. Moreover, in spite of its foundational pantheism, the New Religious Synthesis embraces a host of minor divinities—spirit guides, teaching angels and alien visitors. A consistent message of these voices, delivered via a new class of seers, prophets and magical scientists, is that all faiths express the presence of the numinous sphere just beyond ordinary experience. In addition to advocating religious pluralism, the same entities can usually be counted on to confirm evolutionism and monism. In these ways the New Science and the New Shamanism are completely in sync, their collaboration providing a virtually irrefutable double-barreled argument for the New Religious Synthesis. When angels and scientists agree, who are mere humans to doubt their word?

It has often been noted, and succinctly expressed by Richard Weaver, that ideas have consequences. And no ideas have greater consequences than our religious ideas. As the West moves steadily in the direction of a new spirituality, it becomes imperative to ask whether the New Religious Synthesis provides an adequate account of our human condition and of our spiritual destiny. For instance, what does the resuscitated ancient wisdom have to tell us about who we are as human beings and about our destiny? What is gained and lost in embracing its conception of divinity? Does the New Synthesis adequately address the problem of evil? These are fundamentally religious questions, and the adequacy of the answers they receive

from the Other Spirituality will affect every aspect of our existence. By the same token, does our previous spiritual perspective, what I have termed the Revealed Word, provide better answers to these basic religious questions? Returning briefly to the topics addressed in previous chapters, I would like to offer several implications of our present spiritual direction.

TAKING LEAVE OF HISTORY

In a 1916 interview with Charles N. Wheeler of the *Chicago Tribune*, Henry Ford made the famous statement "History is more or less bunk." While proponents of the New Religious Synthesis do not typically approach history quite so dismissively, they often either express a discomfort with history as a source for spirituality or treat history as an infinitely malleable concept with no grounding in actual events. Instead, personal experience in the realm of the spirit and the insights of experimental science are presented as the fountains from which flows spiritual truth. By contrast, while not denying the validity of individual spiritual experience, advocates of the Revealed Word perspective have always insisted on history—not individual experience—as the ground of religion.

The apostle Paul, by his own account, experienced something that can only be classified as a direct, personal encounter with the divine. A blinding light so powerful that it knocked him to the ground and a voice instructing him about the subsequent course of his life transformed Saul of Tarsus into Paul the apostle. However, despite his own arresting experience, Paul made the physical and historical resurrection of Jesus Christ the sine qua non of Christian theology. "If Christ has not been raised," he wrote in his first letter to the Corinthian church, "our proclamation has been in vain and your faith has been in vain" (1 Cor 15:14). Similarly, the evangelist Luke began his Gospel by insisting that he was writing "an orderly account" of actual events, in order that the reader would "know the truth concerning the things about which you have been instructed"(Lk 1:1-4). Jesus' disciple Peter also insisted that he "did not follow cleverly devised myths," but that he was an "eyewitness" of Christ's "majesty" (2 Pet 1:16; cf. 1 Cor 15:3-4). By the same token, the apostle John affirmed that he and the other disciples "have heard . . . have seen . . . and touched with our hands" the living Jesus (1 Jn 1:3).

This same insistence on the centrality of history to spiritual truth is evident today in Revealed Word proponents. For instance, the Reverend John Stott, a leading contemporary advocate of the perspective, writes that Christianity "does not

rest only on a historical person, Jesus of Nazareth, but on certain historical events which involved him, especially his birth, death, and resurrection."[1]

Should history ground spirituality, as the Revealed Word tradition has insisted? Or should myth, allegory and private spiritual experience—each cut free from external events—provide the basis of our religious commitments? We might say that the advantage and the risk of basing spirituality on history are the same—the possibility of proof and disproof. Vulnerability to historical scrutiny imports openness and candor. When a religious claim can be examined, tested, subjected to critical review, the public being asked to accept the claim is at the very least invited to participate rationally in a process of choice. When, on the other hand, a claim cannot be tested or subjected to any of the ordinary tests of truthfulness, we are left with no recourse but to trust the probity of the claimant.

Two cases may help to illustrate this point. The first occurred more than two hundred and fifty years ago. When the New Testament narratives initially came under sustained public scrutiny in England during the opening years of the eighteenth century, the evidence for the resurrection of Jesus Christ became the focus of particularly intense examination. The Church of England chose not to simply stifle the historical critics, but rather to meet their criticism head on in the public arena. The most famous and successful defense of the resurrection evidences was Bishop Thomas Sherlock's *Tryal of the Witnesses to the Resurrection of Jesus Christ*, first published in 1729. Imagining a trial at which the evidence for and against the resurrection of Jesus was systematically examined, Sherlock masterfully presented the *historical* case for the central Christian miracle in a surprisingly accessible and thorough fashion. Sherlock's book was generally considered an unqualified success, and, remarkably, was not seriously answered in print for nearly fifteen years. Of course, a risk attended Sherlock's efforts, for the church was allowing members of the public to make up their own minds about Christianity's historical evidences. And, predictably, not everyone in the British reading public was convinced by the Bishop's argument.

The famous skeptic Peter Annet proved this point in an especially compelling way in 1744. That year, the first of many editions of Annet's skillful and persuasive response to Sherlock's *Tryal of the Witnesses* appeared in London. Titled *The Resurrection of Jesus Considered by a Moral Philosopher*, Annet's book set out to answer Sherlock argument for argument and to overturn every piece of evidence the Bishop advanced. Like Sherlock's *Tryal*, Annet's *The Resurrection Considered* was wildly popular and controversial. It is impossible to say with any certainty

which author carried the day, but it is possible to say that the public was allowed to consider the evidence and arguments on each side of a crucial historical question: Did the available evidence suggest that Jesus Christ died and then returned to life? The tradition of arguing the historical evidences for and against the Revealed Word's central claims, perhaps launched by Paul's bold statement in his letter to the Corinthians, continues unabated.

My second case is more recent. Shirley MacLaine is famous for describing several of her past lives in the 1985 bestseller *Dancing in the Light*.[2] Among other lives, MacLaine suggests that she was a male actor in ancient Greece and that she was present at the writing of the Constitution and the Declaration of Independence. But perhaps her most riveting and detailed account of a previous existence involves her life as a twelve-year-old orphan girl named Asana who lived with wild elephants "thousands of years ago." "I became known as the princess of the elephants," writes MacLaine. MacLaine/Asana also realizes that she can "communicate with them [the elephants] telepathically."[3] As the elephant princess, MacLaine/Asana "presided over the births of the young, and if one of my friends injured herself, I used more sophisticated human healing techniques to nurse her back to health." MacLaine and the female elephants of the herd also dissuaded a group of male elephants from their plan to kill a man who had murdered a friend of Asana.[4]

It is important to note that MacLaine's "past life incarnations" are not mere diversions related for the sake of entertaining the reader. Rather, they become the factual and experiential basis on which MacLaine develops spiritual principles and techniques that she freely terms "spiritual conjectures."[5] Many of these "I came up with just by being by myself," she writes, though some also involve the assistance of other human beings and a variety of spirit entities.[6] But the past life experiences are particularly important to the spiritual perspective that emerges from the pages of MacLaine's books. For instance, from her time as an elephant princess, MacLaine learned that "we humans should never forget our capacity to connect with the collective spirit of animals."[7]

But unlike Sherlock's claims in *Tryal of the Witnesses*, based as they are on historical documents and developing from allegedly historical events, MacLaine's claims cannot be subjected to any imaginable historical verification. No one can play the critical role of Peter Annet in MacLaine's spiritual cosmos. MacLaine writes within the context of the New Synthesis, a spiritual movement that has taken leave of history, that has severed the spiritual from the physical, the subjective from the

objective and has thus rendered irrelevant any effort to prove or disprove experiential claims as "historically accurate." By the same token, spiritual claims no longer stand or fall on the merits of their attending historical claims. Such a division between claims about events in space and time, on the one hand, and claims about spiritual truths, on the other, is unknown to the Revealed Word. Attending the risk of the Revealed Word's commitment to history is a refreshing honesty before a public being asked to embrace its worldview.

Revealed Word proponents have long argued that history provides their perspective with an objective foundation that serves to ground spiritual claims in verifiable events, a commitment that also serves to limit theological speculation. By contrast, the movement of the New Synthesis away from history and toward myth, away from physical events and toward transcendent symbols, away from verifiable occurrences and toward imaginative narratives, is attended by no commensurate promise to the potential convert. The only promise of spiritual authenticity is that myth somehow conveys timeless and universal religious truths, while history is mired in local events and parochial values. But this dramatic shift in perspective regarding spiritual truth leaves us in an untenable position where the teachings of the historical Jesus recorded in the four New Testament Gospels carry no greater weight than an imagined conversation with Jesus (or an elephant) in one's living room.

I have argued that the Revealed Word tradition's insistence on historical grounding for spiritual truth renders this perspective vulnerable to historical criticism by laying open all of its foundational claims to public scrutiny. Having said this, it is worth noting that arguments against Revealed Word history often reflect, not compelling historical criticism, but an author's more or less personal objections to elements in the historical narrative. Thus, John Shelby Spong asks his readers, "Are we drawn to a Lord who would destroy a herd of pigs and presumably a person's livelihood in order to exorcise a demon (Mark 5:13)?" And again, "Are we impressed when the one we call Lord curses a fig tree because it did not bear fruit out of season (Matt. 21:18, 19)?" The implied criteria for rejecting these stories are not historical, but strictly subjective—the stories do not draw us, do not impress us, by which Spong must mean himself and others already inclined to agree with him.

But do such subjective measures count as tests of the truthfulness of the accounts in question? After all, if Jesus is God incarnate—a central Revealed Word claim—is it reasonable to expect that his actions would consistently strike us as appealing, impressive or even fair? Similarly, Spong rejects the historical Jesus as

someone who "seems to have accepted without question the language of hell employed by his religious contemporaries."[8] Again, this is less an argument against the teachings of the historical Jesus than it is a statement about Spong's revulsion at the idea of hell. Spong's claim says nothing about whether Jesus and his "religious contemporaries" were right or wrong in their views of hell, though it tells us a great deal about Spong's attitude toward such views. Spong's claim is thus better understood as autobiography than as argument.

The New Religious Synthesis dispenses with history, or so its proponents claim, as a means of opening the way to universal religious insights. When obsolete or parochial historical claims are jettisoned, the obstacle to spiritual progress created by a personal and local God is also removed. Biblical narratives can be understood for what they are—metaphors for understanding God. Jesus need no longer be seen as the literal Son of God but rather as a religious philosopher, a mythic hero, a mystic or a symbol for human spiritual aspiration. Religious belief is no longer dependent on outward and historical events in particular locations at remote times, but now finds its source in the ever-contemporary interior life of the spirit, the unfathomable human psyche, the myth-generating subconscious self.

However, may it not also be the case that to sever history from spirituality opens the gate to the self-styled mystic, the spiritual charlatan, the religious expert or just the self-deceived neighbor, each operating in a realm of private interpretation of elusive evidences largely inaccessible to their followers or to any would-be critic? Under the New Religious Synthesis, no longer is the test of actual historical occurrence also a test of truth in religion. Other standards now take history's place as spirituality's foundation, including channeled advice from spirit guides, mystical and hallucinogenic experience, an expert's take-my-word-for-it code-breaking or myth-interpreting, narrative cleverness or the spiritual imagination run amok. History's relative accessibility to the ordinary reader is lost in the mythic mists, tall tales, clouded code and alien advice. Shamans, gurus, scholars of religion and even laboratory scientists now intervene between the public and the divine as a new class of priests. Clearly, the movement away from history has not served to democratize spirituality. Rather, the opposite has occurred. Under the New Religious Synthesis an asymmetrical relationship develops between the gifted few with unaccountable access to spiritual truth and the dependent many incapable of evaluating that truth.

Finally, elevating myth, allegory or narrative turns spirituality inward, inviting us to explore, not the objective external events of human history, but the depths

of our own minds and imaginations. Rather than navigating life's seas by the fixed stars of recorded events, we dive into the "deep well of the psyche" and in these dark waters find, according to our spiritual Jacques Cousteau, Joseph Campbell, "deities [that] are the symbolic personifications of the very energies that are yourself."[9] Because "the symbols of mythology" are "spontaneous productions of the psyche," they are better experienced within our own heads than out in history.[10] Thus, as we saw, Jean Houston led her readers on an interior journey up an imaginary mountain of the psyche where, as in Campbell's well, deities aplenty flourish. But Houston must be trusted as our guide up this mountain, for what we encounter there will never be brought out into the light of external events.

It is interesting to note that the shift from history to myth as the basis for spirituality may find a ready audience among the diverse, far-flung residents of cyberspace. Brenda Brasher writes that "one of the best-kept secrets of cyberspace is the surprising amount of religious practice that takes place there." She adds, "my own explorations have revealed more than a million online religion websites in operation." Mythic forms of spirituality suit the cyberspace experience better than do historical accounts. Brasher writes, "among the genres of human fantasy, cyberspace most closely resembles myth. It is a public story that expresses widely held values and beliefs."[11] Thus, the translation of spiritual truth to a mythic experience may be readily embraced by a new generation of online seekers.

Does spirituality need history? The Revealed Word tradition has always answered *yes;* the New Religious Synthesis says *no.* In the Revealed Word tradition, history has been the scene of God's acts of intervention and ultimately of redemption. A perhaps unrecognized or at least underappreciated fact about this historical grounding is that it has provided an objective, accessible, external foundation for human spiritual experience and religious teaching. As such, appeal to history has tended to restrain theological speculation, and perhaps even the spiritual abuses of leaders inventive enough to manufacture their own internal experiences and clever enough to devise their own myths. The restraint of objective history, however, seldom exerts control over religious thinking or the exercise of spiritual leadership any longer.

THE ADVENT OF REASON

The Revealed Word tradition consistently imbues the human being with extraordinary value, while at the same time reflecting a noteworthy ambivalence about human reason. Clearly, humans are different from the other animals, and much of

this difference has to do with their capacity to think rationally. However, this ancient tradition also cautions against sole reliance on reason for spiritual guidance. The book of Proverbs, for instance, warns the reader to "trust in the LORD with all your heart, and do not rely on your own insight" (Prov 3:5). The mind and rational thought are valued, but nowhere are they presented as adequate to fathom the depths of the human soul, let alone the nature of God.

It is recorded that Jesus himself prayed, "I thank you, Father, Lord of heaven and earth, because you have hidden these things from the wise and the intelligent and revealed them to infants," that is, to those of humble and untrained rational abilities (Lk 10:21). Similarly, the apostle Paul asks the members of the church in the Greek city of Corinth, "Where is the one who is wise? Where is the scribe? Where is the debater of this age? Has not God made foolish the wisdom of this world?" (1 Cor 1:20). This "making foolish" of human wisdom occurs as God surprises the church with a tendency to "reveal to infants" the profoundest of spiritual truths. One wonders how such statements must have sounded to the Greeks, who were prone to find in reason the highest expression of human nature.

Under the New Religious Synthesis, however, this God who reveals profound truths to the simple has been excised from the cosmos and replaced by a very different deity variously described as Reason, Mind, Consciousness or Divine Intellect. This impersonal force that drove the universe's evolutionary destiny was referred to centuries ago in the European magical tradition as the divine *Mens*, or Mind. It was cosmic in scope, and through careful study and practice the magus or magician could control and channel its power. The goal of magical studies was to recreate the cosmic *Mens* within the human mind. Renaissance magi spent their lives training the intellect and the imagination in order to control *Mens* and so transform themselves into virtual deities.[12] Thus, then as now this elevated Reason or Mind is difficult to distinguish from the radically autonomous self seeking its own spiritual advancement. It was always understood that very few members of the human race possessed the discipline, mental capacity and, importantly, spiritual secrets that rendered possible this transformation from human to divinity.

The tension between a spirituality that finds a creating and personal God as the universe's foundational fact, and one that finds that fact in undifferentiated Reason or Consciousness could not be greater. Whereas the apostle John advocated the Revealed Word perspective that "the Word became flesh and dwelt among us"— referring to Jesus as the unique human manifestation of the personal and wholly

other deity—the Deist Peter Annet responded on behalf of a new spirituality that "Reason is God incarnate." In his first epistle, the same John affirmed that "God is light" (1 Jn 1:5). Thomas De Quincey countered for an emerging religion by composing a hymn to "the light of the majestic intellect." The unknown New Testament writer who penned the epistle to the Hebrews urged that "without faith it is impossible to please God" (Heb 11:6). Ayn Rand scolded in *Atlas Shrugged* that the incompetents of the earth had "sacrificed reason to faith."

The New Religious Synthesis calls us to self-adoration as spirituality, to the exaltation of our own rational self-awareness—"the divinity operating within us," according to Annet—as an act or worship. The Other Spirituality's journey away from submission to a personal and sovereign deity, away from moral responsibility before a Creator God, away from community built on worship of the Wholly Other, arrives at no more interesting destination than spiritual narcissism. In Rand, such self-worship is revealed for what it truly is—ruthless self-interest masquerading as rational self-liberation. The less mentally gifted among us—the "incompetents of the earth"—that is, the poor, are punished for the sin of having not enough of the new god.

Perhaps something like Rand's hard-edged elitism is inevitable when Reason becomes a god, particularly in an evolving cosmos. Annet and the Deists argued that Reason was universal. However, they also admitted that most of us never gain sufficient mastery of this internal power to free ourselves from the restraints of conventional morality and the errors of the Revealed Word. Voltaire maintained that a single clear thinking follower of Reason—exemplified in the character Zadig—understood more about true religion than did the masses of the religiously devout. His followers held to the same prejudice; the altar to Reason in Notre Dame bore the busts, not of ordinary citizens, but of four advanced thinkers—Franklin, Rousseau, Montesquieu and, of course, Voltaire himself. Thus, this was not an altar to human reason understood as universal rational ability. Rather, it was an altar to Reason Triumphant, a monument to the rationally gifted members of the human race, the new spiritual vanguard.

Interestingly, De Quincey did not find even the dreams of opium to be available to all. Ordinary existence, "this too intense life of the social instincts," destroys the capacity for great dreams in most people. Only an elite can understand "the mystery of darkness" and "the profound philosophy" that allows Majestic Intellect to escape mundane existence and even history itself. Similarly, the advocates of New

Thought suggested that particular rational gifts and carefully studied techniques are necessary to harness and direct the energy of Mind. Even prayer, that most democratic of spiritual exercises in the Revealed Word, is transformed in New Thought into a rational technique to be mastered. Only the skilled practitioner, not the simple person of faith, can through prayer concentrate mental energy or Mind in such a way as to unleash its healing, life-giving powers.

Reason, it appears, is no egalitarian divinity. But then, an evolving universe cannot afford such a god. Progress in such a universe depends on a determined weeding out of the weak. In this regard, Rand read the face of the future with precision and prescience. The mechanism of evolution always recognizes and rewards the superior members of a species, and, according to the New Synthesis, the most rationally advanced members of the human race are currently being so recognized and so rewarded. The Revealed Word proposed an impartial God, a deity who was, in the biblical phrase, "no respecter of persons" (Acts 10:34 KJV).

Even as sanguine and friendly an analyst of our spiritual destiny as Gary Zukav cannot bring himself to believe that all human beings are equally endowed of the potential for rational advancement. He is aware of the elitism inherent in the idea of self-awareness as the basis of spirituality, and his discomfort with the fact is palpable. "Not all humans are equally aware of their souls." This raises the obvious question, "do all human beings have equal potential?" to which Zukav provides the apparently contradictory answer, "yes and no." Admitting that "this question is complex," he adds that "an individual that is not quite as expanded in his or her awareness is not equal in the sense that we usually mean equal to someone of greater awareness. There is an inequality. Yet it is not an inequality that remains unequal. It is just a temporary level of momentum in the flow of evolution."[13] An unequal equality certainly would be an equality that is not what is usually meant by the term. And yet, this is the best answer the New Religious Synthesis has to offer to the troubling questions raised when any human "potential" is set out as a spiritual hope in a fundamentally evolutionary scheme in which potential or fitness is everything.

It appears, then, that we face a dilemma in the spiritual realm: either all of us are submitted to the uniquely perfect Reason of a personal creator God, or most of us must defer to the more highly evolved reason of some of us. Much science fiction advocates the second option. Time and again space delivers to us our highly evolved alien saviors, advanced intellects whose mission is to enlighten the human race and in this way to help us on to our ultimate destiny—a virtual divinity akin

to their own. By contrast, the Revealed Word proposes the descent from heaven of a single incarnation of the one true God, a single divine person offering salvation universally through grace rather than selectively through rational potential.

THEOLOGICAL SCIENCE

[handwritten: ← study do study metaphysics]

During the modern period, science has taken on greater and greater religious significance. Scientists have become outspoken advocates and devotees of new spiritual systems, while at the same time science has increasingly been employed to prove theological and spiritual propositions. As one writer recently stated the point, the "discoveries of science illuminate both inner and outer experiences," that is, both "physical and nonphysical dynamics."[14] Science, which had always taken the observable world as its only domain, now informs us about the unseen world as well.

The use of scientific experiment to achieve spiritual insight has had a variety of fascinating manifestations in the twentieth century. For instance, at Duke University in 1927, Professor J. B. Rhine created "the first parapsychological lab."[15] Rhine's experiments were intended "to establish the existence of ESP—clairvoyance, precognition, telepathy—and psychokinesis, using experimental methods."[16] He was nurturing a new view of science, one that would have profound implications for a wide range of spiritual thought by the end of the twentieth century.[17] Rhine was not himself an objective scientific observer, but rather "believed that parapsychology was relevant to religion and that it offered a way to reconcile the claims of religion with the principles of science."[18]

Rhine pursued his "seven years of patient work" with a virtually religious commitment to establishing on scientific grounds various unobservable powers of the human mind. Other scientists scoffed, but Rhine countered prophetically that "the stone which a hasty science rejected has sometimes become the corner of its later structure."[19] Rhine hoped to overturn the "psychological dogma" that "*nothing* can enter the mind except through the gateways of the recognized senses" through scientific experiments alone. And he felt he succeeded and that a "new frontier" had been opened "by years of testing and hundreds of thousands of trials." Rhine found in his results nothing less than a revolutionary view of the mind that would displace traditional psychology in the same way that relativity theory had displaced Newtonian mechanics.[20] Science had shown that the human mind has a spiritual dimension.

The tendency to see science as pregnant with spiritual insight is a commonplace of the new spirituality. Thus, dancer and actress Shirley MacLaine bases her belief

in reincarnation in part on an appeal to science. She writes in her bestselling *Dancing in the Light*, "If, as science says, energy never dies, it merely changes form, then life, which is also energy, never dies. It, too, merely changes form." She continues, "Since energy is never still, because nothing remains inert, then energy must continually have a changing form." What does MacLaine conclude from this scientific observation? "There was no doubt in my mind that the life energy simply changed its form from lifetime to lifetime, just as nature did from spring to spring."[21] Thus, the law of the conservation of energy proves reincarnation and past life experiences. In many similar cases science is now a taken-for-granted source of a new theology.

To view science as a religious hope is not new. Nineteenth-century Biblical critic David Strauss prophetically proclaimed that "he embraced 'the Universe' as revealed by science, in which he purported to find an all-pervasive spirit of love."[22] Similarly, Wayne Teasdale has written recently that mystics have long "known and proclaimed the essential interconnectedness of all things."[23] This spiritual insight is for Teasdale himself also supported by science. According to Teasdale, science proves that "consciousness," not a personal God, is "the basis of reality."[24]

Science has birthed a new theology, or, more accurately, rebirthed an old one. "The most powerful transformative ideas from modern science," writes Ferguson, "connect like parts of a puzzle" and "support each other," thus forming "the scaffolding for a wider worldview." This apparently new worldview is really a primitive one that mystics have articulated for centuries. The great scientific discoveries of our own day have "uncanny parallels to ancient poetic and mystical descriptions of nature," she writes. "Science is only now verifying what humankind has known intuitively since the dawn of history."[25]

Throughout the modern period, science has been employed to confirm spiritual truths that hearken back to earlier traditions. Thomas Paine argued that science supported, not the theistic religion of the Revealed Word, but the pantheistic religion of nature and reason. Madame Blavatsky's Victorian occultism—a social movement that paved the way for the revival of shamanism—was founded on the idea that scientific discoveries confirmed occult practices. According to David Strauss, scientific biblical criticism opened the way to mythological readings of the Bible. The naturalist Ernst Haeckel asserted that science proved both pantheism and monism. And by pursuing the science of psychiatry, John Mack concluded that alien entities were seeking contact with a new class of shamans—UFO abductees.

The trend toward confirming ancient spiritual systems through modern science

continues today. Again, Shirley MacLaine affirms the close connection between discoveries in quantum physics and new spiritualities that resemble old ones. She writes, for example, "J. Robert Oppenheimer said that the general notions about human understanding which are illustrated by discoveries in atomic physics were not wholly unfamiliar. They had a history not only in Buddhist and Hindu thought, but also in our own culture. 'What we are finding,' he said, 'is a refinement of old wisdom.'"[26] A characteristic passage in her *Dancing in the Light* moves effortlessly from contact with spiritual entities to a vision of the lost civilization on Atlantis to a discussion of quantum physics.[27]

And this purposeful blurring of the line between science and spirituality is not limited to nonscientists such as MacLaine. David Gergen, editor-at-large for *U.S. News & World Report*, profiled Severino Antinori for his magazine on August 20, 2001. Antinori, one of the leading scientists in the race to clone the first human being, is a man "who suggests that Napoleon and Galileo are his role models." Gergen points out that "one of Antinori's key supporters in his cloning effort is linked to a group that believes that humans are clones in the image of aliens from another solar system."[28] The group referred to is the Raelian UFO religion, which now claims to have cloned two human beings. According to their leader—a Frenchman calling himself Rael who asserts that he was once abducted by aliens—the goal of their cloning experiments is to achieve immortality through continuous cloning of the individual with the mind transferred from one body to another ad infinitum.

At this juncture in Western history, it is perhaps especially important to recall that spiritual values have long guided scientific endeavors, a fact that is clear from the history of alchemy, eugenics and more recent efforts to clone a human being following the religious tenets of the Raelians. And now science is being employed to "prove" spiritual theories as well. In a culture that has trained itself for three centuries to trust the findings of science, such a procedure will certainly lend an advantage to the religious view that could enlist the largest number of scientists, or at least the most persuasive, in its support.

SPIRITUAL EVOLUTION

According to Teilhard de Chardin, the universe operates on the principle of evolution, and reality itself is, to use his term, "evolutive." Matter has, at this point in time, organized itself into consciousness, and consciousness, driven forward by the

force of evolution, is moving inexorably toward the "Omega Point" of pure consciousness.[29] Scientific discoveries are currently providing insights into our "spiritual evolution," as are tribal spiritual traditions steeped in ancient wisdom often ignored in the West.[30]

At the very core of the New Religious Synthesis is a hope in human advancement through evolution. As George Bernard Shaw phrased the point in 1903, reflecting ideas he borrowed from Friedrich Nietzsche, "Our only hope, then, is evolution. We must replace the man by the superman."[31] This fundamental tenet shows up anywhere one cares to look in the literature of the Other Spirituality. Human spiritual transformation via evolution is the promise of Darwin's heirs from the biologist Huxley to the occultist Blavatsky to New Age novelist James Redfield. As we enter a new era of awareness, or so the argument goes, we are taking an inevitable and unprecedented step in human evolution. Marilyn Ferguson calls evolution "the mandate of nature" and the mechanism by which human beings will achieve the great "leap forward" into a new spiritual age. Is this a consummation devoutly to be wished?

Francis Fukuyama, author of the recently published *Our Posthuman Future*, has said in a recent interview that biotechnology may soon be used to "to consciously take an otherwise normal human being and make him or her into something very different." Calling this "the single greatest danger" of advances in biotechnology, Fukuyama foresees "a period completely unprecedented in human history, where human beings will consciously be able to take over the evolutionary process."[32] But "conscious evolution" is not seen as a danger in all quarters. Psychologist Robert Ornstein, today's leading expert on the evolution of consciousness, believes that directed evolution affords a future to be embraced. The time has come for human beings to seize control of evolution, albeit through education rather than biotechnology. Conscious evolution "may be easier, closer at hand, and more liberating than we might normally think."[33] "Conscious selection," as opposed to natural selection, would be employed to "take our evolution in our own hands."[34] A program of conscious evolution should be moved "to the top of the human agenda."[35]

Such assisted progress was clearly the hope of the first generation of evolutionary scientists. T. H. Huxley envisioned a morally improved human race as the result of guided evolution. Thus, the "social progress" of human beings meant "checking the evolutionary process at every step" and encouraging moral evolution from one level of moral attainment to another. But this possibility is precisely what has Fukuyama

worried, particularly if such occurs in the absence of an adequate conception of human nature. "A better cognitive neuroscience," he writes, "will lead to a much better understanding of the biological basis for human behavior, and thus will offer the potential to manipulate human behavior in ways that we haven't been able to do before." For Fukuyama, this greater control of human behavior, this hastening of humanity's moral evolution, "suggests experiments in social engineering—which are likely to be more successful than our previous efforts at social engineering."[36]

Fukuyama's concerns are reminiscent of those expressed prophetically by C. S. Lewis in his 1947 book *The Abolition of Man*.[37] Lewis argued that one generation could wield power over every subsequent generation by altering human nature through psychological conditioning and genetic engineering. In Lewis's own day this was a very remote possibility, but, as Fukuyama and others have noted, today it is not so remote. With an evolutionary understanding of human nature and destiny before us courtesy of the New Synthesis, the basic genetic makeup of the human race may be altered according to the insights of a spiritual and scientific elite. Lewis wrote, "If any one age really attains, by eugenics and scientific education, the power to make its descendants what it pleases, all men who live after it are the patients of that power." As a result of scientific advances, our "conquest of Nature, if the dreams of some scientific planners are realized, means the rule of a few hundreds of men over billions upon billions of men."[38] Advocates of the Revealed Word have been publicly exercised over the biological implications of Darwinian thinking. However, the evolutionary vision animating current scientific and spiritual movements is more moral than biological, more spiritual than physical, and more likely attained by artificial rather than natural means.

The New Religious Synthesis views human spiritual advance as a matter of incremental evolutionary change over time, and not the result of instantaneous rebirth or spiritual transformation described in the Revealed Word tradition. Zukav, for instance, contends that the human soul is continuously engaged in the process of "evolution toward authentic power."[39] New Synthesis writers hold that the cosmos is a place of increasing complexity and that evolution is its omnipresent operative principle, the organizing and complexifying force at the very center of being. As Ferguson puts the point, "All wholes transcend their parts by virtue of internal coherence, cooperation, openness to input." Moreover, "The higher on the evolutionary scale, the more freedom to reorganize. An ant lives out a destiny; a human being shapes one." So human beings are the only entities free to actually choose their evolutionary des-

tiny because we are the only evolving entities consciously aware of our own existence. "Evolution is a continuous breaking and forming to make new, richer wholes," she writes. "If we enlarge our awareness, admit new information, and take advantage of the brain's infinite capacity to integrate and reconcile, we can leap forward."[40]

But, as I have noted more than once, spiritual evolution in the New Synthesis is not particularly democratic, and so there is reason for caution about this hope of the New Synthesis as well. Recall that Sir Julian Huxley finds that "transhumanist" evolutionary advancement takes place in "the best ten-thousandth" among us. The Revealed Word insists that its central principle—spiritual transformation through grace—is available to all. Herbert Spencer and Charles Darwin both recognized that evolutionary theory made advancement the domain of a few survivors. A vanguard, a capable elite, has always been a component of spiritual evolutionary schemes, even before the publication of *On the Origin of the Species*.

Contemporary writers would never embrace spiritual evolution's more sinister consequences, though earlier proponents of the idea happily advocated them as necessary deductions. For instance, racialism is clearly present in such influential works as Houston Stewart Chamberlain's *Foundations of the Nineteenth Century* (1899), in which the author looks forward to a "new era dominated by Aryan spirituality."[41] Aryan spirituality—the persistent notion that northern Europeans are a more *spiritually* advanced people destined to dominate the other peoples of the world in a new spiritual order—was a common theme of spiritual speculation in the nineteenth century. This impulse is far removed from the Revealed Word notion of the kingdom of God consisting of members from "every people, tribe and nation."

Even the embarrassment of eugenics has not been entirely purged from New Religious Synthesis thinking, though most contemporary writers would repudiate the practice. The Other Spirituality often openly advocates the notion that a small vanguard of the human race possessing the necessary capacities will help the race to advance. The Other Spirituality has at times looked back into human history to discover the evolving ones and then traced a trajectory to those presently among us who are specially fitted for spiritual evolution. Jesus may enter the picture at this point. As Joseph Pearce writes, "Jesus [was] a genius with radically new ideas, an evolutionary *Eureka!* development by which life tried to develop a new aspect of potential."[42] R. M. Bucke was also interested in discovering those members of the human race who had taken the next step of spiritual evolution, and also identified Jesus as a member of this elite group.

In his important apologetic work *Mere Christianity*, C. S. Lewis noted that the further evolutionary development of the human race is an idea most clearly represented in the literary genre now called science fiction. He identified the pervasive hypothesis as a rival to, perhaps a counterfeit of, the Christian idea of spiritual transformation. Lewis writes, "The Christian view is precisely that the Next Step has already appeared. And it is really new. It is not a change from brainy men to brainier men: it is a change that goes off in a totally different direction—a change from being creatures of god to being sons of God."[43] Lewis was prophetic in his realization that human evolution to higher moral and spiritual levels would be a theme of religious speculation in the second half of the twentieth century. He was also emphatic that the biblical vision of a human race spiritually redeemed and transformed through Christ was a vastly superior vision of the human future.

PANTHEISM

Recently, Americans were surprised to hear news reports that followers of the Wicca religion had petitioned the army to allow them to use space at an army base for a religious ceremony. It turned out that groups of Wiccans were meeting at American military bases around the country and in Europe. The rise of Wicca, an updated version of pre-Christian European pantheistic spirituality, corresponds to widespread interest in a variety of similar traditions including Druidism and various forms of witchcraft. The revived nature-worshiping religions have in common an underlying pantheism, a belief in the divinity inherent in all things.

Pantheism is not limited, however, to neo-pagan religions and witchcraft. Many contemporary spiritual movements are fundamentally pantheistic, and pantheism is crucial to the New Religious Synthesis. Pantheism rejects the notion of God as personal and sovereign, instead finding divinity to be an impersonal force, energy, spirit, consciousness or mind in all things. Contemporary Western interest in witchcraft, kabbalah, neopaganism, gnosticism, Theosophy, the occult, astrology, the New Age movement, the New Physics and Eastern religious thought all suggest that pantheistic assumptions are rapidly displacing the theology of a rational, sovereign, personal and moral divinity.[44] Interestingly, in Neale Donald Walsch's alleged conversations with "God," Walsch concludes, "if there is no end to bigness, then there is no *biggest*. This means there *is no God!*" To this notion, "God" replies, "Or, perhaps—*all of it is God*, and *there is nothing else.*"[45]

The Other Spirituality's god is a force to be managed, a potential to be tapped,

a consciousness to be experienced. As Ferguson affirms in *The Aquarian Conspiracy*, God is now "the organizing matrix we can experience but not tell, that which enlivens matter."[46] Similarly, John Shelby Spong has recently stated that "god is the ground of being," something best understood by recourse to "non-personal images." Thus, "the theistic understanding of god no longer works."[47] As something "we can experience but not tell," this new god is perhaps best known by mystics or psychics, regardless of the religious or cultural tradition within which they operate.

Science—one of two great sources, along with spirits, of theological insight in the New Religious Synthesis—provides a basis for seeing God as diffuse and within the physical universe rather than as personal and external to that universe. Dana Zohar and Ian Marshall write that "for some people the idea of a transcendent God who creates, and possibly controls, the universe from a vantage point outside the laws of physics, from beyond space and time, will always remain appealing." However, belief in such a Revealed Word God, albeit "appealing," has no scientific support. A more scientifically justifiable theology understands God as "a basic sense of direction" in the universe that is moving everything that exists "towards further and greater ordered coherence." God is "embodied within . . . the laws of physics" and is "an evolving consciousness within the universe."[48] If, in fact, we inhabit a cosmos that is evolving, and if God is a consciousness contained within the very matter of that cosmos, then it stands to reason that God is an evolving consciousness within that cosmos.

What are the consequences of this new, pantheistic conception of God? Perhaps the principal and most dramatic spiritual change as we move from Revealed Word theism to the pantheism of the New Synthesis occurs precisely here—in the fundamental human-divine relationship. An energy, a Life Force, a spirit in all things, an evolving Consciousness, a Divine Intelligence, even an awe-inspiring spiritual-physical universe, are not a divine Person with whom one may enter a living relationship. Nor is the pantheistic deity of the New Synthesis the kind of god who places moral requirements on one's life. On the moral plane, pantheism allows us to create the god we wish—a god incapable of an opinion about human morality.

This last point brings us to the question of what the Other Spirituality's pantheistic theology has to say to the problem of evil. Gary Zukav writes that the highly evolved or "multisensory personality" will understand God as "Divine Intelligence" or "Conscious Light." Evil, then, is simply the absence of such Light. Thus, "understanding evil as the absence of Light requires you to examine the choices you make each moment in terms of whether they move you toward light or away from it."[49]

But this conception of evil as an "absence of Light" provides neither clear direction for avoiding evil, nor a strong mandate for opposing it. "Do you know the meaning of evil?" asks Shirley MacLaine's Spirit Guide. Answering its own question, the Guide comments that "evil is nothing but energy flowing backward rather than forward. . . . Allow all of your energy to flow back to the God source."[50] If God and we are energy, then there is no moral law at all, only correct or incorrect relationships to this divine energy. Thus, evil properly understood is simply an energy flow problem easily corrected through appropriate techniques.

Such accounts of evil hardly seem adequate to either explain or address the evil expressed in even a single act of murder, let alone wickedness on the scale of the Holocaust or the Rwandan massacres. Perhaps this is why Robert Green Ingersoll, a man whose Civil War experience had sharpened his understanding of the human moral predicament, recognized the need to attempt a serious response to the problem of evil. His "Creed of Science" called on each person to act by a rule of love somehow derived from science. But in the absence of a sovereign and personal God whose own ultimate goodness grounds all adequate conceptions of good and evil and who holds us accountable for our actions, even this call to act voluntarily in love is unlikely to serve as a preventative to human evil.

Ultimately the New Synthesis leaves us looking to ourselves for moral guidance, and thus for the spiritual authority to condemn evil and commend good. A god who cannot hold us accountable for our actions and who cannot reveal to us a moral standard grounded on ultimate goodness is a god whose nature provides no answer to the problem of evil. "Identifying God with everything," writes theologian Peter Jones, "effectively removes from God any real and specific identity."[51] Without that personal, sovereign divine identity as ultimate moral guide and judge, that is, without a God active in the universe and yet separate from it, human beings are in the cosmic driver's seat as minor deities. In New Religious Synthesis writers, Pantheism leads repeatedly to the notion of human divinity. Neale Donald Walsch asks his spirit guide, "You mean, I can even become—dare I say it?—a God?" The guide replies, "You are already a God. You simply do not know it."[52] Even a cursory review of human history would lead a reasonable person to question whether we have proven ourselves morally worthy of this great responsibility.

THE NEW GNOSIS

Artist Alexis Smith's striking Snake Path, part of the Stuart Collection, fascinates

visitors to the campus of the University of California, San Diego. The Snake Path is a 560 foot long, 10 foot wide tiled walkway in the shape of a serpent. The snake's head rests on the terrace of the university's Central Library. Along the path one encounters an enormous granite book with a quotation from John Milton's *Paradise Lost:* "Then wilt thou not be loth to leave this Paradise, but shalt possess a Paradise within thee, happier far." The snake's body wraps around a tropical garden intended to represent the Garden of Eden. The snake leading to the library is said to represent both the loss of innocence and the liberation of the self through the acquisition of knowledge. Smith has said that the idea came to her in a dream. The Snake Path reflects the foundational myth of ancient Gnosticism—that the Edenic serpent was a heroic figure bringing spiritually liberating knowledge to the benighted Adam and Eve, trapped in physical bodies and the space-time dungeon of earth by an incompetent and vindictive deity.

Gnosticism teaches the soul's escape from the world, the body and time by means of secret insights into the nature of spiritual reality. Only the individual possessing hidden spiritual knowledge or *gnosis* has any hope of understanding the truth about our human predicament, and thus of being saved from spiritual darkness and the limitations of the physical. In both its ancient and more modern manifestations gnosticism questions the goodness, often even the reality, of physical existence. The soul is eternal and evolving, a manifestation of the divine essence in the highest realm of reality. The body, on the other hand, is merely the vessel of our entrapment to be escaped by means of the secrets of spiritual ascent.

"A soul has no beginning and no end," writes Gary Zukav, adding that "all souls come directly from the Godhead." Moreover, "not all humans are equally aware of their souls."[53] And yet, "the soul is the individual unit of evolution."[54] The body is simply a means of achieving certain ends that heighten awareness of the soul and its evolution, and once the body has served its purpose, the soul moves on to another location, another body or perhaps another planet, to continue its migration back to the Godhead. Here is Neale Donald Walsch on the same point: "The soul has come to the body, and the body to life, for the purpose of evolution."[55] In response to the question, "Where do advanced souls go?" Zukav answers, "There are many forms of life that exist as advancements of this one. There are literally millions of options. There is life in numerous galaxies. There are millions, indeed billions of other life-filled planets."[56]

"The body," writes Zukav, "is the instrument of the soul," the two standing in the

same relationship as a piano and piano player.[57] The soul, then, is the body's animating intelligence, its "daemon," to use the ancient gnostic term. Without its activating intelligence, the body is a barely living drone. Possessed by a daemon, however, the body takes on life and intelligence. The notion is captured well in the popular *His Dark Materials* trilogy for young adults by Phillip Pullman. One exchange between the two principal characters, Will and Lyra, illustrates the point: "'You *have* got a daemon,' she said decisively, 'Inside you.' He didn't know what to say. 'You have,' she went on, 'You wouldn't be human else. You'd be . . . half dead.'"[58] Moreover, the *daemon* has access to the spirit world and the secrets of advancement to be found there.

The gnostic view of the body and physical existence runs consistently against the grain of the Revealed Word, a spiritual outlook that elevates both. According to the Word, a personal God intentionally created the physical universe, and it was from the beginning essentially good. Human physical existence—our embodiment—is purposeful and meaningful, not a cosmic accident. Christian writer Dallas Willard affirms that "people have a body for one reason—that we might have at our disposal the resources that would allow us to be persons in fellowship and cooperation with a personal God."[59] The Other Spirituality's relative disregard for physical experience challenges this view of the body, as well as the possibility of the individual's "fellowship and cooperation with a personal God." Fukuyama's caution about our view of human nature becomes crucial at this point, for if the soul is important and the body merely its dumb instrument, research that advances the soul, the moral component of the human, may be warranted. However, such experiments would, in effect, alter human nature itself. "My own preference, 'Hands off human nature.' You don't want to do things that really change core human behaviors. . . . [Y]ou don't want to do things that turn people into gods, or subhumans, in effect."[60] However, if the ultimate destiny of the human soul is to evolve to divinity, a core tenet of the rapidly advancing New Religious Synthesis, then where will the ethical principle to prevent such genetic alteration in human nature come from?

Gnostic thought is also committed to the notion that spiritual truth is purposely hidden and either unattainable or indecipherable without special assistance. The secrets that comprise *gnosis* must be learned from spiritual masters, spirit guides, super-intelligent aliens, secret texts, scientific experimentation or arduous exploration. Madame Blavatsky claimed direct instruction by ascended Tibetan spiritual masters like Koot Hoomi; Shirley MacLaine is educated by a spirit guide called the Higher Self; and John Mack's clients receive their higher truth from

aliens. Joseph Smith discovered a secret text that could be read only with the assistance of special lenses, while it takes a scanning electron microscope and a Ph.D. in physics to read the hidden spiritual meanings in subatomic particles. Similarly, a mathematician and high-speed computers were required for Michael Drosnin to finally crack "the Bible Code." The hero of James Redfield's *The Celestine Prophecy* must travel to South America and endure various hardships before acquiring his own secret text—the Manuscript—that reveals the hidden knowledge necessary for spiritual deliverance. And it should also be noted that even more arduous trials must sometimes be endured to acquire the new *gnosis*. John Mack's alien abductees often endure what can only be called torture before they are spiritually qualified to convey the messages the rest of us need to hear. Planetary spirits also found it necessary to mistreat Emanuel Swedenborg before he could absorb spiritual wisdom.

Secret arenas into which the New Religious Synthesis leads the spiritual seeker include the subconscious mind, subatomic space, the world of spirits, the realm of myth, the province of dreams, the domain of magic, the system of the stars, and planets beyond earth. Spiritual secrets from such sources promise limitless potential for personal power. Modern practitioners of *gnosis* will claim the capacity to affect the nature of reality, as well as the certainty of eventual divinity. Such mastery is, however, beyond the reach of all but the most capable and determined. The "Way of knowledge" is for those possessing, according to Joseph Pearce, "dramatic abilities and knowledge."[61] Why such effort, such extraordinary gifts and such unusual capacities? Because "extraordinary effort [is] needed to break with the broad stream that makes up the . . . world of the ordinary." That is, lifting oneself beyond the constraints of the body and conventional morality takes great strength of will—a gift most of us do not possess. However, such massive spiritual exertion is worth whatever it costs, for it opens the way to "ever greater levels of growth and power" for the spiritual master.[62] At the same time, however, such secrecy in the spiritual realm always invites the formation of hierarchies of authority and their attendant potential for spiritual abuse.

By contrast to the esoteric media and elusive masters of gnosticism, Jesus Christ was a remarkably open spiritual teacher. "What I say to you in the dark," he is recorded as having said, "tell in the light; and what you hear whispered, proclaim from the housetops"(Mt 10:27). The general openness of the Revealed Word tradition sets it apart from any spiritual system officially embracing secrecy or subtly suggesting that spiritual knowledge is the private domain of the knowing few. In

Revealed Word thinking, the spiritual knowledge necessary to salvation must be made available to everyone regardless of personal circumstance or ability. Regardless of how one feels about Christian missionary endeavors, it is at least clear from these efforts that the Christian message of salvation by grace is to be broadly proclaimed, and it requires for its complete understanding no ascended masters, secret texts or remarkable devices.

Early Christians contended with a spiritual tradition teaching that the path to spiritual enlightenment ran through a maze of carefully guarded secrets known collectively as *gnosis*. Paul wrote against gnosticism in his epistle to the Colossians, while John tackled the problem in his first epistle. These Christian teachers offered a radically different way into spiritual truth. To *gnosis* they responded with *Logos*, a Revealed Word, literally a divine Person who was the eternal Word. Through this Person, salvation was open to all by grace, a divine gift. Such was the message of the Christian gospel, the openly proclaimed message of spiritual deliverance that eschewed the secrets of the gnostic inner circle, that saw the body as redeemable and that venerated the God of the Jews as both Creator and Redeemer.

The New Religious Synthesis has revived several elements in the ancient Gnostic tradition, so long opposed by the Revealed Word. With *gnosis* on the rise, spirituality is again construed as a matter of mastering secrets or techniques that make possible self-deliverance. Because of its commitment to secrets known only by a few, gnostic thinking breeds spiritual elites. Love of secrecy may seem a harmless endeavor in creative religious thought, but such ideology has had its tragic historic consequences. Richard Noll has pointed out that prior to the Nazi era in Europe there were "cries for new spiritual and political elites to lead the Germanic peoples of Central Europe to new 'awakening' through reliance upon the more highly refined 'intuitive' faculties of such specialists."[63] Historically it has often been a short step from the notion of a spiritual elite to the idea of an elite race. As William Covino writes, "The Great Mind" behind the cosmos can be "invoked" by the spiritual master "to restore truth, beauty and justice to humankind," but also to "ordain a master race."[64] Such a spiritual-racial elite may create a perfectly ordered and enlightened society, may "transform the world with its 'higher' values of community and truth," but at what cost?[65]

Nevertheless, because the retrieval of allegedly lost spiritual secrets places their possessors in a commanding spiritual position, the revival of gnosticism is now advocated as an advance beyond the Revealed Word. But gnosticism represents spiritual

progress only if secrecy is valued over openness, elitism preferred to egalitarianism, and hierarchy deemed superior to community. For all of the intrigue associated with gaining insight into the machinery of the cosmos, for all of the ego-elevation that attends belonging to an inner circle of spiritual adepts, a spirituality based on *gnosis* reintroduces dubious spiritual tendencies into the mainstream of Western spirituality.

SHAMANS AND THE SPIRITUAL FUTURE

That spiritual advancement is aided by nonhuman spiritual guides is simply assumed in many contemporary spiritual works. Bestselling author Neale Donald Walsch, for instance, claims that in 1992 he began receiving direct answers from a spirit source to a series of perplexing moral and religious questions.

> To my surprise, as I scribbled out the last of my bitter unanswerable questions and prepared to toss my pen aside, my hand remained poised over the paper, as if held by some invisible source. Abruptly, the pen began *moving on its own*. I had no idea what I was about to write, but an idea seemed to be coming, so I decided to flow with it. Out came ... "Do you really want an answer to all these questions, or are you just venting?"[66]

The result was a three-year dialogue between Walsch and "God"—a spirit interlocutor—that appears in his three-volume *Conversations with God*, which purports to offer direct instruction from God on a large number of topics ranging from reincarnation (it occurs) to the ultimate source of morality (the individual human being). As noted above, however, the "God" with whom Walsch communicates is not the uncreated and eternal God of the Revealed Word, but apparently only a more advanced soul that was once also a human.

Much Western spirituality now embraces the shamanic tendency strongly repudiated by the Revealed Word tradition. In the ancient world *daemons*, angels and minor gods guided spiritual seekers. Centuries later, disembodied voices advised medieval and Renaissance alchemists, while in the nineteenth century otherworldly visitors in the form of ghosts and spirits instructed guests in the parlors of Victorian mediums. Tribal shamans around the world have for millennia claimed to have contact with demons and spirits offering a wide range of instruction and, importantly, power over one's enemies. This interest in guidance by spirit entities has recently reasserted itself with surprising success. Today one reads of alien advisors, Inner Friends, Higher Selves, supernatural teachers and spirit helpers in a vast and popular spiritual literature.

The Other Spirituality is frequently backward looking, as is clearly illustrated in this reintroduction of shamanism into the mainstream of Western religious experience. According to anthropologist Gerardo Reichel-Dolmatoff, it is the shaman in primitive cultures who "establishes contact with the supernatural powers and who, to the mind of his people, has the necessary esoteric knowledge to use this contact for the benefit of society."[67] This idea of human bridges between the spiritual and material worlds is flourishing again, as is the attendant idea of the inevitable benefit of such contact. Reliance on esoteric knowledge (*gnosis*) to achieve spirit contact is also evident in the new shamanism, as is the notion of a spiritual elite possessing such knowledge. "The shaman's satisfaction," writes Reichel-Dolmatoff, comes from "'knowing' things which others are unable to grasp."[68]

Several potential liabilities attend this recent revival of shamanistic practices, however. First, the shamanism of the New Religious Synthesis substitutes contact with spirit entities for a living relationship with the Revealed Word's creating and redeeming God, a relationship that the Revealed Word has always contended brings ultimate purpose and meaning to life. "The LORD is my shepherd," writes the psalmist, "I shall not want" (Ps 23:1). But the Word's foundational commitment to an ultimate deity is itself a mistake according to many New Synthesis writers. Gary Zukav offers one explanation for the erroneous theology of monotheism when he posits "realms upon realms of intelligences" just beyond our immediate awareness," any one of which "we might think of as God."[69] Whereas these intelligences are often affirmed to be highly evolved spirit beings, none is presented by the New Synthesis as sovereign over the others, nor as humanity's creator. And the Other Spirituality never so much as hints that there exists somewhere a relationship-seeking redeemer God.

Second, with the prevalence of shamanism in the New Synthesis, private mystical, trance or hallucinogenic experience become important and authoritative sources of theology. This is true in spite of the fact that the shaman *as* shaman— whether UFO abductee, New Age teacher, occult medium or spiritual mystic— has no important connection to ordinary life lived in the external world. Every shaman, when functioning *as* shaman, enters through some esoteric method—drugs, incantation, fasting, self-inflicted pain, hypnosis, spirit possession—a solitary world of inner spiritual experience where the limitations of daily existence are suspended, and its problems irrelevant. On the basis of such a disconnected interior experience, spiritual knowledge is obtained that provides alleged answers to impor-

tant moral and religious questions arising from daily life. It is important to contrast this approach to spiritual information with the life of Jesus Christ, lived authentically among ordinary people and under the limitations of daily existence in the villages of Palestine. We "have heard . . . have seen . . . and touched with our hands" the living Jesus, writes the apostle John of his and the other disciples' experience (1 Jn 1:3). The disregard for history shown by the New Synthesis becomes particularly pronounced and problematic in its embrace of shamanic insight—for how is the shaman's advice to be tested?

Third, among the most troubling aspects of modern shamanism is its tendency to preclude the possibility of evil intent on the part of the spirit guides. For Zukav it is a taken for granted fact that "there exists a realm that the religious language of the West would call the Angelic kingdom." In this realm are superevolved spirit beings "of numerous frequencies and qualities of consciousness, many of whom guide and interact with us upon the earth."[70] But according to Zukav, our spirit instructors "have evolved beyond" the possibility of doing evil. He writes, "The circumstances cannot be described in which [the inner teacher's] will might be bent in the wrong way, if there were such a way, or in a negative way."[71] This is a leap of faith if ever one has been taken. To submit one's judgment, indeed, one's life to a spiritual entity on the arbitrary assurance that it is incapable of evil seems perilous at best.

As with other components of the New Religious Synthesis, shamanism stands in sharp contrast to the Revealed Word tradition. Various shamanic practices were widespread in the ancient world, often associated with heinous rituals including human sacrifice. It is perhaps for good reason, then, that the biblical book of Deuteronomy expressed the following warning: "There shall not be found among you any one who burns his son or daughter as an offering, any one who practices divination, a soothsayer, or an augur, or a charmer, or a medium, or a wizard, or a necromancer. For whoever does these things is an abomination to the LORD" (Deut 18:10-12 RSV). New Testament sources express similar disdain for such activities, relegating them to the category of the demonic. Luke writes in the book of Acts that as he and Paul were on their way to the house of Lydia in the city of Thyatira, "we met a slave girl who had a spirit of divination and brought her owners a great deal of money by fortune-telling." Paul is reported to have said to the spirit, "'I order you in the name of Jesus Christ to come out of her.' And it came out that very hour" (Acts 16:16, 18).

Direct contact with spirits is viewed as a profound danger in the Revealed Word. Such is not the case in the New Religious Synthesis, where the practice is repeatedly

commended, and almost never with cautions attached. This movement away from a humble approach in prayer to a personal and sovereign God and instead toward a shamanic elite interacting directly with the spirit world is a watershed event in Western spirituality. It marks a return to a repudiated spirituality that has, until recently, maintained a largely subterranean life. Enjoying again the daylight of popular acceptance, the practices of modern shamanism ought at the very least to be critically examined before becoming a fixed part of accepted religious practice.

MYSTICAL PLURALISM

That direct, mystical contact with the divine is the road to pluralism is an emerging consensus among advocates of the New Religious Synthesis. Correspondingly, the creedal pronouncements of the Revealed Word tradition are often seem as obstacles to the advent of an era of religious unity and hope. Theologians defending an authoritative revelation of God's nature must step down. The spirit person, the shaman, the mystic, the UFO abductee and even the drug experimenter are the pioneers of the soul's new way, explorers of the psyche's deeper reaches, heroes of faith pointing the way out of the old exclusionary doctrines and toward religious pluralism.

As he receives messages from "God" about the true nature of everything, Neale Donald Walsch is told, *"religion is your attempt to speak of the unspeakable."*[72] Thus, any and all conceptions of God are simply personal expressions of the unknowable truth that mystics encounter. "I am God, as you understand Him. I am Goddess as you comprehend Her. I am Conceiver and Creator of Everything as you know and experience. . . . [Y]our perception of reality is more limited than you thought, and the Truth is more *un*limited than you can imagine. I am giving you ever-so-small a glimpse of infinity—and infinite love."[73]

As we have already noted, for proponents of a new religious era, god is the undifferentiated consciousness present in all things, or, as Aldous Huxley and John Shelby Spong would have it, "the ground of being." This notion is not contradicted by Walsch's contact with "God," nor by Shirley MacLaine's conversations with a Higher Self, for these are simply highly evolved intelligences that make no claim to be a preexisting and creating divinity like Yahweh of the Revealed Word. Prescribed theology—theological doctrine of the type taught in the Revealed Word tradition—will never open the door into this realm of pure being, this sphere of light and ecstasy. A deeper, more subjective, more direct spiritual experience is needed to find the divine.

278   THE MAKING OF THE NEW SPIRITUALITY

Deepak Chopra writes of the meditative effort to achieve a breakthrough to spiritual unity or ecstasy. "This process of shifting from activity to stillness," he writes, "is a simple yet very deep description of meditation." He adds, "We could modify the biblical injunction to 'Be still and know ecstasy.'" Of course, the biblical phrase is "Be still, and know that I am God" (Ps 46:10). Thus, Chopra makes the individual's experience of spiritual quietude a substitute for the Revealed Word's personal God. *"Expansion of consciousness is the road to ecstasy,"* writes Chopra.[74] And this experience of expanding consciousness is available in a variety of religious traditions, including the Christian when properly understood.

Christian apologist Ravi Zacharias has written, "The Christian faith is often castigated because the contemporary mind-set is infuriated by any claim to ideational elitism in a pluralistic society. How dare one idea be claimed as superior to another?"[75] It is true that Christianity's persistent claim to unique truthfulness offends modern sensibilities, outrages those seeking a rapprochement among the world's many religious systems. In fact, it is precisely Christianity's insistence that it alone is true among all of those systems that has driven the long public effort to unseat it and find a substitute, peace-making spirituality for the contemporary world.

But Christianity *requires* a unique claim to truth, and its internal logic runs dramatically and uncompromisingly at cross-purposes to religious pluralism. That logic states that God entered human history "in the fullness of time" and took on human flesh in the person of Jesus Christ. This event occurred but once and, when properly understood, is neither capable of duplication, nor does it have an equivalent. Christ's redemptive life and death must remain unique for Christianity to substantiate its foundational claims. And the same can be said of Jesus' resurrection—it must be unique if the logic of atonement is to be consistent. Why would God recognize another universal and ultimately sufficient sacrifice for human sin having recognized this one? Again, each of these claims—that Jesus Christ lived as God incarnate, that he died for human redemption, that he rose in conquest of death—is a sine qua non of Christian orthodoxy. Consequently, each makes the broad religious pluralism of the New Religious Synthesis impossible to reconcile with Christian orthodoxy. If Christians are to join the pluralistic parade, they must first jettison the old idea that Jesus is the unique manifestation of God in human form and reinvent their Messiah as one among many participants in the unifying mystic vision, as an-

other highly evolved spiritual guide, a prophet among prophets or, in Marcus Borg's phrase, a spirit person.

The Other Spirituality presents itself as refurbishing the primordial human religious view, the first human spirituality. Mysticism is inherent to this ancient religious view, the core, it is argued, of all important subsequent religious experience and speculation. This notion clashes with the Revealed Word's account of early human spiritual experience. On the Revealed Word view, the very earliest encounter between humans and the supernatural was, indeed, pure and enriching. A sovereign God created human beings, called them good and entered a relationship with them. Humanity encountered the sovereign creator God and knew him intimately. That intimate relationship was, however, ruined through a disastrous fall into sin, a possibility that mystical experience cannot accommodate.

Many New Synthesis writers have suggested the pluralistic path for Christians if they are to enter the new millennium as good faith partners in the quest for a single, unifying spirituality. But again we encounter a problem, for Christians always have claimed that Christianity was just that—the single, true, universal and unifying spiritual view, the good news of God's act of saving people from every tongue, tribe and nation. The choice, then, between Christianity and the Other Spirituality is a stark one: Jesus Christ as the single divine redeemer of a lost human race or Jesus as one among many spirit people seeking to express the inexpressible.

FINAL CONSIDERATIONS: A NEW AND BETTER WAY?

At the center of the New Religious Synthesis is the striving human will seeking desperately to launch itself into minor godhood in an evolving cosmos through the mechanisms of directed spiritual evolution, spiritualized science and spirit contact. This Other Spirituality that now presents itself as the rightful replacement for the Revealed Word proclaims its spiritual liberation from the worldview that informs Christianity and its freedom from that worldview's personal and wholly other God. But this new way of self-salvation may be little more than the refurbishing of an ancient spiritual mistake.

The New Religious Synthesis promises to secure the soul's triumph over external restraints including time, space, evil, other people, conventional morality and especially traditional religion. But in the process it dispenses with a transcendent and personal deity, irrevocable forgiveness of sin, triumph over death, egalitarian spiritual community and the simple joy of accepting our unchangeable status as in-

finitely valuable but fallen creatures of a living and holy God. This "new way" in religion puts us on the path we are inclined to take when left to our own spiritual devices—to proclaim our own divinity, which, in spite of the idea's obvious absurdity when confronted with the undeniable facts of our individual and corporate limitations, will be proven presently once we learn enough secrets. Could this be the broad road leading to spiritual destruction spoken of by Jesus?

The New Synthesis stresses the exertion of the human will in the spiritual realm, the individual psyche throwing off the restraints of revelation and tradition, human reason crafting its own salvation out of the raw materials of psycho-spiritual technique, mysterious *gnosis* or subjective mystical experience. In response to such spiritual seduction, Jesus continues to urge, "Come unto me."

The combination of pantheism and its attendant nature worship, religious secrecy, spiritual elitism and hopes of scientifically assisted evolutionary progress toward a master-species has, at some historical junctures, had sinister consequences. According to Richard Noll, historian R. G. Collingwood "interprets the rise of fascism and National Socialism in the twentieth century as the direct result of the popularity of the neopaganism in the late 1800s that worshipped the power of the human will and that, in turn, arose to fill a spiritual vacuum created by this very eclipse of faith in orthodox Christianity."[76] Other observers of Western culture have warned against the advent of spiritual systems that jettison a sovereign God and elevate a divine man or race. According to A. N. Wilson, Thomas Carlyle held that "if [faith] was not directed towards the true God, it would be directed towards idols. Hence Carlyle's view—as we can now see, a fatal though perfectly accurate one—that the human race, having discarded belief in the unseen God of Israel, would always look towards *Ubermensch* or Superman as its God-substitute."[77] And the self-promoting candidates for this position have never been hard to find, nor have their followers been few.

The book of Genesis records that the first human temptation was to acquire a forbidden knowledge that would make them "like God." In the late sixteenth century the heretical teacher Giordano Bruno propounded a reworked system of Egyptian magic based on pantheism, demonic guidance and *gnosis*. As the first master of his own system, Bruno believed himself to be, in fact, divine. As Frances Yates writes, "Bruno has made the gnostic ascent . . . and so has become divine, with the Powers within him."[78] The advocates of a new way in religion have paid less attention to spiritual truth than they have to the grand project of inventing and

promoting a self-aggrandizing substitute for an authentic religious faith, a faith, moreover, that made them accountable to a God who could not be bribed. M. Craig Barnes has written that "people who have a God do not need to become one themselves. They are too consumed watching the Lord's salvation unfold."[79] It may be time for us to relearn this simple but profound truth.

NOTES

Chapter One: Introduction: A Changing View of the Spiritual World

[1]Gary Zukav, October 2002, <www.zukav.com>.

[2]Gary Zukav, *The Seat of the Soul* (New York: Simon & Schuster, 1989), p. 67.

[3]Ibid., p. 71.

[4]Ibid., p. 83.

[5]Ibid., p. 102.

[6]Ibid., p. 92.

[7]Ibid., p. 97.

[8]Marija Gimbutas, *The Language of the Goddess: Unearthing the Hidden Symbols of Western Civilization* (San Francisco: Harper & Row, 1989), p. xiv.

[9]Marilyn Ferguson, *The Aquarian Conspiracy: Personal and Social Transformation in the 1980's* (Los Angeles: J. P. Tarcher, 1980), p. 25.

[10]Carl Jung, "The Difference Between Eastern and Western Thinking," in *The Portable Jung* (New York: Penguin, 1976), p. 476.

[11]Wayne Teasdale, *The Mystic Heart* (Novato, Calif.: New World Library, 1999), p. 4.

[12]Carl A. Raschke, *The Interruption of Eternity: Modern Gnosticism and the Origins of the New Religious Consciousness* (Chicago: Nelson-Hall, 1980).

[13]Quoted in Winifred Gallagher, *Working on God* (New York: Random House, 1999), p. xx.

[14]Michael D'Antonio, *Heaven on Earth: Dispatches from America's Spiritual Frontier* (New York: Crown , 1992), p. 13.

[15]Ibid., p. 17.

[16]Wade Clark Roof, *Spiritual Marketplace: Baby Boomers and the Remaking of American Religion* (Princeton, N.J.: Princeton University Press, 1999), pp. 37-38.

[17]Ibid., p. 38.

[18]Teasdale, *Mystic Heart*, p. 4.

[19]Ibid., pp. 4-5.

[20]Ibid., p. 5.

[21]Teresa Watanabe, "Spirituality Is One for the Books," *Los Angeles Times*, September 4, 1999, p. 1.

[22]Robert Wuthnow, *After Heaven: Spirituality in America Since the 1950s* (Berkeley: University of California Press, 1998), p. 14.

[23]Ibid., p. 13.

[24]Philip Jenkins, *Mystics and Messiahs: Cults and New Religions in American History* (Oxford: Oxford University Press, 2000), p. 10.

[25]Lisa Napoli, "When the Astrology Zone Aligns with the Internet," *The New York Times*, October 5, 1998, p. C11.

[26]Robert Wuthnow, *Rediscovering the Sacred* (Grand Rapids, Mich.: Eerdmans, 1992), p. 1.

[27]Karen Hoyt, ed., *The New Age Rage* (Old Tappan, N.J.: Revell, 1987), p. 11.

[28]D'Antonio, *Heaven on Earth*, pp. 12-13.

[29]Shirley MacLaine, *Going Within: A Guide for Inner Transformation* (New York: Bantam, 1989), and *Dancing in the Light* (New York: Bantam 1985).

[30]Ibid., p. 100.

[31]D'Antonio, *Heaven on Earth*, pp. 13.

[32]Carlos Castaneda, *The Teachings of Don Juan: A Yaqui Way of Knowledge* (Berkeley: University of California Press, 1969).

[33]Ibid., p. 7.

[34]Ferguson, *Aquarian Conspiracy*, p. 28.

[35]Carol P. Christ, *Rebirth of the Goddess: Finding Meaning in Feminist Spirituality* (New York: Addison Wesley, 1997), p. xiii. Other titles on goddess worship include Starhawk, *The Spiral Dance* (New York: Harper & Row, 1989); Elinor W. Gadon, *The Once and Future Goddess* (New York: HarperCollins, 1989); Zsuzsanna Emese Budapest, *The Holy Book of Women's Mysteries* (Oakland, Calif.: Susan B. Anthony Coven No. 1, 1986); Jean Shinoda Bolen, *Goddesses in Everywoman* (San Francisco: Harper & Row, 1984); Naomi Goldenberg, *Changing of the Gods: Feminism and the End of Traditional Religions* (Boston: Beacon, 1979).

[36]Carol P. Christ, "Why Women Need the Goddess: Phenomenological, Psychological and Political Reflections," in *Womanspring Rising: A Feminist Reader in Religion*, ed. Carol P. Christ and Judith Plaskow (San Francisco: Harper & Row, 1979), p. 277; quoted in Peter Jones, *The Gnostic Empire Strikes Back: An Old Heresy for The New Age* (Phillipsburg, Penn.: Presbyterian & Reformed, 1992), p. 55.

[37]Gimbutas, *Language of the Goddess*. p. xx.

[38]Ibid., p. xxi.

[39]Barbara Walker, *Restoring the Goddess* (Amherst, N.Y.: Prometheus, 2000).

[40]Akasha Gloria Hull, *Soul Talk: The New Spirituality of African American Women* (Rochester, Vt.: Inner Traditions, 2001), p. 1.

[41]Ibid., p. 2.

[42]Rich Poll, *Apologia Update*, winter 1999, p. 1.

[43]Deepti Hajela, Associated Press, June 4, 2000.

[44]See <www.bolt.com> link to Mystic.

[45]Phyllis Curott, *Book of Shadows: A Modern Woman's Journey into the Wisdom and the Magic of the Goddess* (New York: Broadway, 1998).

[46]Ibid., p. xii.

[47]Ibid.

[48]Ashleen O'Gaea, *The Family Wicca Book: The Craft for Parents and Children* (St. Paul, Minn.: Llewellyn, 1994), p. xi.

[49]Ibid., p. 6.

[50]David A. Cooper, *God Is a Verb: Kabbalah and the Practice of Mystical Judaism* (New York: Riverhead, 1997).

[51]Rodger Kamenetz, *The Jew in the Lotus: A Poet's Rediscovery of Jewish Identity in Buddhist India* (San Francisco: Harper SanFrancisco, 1994).

[52]John Heider, *The Tao of Leadership: Leadership Strategies for a New Age* (New York: Bantam, 1986).

[53]Ibid., p. 31.

[54]*O: The Oprah Magazine*, August 2001, p. 174.

[55]*Civilization*, December 1999, p. 61.

[56]*Transforming the Mind: Teachings on Generating Compassion* (London: Thorsuns, 2000); *The Art of Happiness: A Handbook for Living*, authored with Howard C. Cutler, M.D. (New York: Riverhead, 1998); *The Path to Tranquility: Daily Wisdom* (New York: Viking Arkana, 1999).

[57]Diki Tsering, *My Son: A Mother's Story*, ed. Khedroop Thondup (New York: Viking Arkana, 2000).

[58]See "Buddha Boom," *Civilization*, December 1999, pp. 57-71.

[59]Fritjof Capra, *The Tao of Physics* (Berkeley, Calif.: Shambala, 1975); *The Turning Point: Science, Society and the Rising Culture* (New York: Simon & Schuster, 1982).

[60]Fritjof Capra, *The Web of Life: A New Scientific Understanding of Living Systems* (New York: Anchor, 1996), p. 107.

[61]Ibid.

[62]Fred Alan Wolf, *The Dreaming Universe* (New York: Simon & Schuster, 1994), 344.

[63]Ibid., p. 343.

[64]Amit Goswami, *The Self-Aware Universe: How Consciousness Creates the Material World* (New York: Jeremy P. Tharcher, 1995), p. 11.

[65]Gary Zukav, *The Dancing Wu Li Masters: An Overview of the New Physics* (New York: William Morrow, 1979); Fred Alan Wolf, *The Spiritual Universe: How Quantum Physics Proves the Existence of the Soul* (New York: Simon & Schuster, 1996.

[66]Ferguson, *Aquarian Conspiracy*, p. 23.

[67]Jeremy Narby and Francis Huxley, eds., *Shamans Through Time: 500 Years on the Path to Knowledge* (New York: Jeremy Tarcher, 2001), pp. 301-5.

[68]Ibid., p. 302.

[69]Ibid., p. 303.

[70]Mark Epstein, *Going to Pieces Without Falling Apart* (New York: Broadway, 1998), p. xix.

[71]Ibid., p. i.

[72]Richard Noll, *The Jung Cult: Origins of a Charismatic Movement* (Princeton, N.J.: Princeton University Press, 1994).

[73]John E. Mack, *Abduction: Human Encounters with Aliens* (New York: Charles Scribner's Sons, 1995).

[74]Other books in this growing genre include *Summoned. Encounters with Alien Intelligence* by Dana Redfield and Linda Moulton Howe, *The Custodians: Beyond Abduction* by Delores Cannon, *Reaching for Reality: Seven Incredible True Stories of Alien Abduction* by Constance Clear and *The UFO Enigma: A New Review of the Physical Evidence* by Peter A. Sturrock.

[75]Helen Schucman, *A Course in Miracles and Manual for Teachers* (Tiburon, Calif.: Center for Inner Peace, 1975).

[76]Ibid., pp. 57, 63.

[77]Cadonna M. Peyton, "Schools Assist Students in Developing 'Sixth Sense,'" Associated Press, January 16, 2000.

[78]Ruth Walker, "Translating Belief in God into Health and Well-Being," *The Christian Science Monitor*, December 20, 2001, sec. 2, p. 13.

[79]James H. Austin, M.D., *Zen and the Brain* (Cambridge, Mass.: MIT Press, 1998), p. 695.

[80]Carl Jung, "The Spiritual Problem of Modern Man," in *Modern Man in Search of a Soul*, trans. W. S. Dell and Cary F. Baynes (New York: Harcourt Brace, 1933), p. 209.

Chapter Two: Antecedents of the New Religious Synthesis:
A Brief History of Alternative Spirituality in the West

[1]Leonard Levi, *Blasphemy: Verbal Offense Against the Sacred* (New York: Alfred A. Knopf, 1993), p. 55.

[2]Wayne Shumaker, *The Occult Sciences in the Renaissance: A Study in Intellectual Patterns* (Berke-ley: University of California Press, 1972), pp. 211, 209.

[3]Ibid., p. 201.

[4]See Gavin Ashenden, "The Influence of Hermeticism on Myth and Metaphysics in the Life and Works of Charles Williams" (Ph.D. diss., University of Sussex, 1998-1999).

[5]Shumaker, *Occult Sciences*, p. 233.

[6]Ibid., pp. 225, 214.

[7]Ibid., p. 215.

[8]Ibid., p. 220.

[9]Ibid., p. 228.

[10]Ibid., p. 229.

[11]Ibid., p. 230.

[12]Ibid., p. 235.

[13]Adolphe Franck, *The Kabbalah: The Religious Philosophy of the Hebrews* (1843; reprint, Secaucus, N.J.: Citadel Press, 1979), pp. 26-27.

[14]See ibid., chap. 3, "The Authenticity of the Zohar."

[15]Ibid., p. 16.

[16]Ibid., pp. 13-14.

[17]John C. Wilson, editor's introduction to Franck, *Kabbalah*, p. 8.

[18]Shlomo Giora Shoham, *Bridges to Nothingness: Gnosis, Kabala, Existentialism, and the Transcendental Predicament of Man* (London: Associated University Presses, 1994), p. 21.

[19]Franck, *Kabbalah*, p. 23.

[20]Shoham, *Bridges to Nothingness*, p.111.

[21]Ibid., pp. 110-11.

[22]Ibid., p. 112.

[23]Ibid., p. 97.

[24]Ibid., p. 103.

[25]Ibid., p. 72.

[26]Ibid., p. 73.

[27]Ibid., pp. 111-12.

[28]Hugh J. Kearney, *Science and Change: 1500-1700* (New York: McGraw-Hill, 1971), p. 24.

[29]Ibid., p. 100.

[30]Ibid., p. 48.

[31]Ibid., p. 39.

[32]Ibid., p. 37.

[33]Ibid., p. 100.

[34]Ibid., p. 39.

[35]Ibid., p. 110.

[36]Robert E. Sullivan, *John Toland and the Deist Controversy* (Cambridge, Mass.: Harvard University Press, 1982), p. 199.

[37]Carl A. Raschke, *The Interruption of Eternity: Modern Gnosticism and the Origins of the New Religious Consciousness* (Chicago: Nelson-Hall, 1980), p. 49.

[38]Sullivan, *John Toland*, p. 200.

[39]Kearney, *Science and Change*, p. 106.

[40]Franklin Baumer, *Religion and the Rise of Scepticism* (New York: Harcourt Brace & World, 1960), pp. 90-91.

[41]Kearney, *Science and Change*, p. 130.

[42]Ibid., p. 132.

[43]Roland Bainton, *The Reformation of the Sixteenth Century* (Boston: Beacon, 1952), p. 128.

[44]Bradford Verter, "Dark Star Rising: The Emergence of Modern Occultism, 1800-1950" (Ph.D. diss., Princeton University, 1998), p. 33.

[45]Shumaker, *Occult Sciences*, p. 205.

[46]Ibid.

[47]Ibid., p. 204.

[48]Ibid., p. 205.

[49] Quoted in R. W. Southern, *Western Society and the Church in the Middle Ages* (Baltimore: Penguin, 1970), p. 45.

[50] Ibid., p. 48.

[51] Bainton, *Reformation of the Sixteenth Century*, p. 125.

[52] Ibid., p. 124.

[53] George T. Buckley, *Atheism in the English Renaissance* (1932; reprint, New York· Russell & Russell, 1965), p. 17.

[54] Harold Hutcheson, *Lord Herbert of Cherbury's* De Religione Laici (New Haven, Conn.: Yale University Press, 1944), p. 60.

[55] On the nature of the ancient skeptical tradition, see Julia Annas and Jonathan Barnes, *The Modes of Scepticism* (Cambridge: Cambridge University Press, 1985). On more recent treatments of skepticism, see M. Jamie Ferreira, *Scepticism and Reasonable Doubt* (Oxford: Clarendon, 1986). See also P. F. Strawson, *Scepticism and Naturalism: Some Varieties* (New York: Columbia University Press, 1985).

[56] C. B. Schmitt, "The Rediscovery of Ancient Scepticism in Modern Times," in *The Skeptical Tradition* (Berkeley: University of California Press, 1983), pp. 225-51, esp. p. 228.

[57] Buckley, *Atheism in the English Renaissance*, p. 17.

[58] Mark U. Edwards Jr. *Printing, Propaganda, and Martin Luther* (Berkeley: University of California Press, 1994), p. 367.

[59] Buckley, *Atheism in the English Renaissance*, pp. 18-19.

[60] See James A. Herrick, *The Radical Rhetoric of the English Deists: The Discourse of Scepticism, 1680-1750* (Columbia: University of South Carolina Press, 1997).

[61] Benedict de Spinoza, *The Chief Works of Spinoza*, 2 vols. in 1, trans. R. H. M. Elwes (New York: Dover, 1951).

[62] Jonathan Israels, *The Dutch Republic: Its Rise, Greatness and Fall, 1477-1806* (Oxford: Clarendon, 1995), p. 1048.

[63] Spinoza, *Tractatus*, p. 8; quoted in Nigel M. de S. Cameron, *Biblical Higher Criticism and the Defense of Infallibilism in 19th Century Britain* (Lewiston, N.Y.: Edwin Mellon, 1987), p. 16.

[64] Spinoza, *Tractatus* 6.92; also quoted in Cameron, p. 14.

[65] Spinoza, *Tractatus*, chaps. 6-9.

[66] Edgar Krentz, *The History of Critical Method* (Philadelphia: Fortress, 1975), p. 14.

[67] Ibid.

[68] *The Works of Sir Thomas Browne* (London: n.p., 1857).

[69] Rosalie Colie, *Light and Enlightenment* (Cambridge: Cambridge University Press, 1957), p. 40.

[70] H. McLachlan, *Socinianism in Seventeenth Century England* (Oxford: Oxford University Press, 1951), pp. 325-27.

[71] J. C. D. Clark, *English Society: 1688-1832* (Cambridge: Cambridge University Press, 1985), p. 280.

[72] Krentz, *History of Critical Method*, p. 12.

[73] Ibid., p. 13.

[74]Ibid., p.5.

[75]Colin Brown, *Jesus in European Protestant Thought* (Durham, N.C.: Labyrinth, 1985), p. 281 n. 58.

[76]Krentz, *History of Critical Method*, p. 15. The other works included *Histoire critique du texte du Nouveau Testament* (1689), *Histoire critique des versions du Nouveau Testament* (1693) and *Histoire critique des principaux commentaires du Nouveau Testament* (1693).

[77]Krentz, *History of Critical Method*, p. 15.

[78]Ibid., p.16.

[79]Richard Popkin, *The History of Skepticism from Erasmus to Spinoza* (Berkeley: University of California Press, 1979), p. 4.

[80]Roscoe Pound, *The Development of Constitutional Guarantees of Liberty* (New Haven, Conn.: Yale University Press, 1957), p. 30.

[81]S. G. Hefelbower, *The Relation of John Locke to English Deism* (Chicago: University of Chicago Press, 1918), p. 3.

[82]See, for example, the anonymous *Reasons for Not Proceeding Against Mr. Whiston* (London, 1713), p. 15.

Chapter Three: The Rise of Biblical Criticism:
Allegory, Myth, Codes and the End of History

[1]Thomas Woolston, *Fourth Discourse on the Miracles of Our Saviour* (London: 1729), p. 33.

[2]R. M. Burns, *The Great Debate on Miracles* (Lewisberg, Penn.: Bucknell University Press), p. 10.

[3]Jonathan Swift, "Verses on the Death of Dr. Swift," in *The Poems of Jonathan Swift*, 2nd ed., ed. Harold Williams (Oxford: Clarendon, 1958), p. 564; also quoted in Burns, *Great Debate*, p. 10. Swift attacked Woolston in a note, writing that "Woolston was a Clergyman, but for want of Bread, hath in several Treatises, in the most blasphemous Manner, attempted to turn Our Saviour and his Miracles into Ridicule. He is much caressed by many great Courtiers, and by all the Infidels, and his Books read generally by the Court Ladies" (Williams, *Poems of Jonathan Swift*, p. 564).

[4]Peter Gay, *The Enlightenment: An Interpretation* (New York: Alfred Knopf, 1967), p. 375; Henning Graf Reventlow, *The Authority of the Bible, and the Rise of the Modern World* (Philadelphia: Fortress, 1985), p. 149; John Redwood, *Reason, Ridicule, and Religion* (Cambridge, Mass.: Harvard University Press, 1976), p. 149.

[5]Robert M. Grant and David Tracy, *A Short History of the Interpretation of the Bible*, 2nd ed. (Philadelphia: Fortress, 1984), p. 109.

[6]John Shelby Spong, *Rescuing the Bible from Fundamentalism* (San Francisco: HarperSanFrancisco, 1991), p. 21.

[7]Ibid.

[8]Ibid., p. 22.

[9]Ibid., p. 237.

[10]Ibid., p. 24.

[11] Anthony Collins, *A Discourse of Free Thinking* (London: n.p., 1713), p. 44.

[12] Ibid., p. 45.

[13] Henning Graf Reventlow, *The Authority of the Bible and the Rise of the Modern World* (Philadelphia: Fortress, 1985), p. 412.

[14] Thomas Woolston, *Six Discourses on the Miracles of Our Saviour* (London: n.p., 1727-1729), *First Discourse*, p. 4.

[15] Ibid., p. 34.

[16] Woolston, *Fourth Discourse*, p. 7.

[17] Ibid., p. 6.

[18] Ibid., p. 11.

[19] Ibid., p. 22.

[20] Ibid., p. 17.

[21] Ibid., p. 20.

[22] Simon Browne, *A Fit Rebuke to a Ludicrous Infidel in Some Remarks on Mr. Woolston's Fifth Discourse* (London: R. Ford, 1732), p. i.

[23] Bishop Edmund Gibson, *The Bishop of London's Pastoral Letter to the People of His Diocese* (London: Samuel Buckley, 1728), p. 33.

[24] See Colin Brown, *Jesus in European Protestant Thought* (Durham, N.C.: Labyrinth, 1985), chaps. 1 and 2.

[25] Ibid., pp. 51-52. Brown connects the Deists directly to a number of German Enlightenment theologians.

[26] Harold O. J. Brown, *Heresies* (Garden City, N.Y.: Doubleday, 1984), p. 404.

[27] Ibid.

[28] *New International Dictionary of New Testament Theology*, ed. Colin Brown (Exeter, U.K.: Paternoster, 1975-1978), p. 833; Brown, *Jesus in European Protestant Thought*, p. 2.

[29] Brown, *Jesus in European Protestant Thought*, p. 2.

[30] Gay, *The Enlightenment*, p. 381.

[31] C. Brown, *Jesus in European Protestant Thought*, p. 22; Gay, *The Enlightenment*, p. 332.

[32] Gay, *The Enlightenment*, p. 333.

[33] Eliot also translated Feuerbach's *Essence of Christianity* into English in 1854.

[34] Noel Annan, "Science, Religion, and the Critical Mind," in *The Victorian Age: Essays in Fiction and in Social and Literary Criticism*, ed. Robert Langbaum (Greenwich, Conn.: Fawcett Premier, 1967), pp. 69-74; quote p. 72.

[35] Ibid., pp. 71-72.

[36] J. W. Burrow, *The Crisis of Reason: European Thought, 1848-1914* (New Haven, Conn.: Yale University Press, 2000), p. 197.

[37] David Strauss, *Life of Jesus Critically Examined*, 2 vols., trans. Marian Evans (New York: Calvin Blanchard, 1856), 1:3.

[38] Ibid., 1:3-4.

[39] Ibid., 1:4.

[40]Ibid.

[41]Ibid., 1:33.

[42]Ibid., 1:43.

[43]Ibid., 1:47.

[44]Ibid.

[45]Ibid., 1:47-48.

[46]Ibid., 1:61.

[47]Ibid.

[48]Ibid., 1:63.

[49]Ibid., 2:892-93.

[50]Ibid., 2:895.

[51]Ibid., 2:896.

[52]Ibid., 2:898.

[53]Spong, *Rescuing the Bible*, p. 17.

[54]Ibid., p. 20.

[55]Ibid., pp. 16-17.

[56]Ibid., p. 24.

[57]Ibid., pp. 22-23, 21.

[58]Ibid., p. 37.

[59]Ibid., pp. 37-38.

[60]Ibid., pp. 98, 100.

[61]Ibid., p. 101.

[62]Ibid., p. 24.

[63]Ibid., p. 237.

[64]Ibid., p. 242.

[65]Ibid.

[66]Michael Drosnin, *The Bible Code* (New York: Simon & Schuster, 1997).

[67]Ibid., p. 20.

[68]Ibid.

[69]Ibid., p. 21.

[70]Ibid., p. 38.

[71]Ibid., p. 186.

[72]Ibid., p. 182.

[73]Ibid., p. 20.

[74]Ibid., p. 148.

[75]John Stott, *The Contemporary Christian* (Downers Grove, Ill.: InterVarsity Press, 1992), p. 15.

Chapter Four: The Ascent of Reason: Birth of a Deity

[1]Franklin Baumer, *Religion and the Rise of Scepticism* (New York: Harcourt Brace & World, 1960), p. 35.

[2] Ibid., p. 36.

[3] Carl G. Jung, "The Spiritual Problem of Modern Man," in *Modern Man in Search of a Soul,* trans. W. S. Dell and Cary F. Baynes (New York: Harcourt Brace, 1933), p. 209.

[4] Baumer, *Religion and Rise of Scepticism,* p. 74.

[5] Ibid.

[6] Quoted in ibid., p. 75. See Antoine Nicolas de Condorcet, *Sketch of a Historical Picture of the Progress of the Human Mind,* trans. June Barraclough (New York: Noonday, 1955).

[7] Peter Annet, *The Free Inquirer,* October 17, 1761 (reprinted London: R. Carlile, 1826), p. 3.

[8] Peter Annet, *Lectures Corrected and Revised* (London: J. Smith, n.d.), no. 11, p. 113.

[9] Annet, *Free Inquirer,* October 17, 1761, pp. 3-4.

[10] Ibid., p. 4.

[11] Annet, *Free Inquirer,* November 3, 1761, pp. 21-22.

[12] Peter Annet, *Deism Fairly Stated* (London: W. Webb, 1746), p. 9.

[13] Ibid., p. 10.

[14] Thomas Babington Macaulay, quoted in the introduction to Voltaire, *Zadig and Other Stories,* ed. Irving Babbitt (Boston: D. C. Heath, 1905), p. ix.

[15] Wayne Andrews, *Voltaire* (New York: New Directions, 1981), p. 9.

[16] Baumer, *Religion and Rise of Scepticism,* p. 47.

[17] Theodore Besterman, introduction to Voltaire, *Candide and Other Stories,* trans. Joan Spencer, ed. Henri Bénac (London: Oxford University Press, 1966), p. viii.

[18] Babbitt, introduction to Voltaire, *Zadig,* p. vi.

[19] Besterman, introduction to Voltaire, *Candide,* p. xi.

[20] Ibid., p. x.

[21] Ibid., p. 2.

[22] Ibid., pp. 7-8.

[23] Ibid., p. 20.

[24] Ibid.

[25] Ibid., p. 21.

[26] Ibid., p. 36.

[27] Ibid., pp. 39-40.

[28] Robert A. Wagoner, translator's foreword to *Voltaire,* by Gustave Lanson (New York: John Wiley & Sons, 1966), p. viii.

[29] Andrews, *Voltaire,* p. 2.

[30] William Covino, *Rhetoric and Magic* (Albany: State University of New York Press, 1997), p. 71.

[31] Ibid., p. 73.

[32] Ibid., p. 74.

[33] Thomas De Quincey, *Confessions of an English Opium-Eater and Other Writings,* ed. Grevel Lindop (Oxford: Oxford University Press, 1985), pp. 116-17; quoted in Covino, *Rhetoric and Magic,* p. 77.

[34]Covino, *Rhetoric and Magic*, pp. 77-78. Gregory Dart has written, "In his political writings, De Quincey frequently exhibited a violent fear and loathing of the urban mass" (*Times Literary Supplement*, June 1, 2001, p. 4).

[35]Quoted in Covino, *Rhetoric and Magic*, p. 79.

[36]Ibid.

[37]Thomas De Quincey, *Confessions of an English Opium Eater* and *Suspiria profundis* (Boston: Ticknor, Reed & Fields, 1850), p. 55.

[38]Ibid., p. 56.

[39]Ibid.

[40]Ibid., p. 62.

[41]Ibid., p. 57.

[42]Ibid., pp. 67-68.

[43]Ibid., p. 131.

[44]Ibid.

[45]Ibid., p. 132.

[46]Ibid., p. 133.

[47]Richard Kyle, *The Religious Fringe: A History of Alternative Religion in America* (Downers Grove, Ill.: InterVarsity Press, 1993), p. 49.

[48]Stephen Gottschalk, "Christian Science and Harmonialism," in *Encyclopedia of the American Religious Experience* (New York: Scribner, 1988), p. 903.

[49]Dennis Voskuil, *Mountains into Goldmines: Robert Schuller and the Gospel of Success* (Grand Rapids, Mich.: Eerdmans, 1983), p. 118.

[50]Ibid.

[51]Ibid.

[52]On Eddy and her relationship with Quimby and his ideas, see Gillian Gill, *Mary Baker Eddy* (Reading, Mass.: Perseus, 1998), pp. 119ff.

[53]Ibid., p. 119.

[54]From the Alliance's declaration of purpose; quoted in Voskuil, p. 120.

[55]Quoted in Voskuil, *Mountains into Goldmines*, p. 120.

[56]Quoted in ibid.

[57]Ibid., p. 122. Ralph Waldo Trine, *In Tune with the Infinite* (New York: Crowell, 1897).

[58]Quoted in Voskuil, *Mountains into Goldmines*, p. 122.

[59]Ibid., p. 123.

[60]Ibid.

[61]Ayn Rand, *Atlas Shrugged* (New York: Dutton, 1992), p. 1010.

[62]Ibid., p. 1011.

[63]Ibid., p. 1012.

[64]Ibid., p. 1011.

[65]Ibid., p. 1012.

[66]Ibid., p. 1013.

[67] Ibid.

[68] Ibid. For a discussion of how Rand's works are currently being used to provide moral justification for corporate greed, see Del Jones, "Scandals Lead Execs to *Atlas Shrugged*," *USA Today*, September 24, 2002, p. 1.

[69] Ibid.

[70] Ibid., p. 1015.

Chapter Five: Science and Shifting Paradigms: Salvation in a New Cosmos

[1] Edward S. Reed, *From Soul to Mind: The Emergence of Psychology from Erasmus Darwin to William James* (New Haven, Conn.: Yale University Press, 1997), p. 158.

[2] James Turner, *Without God, Without Creed* (Baltimore: Johns Hopkins University Press, 1985), p. 137.

[3] C. Maurice Davies, *Heterodox London: Phases of Free Thought in the Metropolis* (1874; reprint, New York: A. M. Kelley, 1969), 2:254.

[4] Ibid., pp. 256-57.

[5] Jacques Barzun, *From Dawn to Decadence* (New York: Harper Collins, 2000), p. 572.

[6] C. G. Jung, "The Spiritual Problem of Modern Man," in *Modern Man in Search of a Soul,* trans. W. S. Dell and Cary F. Baynes (New York: Harcourt Brace, 1933), p. 204.

[7] Philip Jenkins, *Mystics and Messiahs: Cults and New Religions in American History* (Oxford: Oxford University Press, 2000).

[8] Amit Goswami, *The Self-Aware Universe: How Consciousness Creates the Material World* (New York: Jeremy P. Tharcher, 1995), p. 60.

[9] Fritjof Capra, *The Tao of Physics: An Exploration of the Parallels Between Modern Physics and Eastern Mysticism* (1975; Boston: Shambala, 2000), p. 17.

[10] Thomas Paine, *The Age of Reason* (Secaucus, N.J.: Citadel, 1974), p. 60.

[11] Ibid., p. 70.

[12] Ibid.

[13] Ibid., p. 73.

[14] Ibid., p. 75.

[15] Hugh J. Kearney, *Science and Change: 1500-1700* (New York: McGraw-Hill, 1971), p. 127.

[16] Paine, *Age of Reason*, p. 79.

[17] Ibid., p. 80.

[18] Ibid., p. 80n.

[19] Ibid., p. 84.

[20] Ibid., p. 80.

[21] Ibid., p. 83.

[22] Ibid.

[23] Ibid., p. 82.

[24] Ibid., p. 84 and 84n.

[25] Ibid., p. 86.

[26] Ibid., p. 88.

[27] Ibid., p. 89.

[28] Paine was not the first to posit a number of inhabited worlds. This had been a mainstay of the magical view of science since at least the time of Bruno and had been explicitly argued in France by Fontenelle (1657-1757) in *Conversations About a Plurality of Worlds* (1685).

[29] Paine, *Age of Reason*, p. 90.

[30] Ibid., p. 91.

[31] Ibid., p. 92.

[32] Paine is likely engaged in the practice David Berman has called "theological lying," strategically implying his acceptance of theism while he advocates pantheism. See Berman's "Deism, Immortality, and the Art of Theological Lying," in *Deism, Masonry and the Enlightenment*, ed. J. A. Leo Lamay (Newark: University of Delaware Press, 1987), pp. 61-78.

[33] Paine, *Age of Reason*, p. 89.

[34] Paine's thinking may be rooted in what Hugh J. Kearney calls the "quasi-religious" Pythagorean belief that the universe is structured "in accordance with the laws of mathematics" (*Science and Change*, p. 137).

[35] Kearney, *Science and Change*, p. 215.

[36] Robert G. Ingersoll, *The Truth Seeker* (New York: n.p., 1890), p. 1.

[37] Ibid., p. 2.

[38] Robert G. Ingersoll, "The Mistakes of Moses," in *The Works of Robert G. Ingersoll*, vol. 1 (New York: Dresden Publishing, 1912), p. 98.

[39] Ingersoll, *Truth Seeker*, p. 2.

[40] Ingersoll, "Mistakes," p. 101.

[41] Ibid., p. 105.

[42] Ibid., p. 106.

[43] Ibid., p. 97.

[44] Ibid., p. 99.

[45] Ingersoll, *Truth Seeker*, p. 3.

[46] Robert G. Ingersoll, "The Foundations of Faith," in *The Works of Robert G. Ingersoll*, 12 vols., memorial ed. (New York: Dresden, 1912-1929), 4:290-91.

[47] The SETI project began in 1960 with Frank Drake's first experiment called Project Ozma. See Frank Drake, "Project Ozma," *Physics Today* 14 (1960): 40-46. For a more recent report on the effort to find intelligent life elsewhere in the universe, see P. Horowitz and C. Sagan, "Five Years of Project META: An All Sky Narrowband Radio Search for Extraterrestrial Signals," *Astrophysical Journal* 415 (1993): 218-35. Also of interest is Sagan's obscure early work on communication with alien intelligences, *The Cosmic Connection: An Extraterrestrial Perspective* (New York: Dell, 1973). See also Walter Sullivan's bestseller *We Are Not Alone* (New York: McGraw Hill, 1964).

[48] Carl Sagan, *The Demon-Haunted World: Science as a Candle in the Dark* (New York: Random House, 1995), p. 9.

[49]Ibid., p. 10.

[50]Ibid., p. 12.

[51]Ibid., p. 13.

[52]Ibid., p. 14.

[53]Ibid., p. 27.

[54]Ibid., p. 29.

[55]Ibid., p. 12.

[56]Ibid., p. 31.

[57]Ibid., p. 34.

[58]Ibid., p. 35.

[59]Ibid.

[60]Carl Sagan, *Contact: A Novel* (New York: Simon & Schuster, 1985), pp. 356-57.

[61]Ibid., p. 358.

[62]Ibid., p. 359.

[63]Ibid., p. 363.

[64]Ibid., p. 364.

[65]Ibid., pp. 366-67.

[66]Gordon Plummer, *From Atom to Kosmos: Journey Without End* (Wheaton, Ill.: Theosophical Publishing House, 1989).

[67]Gary Zukav, *The Dancing Wu Li Masters: An Overview of the New Physics* (New York: William Morrow, 1979), p. 331.

[68]Ibid.

[69]Marilyn Ferguson, *The Aquarian Conspiracy: Personal and Social Transformation in the 1980's* (Los Angeles: J. P. Tarcher, 1980), p. 146.

[70]Ibid., p. 148.

[71]Goswami, *Self-Aware Universe*, p. 11.

[72]Ibid.

[73]Fred Alan Wolf, *The Dreaming Universe* (New York: Simon & Schuster, 1994), pp. 343-44.

[74]Capra, *Tao of Physics*, p. 17.

[75]Ibid., p. 81.

[76]Fritjof Capra, *The Web of Life: A New Scientific Understanding of Living Systems* (New York: Anchor, 1996), 7.

[77]Capra, *Web of Life*, p. 295.

[78]Goswami, *Self-Aware Universe*, p. 60.

[79]Jeremy Narby and Francis Huxley, eds., *Shamans Through Time: 500 Years on the Path to Knowledge* (New York: Jeremy Tarcher, 2001), p. 305.

[80]Zukav, *Dancing Wu Li Masters*, p. 337.

Chapter Six: Evolution and Advancement: The Darwins' Spiritual Legacy

[1]Joseph Smith Jr., "King Follett Discourse" (1844) posted on Kingdom of Zion site

<www.kingdomofzion.org>. See also Joseph Smith, *Teachings of the Prophet Joseph Smith* (Salt Lake City: Deseret, 1976), pp. 342-61.

[2]Ibid.

[3]Ibid.

[4]Robert Ornstein, *The Evolution of Consciousness* (New York: Prentice Hall, 1991), p. 279.

[5]Ibid., p. 273.

[6]Robert Ornstein and Paul Ehrlich, *New World, New Mind* (Cambridge Mass.: Malor, 1989), p. 195.

[7]J. W. Burrow, *The Crisis of Reason: European Thought, 1848-1914* (New Haven, Conn.: Yale University Press, 2000), p. 43.

[8]For Rousseau's theory of education, see *Emile or On Education*, trans. Allan Bloom (New York: Basic Books, 1979).

[9]Erasmus Darwin, *Zoonomia*, part 1 (London: J. Johnson, 1794); 2nd ed. parts 1-3, 2 vols. (London: J. Johnson, 1796); 3rd ed., 4 vols. (London: J. Johnson, 1801).

[10]Erasmus Darwin, *The Essential Writings of Erasmus Darwin*, ed. Desmond King-Hele (London: McGibbon & Kee, 1968), p. 11. *The Temple of Nature; or the Origins of Society* (London: J. Johnson, 1803; 2nd ed. 1806-1807; 3rd ed. 1825). Interestingly, this poem was published in the Russian *Journal of the Ministry of National Education* in 1911, and this translation was reissued in book form in Moscow in 1956 and again in 1960.

[11]Edward S. Reed, *From Soul to Mind: The Emergence of Psychology from Erasmus Darwin to William James* (New Haven, Conn.: Yale University Press, 1997), p. 14.

[12]E. Darwin, *Essential Writings*, p. 97.

[13]Ibid.

[14]Reed, *Soul to Mind*, p. 39.

[15]E. Darwin, *Essential Writings*, p. 75.

[16]Ibid., p. 76.

[17]Ibid., p. 173.

[18]Reed, *Soul to Mind*, p. 41.

[19]Ibid., p. 42.

[20]Mary Shelley, *Frankenstein* (1831; reprint, New York: Dover, 1994), p. viii.

[21]E. Darwin, *Essential Writings*, p. 163.

[22]Ibid.

[23]Ibid., p. 165.

[24]A. N. Wilson, *God's Funeral* (New York: W. W. Norton, 1999), p. 162.

[25]John Passmore, *A Hundred Years of Philosophy* (1968; reprint, New York: Viking Penguin, 1978), p. 40.

[26]Wilson, *God's Funeral*, p. 162.

[27]Herbert Spencer, *First Principles* (1863; reprint, Westport, Conn.: Greenwood, 1976), p. 207.

[28]Wilson, *God's Funeral*, p. 158.

[29]Quoted in Adrian Desmond and James Moore, *Darwin: The Life of a Tormented Evolutionist* (New York: W. W. Norton, 1994), p. 315.

[30]Wilson, *God's Funeral*, p. 189.

[31]Frank Burch Brown, *The Evolution of Charles Darwin's Religious Views* (Macon, Ga.: Mercer University Press, 1986).

[32]Franklin Baumer, *Religion and the Rise of Scepticism* (New York: Harcourt Brace & World, 1960), pp. 147-48.

[33]Brown, *Evolution of Charles Darwin's*, pp. 29-30.

[34]Adrian Desmond and James Moore, *Darwin: The Life and Time of a Tormented Evolutionist* (New York: Norton, 1991), p. 293.

[35]Brown, *Evolution of Charles Darwin's*, pp. 29-30.

[36]"De-censoring Darwin's Religion," in *Classics of Free Thought*, ed. Paul Blanshard (Buffalo, N.Y.: Prometheus, 1977), p. 44.

[37]Ibid., p. 47.

[38]Ibid., p. 44.

[39]Ibid., p. 45.

[40]Reed, *Soul to Mind*, p. 169.

[41]John Angus Campbell, "Darwin, Thales, and the Milkmaid: Scientific Revolution and Argument from Common Beliefs and Common Sense," in *Perspectives on Argument*, ed. Robert Trapp and Janice Schuetz (Prospect Heights, Ill.: Waveland, 1990), pp. 207-20.

[42]Ibid., p. 209.

[43]Baumer, *Religion and Rise of Scepticism*, p. 148.

[44]Charles Darwin, *On the Origin of the Species* (1859; Cambridge, Mass.: Harvard University Press, 1964), pp. 201-2.

[45]Ibid., pp. 202-3.

[46]The same argument is advanced today by Stephen J. Gould in his many books. See, for example, *The Panda's Thumb*.

[47]Quoted in Campbell, "Darwin, Thales," p. 213.

[48]Ibid., p. 214.

[49]Baumer, *Religion and Rise of Scepticism*, p. 148.

[50]Robert Richards, *The Meaning of Evolution* (Chicago: University of Chicago Press, 1992), p. 86.

[51]Ibid., p. 87.

[52]Ibid., p. 89.

[53]Ibid., p. 90.

[54]Quoted in "De-Censoring Darwin's Religion," pp. 46-47.

[55]Reed, *Soul to Mind*, p. 173.

[56]Ibid., p. 173.

[57]Quoted in Baumer, *Religion and Rise of Scepticism*, p. 149. See George Bernard Shaw, *Back to Methuselah*.

[58] Quoted in Baumer, *Religion and Rise of Scepticism*, p. 149.

[59] Burrow, *Crisis of Reason*, pp. 99-100.

[60] August Forel, *The Social World of Ants*, trans. C. K. Ogden (New York: Albert & Charles Boni, 1930), 2:350; quoted in Richard Noll, *The Jung Cult: Origins of a Charismatic Movement* (Princeton, N.J.: Princeton University Press, 1994), p. 321n.

[61] Forel, *Social World of Ants*, 2:351; quoted in Noll, *Jung Cult*, p. 321n.

[62] "Transhumanism," in *Classics of Free Thought*, ed. Paul Blanshard (Buffalo, N.Y.: Prometheus, 1977), p. 80.

[63] Ibid.

[64] Julian Huxley, *Evolution: The Modern Synthesis* (1942; reprint, London: Allen & Unwin, 1974).

[65] Ibid., p. 556.

[66] Ibid., p. 561.

[67] Ibid., p. 563.

[68] Ibid., pp. 564-65.

[69] Ibid., pp. 572-73.

[70] Ibid., pp. 573-74.

[71] Ibid.

[72] Ibid., p. 575.

[73] Ibid.

[74] Ibid., p. 576.

[75] Ibid., p. 577.

[76] Ibid., p. 578.

[77] Ibid.

[78] Laurence Brown, Bernard C. Farr and R. Joseph Hoffmann, eds., *Modern Spiritualities* (Amherst, N.Y.: Prometheus, 1997), p. 209.

[79] Ibid., pp. 210-11.

[80] Ibid., p. 212.

[81] Ibid.

[82] Ibid.

[83] Pierre Teilhard de Chardin, *The Future of Man*, trans. Norman Denny (1959; New York: Harper & Row, 1964), p. 80.

[84] Brown, Farr and Hoffmann, *Modern Spiritualities*, p. 213.

[85] Teilhard de Chardin, *Future of Man*, p. 80.

[86] Ibid., p. 120.

[87] James H. Austin, *Zen and the Brain: Toward an Understanding of Meditation and Consciousness* (Boston: MIT Press, 1999).

[88] Ibid., p. 685.

[89] Ibid., p. 686.

[90] Ibid., pp. 686-87.

[91]Ibid., p. 687.

[92]Ibid., p. 688.

[93]Ibid., p. 689.

[94]Ibid., pp. 689-90.

[95]Ibid., p. 691.

[96]Ibid., p. 693.

[97]James Redfield, *The Celestine Prophecy* (New York: Time Warner Books, 1993), p. 98.

[98]Ibid., p. 99.

[99]Ibid., p. 100.

[100]Ibid., p. 120.

[101]Philip Jenkins, *Mystics and Messiahs: Cults and New Religions in American History* (Oxford: Oxford University Press, 2000), p. 73.

[102]Associates claimed that as a young man Hitler was taken with the principal character in Wagner's operatic adaptation of Bulwer-Lytton's *Rienzi*. The German leader acknowledged to Wagner's widow in 1939 that seeing a performance of the opera was the turning point in his life. See Nicholas Goodrick Clark, *The Occult Roots of Nazism: Secret Aryan Cults and Their Influence on Nazi Ideology* (New York: New York University Press, 1985), for a discussion of Bulwer-Lytton, the Victorian occult movement and Nazi ideology.

[103]George Edward Bulwer-Lytton, *The Coming Race* (Santa Barbara, Calif.: Woodbridge, 1989), p. 11.

[104]Ibid., p. 12.

[105]Ibid., pp. 14-15.

[106]Ibid., p. 25.

[107]Ibid.

[108]Bulwer-Lytton was not the first to write of the Aryans as a master race. In 1855, sixteen years prior to the publication of *The Coming Race*, Arthur de Gobineau had published his theory of Aryan racial superiority in *On the Inequality of the Races of Man*.

[109]See Chris Hodenfield, "The Sky Is Full of Questions: Science Fiction in Steven Spielberg's Suburbia," *Rolling Stone*, January 26, 1978, pp. 33-38.

[110]Herbert Spencer, *First Principles* (1863; reprint, Westport, Conn.: Greenwood, 1976), p. 207. On the spiritual impact of *Close Encounters* on another prominent Hollywood director, see *New York Times Magazine*, September 22, 2002, p. 59. Emily Nussbaum writes that the "existential revelation [of Joss Whedon, creator of *Buffy the Vampire Slayer*] arrived during an adolescent viewing of *Close Encounters of the Third Kind*." Whedon "became convinced that the pop genres he loved—sci-fi and horror movies among them—could be more than just entertainment. They could carry subversive ideas into the mainstream" (p. 58).

[111]Daniel Leonard Bernardi, *Star Trek and History: Race-ing Toward a White Future* (Rutgers, N.J.: Rutgers University Press, 1998), p. 56.

[112]Ibid., p. 126.

[113]Ibid., p. 119.

[114]Aldous Huxley, "Further Reflections on Progress," in *Huxley and God: Essays*, ed. Jacqueline Hazard Bridgeman (San Francisco: HarperSanFrancisco, 1992), p. 113.

[115]Marilyn Ferguson, *The Aquarian Conspiracy: Personal and Social Transformation in the 1980's* (Los Angeles: J. P. Tarcher, 1980), p. 159.

[116]Gary Zukav, *The Seat of the Soul* (New York: Simon & Schuster, 1989), p. 182.

[117]Wilson, *God's Funeral*, p. 165.

[118]Baumer, *Religion and Rise of Scepticism*, p. 147.

Chapter Seven: Pantheism in the Modern World: Nature or God

[1]Pierre Teilhard de Chardin, *The Heart of Matter*, trans. Rene Hague (New York: Harcourt Brace Jovanovich, 1978), p. 26.

[2]Ibid., p. 28.

[3]Ibid., p. 19.

[4]Ibid.

[5]Ibid., p. 29.

[6]Ibid., p. 30.

[7]Quoted in Fred Alan Wolf, *The Spiritual Universe* (New York: Simon & Schuster, 1996), p. 104.

[8]Richard Noll, *The Jung Cult: Origins of a Charismatic Movement* (Princeton, N.J.: Princeton University Press, 1994), p. 49.

[9]Ernst Haeckel, *The Riddle of the Universe at the Close of the Nineteenth Century*, trans. Joseph McCabe (New York: Harper & Brothers, 1900), p. 337.

[10]Wolf, *Spiritual Universe*, p. 95.

[11]Ibid., p. 86.

[12]Helen Schucman, *A Course in Miracles: Workbook for Students* (Tiburon, Calif.: Center for Inner Peace, 1975), p. 45.

[13]Hershel Parker, "Ralph Waldo Emerson," in *Norton Anthology of American Literature*, shorter ed. (New York: W. W. Norton, 1980), p. 265.

[14]Daniel C. Dennett, *Darwin's Dangerous Idea: Evolution and the Meanings of Life* (New York: Simon & Schuster, 1995), p. 185. See also Benedict de Spinoza, *Ethics*, in *The Chief Works of Benedict de Spinoza*, trans. R. H. M. Elwers, vol. 2 (New York: Dover, 1951); and Steven Nadler, *Spinoza: A Life* (Cambridge: Cambridge University Press, 1999), pp. 227-33.

[15]Robert E. Sullivan, *John Toland and the Deist Controversy* (Cambridge, Mass.: Harvard University Press, 1982), p. 196.

[16]Ibid., p. 44.

[17]Ibid., p. 175.

[18]Quoted in ibid., p. 182.

[19]Ibid., pp. 182, 183.

[20]John Toland, *Tetradymus* (1720), pp. 85; quoted in Sullivan, *John Toland*, p. 184.

[21]Quoted in Sullivan, *John Toland*, p. 185.

[22]John Toland, *Letters to Serena* (London: Bernard Lintot, 1704), p. 115.

[23]Sullivan, *John Toland*, p. 184.

[24]Ibid., p. 186.

[25]Robert D. Richardson, *Emerson: The Mind on Fire* (Berkeley: University of California Press, 1995), p. 21.

[26]Ibid., p. 23.

[27]Ibid., p. 24.

[28]Ibid., p. 198.

[29]Quoted in ibid., p. 198. See Sampson Reed, *Observations on the Growth of the Mind* (Boston: Cummings Hilliard, 1826).

[30]Guillaume Oegger, *The True Messiah*, trans. Elizabeth Peabody (1832; Boston: Elizabeth Peabody, 1842).

[31]Philip Jenkins, *Mystics and Messiahs: Cults and New Religions in American History* (Oxford: Oxford University Press, 2000), p. 71.

[32]Richardson, *Emerson*, p. 250.

[33]Ibid., p. 258.

[34]Parker, "Ralph Waldo Emerson," p. 266.

[35]Carl Bode, ed., introduction to *The Portable Emerson* (New York: Penguin, 1981), p. xxix.

[36]Ibid., p. xxxi.

[37]Parker, "Ralph Waldo Emerson," p. 263.

[38]Bode, *Portable Emerson*, p. xxx.

[39]Ibid., p. xxxi.

[40]Ibid., p. xxix.

[41]Richardson, *Emerson*, p. 153-54.

[42]Ralph Waldo Emerson, "Nature," in *Norton Anthology of American Literature*, shorter ed. (New York: W. W. Norton, 1980), p. 268.

[43]Ibid., p. 269.

[44]Bode, *Portable Emerson*, p. xxxiv.

[45]Ralph Waldo Emerson, "Divinity School Address," in *Norton Anthology of American Literature*, shorter ed. (New York: W. W. Norton, 1980), p. 287.

[46]Ibid., pp. 287-88.

[47]Ibid., p. 288.

[48]Ibid.

[49]Ibid., p. 289.

[50]Quoted in Bode, *Portable Emerson*, p. xix.

[51]Parker, "Ralph Waldo Emerson," pp. 264-65.

[52]Richardson, *Emerson*, p. 250.

[53]Noll, *Jung Cult*, pp. 43.

[54]Ibid., p. 47.

[55]Ibid., p. 49.

[56]Haeckel, *Riddle of the Universe*, p. 17.

[57]Ibid., p. 19.

[58]Ibid.

[59]Ibid., p. 20.

[60]Ibid., pp. 20-21.

[61]Ibid., pp. 148-49.

[62]Ibid., p. 109.

[63]Ibid., p. 138.

[64]Ibid.

[65]Ibid., p. 143.

[66]Ibid., p. 163.

[67]Ibid., p. 166.

[68]Ibid., p. 171.

[69]Ibid., p. 243.

[70]Ibid., p. 244.

[71]Ibid., p. 280.

[72]Ibid., p. 281.

[73]Ibid., p. 331.

[74]Ibid., pp. 336-37.

[75]Ibid., p. 345.

[76]Ibid., p. 347.

[77]Ibid., p. 353.

[78]Ibid., p. 356.

[79]Ibid., p. 357.

[80]Ibid., pp. 381-82.

[81]Ibid., p. 382.

[82]Noll, *Jung Cult*, p. 49.

[83]Ibid., p. 50.

[84]Ibid., p. 79.

[85]Henri Bergson, *The Two Sources of Morality and Religion* (1935; Notre Dame, Ind.: University of Notre Dame Press, 1977), p. 113.

[86]Ibid., pp. 209-10.

[87]Ibid., p. 210.

[88]George Bernard Shaw, *Man and Superman* (Baltimore, Md.: Penguin, 1955), p. 167.

[89]Ibid., p. 167.

[90]Ibid., p. 153.

[91]Ibid., p. 172.

[92]Ibid., p. 152.

[93] Ibid., p. 241.

[94] Ibid., p. 249.

[95] Ibid., pp. 251-52.

[96] Ibid., p. 252.

[97] Ibid., p. 253.

[98] Ibid., p. 256.

[99] Catherine L. Albanese, *America, Religions and Religion*, 2nd ed. (Belmont, Calif.: Wadsworth, 1992), p. 355.

[100] Danah Zohar and Ian Marshall, *The Quantum Society: Mind, Physics and a New Social Vision* (New York: William Morrow, 1994), p. 231.

[101] Ibid.

[102] Ibid., p. 232.

[103] Ibid., p. 233.

[104] Ibid., p. 235.

[105] Ibid., p. 236.

[106] Ibid., p. 237.

[107] Ibid., p. 238.

[108] Ibid.

[109] Ibid., p. 239.

[110] Ibid.

[111] Ibid., p. 240.

[112] Ibid.

[113] Ibid., pp. 240-41.

[114] Ibid., p. 241.

[115] Ibid., p. 242.

[116] Herman Hesse, *Siddhartha*, trans. Hilda Rosner (New York: New Directions, 1951), p. 117.

[117] Daniel C. Dennett, *Darwin's Dangerous Idea: Evolution and the Meanings of Life* (New York: Simon & Schuster, 1995), p. 520.

[118] Ibid., p. 502.

[119] Wolf, *Spiritual Universe*, p. 86.

[120] Ibid., p. 39.

[121] Ibid.

[122] Ibid., pp. 199-200.

Chapter Eight: The Rebirth of Gnosticism: The Secret Path to Self-Salvation

[1] Steven J. Hedges et al., "www.masssuicide.com," *U.S. News & World Report*, April 7, 1997, p. 28.

[2] Ibid., p. 30.

[3] This conventional view is challenged by scholars including Birger A. Pearson. See his

"The Problem of 'Jewish Gnostic' Literature," in *Nag Hammadi and Early Christianity*, ed. C. W. Hedrick and R. Hodgson (Peabody, Mass.: Hendrickson, 1986), pp. 15-35.

[4]See, for example, Michael Allen Williams, *Rethinking "Gnosticism": An Argument for Dismantling a Dubious Category* (Princeton, N.J.: Princeton University Press, 1996).

[5]Carl A. Raschke, *The Interruption of Eternity: Modern Gnosticism and the Origins of the New Religious Consciousness* (Chicago: Nelson-Hall, 1980), p. 20.

[6]Ibid.

[7]Yuri Stoyanov, *The Hidden Tradition in Europe* (London: Penguin/Arkana, 1994), p. 224.

[8]Hans Jonas, "Gnosticism," *The Encyclopedia of Philosophy,* vol. 3, ed. P. Edwards (New York: Macmillan, 1967), p. 336.

[9]Raschke, *Interruption of Eternity*, p. 24.

[10]Ibid.

[11]Jonas, "Gnosticism," p. 340.

[12]Jack Lindsay, *Origins of Astrology* (New York: Barnes & Noble, 1971), p. 121.

[13]Ibid., p. 120.

[14]Raschke, *Interruption of Eternity*, p. 70.

[15]Jacob Ilive, *The Oration Spoke at Trinity Hall in Aldersgate Street: On Monday, January 9, 1738* (London: J. Wilford, 1738), p. 7.

[16]Jacob Ilive, *The Layman's Vindication of the Christian Religion* (London: n.p., 1730), p. 4.

[17]Ibid., p. 7.

[18]Ilive, *The Oration Spoke at Joyner's Hall* (London: n.p., 1733).

[19]Ibid., pp. 22-23.

[20]Ibid., p. 25.

[21]Ibid., p. 59.

[22]Ibid.

[23]Ibid., p. 60.

[24]Pheme Perkins, *Gnosticism and the New Testament* (Minneapolis: Fortress, 1993), p. 40.

[25]Raschke, *Interruption of Eternity*, p. 73.

[26]Charles Gildon, "Letter to R. B.," in *The Oracles of Reason*, by Charles Blount (London: n.p., 1693), pp. 178-79; quoted in David Berman, "David Hume and the Suppression of Atheism," *Journal of the History of Philosophy* 21, no. 3 (1983): 375-87; quote p. 381.

[27]Charles Blount, *Anima mundi* (London or Amsterdam: n.p., 1678), pp. 63-64.

[28]William Derham, *Astro-Theology, or a Demonstration of the Being and Attributes of God from a Survey of the Heavens* (London: W. Innys, 1715).

[29]Ibid., p. 1.

[30]Ibid., p. 218.

[31]Ibid., p. 220.

[32]Ibid., p. xlix.

[33]Raschke, *Interruption of Eternity*, p. 41.

[34]Jacob Ilive, *A Dialogue Between a Doctor of the Church of England and Mr. Jacob Ilive* (London:

T. Cooper, 1733), p. 28.

[35]Ibid., p. 32.

[36]Ibid., p. 34.

[37]Jacob Ilive, *The Book of Jasher* (London: n.p., 1751), p. 3.

[38]Ibid., p. 3.

[39]Ibid., chap. 3, vv. 17 and following.

[40]Ibid., chap. 3, vv. 12 and following.

[41]For a standard biographical account of Smith, see Fawn Brodie, *No Man Knows My History* (New York: Alfred A. Knopf, 1967). For a more accurate understanding of Smith's spiritual orientation, see Harold Bloom, *The American Religion: The Emergence of the Post-Christian Nation* (New York: Simon & Schuster, 1992).

[42]Bloom, *American Religion*, p. 112.

[43]D. Michael Quinn, *Early Mormonism and the Magic World View* (Salt Lake City: Signature, 1998). See Smith's own account, in which he notes the date September 22: Joseph Smith, *History of the Church*, in *Pearl of Great Price* (Salt Lake City, Utah: Church of Jesus Christ of Latter Day Saints, 1981), p. 55.

[44]Quinn, *Early Mormonism*, pp. 136-77.

[45]Jan Shipps, "The Latter-Day Saints," in *Encyclopedia of American Religious Experience* (New York: Scribner, 1988), p. 652.

[46]Quinn, *Early Mormonism*, p. 70.

[47]Ibid., p. 136.

[48]Ibid., p. 98. On Smith's interest in the magical tradition see Lance S. Owens, "Joseph Smith and Kabbalah: The Occult Connection," *Dialogue: A Journal of Mormon Thought 27*, no. 3 (1994): 117-94. The essay received the Mormon History Association award in 1995.

[49]Ibid., p. 39.

[50]Ibid., p. 72-73. Stars figure prominently in Smith's theology. See, for example, *The Book of Abraham* 3:2-18, in Smith, *Pearl of Great Price*, p. 34.

[51]On the Smith family's involvement with folk-magic, see Quinn, *Early Mormonism*, chap. 4, "Magic Parchments and Occult Mentors," pp. 98-135.

[52]Quinn, *Early Mormonism*, p. 39.

[53]Harry L. Ropp, *Are the Mormon Scriptures Reliable?* (Downers Grove, Ill.: InterVarsity Press, 1987), pp. 39-40.

[54]Ibid., p. 38.

[55]George Arbaugh, author of *Revelation in Mormonism* (Chicago: University of Chicago Press, 1932), calls Rigdon the founder of Mormonism. See Ropp, *Are the Mormon Scriptures Reliable?* pp. 37-38. See also Joseph Smith, *Doctrine and Covenants* (Salt Lake City: Church of Jesus Christ of Latter Day Saints, 1981), sects. 35, 37, 40, for examples of Rigdon's prominence in early Mormonism.

[56]Ropp, *Are the Mormon Scriptures Reliable?* p. 38.

[57]For a detailed discussion of Smith's gnostic cosmology, see John L. Brooke, *The Refiner's*

Fire: The Making of Mormon Cosmology, 1644-1844 (Cambridge: Cambridge University Press, 1999).

[58]Bloom asks, "Is it not likely that Smith left other secret teachings that have been handed down only within the hierarchy?" (*American Religion*, p. 125). Access to Mormon temples remains restricted to Mormons in good standing with the Church.

[59]Bloom, *American Religion*, p. 111. Smith's famous statement is from his "King Follett Discourse," which is available online at <kingdomofzion.org>.

[60]Anthony Hoekema, *The Four Major Cults* (Grand Rapids, Mich.: Eerdmans, 1963), pp. 38-39.

[61]Bloom, *American Religion*, p. 114.

[62]See Quinn, *Early Mormonism*, pp. 70-83.

[63]Hoekema, *Four Major Cults*, p. 45.

[64]Ibid., p. 43.

[65]Joseph Campbell, ed., introduction to *The Portable Jung*, trans. R. F. C. Hull (New York: Penguin, 1976), p. vii.

[66]John P. Dourley, *The Illness We Are: A Jungian Critique of Christianity* (Toronto: Inner City Books, 1984), p. 72.

[67]Richard Noll, *The Jung Cult: Origins of a Charismatic Movement* (Princeton, N.J.: Princeton University Press, 1994), p. 6.

[68]Ibid., p. 23.

[69]Campbell, *Portable Jung*, p. viii.

[70]Noll, *Jung Cult*, p. 28.

[71]Dourley, *Illness We Are*, p. 99.

[72]Ibid., pp. 94, 95.

[73]Ibid., p. 74.

[74]Carl Jung, *The Collected Works of Carl Jung*, trans. R. F. C. Hull, ed. H. Read, M. Fordham, G. Adler, W. McGuire (Princeton, N.J.: Princeton University Press, 1953-1979), *Mysterium coniunctionis*, CW 14, par. 742; quoted in Dourley, *Illness We Are*, p. 98.

[75]Noll, *Jung Cult*, p. 21.

[76]Ibid., p. 18.

[77]Carl Jung, "The Difference Between Eastern and Western Thinking," part 1 of "Psychological Commentary on the Tibetan Book of the Great Liberation," from *Psychology and Religion: West and East* in *Collected Works*, vol. 2, pars. 759-87, in *The Portable Jung*, trans. R. F. C. Hull (New York: Penguin, 1976), p. 475.

[78]Dourley, *Illness We Are*, p. 78.

[79]Jung, "Eastern and Western Thinking," p. 475.

[80]Ibid., p. 476.

[81]Noll, *Jung Cult*, p. 6.

[82]Ibid.

[83]Ibid., p. 7.

[84]Ibid., p. 297. Noll quotes Edward Edinger, *The Creation of Consciousness: Jung's Myth for*

Modern Man (Toronto: Inner City Books, 1984), p. 90.

[85]Jean Houston, *A Passion for the Possible: A Guide to Realizing Your True Potential* (San Francisco: HarperSanFrancisco: 1997), p. 20.

[86]Ibid., p. 21.

[87]Ibid., p. 24.

[88]Ibid., p. 25.

[89]Ibid., p. 28.

[90]Ibid., p. 31. Similarly, Carl Jung entertained the possibility of "a quasi-spiritualist, quasi-biological idea . . . ancestor possession—that is, literally, spiritual possession by one's ancestors." Noll, *Jung Cult*, p. 23.

[91]Houston, *Passion for the Possible*, p. 32.

[92]Ibid.

[93]Ibid., p. 34.

[94]Ibid., p. 35.

[95]Ibid., p. 115.

[96]Ibid., p. 113.

[97]Ibid., pp. 116, 118.

[98]Ibid., p. 133.

[99]Ibid., p. 138.

[100]Ibid., p. 140.

[101]Ibid., p. 142.

[102]Ibid., p. 144.

[103]Ibid., p. 155.

[104]Ibid., p. 161.

[105]Ibid., p. 167.

[106]Ibid., p. 162.

[107]Catherine L. Albanese, *America, Religions and Religion*, 2nd ed. (Belmont, Calif.: Wadsworth, 1992), p. 357. Madame Blavatsky and her sources of spiritual information are discussed in my chapter nine.

[108]Ibid.

[109]Steve Kellmeyer, "The Gnostix," *Envoy* 4, no. 5 (2000): 34-39, quote p. 39.

[110]Ibid., p. 37.

[111]Carlos Castaneda, *The Teachings of Don Juan: A Yaqui Way of Knowledge* (Berkeley: University of California Press, 1969), p. 145.

[112]Raschke, *Interruption of Eternity*, p. 34.

[113]Theodor W. Adorno, "Theses Against Occultism," in *Minima Moralia: Reflexionen aus dem beschädigten Leben* (Berlin: Suhrkamp Verlag, 1951), pp. 238-41 (English translation *Minima Moralia: Reflections from Damaged Life*, trans. E. F. N. Jephcott (London: New Left, 1978).

[114]William Covino, *Rhetoric and Magic* (Albany: State University of New York Press, 1997), p. 90.

Chapter Nine: Modern Shamanism: Spirit Contact and Spiritual Progress

[1]Jeremy Narby and Francis Huxley, eds. *Shamans Through Time: 500 Years on the Path to Knowledge* (New York: Jeremy Tarcher, 2001), p. 1.

[2]Philip Jenkins, *Mystics and Messiahs: Cults and New Religions in American History* (Oxford: Oxford University Press, 2000), p. 170.

[3]Narby and Huxley, *Shamans Through Time*, p. 5.

[4]Ibid.

[5]Ibid., p. 6.

[6]Emanuel Swedenborg, *The Worlds in Space* (1758; reprint, London: The Swedenborg Society, 1998), p. 1.

[7]Ibid., p. 113.

[8]Ibid., p. 14.

[9]Ibid., p. 86.

[10]Ibid., p. 111.

[11]Ibid., p. 14.

[12]Ibid., p. 50.

[13]Ibid., p. 73.

[14]Ibid., p. 47.

[15]Ibid., p. 33.

[16]Ibid., p. 34.

[17]Ibid., p. 104.

[18]Again I am reminded here of the closing scenes of Steven Spielberg's *Close Encounters of the Third Kind*, in which the delicate features of advanced aliens are juxtaposed with shots of human beings exhibiting similar features. The suggestion is that some of us have already taken the next evolutionary step. Unfortunately, as our faces reveal, some of us have not.

[19]Swedenborg, *Worlds in Space*, p. 44.

[20]Ibid., p. 99.

[21]Ibid., p. 65.

[22]Ibid., p. 46.

[23]Ibid., p. 89.

[24]Ibid., p. 93.

[25]Bradford Verter, "Dark Star Rising: The Emergence of Modern Occultism, 1880-1950" (Ph.D. diss., Princeton University, 1998), p. 135n.

[26]Ibid., p.134.

[27]Ibid.

[28]Jenkins, *Mystics and Messiahs*, p. 73.

[29]Lawrence Sutin has recently published an extensive biography of Crowley: *Do What Thou Wilt: A Life of Aleister Crowley* (New York: St. Martin's Griffin, 2000).

[30]Ibid., pp. 2-3.

[31]Ibid., p. 4.

[32] Verter, "Dark Star Rising," p. 139.

[33] Ibid.

[34] See ibid., pp. 129-30n: "During the early and mid-nineteenth century, sensational yarns, ghost stories and Oriental tales were everywhere: newspapers, magazines, chapbooks, serial pamphlets, and books."

[35] Jenkins, *Mystics and Messiahs*, pp. 76-77.

[36] Carl Jung, "The Spiritual Problem of Modern Man," in *Modern Man in Search of a Soul*, trans. W. S. Dell and Cary F. Baynes (New York: Harcourt Brace, 1933), pp. 210-11.

[37] H. P. Blavatsky, *Isis Unveiled* (1877; reprint, Pasadena, Calif.: Theosophical University Press, 1998), 1:282.

[38] Judge Henry Steele Olcott, *The Sun*, September 26, 1892; quoted in Warren Sylvester Smith, *The London Heretics 1870-1914* (New York: Dodd Mead, 1968), p. 159.

[39] On Blavatsky see John Symnonds, *Madame Blavatsky, Medium and Magician* (London: n.p., 1959).

[40] Smith, *London Heretics*, p. 247.

[41] Ibid., 146.

[42] Mary K. Kneff, *Personal Memoirs of H. P. Blavatsky* (New York: n.p., 1937), p. 54; quoted in Smith, *London Heretics*, p. 147.

[43] Richard Noll, *The Jung Cult: Origins of a Charismatic Movement* (Princeton, N.J.: Princeton University Press, 1994), p. 65.

[44] Ibid.

[45] Ibid., p. 64.

[46] Jenkins, *Mystics and Messiahs*, p. 41.

[47] Blavatsky, *Isis Unveiled*, 1:93.

[48] Ibid., 1:94.

[49] Jenkins, *Mystics and Messiahs*, p. 84.

[50] Noll, *Jung Cult*, p. 83.

[51] Jenkins, *Mystics and Messiahs*, p. 96.

[52] Noll, *Jung Cult*, p. 83.

[53] Catherine L. Albanese, *America, Religions and Religion*, 2nd ed. (Belmont, Calif.: Wadsworth, 1992), p. 356.

[54] Blavatsky, *Isis Unveiled*, 1:296.

[55] Ibid.

[56] Adrian Desmond and James Moore, *Darwin: The Life of a Tormented Evolutionist* (New York: W. W. Norton, 1994), p. 538.

[57] Blavatsky, *Isis Unveiled*, 1:296, emphasis in original.

[58] Ibid.

[59] Jenkins, *Mystics and Messiahs*, p. 72.

[60] Blavatsky, *Isis Unveiled*, 1:296.

[61] See, for example, Jenkins's discussion of The Silver Shirts who followed self-styled as-

cended master William Dudley Pelley (1885-1965) in America of the 1930s and 1940s (*Mystics and Messiahs*, pp. 95-96). Many neopagan groups, e.g., Asatru organizations, teach a thinly veiled racialist philosophy.

[62]John E. Mack, *Abduction: Human Encounters with Aliens* (New York: Charles Scribner's Sons, 1994).

[63]Other books in the abduction genre include Dana Redfield, *Summoned: Encounters with Alien Intelligence*; Dolores Cannon, *The Custodians: Beyond Abduction* and Constance Clear, *Reaching for Reality: Seven Incredible True Stories of Alien Abduction*.

[64]Mack, *Abduction*, preface.

[65]Ibid., p. 3.

[66]Ibid., pp. 3-4.

[67]Ibid., p. 4.

[68]Ibid.

[69]Ibid., pp. 4-5.

[70]Ibid., pp. 6-7.

[71]Ibid., p. 8.

[72]Ibid.

[73]Ibid.

[74]Ibid., p. 9.

[75]Ibid., p. 32.

[76]Joseph Campbell, "Myths from West to East" in *The Universal Myths: Heroes, Gods, Tricksters and Others* (New York: Penguin, 1990), p. 59.

[77]Mack, *Abduction*, p. 18.

[78]Ibid., p. 17.

[79]Jenkins, *Mystics and Messiahs*, p. 172. See also Brad Gooch, " 'He's Only a Thought Away': Sleuthing *The Urantia Book*," in *Godtalk: Travels in Spiritual America* (New York: Alfred A. Knopf, 2002), pp. 3-62.

[80]Mack, *Abduction*, p. 32.

[81]Whitley Streiber, *Communion* (New York: Beech Tree, 1987); *Transformation: The Breakthrough* (New York: Beech Tree, 1988); *Confirmation: The Hard Evidence for Aliens Among Us* (New York: St. Martin's, 1998).

[82]Streiber, *Transformation*, p. 237.

[83]Paul Ferrini, *Love Without Conditions: Reflections of the Christ Mind* (South Dearfield, Mass.: Heartways, 1997).

[84]Ibid., p. 7.

[85]Ibid., p. 8.

[86]Ibid.

[87]Ibid.

[88]Ibid., p. 9.

[89]Ibid., p. 16.

[90]Ibid.

[91]Ibid., p. 18.

[92]Ibid.

[93]Ibid., p. 20.

[94]Gary Zukav, *The Seat of the Soul* (New York: Simon & Schuster, 1989), p. 180.

[95]Ibid., p. 181.

[96]Ibid.

[97]Ibid., p. 182.

[98]Neale Donald Walsch, *Conversations with God: An Uncommon Dialogue*, vol. 1 (New York: G. P. Putnam & Sons, 1995), p. 208.

[99]Narby and Huxley, *Shamans Through Time*, p. 305.

Chapter Ten: The Mystical Path to Pluralism: Discovering That All Is One in Religion

[1]Wayne Teasdale, *The Mystic Heart* (Novato, Calif.: New World Library, 1999), p. 72.

[2]Ibid., p. 75; emphasis in original.

[3]Ibid., p. 74.

[4]Ibid., p. 26.

[5]Ibid., p. 25.

[6]Ibid.

[7]Ibid., p. 45.

[8]Ibid., p. 46.

[9]Ibid., p. 47.

[10]Ibid., p. 48.

[11]Mircea Eliade, *A History of Religious Ideas*, vol. 1, trans. Willard Trask (Chicago: University of Chicago Press, 1978), p. xv; emphasis in original.

[12]Harold Hutcheson, *Lord Herbert of Cherbury's* De religioni laici (New Haven, Conn.: Yale University Press, 1944), p. 87.

[13]Franz Cumont, *Astrology and Religion Among the Greeks and Romans* (New York: Valor Publications, 1960), p. 3.

[14]Kenneth Scott Latourette, *A History of Christianity* (New York: Harper & Row, 1953; rev. 1975), 2:1123.

[15]Franklin L. Baumer, *Religion and the Rise of Scepticism* (New York: Harcourt Brace & World, 1960), p. 154.

[16]Rudolf Otto, *The Idea of the Holy*, trans. John W. Harvey (London: Oxford University Press, 1927), p. 52.

[17]Ibid., p. 6.

[18]Ibid., p. 17.

[19]Sigmund Freud, *The Future of an Illusion*, trans. W. D. Robson-Scott (London: Hogarth Press and the Institute of Psychoanalysis, 1928), p. 28.

[20]Ibid., pp. 33-34.

[21]John P. Dourley, *The Illness We Are: A Jungian Critique of Christianity* (Toronto: Inner City Books, 1984), p. 9.

[22]Peter Miller, "Jane Goodall," *National Geographic*, December 1995, p. 110.

[23]Eugene G. D'Aquili and Andrew B. Newberg, *The Mystical Mind: Probing the Biology of Religious Experience* (Philadelphia: Fortress, 1999).

[24]Roland Bainton, *The Reformation of the Sixteenth Century* (Boston: Beacon, 1952), p. 128.

[25]Ibid.

[26]Bradford Verter, "Dark Star Rising: The Emergence of Modern Occultism, 1800-1950" (Ph.D. diss., Princeton University, 1998), p. 30.

[27]Wayne Shumaker, *The Occult Sciences in the Renaissance: A Study in Intellectual Patterns* (Berke-ley: University of California Press, 1972), p. 205.

[28]Ibid.

[29]Charles Blount, *Anima mundi* (Amsterdam or London: n.p., 1678).

[30]Robert Hurlbutt, *Hume, Newton and the Design Argument* (Lincoln: University of Nebraska Press, 1965), p. 70.

[31]Ibid.

[32]Ibid.

[33]Blount, *Anima mundi*, preface.

[34]Ibid.

[35]*A Speech Delivered by an Indian Chief* (London: n.p., 1753), p. 4.

[36]Carl Jung, "The Modern Spiritual Problem," in *Modern Man in Search of a Soul*, trans. W. S. Dell and Cary F. Baynes (New York: Harcourt Brace, 1933), pp. 209-10.

[37]R. M. Bucke, *Cosmic Consciousness: A Study in the Evolution of the Human Mind* (1901; New York: Dutton, 1966), p. 17.

[38]Ibid.

[39]Ibid., p. 18.

[40]Ibid. See a similar discussion of mystical states in Andrew Newberg and Eugene D'Aquili, *Why God Won't Go Away* (New York: Ballantine, 2002), pp. 98-127.

[41]Bucke, *Cosmic Consciousness*, p. 18.

[42]Ibid., p. 22.

[43]Ibid., pp. 40-41.

[44]Ibid., p. 41.

[45]Ibid., p. 42.

[46]Ibid.

[47]Ibid., p. 52.

[48]Ibid.; emphasis in original.

[49]Ibid., p. 59.

[50]Ibid., p. 67.

[51]Ibid.

[52] Ibid., p. 69.

[53] Ibid., p. 71.

[54] Ibid., p. 96.

[55] Ibid., p. 99.

[56] Ibid., p. 72.

[57] Ibid.

[58] Ibid., p. 73.

[59] Ibid.

[60] Ibid.

[61] Ibid., p. 74.

[62] Ibid., p. 100.

[63] Huston Smith, introduction to *The Transcendent Unity of Religions,* by Frithjof Schuon (1957; Wheaton, Ill.: Theosophical Publishing House, 1984), pp. ix-xxvii.

[64] Ibid., p. xv.

[65] Ibid., p. xvi.

[66] Ibid., p. xxvi.

[67] Frithjof Schuon, *The Transcendent Unity of Religions* (1957; Wheaton, Ill.: Theosophical Publishing House, 1984), p. 47.

[68] Ibid., p. 14.

[69] Ibid., p. 38.

[70] Ibid., p. 21.

[71] Ibid.

[72] Ibid., p. 23.

[73] Ibid., p. 25.

[74] Ibid., p. 20.

[75] Ibid., p. 19.

[76] Ibid.

[77] Ibid., p. 26.

[78] Ibid., p. 27.

[79] Ibid., p. 33.

[80] Ibid., p. 81.

[81] Ibid., p. 125.

[82] Ibid., p. 125n.

[83] Ibid., p. 39.

[84] Ibid., p. 35.

[85] Joseph Campbell, *Transformations of Myth Through Time* (New York: Harper & Row, 1990), p. 93.

[86] Joseph Campbell, "Myths from West to East," in *The Universal Myths: Heroes, Gods, Tricksters and Others* (New York: Penguin, 1990), p. 43.

[87] Campbell, *Transformations of Myth,* p. 95.

[88]Ibid., p. 102.

[89]Ibid., pp. 104-5.

[90]Ibid., p. 106.

[91]Ibid.

[92]Ibid., p. 102.

[93]Ibid., p. 176.

[94]Campbell, "Myths from West to East," p. 45.

[95]Ibid., pp. 45-46.

[96]Huston Smith, *Cleansing the Doors of Perception* (New York: Tarcher/Putnam, 2000), pp. xvi-xvii.

[97]Ibid., p. 80.

[98]Campbell, *Transformations of Myth,* p. 94.

[99]Campbell, "Myths from West to East," p. 49.

[100]Ibid., p. 50.

[101]Marcus J. Borg, *Meeting Jesus Again for the First Time: The Historical Jesus and the Heart of Contemporary Faith* (San Francisco: HarperSanFrancisco: 1994), p. 29.

[102]Ibid., p. 14.

[103]Ibid., p. 15.

[104]Ibid., p. 17.

[105]Ibid., pp. 31-32.

[106]Ibid., p. 32.

[107]Ibid.

[108]Ibid., p. 33.

[109]Mack, *Abduction,* p. 9.

[110]Borg, *Meeting Jesus Again,* p. 34.

[111]Ibid., p. 36.

[112]Ibid., p. 37.

[113]Ibid.

[114]Ibid., p. 87.

[115]Ibid., p. 110.

[116]Ibid., p. 119.

[117]Ibid., p. 120.

[118]John G. Burke, "Hermetism as a Renaissance World View," in *The Darker Vision of the Renaissance,* ed. Robert S. Kinsman (Berkeley: University of California Press, 1974), p. 115.

[119]Peter Annet, *Judging for Ourselves* (London: n.p., 1747), p. 5.

[120]Teasdale, *Mystic Heart,* p. 26.

[121]Ibid.

[122]Ibid., p. 25.

[123]Gary Zukav, *The Seat of the Soul* (New York: Simon & Schuster, 1989), p. 182.

Chapter Eleven: Conclusion: A New Spirituality for a New Age

[1]John Stott, *The Contemporary Christian* (Downers Grove, Ill.: InterVarsity Press, 1992), p. 15.

[2]Shirley MacLaine, *Dancing in the Light* (New York: Bantam, 1985).

[3]Ibid., pp. 370-71.

[4]Ibid., pp. 372-73.

[5]Ibid., p. 113.

[6]Ibid., p. 112.

[7]Ibid., p. 375.

[8]John Shelby Spong, *Rescuing the Bible from Fundamentalism* (San Francisco: HarperSanFrancisco, 1991), p. 21.

[9]Joseph Campbell, *Transformations of Myth Through Time* (New York: Harper & Row, 1990), p. 106.

[10]Joseph Campbell, *The Hero with a Thousand Faces* (New York: MJF Books, 1949), p. 4.

[11]Brenda Brasher, *Give Me That Online Religion* (San Francisco: Jossey-Bass, 2001), p. 6.

[12]On the divine *Mens* and the Renaissance magical tradition, see Frances Yates's excellent study *Giordano Bruno and the Hermetic Tradition* (Chicago: University of Chicago Press, 1964).

[13]Gary Zukav, *The Seat of the Soul* (New York: Simon & Schuster, 1990), p. 185.

[14]Ibid., p. 67.

[15]Laurence Brown, Bernard C. Farr and R. Joseph Hoffmann, eds., *Modern Spiritualities* (Amherst, N.Y.: Prometheus, 1997), p. 224.

[16]Ibid., p. 226.

[17]Ibid.

[18]Ibid., p. 227.

[19]Joseph Banks Rhine, *New Frontiers of the Mind: The Story of the Duke Experiments* (New York: Farrar & Rinehart, 1937), pp. 3, 5.

[20]Ibid., p. 269.

[21]MacLaine, *Dancing in the Light*, p. 369.

[22]J. W. Burrow, *The Crisis of Reason: European Thought, 1848-1914* (New Haven, Conn.: Yale University Press, 2000), p. 198.

[23]Wayne Teasdale, *The Mystic Heart* (Novato, Calif.: New World Library, 1999), p. 72.

[24]Ibid., p. 74.

[25]Marilyn Ferguson, *The Aquarian Conspiracy: Personal and Social Transformation in the 1980's* (Los Angeles: J. P. Tarcher, 1980), p. 152.

[26]MacLaine, *Dancing in the Light*, p. 342.

[27]Ibid., pp. 341-42.

[28]David Gergen, "Trouble in Paradise," *U.S. News & World Report*, August 20, 2001, p. 80.

[29]Pierre Teilhard de Chardin, *The Heart of Matter*, trans. Rene Hague (New York: Harcourt Brace Jovanovich, 1978), p. 10.

[30]Pierre Teilhard de Chardin, *The Future of Man*, trans. Norman Denny (1959; reprint, New York: Harper & Row, 1964), pp. 190-91.

[31]George Bernard Shaw, "The Revolutionist's Handbook," in *Man and Superman* (Baltimore: Penguin, 1955), p. 251.

[32]Michael Cromarty, "A Conversation with Francis Fukuyama," in *Books and Culture*, July/ August 2002, p. 9. Francis Fukuyama, *Our Posthuman Future: Consequences of the Biotechnology Revolution* (New York: Farrar, Straus & Giroux, 2002).

[33]Robert Ornstein, *The Evolution of Consciousness* (New York: Prentice Hall, 1991), p. 279.

[34]Ibid., p. 273.

[35]Robert Onstein and Paul Ehrlich, *New World, New Mind* (Cambridge Mass.: Malor, 1989), p. 195.

[36]Cromarty, "Conversation with Francis Fukuyama," p. 9.

[37]C. S. Lewis, *The Abolition of Man* (New York: Macmillan, 1947).

[38]Ibid., pp. 36, 37.

[39]Zukav, *Seat of the Soul*, p. 174.

[40]Ferguson, *Aquarian Conspiracy*, pp. 169-70.

[41]Burrow, *Crisis of Reason*, p. 215.

[42]Joseph Chilton Pearce, *The Crack in the Cosmic Egg: Challenging Constructs of Mind and Reality* (New York: Washington Square Press, 1971), p. 180.

[43]C. S. Lewis, *Mere Christianity* (New York: Macmillan, 1960), p. 185.

[44]Stuart Clark, *Thinking with Demons: The Idea of Witchcraft in Early Modern Europe* (Oxford: Clarendon, 1997), pp. 11-12.

[45]Neale Donald Walsch, *Conversations with God: An Uncommon Dialogue*, vol. 1 (New York: G. P. Putnam & Sons, 1995), p. 200; emphasis in original.

[46]Ferguson, *Aquarian Conspiracy*, p. 382.

[47]John Shelby Spong, lecture at Christ Community Church, Spring Lake, Mich., September 28, 2001.

[48]Dana Zohar and Ian Marshall, *The Quantum Self: Human Nature and Consciousness Defined by the New Physics* (New York: William Morrow, 1990), p. 226.

[49]Zukav, *Seat of the Soul*, pp. 71-72.

[50]MacLaine, *Dancing in the Light*, p. 360.

[51]Peter Jones, *The Gnostic Empire Strikes Back: An Old Heresy for the New Age* (Phillipsburg, N.J.: Presbyterian & Reformed, 1992), p. 59.

[52]Walsch, *Conversations with God*, pp. 201-2.

[53]Zukav, *Seat of the Soul*, p. 185.

[54]Ibid., p. 186.

[55]Walsch, *Conversations with God*, p. 126.

[56]Zukav, *Seat of the Soul*, p. 181.

[57]Ibid., p. 188.

[58]Phillip Pullman, *The Subtle Knife* (New York: William Knopf, 1997), p. 25.

[59]Dallas Willard, *The Spirit of the Disciplines: Understanding How God Changes Lives* (San Francisco: HarperSanFrancisco, 1991), p. 92.

[60]Cromarty, "Conversation with Francis Fukuyama," p. 9.

[61]Pearce, *Crack in the Cosmic Egg,* pp. 169, 168.

[62]Ibid., p. 166.

[63]Richard Noll, *The Jung Cult: Origins of a Charismatic Movement* (Princeton, N.J.: Princeton University Press, 1994), p. 39.

[64]William Covino, *Rhetoric and Magic* (Albany, N.Y.: State University of New York Press: 1997), p. 90.

[65]Noll, *Jung Cult,* p. 35.

[66]Walsch, *Conversations with God,* p. 1.

[67]Gerardo Reichel-Dolmatoff, "Shamans Are Intellectuals, Translators, and Shrewd Dealers," in *Shamans Through Time: 500 Years on the Path to Knowledge,* ed. Jeremy Narby and Francis Huxley (New York: Jeremy Tarcher, 2001), pp. 216-22, quote p. 216.

[68]Ibid., p. 222.

[69]Zukav, *Seat of the Soul,* p. 185.

[70]Ibid., p. 182.

[71]Ibid., p. 183.

[72]Walsch, *Conversations with God,* p. 195; emphasis in original.

[73]Ibid., pp. 197-98.

[74]Deepak Chopra, *The Path to Love: Renewing the Power of Spirit in Your Life* (New York: Harmony, 1997), p. 290; emphasis in original.

[75]Ravi Zacharias, *Can Man Live Without God?* (Dallas: Word, 1994), p. 121.

[76]Noll, *Jung Cult,* p. 38.

[77]A. N. Wilson, *God's Funeral* (New York: W. W. Norton, 1999), p. 59.

[78]Yates, *Giordano Bruno,* p. 239.

[79]M. Craig Barnes, *When God Interrupts: Finding New Life Through Unwanted Change* (Downers Grove, Ill.: InterVarsity Press, 1996), p. 158.

Index of Names

Adams, Samuel, 99
Adorno, Theodore, 202
Agrippa, Cornelius, 47
Albanese, Catherine, 170, 199
Annet, Peter, 58, 77-79, 85, 87-89, 95, 184, 253-54, 259
Antinori, Severino, 263
Applewhite, Marshall, 177-78, 199
Augustine, 178
Austin, James H., 30, 141-43
Bach, Richard, 22
Bacon, Francis, 232, 235
Bainton, Roland, 46, 49, 230-31
Balzac, Honore de, 235
Barnes, M. Craig, 281
Barzun, Jacques, 97
Baumer, Frank, 75-76, 129, 150
Bergson, Henri, 140, 167-69, 174
Bernardi, Daniel, 148
Besant, Annie, 215
Besterman, Theodore, 82
Blake, William, 85, 122-23, 235
Blavatsky, Madame H. P., 145, 211-17, 224, 262, 264, 271
Bloom, Harold, 185, 189-90
Blount, Charles, 50, 183, 231-32, 248
Borg, Marcus, 215, 230, 244-48, 279

Braschler, Von, 23
Brasher, Brenda, 257
Brown, Simon, 59
Brown, Sir Thomas, 52
Bruno, Giordano, 38, 45-46, 48, 102, 155, 215, 248, 280
Buckley, George T., 50
Bulwer-Lytton, George Edward, 145-46, 200, 210-12, 217
Burke, John G., 248
Butler, Samuel, 132
Byron, Lord, 123
Campbell, John, 129, 131
Campbell, Joseph, 15, 191, 194, 197, 220, 230, 240-43, 248, 257
Capra, Fritjof, 26, 98, 115-16
Carlyle, Thomas, 158, 280
Castellio, Sebastiani, 50
Celsus, 232
Chillingworth, William, 50
Chopra, Deepak, 29, 278
Chubb, Thomas, 58
Cicero, 50, 232
Clark, Glen, 92
Clark, J. C. D., 52
Clarke, Arthur C., 145
Clifford, W. K., 134
Coleridge, Samuel Taylor, 85, 122, 156, 158
Collins, Anthony, 52, 58, 80
Comte, August, 96-97
Condorcet, Marquis de, 76
Confucius, 214
Cooper, David, 24
Cope, Stephen, 29
Cordovero, Rabbi Moses, 154
Covey, Stephen, 25

Covino, William, 85, 87, 273
Cowdery, Oliver, 188-89
Crowley, Aleister, 88, 210-12
Curott, Phyllis, 23
Dalai Lama, 25, 143
Darab, Dastur, 233
Darwin, Charles, 120-21, 123-35, 139, 141, 149, 150, 156, 163, 174-75, 215-16, 264, 266
Darwin, Erasmus, 120-23, 125, 132, 143
Darwin, Robert Waring, 125
Dennett, Daniel, 154, 174, 175
Derham, William, 183
Desmond, Adrian, 127
Dickens, Charles, 126
Drosnin, Michael, 58, 69-73, 272
du Perron, Antequil Dupuis, 233
Eckhart, Meister, 47-49, 215
Eddy, Mary Baker, 90-91, 98, 156
Edgeworth, Richard, 120
Edinger, Edward, 194
Ehrlich, Paul, 119
Eliade, Mercia, 228
Eliot, George, 61
Emerson, Mary Moody, 156
Emerson, Ralph Waldo, 103, 153, 156-62, 169-70, 174, 194, 206
Epstein, Mark, 27
Erasmus, 120-23, 125, 128, 132, 143, 149, 232
Ernesti, Johann August, 60
Evans, Warren Felt, 90-91
Fenton, Peter, 29

Ferguson, Marilyn, 15, 21-22, 26, 101, 115, 149, 262, 264-65, 268

Feuerbach, Ludwig, 228

Ficino, Marsilio, 38, 42, 47

Fillmore, Charles, 91

Fillmore, Myrtle, 91

Fontenelle, Bernard, 207

Forel, August, 136

Foster, Jodi, 107

Fox, Emmet, 92

Franck, Adolphe, 41

Franklin, Benjamin, 75, 98, 121, 129, 150, 259

Free, William, 240

Freud, Sigmund, 28, 193, 229

Fukuyama, Francis, 264-65, 271

Funk, Robert W., 244

Galileo, 45, 263

Galton, Francis, 135-36

Gates, Bill, 25

George I, King, 56

Gergen, David, 263

Gibson, Bishop Edmund, 56, 59-60

Gildon, Charles, 183

Gimbutas, Marija, 22-23

Goethe, Johann Wolfgang von, 156, 163, 214

Goodall, Jane, 229

Goswami, Amit, 26, 98, 115-16, 226

Gottschalk, Stephen, 90

Haeckel, Ernst, 120, 135-36, 152-53, 162-66, 169, 262

Harris, Martin, 187

Hartley, David, 121

Hefelbower, S. G., 53

Heider, John, 25

Henslow, John Stevens, 126

Herbert, Lord, 52, 228

Hermes Trismegistus, 38, 44, 46, 231

Hesse, Herman, 174

Hobbes, Thomas, 232

Hoekema, Anthony, 190

Hooker, James, 126

Houston, Jean, 18, 194-98, 202-3, 218, 221, 257

Hubbard, L. Ron, 199

Hull, Akasha Gloria, 23

Huxley, Aldous, 86, 88, 136-38, 140, 148-50, 240, 277

Huxley, Francis, 205

Huxley, Julian Sorell, 136-39, 144-46, 264, 266

Huxley, T. H., 120, 134-36, 168, 264

Huygens, Christiaan, 183

Ilive, Jacob, 181-85, 187, 190, 198-99, 201, 203

Ingersoll, Robert Green, 103-7, 109-10, 114, 117, 136, 269

Israel, Jonathan, 52

Jenkins, Philip, 19, 98, 158, 205, 211, 214-16

John the apostle, 258-59, 276

John XXII, Pope, 47

Jonas, Hans, 180

Jones, Peter, 269

Judge, William Q., 213

Jung, Carl, 16, 28, 35, 55, 76, 97, 191-94, 202-3, 212, 220, 229, 233

Kamenetz, Roger, 25

Kearney, Hugh, 43, 100

Keats, John, 122

Kelley, Edmund, 45

Kellmeyer, Steve, 200

Kellogg, Wilfred, 220

Kepler, Johann, 46

King, George, 199

King, Stephen, 210

King-Hele, Desmond, 122

Koot Hoomi, 271

Krentz, Edgar, 53

Lamarck, Jean Baptiste, 123-24, 132

Lao Tze, 221

Las Casas, 235

Law, William, 122, 156

Leibniz, Gottfried Wilhelm von, 81

Lessing, Gotthold Ephraim, 60-61

Levi, Leonard, 36-37

Lewis, C. S., 265, 267

Lindsay, Jack, 181

Locke, John, 52, 58, 157, 232

Lucas, George, 22, 24, 200

Luther, Martin, 53-54

Macaulay, Thomas Darbington, 79

Mack, John, 28, 206, 217-20, 224, 246, 262, 271-72

MacLaine, Shirley, 21, 254, 261-63, 269, 271, 277

Malthus, Thomas Robert, 129

Marcion, 178

Marshall, Ian, 170-74, 177-78, 268

Mesmer, Franz, 90, 214

Michaelis, Johann David, 60

Milton, John, 270

Mirandola, Pico della, 38, 231

Montaigne, Michel de, 232

Montesquieu, Baron de, 75, 80, 259

Moore, James, 127

Muhammad, 51, 221, 235, 239

Mulford, Prentice, 91

Narby, Jeremy, 27, 117, 205, 224

Newton, Sir Isaac, 43, 46, 70, 80-81, 114

Nicholas of Cusa, 47, 231

Nietzsche, Friedrich, 93, 165, 175, 191-92, 264

Noll, Richard, 28, 152, 162, 192-94, 216, 273, 280

Noyes, John Humphrey, 134, 143

Oegger, Guillaume, 158

Olcott, Colonel Henry Steele, 213-15

Ornstein, Robert, 119, 264

Otto, Rudolf, 228-29

Owens, Lance S., 30

Paine, Thomas, 98-103, 109-10, 113-14, 117, 156, 165, 262

Paley, William, 127, 157

Parker, Hershel, 161

Pascal, Blaise, 81

Passmore, John, 123

Peale, Norman Vincent, 92

Pearce, Joseph Chilton, 266, 272

Philostratus, 232

Planck, Max, 170

Plato, 43, 179

Plotinus, 152, 156, 179, 235

Plummer, Gordon, 114

Pollock, Frederick, 134

Popkin, Richard, 53

Porphyry, 43, 51, 232

Pound, Roscoe, 53

Priestley, Joseph, 156

Proclus, 179

Puech, Henri Charles, 179

Pullman, Philip, 271

Pythagoras, 38, 114, 179, 215

Quimby, Phineas Parkhurst, 90-91

Quinn, D. Michael, 186-87, 190

Raleigh, Sir Walter, 52

Rand, Ayn, 77, 89, 92-95, 165, 259-60

Raschke, Carl, 16, 45, 180-81, 201

Redfield, James, 22, 143-44, 264, 272

Reed, Sampson, 157

Reichel-Dolmatoff, Gerardo, 275

Reimarus, Hermann Samuel, 60-61

Renan, Joseph Ernst, 97

Rhine, J. B., 261

Richards, Robert, 132-33

Rigdon, Sidney, 189

Rips, Iliyahu, 69-70

Rodenberry, Gene, 148

Rojcewicz, Peter, 219

Roof, Wade Clark, 18

Ropp, Harry L., 188-89

Rousseau, Jean-Jacques, 75, 120, 259

Rowling, J. K., 24

Rush, Benjamin, 99

Sagan, Carl, 107-14, 117, 207

Schleicher, August, 216

Schleiermacher, Friedrich, 157, 228

Schmitt, C. B., 50

Scholem, Gershom, 41

Schucman, Helen, 28, 153

Schuon, Frithjof, 230, 237-40, 248

Seneca, 50, 232

Sextus Empiricus, 50

Shakespeare, William, 167

Shaw, George Bernard, 133, 153, 167-69, 174, 264

Shelley, Mary, 121-22

Shelley, Percy, 122-23

Sherlock, Thomas, 253-54

Shipps, Jan, 186-87

Shoham, Shlomo, 41-42

Siegel, Bernie, 29

Simon, Richard, 53

Sinnett, A. P., 216

Smith, Alexis, 269-70

Smith, Ethan, 188-89

Smith, Huston, 230, 238, 242-43, 248

Smith, Joseph, 119-20, 156, 185-91, 199, 202-3, 206, 212, 272

Southern, R. W., 48, 66

Spaulding, Solomon, 188-89

Spencer, Herbert, 120, 123-24, 147, 149-50, 266

Spinoza, Benedict de (Baruch), 46, 51-52, 152-56, 171, 174, 215, 232

Spong, J. S., 56-58, 66-69, 71-73, 255-56, 268, 277

Stapledon, Olaf, 145

Steiner, Rudolf, 214

Stewart, Dugald, 157

Stott, John, 72, 252

Stoyanov, Yuri, 179

Strauss, David, 58, 60-66, 68-69, 71-73, 179, 247, 262

Streiber, Whitley, 220-21

Sullivan, Robert, 45, 155-56

Sutin, Lawrence, 211

Swedenborg, Emanuel, 157, 206-10, 218, 224, 272

Swift, Jonathan, 56

Teasdale, Wayne, 16, 18-19, 226-27, 248, 262

Teilhard de Chardin, Pierre, 139-41, 144, 151, 263

Tennyson, Alfred Lord, 214

Thetford, William, 28

Thoreau, Henry David, 157

Tindal, John, 58

Toland, John, 50-52, 58, 152-56, 169, 174

Trine, Ralph Waldo, 90-92, 95

Tucker, Ellen, 157-58

Valentinus, 178, 215

Vaux, Madame Clotilde de, 97

Verter, Bradford, 47, 211-12, 231

Voltaire, 75-77, 79-85, 89, 93, 95, 99, 128, 259

Voskuil, Dennis, 90-92

Walker, Barbara, 23

Walker, Ruth, 29

Wallace, Alfred Russel, 126, 128, 139, 216-17

Walsch, Neale Donald, 224, 267, 269-70, 274, 277

Walter, Luman, 187

Wasson, Gordon, 205

Watanabe, Teresa, 19

Weaver, Richard, 251

Weigel, Valentin, 48

Weil, Andrew, 29

Weissmandel, H. M. D., 70

Wells, H. G., 145

Wheeler, Charles N., 252

Whitman, Walt, 235

Willard, Dallas, 271

Wilson, A. N., 124, 149, 280

Winfrey, Oprah, 14-15, 25, 223

Wolf, Fred Alan, 26, 115, 152-53, 175-76

Wolf, Leibl, 24

Woolston, Thomas, 55-63, 66, 68-69, 71, 73, 80-81, 179, 207, 215

Wordsworth, William, 85, 122-23, 158

Wuthnow, Robert, 19-20

Yates, Frances, 280

Yeats, W. B., 214

Yepes, John, 235

Zacharias, Ravi, 278

Zohar, Dana, 170-74, 268

Zukav, Gary, 14-15, 26, 114, 117, 149, 223-24, 248, 260, 265, 268, 270, 275-76

Index of Subjects

*Abduction: Human Encounters
  with Aliens*, 28, 217, 219-20
Abel, 184-85
Abolition of Man, The, 265
Abraham, 41, 66, 185
abyss, 48
Adam and Eve, 41, 52-53, 78-
  79, 105, 181, 184, 190, 199,
  270
adepts, 180
Advanced Metaphysical
  Study Center, 29
Aetherius Society, 199
Age of Reason, The, 99-100,
  103, 165
Ageless Body, Timeless Mind, 29
Albigensians, 37
alchemy, alchemists, 45, 47,
  117, 191-92, 205, 208, 243,
  263, 274
alcohol, 87
Alexandria, 38
alien, aliens, 27-28, 30, 107,
  112-13, 124, 141, 147-48,
  178, 199, 207-9, 217-21, 224,
  251, 256, 260 262-63, 271-
  72, 274
Allah, 245
allegory, 49, 56, 59, 63, 253,
  256
America, 19, 25, 90, 93, 98,
  103-4, 126, 137, 153, 158-59,
  174, 185-86, 188, 191, 193,
  200, 204, 206, 211-12, 214,
  237, 272
American Book Club, 14

American colonies, 56, 59
amino acids, 144
Amsterdam, 153
ancient religions, 136, 231
ancient spiritual traditions,
  26
ancient wisdom, 114-15, 117,
  193, 251, 264
angels, 18, 41, 147, 181-82,
  186, 206-7, 210, 221, 251,
  274
  fallen, 177, 182-83, 201
  Michael, 7, 17, 58, 69, 72-
    73, 186-87, 190, 226, 248,
    262, 272
animal magnetism, 90
Anthroposophy, 214
antisemitism, 57
Aquarian Conspiracy, The, 15,
  21-22, 26, 115, 149, 268
archetypes of the
  unconscious, 220
Armageddon, 71
Art of Happiness, The, 25
Aryans, Aryan spirituality,
  145, 215, 266
Asana, 254
Asclepius, 39-40, 181
astral fatalism, 181
astrology, 18-19, 44, 46-47,
  187, 194, 228, 267
AstroNet, 19
astronomers, astronomy, 46,
  101, 105, 114, 172, 183, 209
Astro-Theology, 183
atheism, 154, 227
Atlantis, 263
Atlas Shrugged, 92-93, 259
Atman, 245
atonement, 49, 105, 250, 278

Aurora, 48, 158
authority as source of truth,
  238
Averroes, 232
Avesta, 233
Babylon, 82
Bacchus, 56
Balkans, 37
Beast, the, 211
Beghards, 37
Beguines, 37
Berkeley Psychic Institute, 29
Bible, 32, 34, 45, 49-58, 60-63,
  66-74, 77, 80, 99-100, 104-5,
  154, 185-86, 189, 192, 232,
  237, 245, 247, 262, 272
Bible Code, The, 58, 69, 71-72,
  272
biblical criticism, 20, 51-54,
  56, 58, 60-61, 66, 69, 72-73,
  81, 99, 160, 244, 262
Biographia, 85
biology, biologists, 27, 46,
  105, 124, 129, 137, 220
Black Elk, 205, 243
black holes, 112
blasphemy, 56, 99
body, 28-29, 37-39, 41, 43-44,
  68, 84-85, 91, 118, 120-21,
  124, 151, 163-64, 181, 184,
  191-92, 201, 204-5, 208-9,
  222-23, 242, 263, 270-73
Bogomiles, 37
Bologna, 50
Bolt.com, 23
Book of Divine Consolation, 48
Book of Lies, 211
Book of Mormon, 186-89
boson, 171
Brahmans, 155, 215, 222,

241, 245

brain, 30, 87, 89, 107, 118, 124, 138, 141, 143, 147, 164, 196, 198, 230, 266

Buddha, 25, 29, 141-42, 174, 214, 216, 221-22, 236

Buddhism and the Way of Change, 27

Buddhism, 24, 27, 116, 141, 215, 227

Buddhist Catechism, 215

Cagliostro, 214

Cain, 184

Caleb, 183-84

Cambridge Platonists, 43

Cambridge University, 55, 125

Candide, 80-82

carbon, 144

Castle of the Heavens, 46

Cathars, 37

Catholicism, 24, 45

Celestine Prophecy, The, 22, 143-44, 272

chakra, 23

Chaldeans, 38, 183

Chandogya, 241

channeling, 215, 220, 222

Chase, The, 148

chemistry, 46, 209

China, 161

Christ Mind, 221-23

Christian Science, 29, 98

Christianity Not Mysterious, 154

Christianity, 38, 45-48, 50-52, 54-55, 57-61, 63, 65, 68, 72-73, 75-77, 79-80, 85, 96, 99-102, 104, 120, 125, 127-28, 139, 150, 152, 154, 157, 160,

162, 165-66, 179, 185, 192, 194, 215, 222, 224, 227, 229-31, 239, 246-47, 252-53, 278-80

Christology, 65, 247

Church of England, 253

Civil War, 104, 107, 269

clairvoyance, 261

classical languages, 51

cloning, 263

Close Encounters of the Third Kind, 147

comets, 183

Coming Race, The, 145-46, 217

Common Sense, 98

Communion, 220

community, 18, 25, 32, 44, 63, 69, 108, 117, 169, 192, 200, 226, 259, 273-74, 279

complementarity, 114

computers, 115, 200, 272

Conduct of Life, 161

Confessions of a Drug Fiend, 211, 212

Confessions of an English Opium Eater, 86

Confirmation, 221

conscious evolution, 119, 150, 264

consciousness, 15-16, 18, 22, 26, 34, 39, 55, 62, 64-66, 68, 77, 99, 103, 111, 114-15, 119, 137, 140-42, 144, 149-53, 157, 159-60, 163-64, 167, 171-73, 180, 193, 198, 202, 218-19, 221, 224, 226-29, 233-36, 240-43, 245, 248, 251, 262-64, 267-68, 276-78

Contact, 107, 111, 113, 204, 207

Continuum, The, 148

Conversations with God, 224, 274

Copernicanism, 45

Corinth, 258

Cornell University, 107

Corpus Hermeticum, 38-39, 42, 44

Cosmic Consciousness, 233-38

Cosmos, 96, 107

Course in Miracles, A, 28, 153, 250

Creative Evolution, 140

Creed of Science, The, 106

culture war, 96, 166

Dachau, 57

daemons, 39-40, 43, 274

Dancing in the Light, 21, 254, 263

Darwinism, 130, 133, 135, 162, 194

death, 28, 33, 38, 45, 49, 57, 61, 68, 72, 76, 83, 88, 94, 107, 114, 118, 125, 140, 145, 152, 154, 156, 181, 196, 201, 208-10, 213-14, 222, 232, 234, 237-38, 240, 242, 249, 253, 278-79

Declaration of Independence, 254

deep massage, 29

deists, deism, 51, 54, 58, 60-61, 66, 72, 77-78, 80-81, 84, 87, 99, 101, 106, 128, 181, 184, 228, 232, 259

Deitas, 48

Demon-Haunted World, 107-10

demons, demonic, 56, 108,

117, 204-5, 210, 212, 235, 274, 276, 280
Dianetics, 199
Diary of a Drug Fiend, 88
dinosaurs, 71
divina sapientia, 215
divination, 187, 276
divine energy, 19, 34, 43, 152-53, 163, 212, 269
Divine Other, 197
DNA, 148
Dominicans, 47
don Juan, 21, 201, 205
dreams, dreaming, 28, 86-89, 112, 115, 259, 265, 272
Druids, Druidism, 22, 155, 267
dualism, 26, 115, 151, 162-64, 223
Duke University, 66, 261
dukha, 116
earth, 182, 190, 220
Edinburgh University, 120, 125
education, 19, 80, 104, 120, 125, 142, 158, 264-65
egoism, 92, 133, 166
Egypt, Egyptians, 25, 38, 84, 145, 156, 161, 183-84, 248
Ein Sof, 24
electricity, 121
electrons, 171
elemental spirits, 182
Elementargedanken (elementary ideas), 240, 243
elites, 178, 198, 202, 239, 273
emanations, 172
emotions, 32, 64, 111
energy, 35, 42, 91, 112, 115, 140, 144, 146, 153, 163, 165,

167, 170, 172, 195, 213, 219, 241, 260, 262, 267-69
England, 56, 59-62, 69, 77, 81, 86, 98-99, 120, 126, 129, 137, 146, 153, 156-57, 206, 210, 213, 253
enlightened self-interest, 92
Enlightenment, 20, 48, 52, 77, 79-80, 85, 87, 95, 103, 125, 181-83, 201, 204
Enoch, 190
Enos, 184
entertainment, 19, 103, 158
entheogens, 242
eros, 164
Eskimos, 64
ESP, 261
Essence of Christianity, The, 228
eternity, 89, 119, 201
ethical process, 135
eugenics, 134-36, 143, 263, 265-66
Europe, Europeans, 20, 23, 36-38, 40, 43, 46, 50, 53-54, 76, 79, 124, 133, 135-36, 150, 152-53, 156, 158, 162, 164, 166, 174, 178, 188, 193, 213-14, 216-17, 232-33, 266-67, 273
evil, 37, 56, 66, 79, 81, 94, 144, 157, 178, 182-83, 185, 200, 222, 234, 251, 268-69, 276, 279
evolution, 14-15, 23, 34, 49-50, 64-65, 71, 118-21, 123-44, 147-50, 152, 163-65, 167-69, 171, 173-75, 197-98, 203, 215-17, 223-24, 227, 230, 233-35, 245, 251, 260, 263-65, 267, 270

of consciousness, 174, 264
Evolution and Ethics, 135
Evolution: The Modern Synthesis, 137
evolving universe, 140, 251, 260
exodus, 70, 105
extraterrestrials, 114, 183
faith, 22, 47, 51, 54, 57, 60, 66, 68, 77, 81, 89, 93, 97, 100-105, 109-10, 121, 127-28, 131, 142, 164-65, 169, 175, 179, 181, 193-94, 199, 202-3, 210, 227-28, 235, 237, 239, 247-49, 251-52, 259-60, 276-81
Fall, the, 33, 52, 78, 81, 93, 179, 184
Family Wicca Book, 24
fasting, 275
fermions, 171
Festival of Liberty and Reason, 75
Final End, 149-50
First Principles, 124
Foundations of Faith, The, 106
Foundations of the Nineteenth Century, 266
Fountainhead, The, 92
France, 51, 69, 80, 97, 153, 237
Frankenstein, 121-22
Frederick II of Denmark, 46
Free Inquirer, The, 78
Free Spirits, 37
freethinking, 82, 87-88, 104, 137
French Revolution, 76, 123, 211
From Atom to Kosmos, 114

Future of an Illusion, The, 229

Future of Man, The, 140

Gaia, 23

galactogenesis, 113

Garden of Eden, 184, 190, 270

Garden of Pomegranates, 154

Gefühl, 157

Genesis, 41, 66, 70-71, 78-79, 105, 184-85, 201-2, 280

genius, 145

genome, 142

Germany, 47, 60-62, 69, 120, 135, 153, 162, 193

gnosis, 37-38, 73, 173, 179-80, 182, 184, 187, 189, 191, 196-97, 200-203, 251, 270-75, 280

Gnostic Church, 194

Gnosticism, Gnostics, 37, 41, 43, 178-83, 185, 187, 189, 191-95, 197, 199, 201, 203, 243, 270

God
  creation, 25-26, 28, 32, 37, 41-42, 45, 71, 78-79, 95, 100-101, 103, 105, 113-14, 125-26, 129, 138, 150, 153, 161, 164, 170-71, 173, 175, 180-81, 190, 200-201
  creator, 41, 84, 103, 148, 160, 170, 175-76, 180, 200, 260, 275, 279
  origin of idea, 229
  rejection of Christian conception, 37, 62, 73, 79-80, 109, 127, 152, 169, 192, 212

God Is a Verb, 24, 285

goddess, 22-23, 76, 277

Godhead, 48-49, 173, 270

God-men, 239

Godolphin, 211

Going to Pieces Without Falling Apart, 27

Going Within, 21

golden plates, 186-89

gospel, 40, 63, 73, 106, 119, 224, 232, 247, 273

Gospels, 61-62, 67, 255

grace, 123, 144, 203, 239, 251, 261, 266, 273

Grand Man, 208

gravity, 70

Great Life, 197

Great Mother, 24

Great Spirit, 245

Great White Brotherhood, 214

Greece, Greeks, 152, 155, 173, 181, 254, 258

guardians, 197

guilt, 106, 183, 223

Hale-Bopp comet, 177

hallucinogens, 139, 242

Harmonialism, 90

Harry Potter, 24

Harvard University, 108

healing, 19, 27, 29, 59, 77, 88, 90, 204, 254, 260

health, 20, 29, 90, 236, 254

heaven, 41, 76, 83, 94, 101, 139, 149, 181-82, 198, 207-10, 241, 244, 250, 258, 261

Heavenly Partner, 197

Hebrew alphabet, 40

Hebrews, letter to the, 67, 71, 156, 188, 259

helium, 143, 144

hell, 38, 57, 106, 121, 182, 256

Henriade, 80

Henry IV, king of France, 80

Hereditary Genius, 135

heretics, 50, 178, 232

hermeticism, hermetic tradition, 38-41, 44, 47, 208, 231, 248

Hero and the Goddess, 194

Hero with a Thousand Faces, 240

hierarchy, 79, 274

higher self, 271, 277

Hindu, Hinduism, 30, 115, 158, 172, 192, 213-15, 220, 232-33, 263

Historical Atlas of World Mythology, 240

history, 16, 34, 38, 41-42, 49, 51-53, 55-62, 64-68, 71-74, 76, 87, 94, 99, 133, 137, 141, 144-45, 152, 171, 174-75, 178-81, 184-89, 191-92, 194, 200-202, 214, 218, 220, 222, 228, 232, 235, 239-40, 245-47, 249-57, 259, 262-64, 266, 269, 276, 278

History of the World, 52

Hitler, Adolf, 145, 147

Holy Spirit, 78, 222

humanism, humanists, 7, 43, 49-51, 232

Hveen, 46

hydrogen, 144

hypnosis, 90, 196, 275

I Ching, 194

Idea of the Holy, 228

illumination, 45, 48, 78, 143-44, 158

illusion, 28, 115-16, 169, 200, 222

imagination, 34, 64, 77, 85, 108, 122, 131, 247, 256, 258

immortality, 38, 157, 161, 166, 263

impermanence, 26, 116

In Tune with the Infinite, 91

incantation, 275

India, 39, 41, 114, 155, 161, 213-14, 233, 237, 240

Industrial Revolution, 120

Indwelling Presence, 91

Ingram Book Company, 19

Inner Friend, 197, 221

Inquisition, 37

insanity, 121, 235

inspiration, 52, 63, 111, 123, 205

intellect, 14, 34, 62, 77, 83, 88-89, 95, 155, 168, 258-59

Interspiritual Age, 13, 18

interventionism, 73

intolerance, 80, 82-83, 85

Iraq, 242

Isaac, 43, 46, 53, 66, 70, 80, 114, 185

Isaiah, 63, 71

Isis Unveiled, 212, 215, 217

Islam, 232, 237

Israel, Israelites, 32, 52, 69, 72, 186, 188, 247, 280

Italian Humanists, 51

Italy, 45, 50

Jasher, The Book of, 184-85, 187

Jesuits, 80

Jesus Christ, 28, 32-33, 40, 50, 119, 185, 209, 221, 226, 228, 238, 247, 249, 252-54, 272, 276, 278-79
    miracles, 51-52, 55-56, 58-

59, 61-62, 65, 73, 81, 105, 111, 127, 146
    "mistakes of Moses," 104-5
    as spirit person, 245-48, 277, 279

Jet Propulsion Laboratory, 107

Jew in the Lotus, The, 25

Jews, Judaism, 19, 24-25, 32, 38, 41, 67, 154, 183-84, 229, 246, 273

Job, book of, 100

Judeo-Christian tradition, 14, 20, 250

judgment, 33, 53, 94, 106, 133, 246, 276

Jung Cult, The, 28

Jungian analysis, 192

Jupiter, 207-8

kabbalah, 24, 40-41

Kolob, 190, 199

Krishna, 221-22

Krishnamurti, 143

Krystallnacht, 57

Kundun, 25

Lamanites, 186

Language of the Goddess, The, 22

Leipzig, 53

Lemuria, 215

Letters to Serena, 156

Liberating the Gospels, 66

Life Force, 146, 168-69, 268

Life of Jesus (Renan), 97

Life of Jesus (Strauss), 58, 61-62, 65, 69,

life-energy, 193

life-principle, 166

light, 14, 37, 44, 70, 82, 88, 105, 108-10, 112, 146-47,

165, 170, 195, 209, 220, 222, 242, 252, 257, 259, 268, 272, 277

literalism, 63, 66, 245

literature, 50, 92, 97, 141, 206, 208, 212, 248, 264, 274

London, 86, 97-98, 145, 181-82, 199, 201, 206, 213, 217, 232, 253

London School of Science, 145

love, 37, 49, 93-94, 106, 122, 140, 145, 157, 165-66, 196-97, 210, 213, 262, 269, 277

Love Without Conditions, 221-23

Lucifer, 182-83

Luke, the evangelist, 200, 252, 276

Lunar Society, 120

lunatics, 235

Lyceum movement, 158

lying, 102, 123

Madras, 213

magi, 180, 248, 258

magic, 21, 24, 40, 42, 67, 91, 179, 187, 202, 208, 210-11, 213, 272, 280

magical imagination, 85, 87

magical science, 47, 54

magus, 36, 44, 258

Mahatmas, 214, 216

Majestic Intellect, 77, 95, 259

Man and Superman, 168

Man of Philosophy, 168

Mani, 178

Manuscript, the, 144, 272

Maria Sabina, 205

Marriage of Heaven and Hell, The, 122

Mars, 207

Mary, 37, 56, 90, 98, 121-22, 156

Masks of God, The, 240

mass media, 31, 103

Masters, 14, 26, 114, 212, 214

Matrix, The, 199-200

matter, 26, 43-44, 49, 51, 90, 94, 102, 110, 113, 115, 117, 122, 127, 140, 143-44, 146, 151, 154-55, 157, 163-67, 170-71, 180, 186, 190-91, 203, 233, 235, 251, 265, 268, 273

maya, 92, 115-16

Meaning of Evolution, The, 132

medicine, 19, 21, 27, 29, 46, 88, 90, 109, 125, 200, 209, 243

meditation, 29, 96, 117, 194, 196, 278

Mediterranean Sea, 188

mediums, 34, 205, 274

memory, 16, 25, 97, 207-8, 218, 229, 235

Menander, 178

Mens, 59, 258

Mental Cure, The, 91

Mercury, 204, 207

Mere Christianity, 267

mesmerism, 90

Messiah, 59, 245, 278

META/Sentinel, 108

Middle Ages, 36

Middle East, 24, 70

Milky Way, 112

Mind Games, 194

mind, 38-39, 77, 90-91, 93-95, 152, 155, 157, 161, 194, 222, 230, 233, 251, 258, 260, 273

miracles, 51-52, 55-56, 58-59, 61-62, 65, 73, 81, 105, 111, 127, 146

Mithra, 83, 192

Monism, 162-63

Monistenbund (Monistic Alliance), 166

moral nature, 234-36

morality, 37, 73, 87, 92-95, 103, 106, 135, 180, 201, 259, 268, 272, 274, 279

Mormon Church, 185-86

Moroni, 186, 190

Morpheus, 200

Morya, 216

Moses, 41, 51, 63, 66, 78-79, 105, 154, 183-84, 221

multisensory humanity, 14

multisensory personality, 268

Munich, 147

music, 16, 30-31, 44, 112

My Son: A Mother's Story, 25

Mystery School, 194

mystics, mysticism, 21, 34, 37-39, 46-49, 94, 96, 98, 116, 138, 154, 160-61, 172-73, 180, 192, 212-14, 219, 226-27, 230-31, 235-37, 241-43, 245-48, 251, 262, 268, 277

mythi, 62, 64-65, 247

Mythic Life, 194

myth-making function, 167

myths, mythology, 40, 57, 60, 63-65, 68-69, 73, 101, 104, 113, 179, 191, 194, 197-98, 218, 240, 242, 252, 257

Napoleon, 263

Nara, 142

narrative, 21, 64, 68, 82, 84, 92, 184-86, 199-200, 207,

247, 255-56

NASA, 108

Nathan the Wise, 61

Native American religions, 22

Native Americans, 188

natural selection, 134, 216

nature, 18, 20, 22-23, 26, 33-34, 39, 44, 47, 52, 64-65, 88, 94, 100-101, 104-6, 114-15, 117-18, 121-23, 127, 129-31, 144, 150, 152, 154-55, 157, 159-66, 168, 170-72, 174-75, 178, 188, 190, 199, 202, 207, 209, 213, 217-18, 223-24, 227, 229, 232, 236, 239, 241, 245, 258, 262, 264-65, 267, 269-72, 277, 280

Nature, 23, 34, 83, 88, 101-2, 123, 151-52, 154, 156, 158-61, 168, 174, 229, 265

Nauvoo, Illinois, 119

Nazis, Nazism, 193

Neo-Platonism, 7, 42-44, 47, 231

Nephites, 186

nerve therapy, 122

Netanyahu, Benjamin, 70

Netherlands, 51, 153

New Age, 17-20, 22-23, 25, 92, 142, 192, 194, 205-6, 250, 264, 267, 275

New Bottles for New Wine, 137

New Physics, 26, 114, 169, 171, 173, 267

New Science, 26, 30, 114-15, 117, 152-53, 174, 234, 251

New Testament, 15, 37, 56-63, 68, 73, 185, 194, 223, 247, 253, 255, 259, 276

New Thought, 8, 77, 90-91, 95, 260

New World, New Mind, 119

New York, 22, 25, 28-29, 104, 186-88, 194, 213

Noah, 185, 190

nonphysical Teachers, 14, 223

noosphere, 152

Norse gods, 22

North Africa, 237

Nous, 38

nuclear holocaust, 70-71

numbers, numerology, 22-24, 43-44, 47, 111, 113, 115, 193, 239

numinous, 57, 113-14, 229, 251

O: The Oprah Magazine, 14-15, 25, 223

Observations on the Zoonomia, 123

occult, occultism, 23, 36, 38, 40, 43-44, 91, 98, 108, 135, 158, 178, 191-92, 194, 202, 206, 208, 210-16, 248, 262, 267, 275

Ocrated Medal, 107

Of Truth, 228

Office of Galactic Census, 112

Old Testament, 37, 41, 52, 60, 69, 179-80, 183-84

Omega Point, 139-41, 264

On Detachment, 48

opium, 86-89, 95, 259

Oppenheimer, 263

Oracles of Reason, 231

Order of the Golden Dawn, 211

Oregon State University, 244

Organians, 148

Origin of the Species, 120, 123, 125-26, 130, 134, 266

Orpheus, 43

Our Posthuman Future, 264

Out on a Limb, 21

Oxford University, 45, 50, 58, 86, 137, 244

Palestine, 161, 246, 276

pantheism, 101, 103, 153, 155, 157, 159, 161, 163, 165, 167, 169, 171, 173-75, 267, 269

Pantheisticon, 154, 155

parapsychological phenomena, 191

Paris, 45, 47, 75, 80

Parsee sect, 233

Passion for the Possible, A, 177, 194, 196, 198

Passport to the Cosmos, 28, 217

Paul the apostle, 252

Peabody Award, 107

peepstones, 186

Pentateuch, 40, 104

Perennial Philosophy, 240-43

Peres, 70

perfection, 76, 130, 133, 136, 146, 149-50, 209, 228

Persia, Persians, 156, 161

Persian Letters, 80

persuasion, 35, 158

peyote, 205

philosophy, 22, 26, 47, 81, 87-88, 90, 92-93, 97-98, 103, 114-17, 121, 123, 140-41, 149, 151, 153, 157, 159, 163, 165, 209, 211, 215, 232, 243, 259

physics, 26, 96, 98, 114-17, 170-73, 209, 220, 227, 263, 268, 272

pi, 113

Pilgrims of the Rhine, 211

Planetary Society, 107

planetization, 152

planets, 40, 44-45, 100, 102, 108, 113, 115, 127, 182-83, 190, 198-99, 206 8, 218, 220, 224, 270, 272

pleroma, 180

pluralism, 20, 34-35, 60, 82, 116, 221-25, 227-28, 230-33, 235, 237, 240-42, 244-48, 251, 277-78

plurality of worlds, 102

pneumatikoi, 180, 200

Possible Human, The, 194

potential energies, 163

Power of Myth, The, 240

Prae-adamitten, 53

prayer, 33, 91, 260, 277

precognition, 261

prehistory, 181

priestcraft, 232

Primary Terrestrial Mental Channel, 199

Primitive Mind Cure, The, 91

primitive religion, 155

Principia, 81

Prometheus Unbound, 123

prophets, 150, 180, 212, 246, 251, 279

Protestantism, 24, 157

protons, 171

Proverbs, book of, 258

Psalm 19, 100

pseudo-science, 108-9

psuchikoi, 180

psychiatry, 27-28, 217, 262

psychic magic, 192

psychoanalysis, 28, 191, 193

psychokinesis, 261

psychology of religion, 191

psychology, 20, 27, 30, 163, 170, 191, 220, 261

psychoplasm, 163

Public Broadcasting System, 240

Pulitzer Prize, 107

pyramids, 196

Pythagoreans, 155, 183

Quakers, 49

quanta, 170

quantum physics, 14, 96, 173-74, 263

Quantum Society, 170

quantum vacuum, 172

racialism, 266

racism, 133, 216

Rael, Raelians, 263

Rahab, 71

Reagan, Nancy, 17

Reagan, Ronald, 17

Reason, 34, 50, 59, 61, 75-95, 97, 99, 106, 122, 162, 181, 228, 251, 257-60

Reasonableness of Christianity, The, 52

Red Sea, 105

redemption, 41, 43, 125, 179, 182, 203, 250, 257, 278

Reformation, 53

reincarnation, 18-19, 24, 142, 214, 262, 274

relativity, 116, 261

Religion of Humanity, 97

Religion of Protestants, 50

Religion Without Revelation, 137

religious imagination, 57

Renaissance, 36, 38, 40, 42-47, 50-51, 100, 114, 117, 215, 231, 248, 258, 274

repentance, 169, 228

Rescuing the Bible from Fundamentalism, 56, 58, 66

resurrection, 253

Resurrection of Jesus Considered, The, 77

Riddle of the Universe, The, 136, 162-63

ridicule, 55, 63, 121

ritual magic, 202, 211

romantics, romanticism, 85, 122-23, 160-61, 163

Roosevelt, Eleanor, 17

root races, 215

Rosicrucians, 184

Rwandan massacre, 269

Sacred Union, 140

salvation, 33, 41, 46, 50, 79, 90, 105, 150, 169, 180, 200, 202, 226, 232, 236, 238, 246, 261, 273, 280-81

Sanskrit, 241

Satan, Satanism, 37, 210

Saturn, 101, 207

Schechina, 41

schools for psychic development, 28

science fiction, 107, 111-12, 145, 147-48, 198-99, 203, 207, 260, 267

scientific religion, 26, 101-3, 110, 136, 162, 164, 166

Search for the Beloved, 194

Seat of the Soul, The, 223

secrecy, 40, 43, 155, 272-74, 280

Secret Chiefs, 212

Secret Doctrine, The, 214

secret knowledge, 37, 89, 178-81, 187, 200-201, 203, 212

Secret Life, 28, 217

secret teachings, 41, 178

seers, 180, 246, 251

selective breeding, 135

Self-Aware Universe, The, 98

self-awareness, 77, 137, 251, 259-60

self-consciousness, 45, 234

self-salvation, 94, 179, 279

Semitic people, 186

serpent, 78-79, 184, 270

SETI, 108, 295

Seven Years in Tibet, 25

sexual cells, 163

shamans, shamanism, 27, 117, 178, 204-6, 210-12, 214, 225, 256, 262, 274-77

Siddhartha, 174

Signs from the Depths, 86

Simon Magus, 178

sin, 28, 33, 38, 49, 81, 93-94, 105-6, 144, 184-85, 222, 237, 259, 278-79

Sketch of the Progress of the Human Mind, 76

Snake Path, 269-70

Social Statics, 124

sola scriptura, 53

Son of God, 73, 237, 246-47, 256

Sophia, 41

soul, 14, 26, 45, 160, 196

Soul of the Universe, 155

Soul Talk, 23

space, 42, 107, 175, 207-8

Speech Delivered by an Indian Chief, 232

spirit guides, spirit teachers, 186

Spirit Person, 9, 244

spirit possession, 275

spiritual evolution, 13-14, 34, 40, 49, 139-40, 142-44, 151, 168, 173, 178, 190, 194, 196-98, 205, 209, 212, 220, 224, 233-35, 247, 264, 266, 279

spiritual fiction, 143

spiritual knowledge, 34, 73, 178, 212, 241, 270, 272-73, 275

Spiritual Marketplace, 18

Spiritual Universe, The, 26

Spontaneous Healing, 29

sruti, 241

Star Trek, 147-48, 177

Star Wars, 24, 199-200

stars, 40, 45-46, 100, 111, 113, 115, 144, 177, 181-83, 190, 195, 228, 257, 272

srirpiculture, 134, 142

Stoics, 50

subatomic physics, 116

success, 18-19, 24-25, 30, 46, 91, 95, 128-29, 131, 136, 253, 274

suffering, 42, 49, 81, 106, 116, 128, 168, 176

suicide, 37, 177

sun, sun worship, 44, 64, 106-7, 162, 164-66, 229

Sunyata, 172

Superman, 168-69, 280

superstition, 73, 79, 82, 100, 108, 114, 164

survival of the fittest, 124, 135, 217

Swedenborg Society, 206

Switzerland, 192, 237

symbols, 40, 46, 61, 75, 201, 231, 237-40, 243, 255, 257

syncretism, 47

talisman, 40

Tantric Toning, 30

Tao of Physics, The, 26, 115

Tarot, 23

Teachings of Don Juan, 200, 205

telepathy, 138, 261

Temple of Nature, 121, 123

Temple of Reason, 75-76

theism, 101, 127, 131, 155, 163, 165, 227, 268

Theosophist, The, 213

theosophy, 210, 212-15, 267

Thetans, 199

Tibet, 114, 212, 214

Tibetan Book of the Dead, 241

Tibetan Healing, 29

Time Warner Electronic Publishing, 19

tobacco, 204

Torah, 70

transcendence, 21, 42, 57, 68, 75, 97, 98, 102-3, 108, 110-11, 114, 117, 164, 238

Transcendent Unity of Religions, The, 238

Transcendentalism, 158, 161-62

transfiguration, 63

transformation, 15-16, 19, 117, 169, 258, 264-67

Transforming the Mind, 25

Transhumanism, 8, 136

treasure-digging, 187

Treatise of the Three Impostors, 51, 154

Tree of Life, 175

Trinity, 48, 78, 207

True Messiah, 158

Tryal of the Witnesses, 253, 254

Tübingen, 62

Tufts University, 174

Tungus, 204

tyranny, 80, 100

UFO abductees, 206, 218-19, 221, 262

Ultimate Reality, 227, 238-43, 247

UNESCO, 137

Unitarianism, Unitarians, 19, 127

Unity Christian School, 91

Universal Being, 160

University of Chicago, 132

University of Colorado, 141

University of Jena, 162

Upanishads, 158, 215, 233, 237

Urantia Book, 220

ushnisha, 142

Valentinus, 178, 215

Vedas, 215, 241

Vega star system, 111

Venus, 197, 207

vibration, 144

View of the Hebrews, 188-89

Virtue of Selfishness, The, 92

virtue, 51, 76, 92-94, 149, 265

visualization, 91

vitalism, 143

void, 102, 172, 175

Volkish movement, 162, 164, 192-93

Vril, Vrilya, 145, 146, 147, 200, 217

Way of Knowledge, 205

We the Living, 92

wealth, 82, 93, 124

Web of Life, The, 26

Westar Institute, 244

Wicca, 22, 23, 24, 267

wisdom, 21, 25, 28, 32, 83, 100-101, 103, 115-16, 173, 180, 214, 221, 243, 258, 263, 272

witches, witchcraft, 23-24, 205, 210, 267

World Parliament of Religions, 46, 231

Worlds in Space, The, 206-8

wormholes, 112

worship, 22-24, 30, 47, 64, 66-67, 76, 78, 84-85, 97, 101, 103, 110, 152, 155, 161-62, 164-66, 174-75, 184, 228, 231, 241, 248, 259, 280

Wyoming, 147

Xenu, 199

Yahweh, 20, 24, 78-79, 183, 245, 277

Yoga and the Quest for the True Self, 29

yoga, 29, 199

Zadig, 82-85, 259

Zanoni, 211, 217

Zarathustra, 233

Zen and the Brain, 141

Zohar, 40

Zoroaster, Zoroastrianism, 38, 43, 46, 231-33

Conclusion. 174

8 THE REBIRTH OF GNOSTICISM:
   THE SECRET PATH TO SELF-SALVATION 177
   The Fundamentals of Gnosticism 178
   Jacob Ilive: Enlightenment Gnostic. .181
   Joseph Smith's Yankee Gnosticism 185
   Carl Jung and the Gnostic Impulse. .191
   Jean Houston: Gnosticism and the New Age 194
   Science Fiction: The Final Gnostic Frontier 198
   Conclusion. 200

9 MODERN SHAMANISM:
   SPIRIT CONTACT AND SPIRITUAL PROGRESS 204
   Emanuel Swedenborg 206
   Victorian Shamans: Occultism, Theosophy and Spiritualism. 210
   John Mack and UFO Abduction 217
   Paul Ferrini and the Jesus Phenomenon 221
   Conclusion. 223

10 THE MYSTICAL PATH TO PLURALISM:
   DISCOVERING THAT ALL IS ONE IN RELIGION 226
   An Original Religion. 231
   R. M. Bucke 233
   Frithjof Schuon and Transcendent Religious Unity. 237
   Joseph Campbell: The Perennial Philosophy as Pluralistic Hope 240
   Marcus Borg and Jesus the Spirit Person 244
   Conclusion. 247

11 CONCLUSION: A NEW SPIRITUALITY FOR A NEW AGE. 250
   Taking Leave of History 252
   The Advent of Reason 257
   Theological Science 261
   Spiritual Evolution. 263
   Pantheism 267

4 THE ASCENT OF REASON: BIRTH OF A DEITY 75
    Peter Annet 77
    Voltaire and Liberated Reason 79
    Thomas De Quincey. 85
    American New Thought: Mind as Divine Healing Force 90
    Ayn Rand's Argument for Reason 92
    Conclusion. 94

5 SCIENCE AND SHIFTING PARADIGMS:
   SALVATION IN A NEW COSMOS. 96
    Thomas Paine on the Hope of Science 98
    Robert Green Ingersoll: Science and Deliverance 103
    Carl Sagan: From *The Demon-Haunted World* to *Alien Contact* 107
    The New Physics: Science and Ancient Wisdom 114
    Conclusion. 117

6 EVOLUTION AND ADVANCEMENT:
   THE DARWINS' SPIRITUAL LEGACY 118
    Erasmus Darwin. 120
    Lamarck and Spencer 123
    Charles Darwin: Naturalist Prophet 125
    The Spiritual Vision of Darwin's Early Defenders 134
    Julian Huxley: Transhumanism and the Moral Elite 136
    Pierre Teilhard de Chardin: Reaching the Omega Point 139
    James H. Austin: Evolving Brain, Evolving Spirit 141
    James Redfield: The Celestine Prophet 143
    Science Fiction and Human Evolutionary Destiny 145
    Conclusion. 148

7 PANTHEISM IN THE MODERN WORLD: NATURE OR GOD 151
    Spinoza and Toland 153
    Ralph Waldo Emerson. 156
    Ernst Haeckel and *The Riddle of the Universe*. 162
    Bergson and Shaw 167
    A New Pantheistic Physics. 170

CONTENTS

Acknowledgments 11

1 INTRODUCTION: A CHANGING VIEW
   OF THE SPIRITUAL WORLD 13
   Spiritual Changes: A New Age of Belief? 17
   Bestsellers and Blockbusters: Spirituality Goes Public 20
   Talking About Spirituality 30
   The Revealed Word and the New Religious Synthesis 31
   Goals of the Study 35

2 ANTECEDENTS OF THE NEW RELIGIOUS SYNTHESIS:
   A BRIEF HISTORY OF ALTERNATIVE SPIRITUALITY
   IN THE WEST 36
   Spiritual Communities in the Middle Ages 36
   Magic and the Hermetic Tradition 38
   Kabbalah: Secrets in the Pentateuch 40
   Neo-Platonism and Magical Science 42
   European Mysticism 47
   Humanism and the Rise of Biblical Criticism 49
   Conclusion 54

3 THE RISE OF BIBLICAL CRITICISM:
   ALLEGORY, MYTH, CODES AND THE END OF HISTORY 55
   Thomas Woolston and the English Deists 58
   Lessing, Strauss and German Criticism 60
   John Shelby Spong Rescues the Bible 66
   Michael Drosnin's *The Bible Code* 69
   Conclusion 72

for

RUSSEL HIRST

InterVarsity Press
P.O. Box 1400, Downers Grove, IL 60515-1426
World Wide Web: www.ivpress.com
E-mail: mail@ivpress.com

InterVarsity Press® is the book-publishing division of InterVarsity Christian Fellowship/USA®, a student movement active on campus at hundreds of universities, colleges and schools of nursing in the United States of America, and a member movement of the International Fellowship of Evangelical Students. For information about local and regional activities, write Public Relations Dept., InterVarsity Christian Fellowship/USA, 6400 Schroeder Rd., P.O. Box 7895, Madison, WI 53707-7895, or visit the IVCF website at <www.ivcf.org>.

Scripture quotations, unless otherwise noted, are from the New Revised Standard Version of the Bible, copyright 1989 by the Division of Christian Education of the National Council of the Churches of Christ in the USA. Used by permission. All rights reserved.

Cover design: Cindy Kiple

Cover image: Howard Berman/Getty Images

ISBN 0-8308-2398-0

Printed in the United States of America ∞

Library of Congress Cataloging-in-Publication Data

Herrick, James A.
    The making of the new spirituality: the eclipse of the Western
religious tradition/James A. Herrick.
        p. cm.
Includes bibliographical references and index.
    ISBN 0-8308-2398-0 (alk. paper)
    1. Christianity and other religions. 2. Religion and
science—History. 3. Spirituality—History. I. Title
    BR127.H47 2003
    261.2'993—dc21
                                                                                        2002156376

P	20	19	18	17	16	15	14	13	12	11	10	9	8	7	6	5	4	3	2	1
Y	20	19	18	17	16	15	14	13	12	11	10	09	08	07	06	05	04	03

THE MAKING OF THE

NEW SPIRITUALITY

The Eclipse of the
Western Religious Tradition

JAMES A. HERRICK

InterVarsity Press
Downers Grove, Illinois

4 Computer Program Design

The structure of the computer software is a neglected topic in most discussions of analytical systems, despite the fact that the implementation of the software can be the most problematic of the tasks involved. Most failures to meet deadlines can be traced to programming, rather than to conceptual or data bottlenecks. This chapter contains a description of the Simpact software. It is not suggested that the Simpact software represents the best approach for large-scale analytical systems. Instead, the purpose in discussing the software is to give the reader some idea of the specialized procedures, such as hierarchical coding, that are involved in computerizing large-scale analytical systems. The discussion is detailed, and thus the chapter may appear to be specific to the Simpact project. The purpose of such detail is to provide a complete illustration of the principles and procedures involved; without specific illustrations these concepts cannot be adequately explained.

It should be emphasized that discussion of the program design has been restricted to the forecasting system. No attempt has been made to describe programs that are used to derive the parameters or input variables that go into the system. In many cases, these parameters are not the end result of mathematical operations. Where they are, the operation is usually regression analysis, a procedure for which numerous, easy-to-use, prewritten computer packages are available.

The chapter has been organized into three sections. The first section describes the objectives for which the program design was formulated. The second explains the procedures a user must follow in running a job. The third discusses the logic of the programs and the data files, focusing for illustrative purposes on the preprocessing component of Simpact. The material is presented in an informal and simplified manner and should be understandable by a reader with only minimal prior computer experience. However, it should be noted that a reader could skip the chapter with little loss in continuity.

Design Objectives

Very often programming starts without the benefit of a preliminary design phase, and the end product in such cases is almost invariably disappointing to the ultimate users. Chapter 2 has already touched on some of the institutional considerations involved in program design. In this section, the objectives behind the design are described and rationalized.

In designing the Simpact system, there were four major objectives: minimization of cost, simplicity of use, selectivity, and clarity of output. Unfortunately, realizing these objectives involves tradeoffs, chiefly between simplicity and cost. Because of the existence of these tradeoffs, it is necessary to list the design objectives by priority. In designing Simpact, top priority was given to cost minimization, since for a large-scale analytical system, an inappropriate design can easily result in a set of programs that are prohibitively expensive to run.

The cost of running a system is influenced by the language in which it is written. A Fortran-written program, for example, is usually cheaper to execute than an equivalent program written in Apl. Given the language and the purpose of the program, run costs become dependent on the degree of efficiency with which the program has been written. A skillful Fortran programmer will, for example, utilize overlay techniques to minimize core requirements and, therefore, execution costs. Simpact is, for its size, surprisingly inexpensive to run. It is programmed in Fortran and Cobol and incorporates various cost-saving techniques.

A major disadvantage with languages like Fortran and Cobol, however, is that programs written in these languages usually require some programming background to run. Having selected Fortran and Cobol for cost-minimizing reasons, the second-order design objective became simplicity in use or, as it is often termed, user-orientation. The use of Wylbur provided the answer. Wylbur is a text-editing language, and so-called Exec programs written in Wylbur create a pseudo-interactive environment. The user is prompted in English-language questions made by the Wylbur Exec as to the options wanted. Answers thus elicited are translated by the Wylbur Exec and then used to manipulate the data files and the system-control cards controlling the Fortran and Cobol programs. Thus the Wylbur Exec provides the interface between the nonprogramming-oriented user and the files and the programs.

While Wylbur does lessen the awkwardness of the Fortran- and Cobol-written programs, it does have some disadvantages. The use of Wylbur increases run costs, and its painstaking prompts can be quite annoying to the experienced user. For all this, the utilization of text-editing languages, such as Wylbur, offers a neat way of surmounting the major objection to the use of efficient languages like Fortran.

The third design objective of Simpact—selectivity—is related to cost minimization. The cost of printing the entire output from Simpact is many times in excess of the cost of executing the job. Given that a user may be interested in only a small segment of the output, it becomes apparent that the option to retrieve a selected output table and suppress all other printing is crucial. In connection with input, *selectivity* refers to the capability of easily and cheaply modifying a specific data input. Simpact was designed to facilitate selectivity in both input modification and output retrieval. Each input and output variable is uniquely identified by a code. By referring to the appropriate input code, the user can bring the data up onto his terminal screen. There he can modify it, after which he can instruct the machine to replace the original value with its modified counterpart. To select a particular output variable, the user need only type in its code; the machine will then restrict itself to printing out the identified variable.

In seeking to achieve the last design objective—clarity of output—programmers were given no significant role. Output formats designed by programmers, besides their lack of artistic appeal, are often unintelligible to the lay user. The Simpact output format was designed by myself in conjunction with those individuals who would be using the output. Each output variable is printed in the form of a time-series table accompanied by headings and footnotes. The headings and footnotes for each table, selected by the lay users, are input to the program and can be changed at any time. In general, the Simpact output is structured to go directly into a report.

User Procedures

A job can be run in many ways. Earlier large-scale systems tended to be run in batch mode. Cards were fed through a reader and the output came out on a high-speed line printer. Simpact is run in a so-called remote batch mode. The user requests a job run by typing in commands at a portable terminal. After an interval of time, typically 10 minutes, the machine indicates that the job is completed, and the user can, at this point, type in commands requesting that the output be printed either at the terminal or on a high-speed line printer.

Simpact, therefore, involves two stages: generating the output and retrieving the output. The first stage entails two separate, but practically identical steps. In the first step, the user runs programs which compute the output corresponding to the construction of the facility, and in the second step, programs are run to compute the output corresponding to the operation of the facility. In the second stage, output tables which show both construction and operation impacts are retrieved.

It should be noted that the stages are independent of each other, in that the user can retrieve output, even if he has not run the programs that compute the output. This is possible because the output from the last run is stored on a disk. When a new run is made, its solutions automatically replace the values of the last run. This feature allows the user tremendous flexibility. For example, he can go back a month after the job has been run and, assuming no jobs have been run in the interim, retrieve output that he has suddenly decided he wants.

Associated with each stage is a Wylbur Exec program. The first stage is performed with the Inpt Exec program and the second stage uses the Otpt Exec program. These Exec programs, once they are "called in" by the user, conduct a dialogue to ascertain the user's needs and then perform the functions—editing the files and running the programs—that will effect these needs.

Accessing an Exec Program

Before the user can access an Exec program, he must sign on, that is, establish communications with the computer and identify himself to it. In establishing communications between the terminal and the computer, the phone provides the linkage. The terminal is accompanied by an acoustic coupler and a telephone. The user turns on a switch on the terminal and the coupler and then dials a designated phone number; when a high-pitched whine is heard on the receiver, the phone is inserted into the coupler. Next, the carriage-return key on the terminal is hit twice, at which point the computer will type a message indicating that communications have been established and start prompting the user for identification.

The type of identification information required depends on the computer system involved. Typically, the information includes a password and an account number: the password, used for identification purposes, has been selected by the user at some prior time; the account number provides the mechanism for billing the user.

Once the user has "signed on," accessing an Exec program would involve typing in at the terminal "Exec from Inpt," where *Inpt* is the name of the Exec program he wants to use.

Generating Output (Stage 1)

In stage 1, the Inpt Exec must be run twice, once to compute the impacts created by the construction of the facility and then again to get the operation impacts. The procedures for the two runs are identical, except that in a construction run, a construction-input file, Conin, is specified by the user to Inpt, and in an operation run, the operation-input file, Oprin, is specified. Since these procedures are identical, the discussion will assume a construction run.

In making a run, there are three Inpt options. Each option corresponds to a specific type of scenario capability, with the term *scenario* used here to mean a run in which input values of the construction-input file are changed.

Option 1. In this option, the user runs the permanent data file, which contains the input values submitted by the functional specialist and represents the most likely scenario. If new information becomes available, the permanent data files are changed, but otherwise they are left untouched.

Using the first option is very straightforward because it does not involve changing any input values. After the user has signed on and typed in Exec from Inpt, the following dialogue will ensue:

Q1: Do you want instructions?
A1: No

Q2: Do you want to run Conin or Oprin?
A2: Conin
Q3: Do you want to use scenario features?
A3: No
Q4: What priority do you want: priority, standard, night?
A4: Standard
Q5: Sign off?
A5: Yes

The preceding dialogue is more or less self-explanatory. The user makes a construction run and requests that the job run at standard priority.

Option 2. In this option, the user runs one of the many previously created scenario files. These scenario files, which represent some modification of the permanent data file, have been created in a previous run. Since they were saved at that time, they are thus available for future runs.

Exercising Option 2 is only slightly more complicated than running Option 1. In response to question 3, the user indicates that he does want to use scenario capabilities. At this point, the dialogue involves the following exchanges:

Q4: Which scenario file do you want: Highmig, Taxcut, Alocal?
A4: Highmig
Q5: What priority do you want: priority, standard, night?
A5: Priority

In this run, the user submits for execution the previously created scenario file Highmig. The job is submitted at priority.

Option 3. It may well be that none of the previously created scenario files meets the user's needs. In such an instance, the user can create his own scenario file by editing the permanent data file. To create a new scenario file, the response to question 4 changes. The new dialogue is as follows:

Q4: Which scenario file do you want: Highmig, Taxcut, Alocal?
A4: None
Q5: Which file do you want to edit?
A5: Conin
Q6: What name do you want to give the new file?
A6: Lotax

At this point, the user types in codes to retrieve the specific input elements of Conin that are to be changed. New values are typed in to replace the old, and the file thus created is stored under the name Lotax. This file is then submitted for execution. In subsequent runs, Lotax is listed in question 4 as one of the files available for use.

Retrieving Output (Stage 2)

In stage 2, the user specifies the output variable he wants printed out. This output can be retrieved either at the terminal or at a high-speed printer. Stage 2 is performed through the Otpt Exec program. This program has two basic options: a "Group" and a "Select."

Option 1. This is an easy-to-use alternative under which the user selects a predefined group of output variables. Each group has a name associated with it; for example, one group could be a list of twenty fiscal variables stored under the name Tax. When the user specifies the name Tax, this automatically causes the program to print out the latest values for the twenty fiscal variables.

Once the Otpt Exec has been called in, using the first option would involve the following dialogue:

Q1: Do you want Group or Select?
A1: Group
Q2: Which group do you want: Execut, House, Enviro, Tax?
A2: Enviro
Q3: Do you want graphs?
A3: No
Q4: Do you want terminal output?
A4: No
Q5: What priority do you want: priority, standard, night?
A5: Standard
Q6: Sign off?
A6: Yes

In this session, the user picks the Enviro group, a set of environmental variables, for printing. He indicates that he does not want graphs or terminal printout and that the job is to be submitted at standard priority.

Option 2. Under this option, the user has greater flexibility than was afforded by the first alternative. He can select any single variable that he wants printed out. An Option 2 dialogue with Otpt follows:

Q1: Do you want Group or Select?
A1: Select
Q2: What is the model number?
A2: 3
Q3: What is the variable number?
A3: 4
Q4: Do you want another variable?

A4: No
Q5: Do you want graphs?
A5: No
Q6: Do you want terminal output?
A6: No
Q7: What priority do you want: priority, standard, night?
A7: Priority
Q8: Sign off?
A8: Yes

In the preceding dialogue, the user indicates that he wants the fourth variable of the third model printed out. He further indicates in response to question 4 that he does not wish any further variables printed out. If the response to question 4 had been affirmative, questions 2 and 3 would have been repeated.

Program and File Structure

Turning now to the inner workings of programmed Simpact, as distinct from the user's interface with it, three stages can be clearly delineated: preprocessing, computation, and report-generation. The preprocessing and computational stages correspond to stage 1 of the user procedures, that is, generating output. The report-generation stage corresponds to stage 2 of the user procedures, that is, retrieving output.

Preprocessing involves preliminary operations on the input file, such as checking it for completeness. In the *computational stage*, the checked input file is used to compute the solutions which are then written out to a file. In the *report-generation stage*, selected variables from the solution file are printed or graphed out.

Overview

Associated with each stage is a functional program, written in Fortran or Cobol, and input and output files. Also associated with the preprocessing and report-generation stages are Wylbur Exec programs. Figure 4-1 depicts the interrelationships between programs and files.

Preprocessing. This stage involves two programs: the Wylbur Exec program Inpt and the Fortran program Preproc. Inpt performs an interface function, while the actual preprocessing is done by Preproc.

The Inpt program is the mechanism by which the user requests a construction or operation run of the model. The program thus acts as an activating

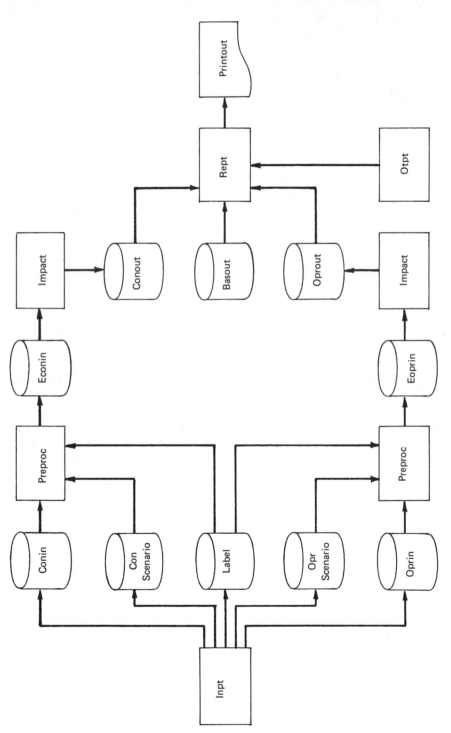

Figure 4-1. Simpact Program Overview

device. If a construction run has been specified by the user, the Inpt program feeds the construction input file, Conin, and a text file, Label, to the functional Fortran program, Preproc.

The operations performed by Preproc involve data checking and reformatting. Data checking involves comparing Conin with Label. Conin contains data values and Label contains a list of names for the variables that Conin should have. Conin is defined to be correct if it contains values for all the variables listed in Label. Once Conin is checked, it is reformatted into an expanded form and written out under the name Econin.

Computation. This stage constitutes the analytical core of Simpact. The Fortran program, Impact, contains a programmatic representation of the mathematical structure of Simpact. It reads in Econin, the file containing the values for the input variables for the construction phase, and performs the manipulations necessary to create the construction-output solutions. These solutions are written out in a coded, densely formatted file called Conout.

Report Generation. In this stage, the output variables requested by the user are printed out, each in a time-series table. The table contains the impacts created by the construction phase, the impacts created in the operation phase, and the baseline values for the variable.

Report generation is performed by a Cobol program called Rept. This program reads in four files: Reqst, Conout, Oprout, and Basout. Reqst tells Rept what variables the user wants printed. Conout, Oprout, and Basout constitute a complete data base on construction impacts, operation impacts, and baseline values, respectively. The file Reqst is the output of the Wylbur program Otpt. Conout and Oprout are created by the Impact program. Basout is a user-entered file.

The objective of the Rept program is to create a table with the same variable drawn from the three data files. The variables that Rept selects depend on the names stored in the Reqst file. Once the Rept program has selected the variables, it performs some elementary mathematical operations on the collected variables—for example, values in Conout and Oprout are added—and then prints out the time-series tables.

Conin File

The Conin file contains the input variables used to compute the impacts created by the construction of the facility. It is identical in format with the Oprin file, which contains the input variables for the operation run. Conin is stored on magnetic disks, with each line, or record, in the format of the eighty-column punchcard.

Simpact is an annual multiregional system. For the purpose of this exposition, let it be assumed that there are 5 years and that impacts are computed for each of seven subregions. Then for each input variable, thirty-five values must be provided; for example, the values for the input variable policemen per capita must be entered for each of 5 years and for each of seven regions.

The way in which Conin is set up allows each line to contain the entire set of values for 1 year. For example, a line could contain the seven regional input values for the policemen-per-capita variable for the year 1979. In addition to data, the line would also contain a code. The overall layout of a line would be as follows:

1. Columns 1 through 8 contain the code.
2. Columns 9 and 10 are blank.
3. Columns 11 through 20 contain the input value for the first subregion.
4. Columns 21 through 30 contain the input value for the second subregion.
5. Columns 31 through 80 contain the input value for the remaining five subregions, with each value in a field of ten columns.

The purpose of the code in columns 1 through 8 is to uniquely identify each line to allow its retrieval. The code setup is as follows:

1. Columns 1 and 2 are used to identify the model in which the variable belongs; for example, a 03 indicates that the variable belongs to the third model of the system.
2. Columns 3 through 5 are used to identify the position of the variable within the model; for example, a 016 indicates that the variable is the sixteenth in the model.
3. Column 6 is used to identify whether or not the value of the variable differs by region; for example, a 0 indicates no variation and a 1 indicates variation.
4. Columns 7 and 8 are used to identify the year; for example, an 83 would indicate the year 1983.

If the user has typed in a 0 in column 6, indicating no spatial variation, all the fields in the card need not be filled. Columns 11 through 20 will contain the value that is to apply to all regions. Similarly, if there are 0s in columns 7 and 8, indicating that the values do not vary temporally, then there would be only one card for the input variable rather than the usual one card per year.

Label File

The Label file contains a list of identifiers for the variables in the Conin and Oprin files. There is one line in the file for each input variable, and the line is in the form of the eighty-column punchcard. The layout is as follows:

1. Columns 1 through 6 contain the code, which is the same as the one used in Conin.
2. Columns 7 through 10 are blank.
3. Columns 11 through 80 contain a textual identifier for the input variable.

Scenario Files

Scenario files, such as the Lotax file described in the user procedures, are created by editing. These scenario files are very sparse. Assume that the user, in creating Lotax, has replaced 14 lines of the 2000-line Conin file. In such a case, the Lotax file would contain only the 14 edited lines. The 1986 unchanged lines would not be transferred from Conin to Lotax.

The sparse storage mode of the scenario files has been set up to minimize storage costs. Scenario files created in one run are stored and become available in subsequent runs. If the scenario files are stored in the same detail as Conin, that is, they contain 2000 lines, this would increase storage costs enormously.

Econin File

The Econin file is created by the Preproc program by expanding the Conin file and merging it with a scenario file, if one has been created. If there is no scenario file, Econin will contain exactly the same data as Conin, but stored in an expanded mode. Conin stores its data in an efficient manner, that is, in a format designed to avoid spatial and temporal redundancy. Where the same value applies across regions or years, separate values need not be provided in Conin for each region and year. However, the computational program requires a value for each year and each region. Econin provides such a file. Since Econin is a temporary file, inefficient storage is not of concern. After the Impact program has read in Econin, it deletes it.

Inpt Exec Program

The Inpt Exec program is written in the Wylbur language and is used both for creating scenario files and for submitting a permanent data file or scenario file for execution. The program is made up of three major segments: file selection, file editing, and file submission.

The *file-selection segment* determines whether the user wants to run Conin or Oprin and whether scenario capabilities are required. If no scenario capabilities are desired, the program branches to the file-submission segment to submit Conin or Oprin for a run. If the answer is yes, the program continues to the editing segment.

The purposes of the *file-editing segment* is to create scenario files. This segment prompts the user as to the name to be assigned to the to-be-created file, the code of the data items to be replaced, and the new values for these items. It performs the necessary replacements and then transfers control to the file-submission segment.

The *file-submission segment* will submit the appropriate file for execution at the priority level selected by the user. Once this has been done, it will sign the user off.

Preproc Program

The Fortran program, Preproc, does the actual preprocessing associated with this stage. If it is a construction run, Preproc will read in the permanent data file, Conin; the scenario file, let us say Lotax; and the textual file, Label. Preproc will, after processing, write out the expanded data file, Econin, a file which is the input to the computational program, Impact.

The Preproc program consists of a mainline control program and various subroutines. The control program coordinates the operation of the subroutines but does not have any distinct functional role. Control is exercised by making calls to the various subroutines. When a call is made to a subroutine, it executes and then passes control back to the main program. The order in which the subroutines are executed depends on the order in which the call statements are arranged in the mainline program. Apart from read-and-write subroutines, Preproc contains subroutines which perform expansion, error-checking, and merging functions.

The expansion function is based on a scan on Conin. The Preproc program first locates those codes which indicate that only one value has been entered for a given year because there is no regional variation. It then writes out the value as many times as there are regions. Next the program locates those codes which indicate that only one line of data has been provided because no temporal variation exists. It writes out that line as many times as there are years.

The error-checking function is performed by comparing Conin to Label. Based on the codes that appear in each file, the program can determine which variables in Conin are missing. In such cases it will print out the line of text from Label to identify the missing variables. If there are missing variables, the program stops all further processing.

In the merging function, the scenario file, Lotax, is combined with the permanent data file, Conin, to give Econin. Merging involves replacing the values in Conin with their edited counterparts. The Preproc program scans the two files, searching for a code match. When it finds such a match, it replaces the line in Conin with the corresponding line in Lotax. At this point, the program writes out the expanded merged file, Econin, and this terminates the preprocessing stage.

5 Economic and Demographic Model

Certainly among the most important issues surrounding the construction and operation of a new facility are the economic and demographic impacts it will create. From the point of view of the host community, the major benefit of a new plant is the jobs that it will create, and the chief problem, as perceived by the local citizenry, is the arrival of in-migrants.

Computing the number of new jobs and in-migrants requires a sophisticated, interdisciplinary approach. However, the usual method of analysis has been the application of the simple and highly aggregative economic base multiplier method. In the Simpact Economic and Demographic Model, a uniquely integrated approach synthesizing the complex input-output technique with sociological factors has been developed. The number of new jobs at the primary facility, that is, the plant whose construction has necessitated the study, is of course known. Calculating the spinoff production and jobs is performed in Simpact using input-output multipliers. The number of in-migrants is calculated by taking into account jobs created, local labor availability, and the sociological characteristics of the potential employees.

The purpose of this chapter is to describe the Economic and Demographic Model. The chapter has been organized into three sections and is complemented by an appendix. The first section presents an overview of the model, using flowcharts to illustrate the basic concepts involved. The second section explains the economic analysis equation by equation, and the third section performs a similar role with respect to the demographic analysis. The equations are listed in appendix 5A. Both the appendix and the text, to a large extent, are self-contained. A reader who is familiar with economic and demographic impact modeling could probably read the equations without referring to the text. Similarly, a reader could acquire an understanding of how the model works by confining himself to the text.

Overview of the Model

The Economic and Demographic Model is basically concerned with predicting three classes of variables: production, employment, and population. Specifically, the model's objective is to predict how the levels of these variables will change when a large-scale facility is constructed and operated in the region of analysis. Of these three variable classes, production is the most important conceptually.

49

Employment depends on production, and in-migrating population is, in turn, a function of employment opportunities.

Figure 5-1 presents an overview of the components of the production variable and their interrelationships. *Total production* is equal to the sum of the production at the primary facility and secondary production. *Secondary production* is defined as that which results from the advent of the primary facility and includes supplier, indirect, and induced production.

Supplier production refers to the changes in regional production that occur as a result of the local procurement of the primary facility. For example, a steel facility requires as inputs iron ore, coking coal, limestone, and refractory materials, some of which are acquired from suppliers located in the region. Of course, a substantial percentage of the inputs are externally purchased, and in the case of the steel facility, refractory linings are probably the only significant local purchase.

Indirect production refers to the entire cycle of so-called interindustry effects generated when the supplier industries—in the preceding example, the refractories—start to increase their own local purchases. In theory, this sets off

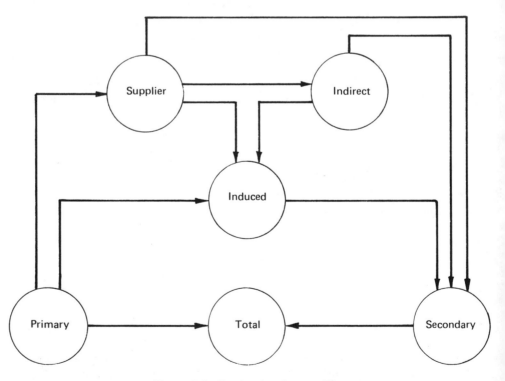

Figure 5-1. Production Impact Flow

round after round of activity. However, the value of these rounds very quickly diminishes, and their final aggregated value can be determined by the use of input-output multipliers.

Induced production refers to those effects created by the consumption expenditures of the primary employees, supplier employees, and indirect employees. These production changes occur mainly in wholesale and retail trade and in other service sectors. In nonurbanized regions, induced production is likely to exceed both supplier and indirect production considerably.

Figure 5-2 presents a simplified schematic depiction of the overall economic and demographic analysis. The starting point of the model is the production at the primary facility. This number is exogenous to the model and is provided by the builder of the facility. Primary production forms the basis for calculating supplier production and indirect production. After these have been calculated, production is translated to employment; and the sum of primary, supplier, and indirect employee expenditures is used to compute induced production. The supplier, indirect, and induced production values are then aggregated to give secondary production. Total production is the sum of primary and secondary production.

Both the primary and secondary employees in the model are disaggregated into four demographic classes: original residents, commuters, weeklies, and movers. *Original residents* are those employees who are living in the area prior to project start-up. *Commuters* are defined as workers who drive to work daily from homes located outside the study area. *Weeklies* are in-migrants who spend the week in the regional study area in "singles" quarters, but spend the weekend with their families in residences located outside the study area. *Movers* are in-migrants who move into the region with their families and establish permanent residence.

In-migrating households are calculated solely as a function of the number of weeklies and mover employees. Since original residents and commuters are not in-migrants, they are excluded. Households become the basis for determining in-migrant population.

Production and Employment

This section explains the equations used to compute production and employment in the model. The material presented in this section covers what is, in many ways, the most complicated segment of the Simpact system. The first reason for this complexity is the use of multipliers produced by the mathematical technique of input-output analysis, although input-output itself is not conducted in the system. Second, there is the dramatic difference in the values of the input variables used in the construction and operation runs, a situation which does not occur in the other models that constitute the system. A third

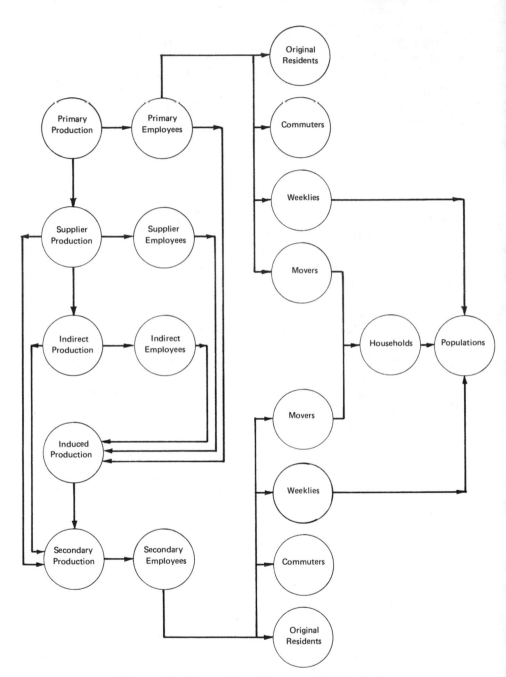

Figure 5-2. Economic and Demographic Analysis

reason for the complexity of this segment is the existence of particularly strong linkages between the equations, in that the solutions from earlier equations become inputs in the deriving solution of the latter equations.

Equation 5.1: Primary Employee Demographic Mix. The purpose of this equation is to calculate the number of primary employees falling in each of the four demographic groups: original residents, commuters, weeklies, and movers. The allocation of employees to a particular demographic group is performed separately for each occupational category. The occupational disaggregation is important because there can be substantial variation between the percentage of a particular occupational group falling in a given demographic class. For example, highly skilled construction workers, such as millwrights, could well be in short supply in a given region, which means that the percentage of original residents will be low for this occupational group. At the same time, the number of unemployed laborers in the region could be quite high

The system user has to develop input variables that define the percentages falling in the four demographic classes for each occupational group. In developing such values, a useful source is the Tennessee Valley Authority (TVA), which has been conducting surveys at construction sites since 1968 to determine the demographic mix of construction workers. The procedures, described later along with TVA surveys, can be used in selecting input values for the construction run. Since the procedures for selecting values for an operation run are relatively straightforward, they will not be discussed here.

In determining the number of original residents, the local union is an important contact. In the construction industry, the contractor has to work through the local union in obtaining the manpower required, since the local union has primary jurisdiction in placing its members on the job. When its supply of labor is exhausted, it calls in the closest sister local. Additionally, in skill categories where apprenticeships are of short duration, in times of high demand unions are likely to open their membership to area residents on a temporary basis. However, not all members of the local union working at the site are going to be considered original residents of the region. Only those members who actually live in the region of analysis are so classified.

Selecting the allocation percentage for the commuters involves drawing a commuting boundary, which defines the area from which workers will commute to the site. In drawing the ring, driving time is the criterion. For example, all areas which are a one-way 2-hour drive or less from the site could be considered as being within the commuting circle. As a practical alternative, a 100-mile radius could be used. Once the commuting circle is defined, all available workers within the circle but outside the study region could be regarded as potential commuters.

To calculate the number of weeklies—the workers who live at the site during the week and return home on the weekend—another circle must be drawn. The area between the two concentric circles will define the weeklies pool. For example, if the new circle had a radius of 400 miles, then all available workers who live more than 100 miles from the site but less than 400 would be potential weeklies. In defining the radius of the outer circle, the relevant criterion is weekend commuting distance. A radius of 400 miles would assume that the worker is willing to make weekend journeys taking as long as 8 hours one way.

If the supply of original residents, commuters, and weeklies is not sufficient, it is assumed that movers will in-migrate to the study region. These permanent in-migrants are individuals who cannot, or do not want to, live the weeklies' lifestyle. They are assumed to come from regions outside the weeklies' circle; that is, they live more than 400 miles from the site. In general, construction workers are reluctant movers and will do their utmost to avoid uprooting their families. Conditions that encourage them to consider moving are the potential for extended employment at the project and the availability of good housing and public services in the vicinity of the site.

Equation 5.2: Supplier Production. The purpose of this equation is to calculate the supplier production resulting from the local procurement of the primary facility. Supplier production by sector is calculated by multiplying the primary-activity variable by a set of supplier coefficients. The primary-activity variable for the construction run is the primary facility's construction cost; for the operation run, it is the value added at the facility.

To derive the supplier coefficients, the purchasing department at the corporate headquarters of the proposed facility can be consulted, for it can indicate the probable purchases that will be made in the region of analysis.

Alternatively, the direct multipliers of an input-output table can be used. Very often there will be no input-output table for the region of analysis, and deriving one is prohibited by the high cost of such an effort. In such cases, a number of input-output tables must be consulted. These multipliers will exhibit a pattern, with the size of the multiplier positively correlated to the economic base of the region. Based on this pattern, multiplier values that correspond approximately to the economic structure of the region of analysis can be selected.

The procedure for selecting supplier coefficients from an input-output table will be illustrated for a construction run, using the construction of a petroleum refinery in the Houston-Galveston area as an example. A 151-sector input-output table of the region has been developed for the Department of Housing and Urban Development by Louis H. Stern and others at the University of Houston and is described in a June 1972 report entitled *Houston-Galveston Regional Input-Output Study for 1967.*

In the table, there is for each sector a set of supplier coefficients or, as they are more traditionally called, direct multipliers. These multipliers indicate the various components of a dollar of production. The relevant sector for the construction of a petroleum refinery, or other heavy facility, is sector 22—industrial construction. For this sector, according to the table, every dollar of its production will require 38 cents of local business inputs, with local valve and pipe-fitting producers the largest recipients, enjoying a 7.4 cent increase in production. The remaining 62 cents go to households in the form of wages and profits and to pay for imports of material from other areas, federal taxes, and local taxes. This implies that 0.38 is the sum of the supplier coefficients, and that the supplier coefficient for the valve and pipe-fitting sector is equal to 0.074.

Equation 5.3: Indirect Production. The purpose of this equation is to calculate the indirect-production effects created by the supplier-industry purchases. It should be emphasized that these indirect effects do take into account the entire cycle of interindustry linkages.

While indirect production is caused by supplier production, in practice it is calculated from primary production. A full explanation of the reason would require a lengthy digression into regional input-output modeling, on which there are many excellent texts, and consequently has been omitted. In equation 5.3, primary production is multiplied by a set of indirect coefficients to give indirect production by sector.

The indirect coefficients or multipliers can be read from an input-output table. These table multipliers give the indirect effect of a $1 increase in production in one sector on each of the other sectors. For the industrial construction sector of the Houston-Galveston region, the total indirect multiplier is 11 cents, with the valve and pipe-fitting sector getting 0.2 cents. Thus a $1 increase in industrial construction would cause production of the local valve and pipe-fitting producers to go up 7.6 cents, 7.4 cents because of direct or supplier effects and 0.2 cents because of the indirect cycle.

Equation 5.4: Supplier and Indirect Production. This equation sums the solutions from the two preceding equations. In these earlier equations, the supplier- and indirect-production changes had been calculated for a variety of sectors. In this equation, these effects are summed across sector.

Equations 5.5 through 5.7: Supplier and Indirect Employment. In the first of these three equations, aggregated supplier and indirect production, solved in equation 5.4, is multiplied by an employment-to-production ratio to give employment. This operation is performed by sector, and consequently, the output of equation 5.5 is the employment in each sector that is created by supplier and indirect effects.

In equation 5.6, employment is converted from a sectoral classification to an occupational classification. To perform this conversion, the user must input variables defining the occupational composition of each sector.

In equation 5.7, the occupationally arranged employees are disaggregated by demographic group. To perform this disaggregation, input variables indicating the percentage of each occupational group falling into the demographic categories of original residents, commuters, weeklies, and movers have to be used.

Equations 5.8 and 5.9: Induced Production. The first of these two equations derives the employment base for calculating induced production, and the second equation calculates this production. Earlier equations have developed occupational-demographic classifications of primary employment (equation 5.1) and supplier and indirect employment (equation 5.7). In equation 5.8, the solutions from equations 5.1 and 5.7 are aggregated to give total primary, supplier, and indirect employees cross-classified by occupational and demographic group.

Induced production is assumed to be created by the local expenditures of the primary, supplier, and indirect employees. Clearly, the local expenditures of a commuter will be considerably smaller than those of a mover, which is why the demographic delineation is necessary. Similarly, for a given demographic group, a worker in a low-paying occupational group will spend less than one who is in a better-paid category, a fact which necessitates occupational disaggregation.

In equation 5.8, induced production is calculated by multiplying employees in each occupational-demographic group by a corresponding induced-production-per-employee input variable. This input variable gives the amount of local production that will be created by the expenditures of a single worker.

Deriving a value for the induced-worker multipliers involves two steps: (1) determination of the consumption expenditures of a worker, a function of his or her occupation, using a consumption function; and (2) reading the local production effect of this expenditure from an input-output table.

A "closed" input-output table contains a household column. This column gives the effect of the entire round of production effects created by $1 of expenditure by a consumer resident of the region. In the Houston-Galveston region, the effect of $1 of consumer expenditure is to increase local department and variety store sales by 7.3 cents, food and grocery store sales by 6.2 cents, service station sales by 3.1 cents, and so on. As the preceding example demonstrates, induced multipliers tend to be high in the service sectors.

Equations 5.10 through 5.12: Induced Employment. These three equations are the induced analogues to equations 5.5 through 5.7. In equation 5.10, induced production by sector is converted to induced employment by sector. In equation 5.11, induced employment by sector is transformed into induced employment by occupation group, and the output of equation 5.12 is induced employment cross-classified by occupational and demographic category.

Equations 5.13 and 5.14: Secondary Totals. At this point, all the supplier, indirect, and induced computations have been completed, and it is possible to generate the secondary totals by summing these earlier solutions. Equation 5.13

computes secondary production, and equation 5.14 computes secondary employment.

Equations 5.15 through 5.17: Grand Totals. These three equations conclude the production and employment analysis. Equation 5.15 sums primary and secondary production to give total production, and equation 5.16 performs a similar function with respect to employment.

The output of equation 5.16 is more specifically total employment cross-classified by occupational and demographic group, a variable which needs further processing. In equation 5.17, the classificatory scheme of the solution of equation 5.16 is rearranged from an occupational-demographic grouping to an income-demographic grouping. To perform this rearrangement, input values defining the income structure of each occupational group are needed. The solution of equation 5.17 is total employees cross-classified by income and demographic groups.

Households and Population

The objective of the households and population analysis is to provide the demographic base for the Community Planning Model. In estimating infrastructure requirements, because of inadequate demographic information, there is a tendency to overestimate the needs. The households and population analysis of Simpact seeks to overcome this problem by identifying those segments of the population with specific infrastructure needs.

Infrastructure requirements depend, in part, on income levels, with the type of housing requirements, in particular, most dependent on income. Public infrastructure tends to be less dependent on income, but is very sensitive to the demographic mix of the new employment, since the four demographic employee groups have very different infrastructure needs. Original residents have been living in the region prior to the construction of the plant and consequently require no new housing or other infrastructure. Commuters travel daily to work from areas located outside the region and also do not need any infrastructure. Weeklies, who live in the study region during the week but return home to their families on the weekend, require only limited infrastructure. It is the movers, who migrate into the study region with their families, who have the greatest infrastructure requirements.

Equations 5.18 and 5.19: Movers' and Weeklies' Employment. The households and population segment of the Economic and Demographic Model uses as input the solution from equation 5.17, that is, total employees cross-classified by income group and by the four demographic groups. This variable constitutes the only input to the households and population analysis from the production and employment modeling.

Of the four demographic groups, only the two in-migrating categories of weeklies and movers are of interest. Equation 5.18 merely selects from the total-employee variables of equation 5.17 that partition corresponding to movers. This operation gives total mover employees classified by income group. Equation 5.19 performs a similar operation with respect to weeklies, and its output is weeklies classified by income group.

Equations 5.20 through 5.23: Mover Households. Transforming employees to households is a complicated task in today's world of two-working-member households. In equations 5.20 through 5.23, mover employment is converted to mover households by focusing on the three constituent elements: singles, one-working-member households, and two-working-member households.

The first step involves dividing mover employees into singles and marrieds. The solution to equation 5.20 is single-mover employees classified by income group, and the solution to equation 5.21 is married movers classified by income group. To perform this disaggregation, a variable defining that fraction of mover employees in each income group who are married has to be input.

In the case of single movers, the number of employees classified by income group is equal to the number of households classified by income group. For married movers, this need not be the case, since mover employees could be married to each other. In the model, married-mover households are solved as a function of married-mover employees, with the function equal to the fraction of mover employees married to each other. Converting married employees to households does not constitute the end of the problem. The income classification must be rearranged to allow for the fact that the income of a two-working-member household is higher than that of a single-working-member household. There is no clearcut manner in which to incorporate this. In the model, two-working-member households are somewhat arbitrarily shifted to an income grouping two slots higher than that of the head of the family. The process of converting married-mover employees by income group to mover households by income group is performed in equation 5.22.

In equation 5.23, married-mover households by income group are further disaggregated by family size. To perform this disaggregation, it is necessary to input values that define, for each household income group, the percentages falling in each of the different family-size groups.

Equations 5.24 through 5.27: Population. At this stage in the model, it is possible to calculate the in-migrating population. The components that go into these calculations are weeklies, single-mover employees, and married-mover households classified by family size. Weeklies and single movers constitute a one-to-one transferral to population. For households, the number falling in each size category must be multiplied by the corresponding family size to give population. These calculations are performed in equation 5.24.

For the purpose of the education component of the Community Planning Model, it is necessary to have more detailed population data than that provided by equation 5.24. Specifically, a children-by-age-group variable is required. In equation 5.26, the number of in-migrating children is calculated by multiplying mover households, classified by family-size group, by the number of children associated with a household in a given family-size group. Next, in equation 5.27, children are disaggregated into various age classifications, with the age classifications corresponding to school systems. To perform the cohort-like disaggregation, it is necessary to input a variable defining the percentage of children falling in each age group. Equation 5.27 concludes the Economic and Demographic Model.

Appendix 5A: Equations

Listed here are the equations in the Economic and Demographic Model. In naming the variables in the model, the following conventions have been followed. The output variables are denoted by the symbol YE, the Y indicating output and the E standing for Economic and Demographic Model. The variables are numbered by their order of appearance: the first output variable is YE_1, the second YE_2, and so on. Input variables are named and numbered analogously. They are denoted by XE, with the X indicating input and the E standing for Economic and Demographic Model.

Most of the variables in the model are vectors or matrices and are consequently subscripted. For example, $YE_{1(b)}$ indicates that the first output variable is a vector containing b elements and $XE_{2(a,b)}$ indicates that the second input variable is a matrix containing a rows and b columns. The variables are dimensioned by letter subscripts, rather than numerics, because they will vary by study. For example, the subscript a, which denotes labor occupation group, was equal to 9 in the last Simpact application, but would probably be lower in less-well-funded projects.

The equations of the model involve simple matrix manipulations. These manipulations are not those used in linear algebra—to have expressed them in such a form would have been unnecessarily cumbersome—but involve parallel processing. In general, the operations are straightforward in nature, and a look at the definition of the variable names should make the function performed by the equation clear.

$$YE_{1(a,b)} = XE_{1(a)} \times XE_{2(a,b)} \tag{5.1}$$

where $YE_{1(a,b)}$ = Primary employees in occupation group a who are in demographic group b

$XE_{1(a)}$ = Primary employees in occupation group a

$XE_{2(a,b)}$ = Percentage of primary employees in occupation group a who are in demographic group b

$$YE_{2(c)} = XE_3 \times XE_{4(c)} \tag{5.2}$$

where $YE_{2(c)}$ = Supplier production in sector c

XE_3 = Primary production

$XE_{4(c)}$ = Supplier multipliers for sector c

61

$$YE_{3(c)} = XE_3 \times XE_{5(c)} \qquad (5.3)$$

where $YE_{3(c)}$ = Indirect production in sector c

XE_3 = Primary production

$XE_{5(c)}$ = Indirect multipliers for sector c

$$YE_{4(c)} = YE_{2(c)} + YE_{3(c)} \qquad (5.4)$$

where $YE_{4(c)}$ = Supplier and indirect production in sector c

$YE_{2(c)}$ = Supplier production in sector c

$YE_{3(c)}$ = Indirect production in sector c

$$YE_{5(c)} = YE_{4(c)} \times XE_{6(c)} \qquad (5.5)$$

where $YE_{5(c)}$ = Supplier and indirect employees in sector c

$YE_{4(c)}$ = Supplier and indirect production in sector c

$XE_{6(c)}$ = Number of jobs in sector c per dollar of production

$$YE_{6(a)} = \overset{c}{\Sigma} (YE_{5(c)} \times XE_{7(c,a)}) \qquad (5.6)$$

where $YE_{6(a)}$ = Supplier and indirect employees in occupation group a

$YE_{5(c)}$ = Supplier and indirect employees in sector c

$XE_{7(c,a)}$ = Percentage of employees in sector c who are in occupation group a

$$YE_{7(a,b)} = YE_{6(a)} \times XE_{8(a,b)} \qquad (5.7)$$

where $YE_{7(a,b)}$ = Supplier and indirect employees in occupation group a who are in demographic group b

$YE_{6(a)}$ = Supplier and indirect employees in occupation group a

$XE_{8(a,b)}$ = Percentage of employees in occupation group a who are in demographic group b

$$YE_{8(a,b)} = YE_{1(a,b)} + YE_{7(a,b)} \qquad (5.8)$$

where $YE_{8(a,b)}$ = Primary, supplier, and indirect employees in occupation group a who are in demographic group b

$YE_{1(a,b)}$ = Primary employees in occupation group a who are in demographic group b

$YE_{7(a,b)}$ = Supplier and indirect employees in occupation group a who are in demographic group b

$$YE_{9(c)} = \overset{a\,b}{\Sigma\Sigma} \, (YE_{8(a,b)} \times XE_{9(a,b,c)}) \qquad (5.9)$$

where $YE_{9(c)}$ = Induced production in sector c

$YE_{8(a,b)}$ = Primary supplier and indirect employees in occupation group a who are in demographic group b

$XE_{9(a,b,c)}$ = Induced multipliers by occupation group a and demographic group b for each of c sectors

$$YE_{10(c)} = YE_{9(c)} \times XE_{6(c)} \qquad (5.10)$$

where $YE_{10(c)}$ = Induced employees in sector c

$YE_{9(c)}$ = Induced production in sector c

$XE_{6(c)}$ = Number of jobs in sector c per dollar of production

$$YE_{11(a)} = \overset{c}{\Sigma} \, (YE_{10(c)} \times XE_{7(c,a)}) \qquad (5.11)$$

where $YE_{11(a)}$ = Induced employees in occupation group a

$YE_{10(c)}$ = Induced employees in sector c

$XE_{7(c,a)}$ = Percentage of employees in sector c who are in occupation group a

$$YE_{12(a,b)} = YE_{11(a)} \times XE_{8(a,b)} \qquad (5.12)$$

where $YE_{12(a,b)}$ = Induced employees in occupation group a who are in demographic group b

$YE_{11(a)}$ = Induced employees in occupation group a

$XE_{8(a,b)}$ = Percentage of employees in occupation group a who are in demographic group b

$$YE_{13(c)} = YE_{4(c)} + YE_{9(c)} \qquad (5.13)$$

where $YE_{13(c)}$ = Secondary production in sector c

$YE_{4(c)}$ = Supplier and indirect production in sector c

$YE_{9(c)}$ = Induced production in sector c

$$YE_{14(c)} = YE_{5(c)} + YE_{10(c)} \tag{5.14}$$

where $YE_{14(c)}$ = Secondary employees in sector c

$YE_{5(c)}$ = Supplier and indirect employees in sector c

$YE_{10(c)}$ = Induced employees in sector c

$$YE_{15} = (\overset{c}{\Sigma} YE_{13(c)}) + XE_3 \tag{5.15}$$

where YE_{15} = Total production

$YE_{13(c)}$ = Secondary production in sector c

XE_3 = Primary production

$$YE_{16(a,b)} = YE_{8(a,b)} + YE_{12(a,b)} \tag{5.16}$$

where $YE_{16(a,b)}$ = Total employees in occupation group a who are in demographic group b

$YE_{8(a,b)}$ = Primary, supplier, and indirect employees in occupation group a who are in demographic group b

$YE_{12(a,b)}$ = Induced employees in occupation group a who are in demographic group b

$$YE_{17(b,d)} = \overset{a}{\Sigma} (YE_{16(a,b)} \times XE_{9(a,d)}) \tag{5.17}$$

where $YE_{17(b,d)}$ = Total employees in demographic group b who are in income group d

$YE_{16(a,b)}$ = Total employees in occupation group a who are in demographic group b

$XE_{9(a,d)}$ = Percentage of employees in occupation group a who are in income group d

$$YE_{18(d)} = YE_{17(b=1,d)} \tag{5.18}$$

where $YE_{18(d)}$ = Mover employees in income group d

$YE_{17(b=1,d)}$ = Subset of YE_{16} corresponding to movers

$$YE_{19(d)} = YE_{17(b=2,d)} \tag{5.19}$$

where $YE_{19(d)}$ = Weeklies in income group d

$YE_{17(b=2,d)}$ = Subset of YE_{16} corresponding to weeklies

$$YE_{20(d)} = YE_{18(d)} \times XE_{10(d)} \tag{5.20}$$

where $YE_{20(d)}$ = Single-mover employees in income group d

$YE_{18(d)}$ = Mover employees in income group d

$XE_{10(d)}$ = Percentage of mover employees in income group d who are single

$$YE_{21(d)} = YE_{18(d)} - YE_{20(d)} \tag{5.21}$$

where $YE_{21(d)}$ = Married-mover employees in income group d

$YE_{18(d)}$ = Mover employees in income group d

$YE_{20(d)}$ = Single-mover employees in income group d

$$YE_{22(d)} = f_{21}(YE_{21(d)}) \tag{5.22}$$

where $YE_{22(d)}$ = Married-mover households in income group d

f_{21} = Nonlinear transformation function designed to take into account that some movers have working spouses

$YE_{21(d)}$ = Married-mover employees in income group d

$$YE_{23(d,e)} = (YE_{22(d)} \times XE_{11(d,e)}); YE_{19(d)} \tag{5.23}$$

where $YE_{23(d,e)}$ = Mover households in income group d and family group e

$YE_{22(d)}$ = Married-mover households in income group d

$XE_{11(d,e)}$ = Percentage of married-mover households in income group d who are in size group e

$YE_{19(d)}$ = Single-mover employees in income group d

$$YE_{24} = (\overset{d}{\Sigma} YE_{23(d,e)}) \times e \tag{5.24}$$

where YE_{24} = Mover population

$YE_{23(d,e)}$ = Mover households in income group d and family group e

e = Family size

$$YE_{25} = (\overset{d}{\Sigma} YE_{19(d)}) + YE_{24} \tag{5.25}$$

where YE_{25} = Total in-migrating population

$YE_{19(d)}$ = Weeklies employees income group d

YE_{24} = Mover population

$$YE_{26(f)} = (\overset{d}{\Sigma} YE_{22(d,e)}) \times XE_{13(e)} \tag{5.26}$$

where $YE_{26(f)}$ = Number of in-migrating children

$YE_{22(d,e)}$ = Mover households in income group d and family group e

$XE_{13(e)}$ = Number of children associated with a household in family group e

$$YE_{27(f)} = YE_{26} \times XE_{14(f)} \tag{5.27}$$

where $YE_{27(f)}$ = In-migrating children in educational group f

YE_{26} = Number of in-migrating children

$XE_{14(f)}$ = Percentage of in-migrating children in school-age group f

6

Community Planning Model

Very often large-scale projects are developed in remote areas where little or no infrastructure exists. At other times, they may be developed in small communities. In both cases, a relatively substantial investment in supporting infrastructure is necessary. Predicting the nature of the infrastructure requirements is the domain of the so-called new town or community planning models. Simpact contains a fairly elaborate Community Planning Model, which is explained and documented in this chapter. The first section contains an overview of the model, and the following sections describe the equations used to compute infrastructure requirements and costs. The equations, themselves, are contained in appendix 6A.

Overview of the Model

The type of infrastructure required to support a large project can be categorized by the source used to finance it. Using this taxonomy, one would have both privately financed and publicly financed infrastructures. Private infrastructure includes the factories, offices, and stores associated with the secondary economic activity, as well as the homes, apartments, and motels required to house the in-migrating primary and secondary workers. Public infrastructure, on the other hand, consists of schools, police stations, fire stations, streets, water supply and sanitation facilities, and solid-waste landfills.

Figure 6-1 presents a schematic overview of the economics, housing, and social infrastructure analysis of the Community Planning Model. Circles in the figure denote variables from the Economic and Demographic Model, and the rectangles identify the variables of the Community Planning Model. The figure shows that for each infrastructure category, floor space, construction costs, and land areas are calculated. The manner in which these variables is computed is very straightforward and does not vary much among the categories.

For secondary economic infrastructure, floor space is calculated by multiplying employment by a floor-space-per-employee variable, and land-area requirements are computed analogously. Construction cost is calculated as a function of floor space.

In the housing analysis, the number of housing units demanded is predicted as a function of the number of households. Housing units become the basis for computing floor space and land area, and floor space is used in determining housing construction costs.

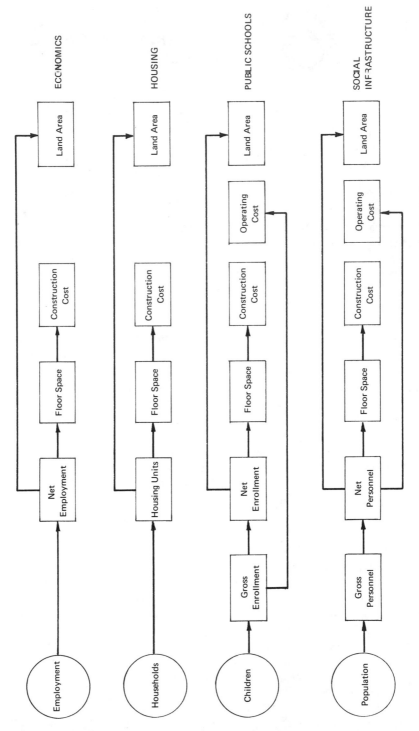

Figure 6-1. Economic, Housing, and Social Infrastructure Analysis

In the educational infrastructure analysis, public school enrollment is a function of population. Enrollment is used to compute floor space, operating costs, and land area, with construction cost, as usual, calculated from floor space.

For social infrastructure, a category which includes such services as fire protection, personnel requirements are solved as a function of population. The number of personnel is then used in calculating floor space, operating cost, and land area. Construction cost is calculated on the basis of floor space.

Figure 6-2 graphically depicts the physical infrastructure analysis of the Community Planning Model. Physical infrastructure is used here to include local streets, storm sewers, water-treatment works and pipe networks, and solid-waste landfills.

The miles of local street required is determined as a function of new housing developments. The associated construction cost, operating cost, and land area are computed from miles of required street. The length of the storm sewer network, water-pipe network, and sewer-pipe network are all computed as a function of street length. The associated construction and operating costs are based on the length of the pipe required.

The required capacities of water-treatment and sewer-treatment works are based on water consumption and sewage generation, respectively, variables which are themselves functions of the population and employment solutions of the Economic and Demographic Model. Construction and operating costs for the treatment works are based on the required capacity.

The procedures used to calculate solid-waste disposal facilities are similar to those used for water-treatment and sewer-treatment works. Solid waste generated is determined as a function of population and employment. Landfill acreage required is based on the solid-waste generated, and the associated construction and operating costs are calculated as a function of landfill acreage.

Private Infrastructure

The building of economic infrastructure is solely the responsibility of the businesses enjoying the sales expansion, while the responsibility for housing construction will be shared by various entities. Conventional housing is typically erected by private developers, but where private developers are not forthcoming in sufficient numbers, the management of the primary project may set up a housing subsidiary. In this section, the procedures used to estimate and cost-out economic and housing infrastructure requirements are explained.

Secondary Economic Infrastructure

Equation 6.1: Net Employment. In this equation, employment, a solution from the Economic and Demographic Model, is converted from a "gross" to a "net"

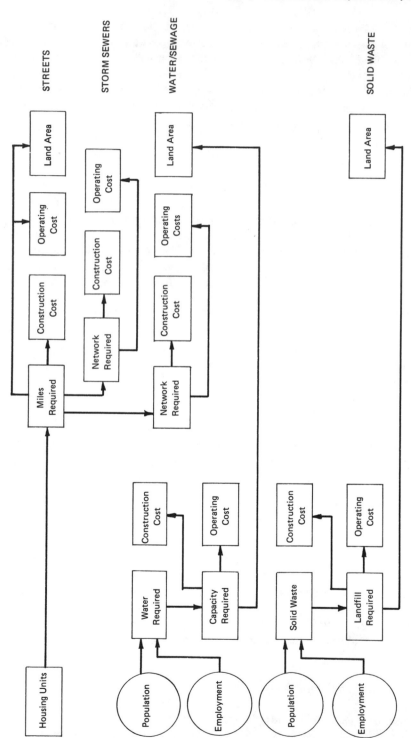

Figure 6-2. Physical Infrastructure Analysis

basis. *Net employment* is defined as the excess of gross employment over baseline surplus employment. *Baseline surplus employment* is an exogenous input which is designed to incorporate the fact that an increase in employment will not automatically lead to the construction of new space. It represents the number of new employees who will work in existing facilities and is highly region- and sector-specific. For example, in a region that has experienced an economic downturn, or in a region that has built a new shopping mall, the number of additional employees in the trade sector who can be accommodated in existing stores is likely to be quite significant. Because of this site specificity, it is necessary to survey local conditions before selecting a value for the baseline surplus variable.

Equations 6.2 and 6.3: Cost Requirements. In equation 6.2, floor space required is calculated by multiplying net employment by a floor-space-per-employee variable. In equation 6.3, construction cost is calculated by multiplying required floor space by a construction-cost-per-square-foot variable.

A good source of data on the cost-input variable in equation 6.3 is the annual publication by the Robert Snow Means Company, Inc., entitled *Building Construction Cost Data.* The Means Company publishes its estimates based on surveys that it conducts of the construction industry. Estimates for various building types are published. The published construction-cost estimates include the costs of site preparation, building construction, heating, ventilation, and air conditioning. Cost for special capital equipment (for example, x-ray machines for hospitals) is not included in the Means Company estimates.

Equations 6.4 and 6.5: Spatial Requirements. In equation 6.4, land area requirements are calculated by multiplying net employment by a land-area-per-employee variable. In equation 6.5, the open and paved land area is calculated by multiplying the land-area solution from equation 6.4 by an input variable, defining the percentage which is open and paved. It should be noted that all the secondary economic infrastructure computations are performed separately for each industrial and commercial sector.

Housing

Equation 6.6: Housing Units for Movers. In this equation, the number of units of each housing type that will be required by mover households is estimated. There are a variety of housing types built into the model. The categories include townhouses, low-rise apartments, high-rise apartments, single-family homes on quarter-acre lots, single-family homes on half-acre lots, and single-family homes on acre lots. In allocating a household group to a housing type, a key factor is the household's income, which determines what the household can afford by way of mortgage payments or rent. It has been traditionally assumed that the price of the house can be 2.5 times a family's annual gross income. However, studies have indicated that this ratio varies by income group. For example, the 1977 publication of the Realtors National Marketing Institute, entitled *Profile of the Single-Family Homeowner*, states that for families with high incomes, the ratio was lower. For households with incomes between $10,000 and $15,000, the ratio was 2.0, and for families with incomes greater than $15,000, the ratio was under 2.0. The study also found that the ratio was higher for previous homeowners than for those buying their first home. For example, households with incomes between $20,000 and $25,000 who were previous homeowners spent 2.0 times their gross incomes when buying a house, while families who were previously renting spent only 1.5 times their incomes. The greater value-income ratio for previous owners is due to the equity these individuals realized from the sale of their former residences, which enabled them to afford more expensive homes than those who previously had rented.

After the amount of money a household group can afford to spend in buying a home has been determined, the housing types it can purchase can be identified. For example, a household in the income group of $20,000 to $25,000 can afford a home costing about $40,000. Such an amount could cover a single-family quarter-acre home or a townhouse, but not a larger single-family home. The choice between the single-family quarter-acre home and the townhouse would be influenced by family size, with the larger families opting for the home.

Equation 6.7: Housing Units for Weeklies. In estimating the housing requirements of weeklies, the same type of equation is used, but the value-income approach used for determining housing-choice input values is not appropriate. Weeklies generally seek out the least costly accommodation. They stay in inexpensive local motels, rent rooms, or occupy mobile homes. Weeklies also occupy more conventional housing, but usually on a shared basis.

Equation 6.8: Total Housing Units. In this equation, total housing requirements are computed by summing the mover and weeklies demand across housing type.

Equations 6.9 through 6.10: Cost Requirements. In equation 6.9, the floor-space requirements are calculated by multiplying housing units by the floor space per unit. This operation is performed separately for each housing type. The floor space per unit is based on a particular design. For townhouses, the number of bedrooms affects the square footage. Townhouses come in two-bedroom and three-bedroom units, with three-bedroom units containing 15 to 20 percent more floor space. In equation 6.5, construction cost is calculated by multiplying floor space by construction cost per square foot.

Equations 6.11 and 6.12: Spatial Requirements. In equation 6.11, the land area associated with housing is calculated by multiplying housing units demanded by the land area per unit. In equation 6.12, the solution of equation 6.11 is multiplied by the percentage of land which is open and paved.

In developing values for the land-area-per-housing-unit input variable, the procedure differs according to whether it is a single-family or multifamily accommodation. In the case of single-family homes, the lot size is given by definition—for a single-family, quarter-acre home, the lot size is 0.25 acre. For multifamily accommodations, lot size per unit is obtained by dividing the gross acreage of the building by the number of units in the building. Gross acreage is defined as including land for entrance drive, parking spaces, and recreation. If, for example, the building is on a 1-acre lot and contains 10 units, the lot size per unit would be 0.1 acre.

In developing a value for the input variable, percentage of the land which is open and paved, the layout of the lot must be carefully considered. In the case of a single-family home on a quarter acre, the lot size is 10,890 square feet. Part of the lot will be covered by building, part of it will be seeded, planted, or otherwise undisturbed, and part of it will be paved. The open and paved segment will consist of a driveway and a patio. If one assumes that the driveway is 10 feet wide, the square footage of a 75-foot driveway would be 750 square feet. With a patio of 250 square feet, this would give an open and paved area of 1,000 square feet, which means that approximately 9 percent of the quarter-acre lot would be open and paved.

Educational Infrastructure

In the Simpact system, the publicly financed educational infrastructure that must be provided to meet the needs of the in-migrants is estimated, but privately financed schools are ignored. Such institutions have experienced declining enrollment in recent years and suffer from excess capacity. Consequently, it can be assumed that those in-migrating children who want to attend private schools can be accommodated within existing facilities.

Educational facilities in Simpact fall into two categories: general and vocational. General education encompasses public instruction for grades from kindergarten through 12. There are various ways in which grades can be grouped into facilities. For example, an elementary school can include classes up to grade 5, a middle school can cover grades 6 through 8, and a senior high school can cover grades 9 through 12. Vocational schools offer a technical alternative to senior high schools. Therefore, in estimating the senior high school requirements, students attending vocational schools must be subtracted from the senior high school population.

Equations 6.13 and 6.14: Enrollment. In equation 6.13, gross public school enrollment is computed by multiplying children classified by age group, a solution of the Economic and Demographic Model, by the percentage who attend public schools. The proportion is less than 1.0, reflecting the fact that students also attend private schools.

An increase in enrollment does not automatically mean that new schools must be built. In many instances, there may be excess capacity in existing schools. To allow for this, in equation 6.14, gross enrollment is converted to net enrollment by subtracting baseline surplus from gross enrollment.

Baseline surplus enrollment is defined as the number of additional pupils who can be accommodated within existing facilities. To obtain a value for the baseline surplus, the baseline enrollment of existing facilities must be subtracted from the standard enrollment. *Standard enrollment* is calculated by multiplying the number of classrooms by the recommended pupils per classroom and by a utilization factor.

An example may help clarify this approach. If a school has 40 classrooms, a utilization factor of 0.85, and a recommended pupil per classroom size of 25, it would have a standard enrollment of 850. If the actual enrollment were 750, this would mean a baseline surplus of 100 pupils.

Equations 6.15 and 6.16: Construction-Cost Requirements. In equation 6.15, required educational floor space is calculated by multiplying net enrollment by floor space per pupil. In equation 6.16, construction cost is computed by multiplying floor space by construction cost per square foot.

It should be noted that the floor-space solutions of equation 6.15 are "externally" compared with the floor space associated with a typical facility. In this external comparison, the total floor space required is divided by the floor space of a typical facility to give the number of required facilities. For example, if 90,000 square feet of elementary school space is required and 60,000 square feet is the size of a typical facility, this would imply that 1.5 new elementary schools would be needed. This could mean that one new facility would be built and a wing added to an existing school.

Equations 6.17 and 6.18: Spatial Requirements. In equation 6.17, land-area requirements are computed by multiplying net enrollment by land area per pupil. In equation 6.18, the solution from equation 6.17 is multiplied by an input variable defining the percentage of the land which is open and paved.

Land area per pupil can be calculated by dividing recommended land area for a school facility by the recommended number of students. For example, an elementary school of 600 pupils with an area of 15 acres would work out to 0.025 acre per pupil.

The percentage of the lot which is open and paved is a function of the plot layout. In calculating this percentage, allowance must be made for parking lots, roads, paved play areas such as basketball courts, and so on.

Equation 6.19: Operating-Cost Requirements. In equation 6.19, operating costs are calculated by multiplying gross enrollment by operating cost per pupil. Operating costs are a function of gross enrollment, rather than net, because new students—whether or not they require new facilities—do need materials, transportation, and other educational services.

The operating costs include outlays for instruction, administration, maintenance of the facility, bus services, materials, and student recreation. The operating cost per pupil may vary by state and by school district. Thus, in selecting a value, the school districts in the region of analysis should be consulted.

Social Infrastructure

The manner in which the requirements for other social infrastructure categories are projected is highly symmetrical. For instance, exactly the same type of equations can be used to project law-enforcement requirements as are used to project fire-protection requirements. This section describes the "generic" social infrastructure equations, after which the characteristics of various social infrastructure categories are described.

Equations

There are seven equations—6.20 through 6.26—which must be applied for each social infrastructure category. In equation 6.20, gross personnel requirements are estimated by multiplying population by personnel requirements per capita. In equation 6.21, gross personnel is converted to net personnel by deducting baseline surplus. In equation 6.22, the floor-space requirements are estimated by multiplying net personnel by floor space per personnel. In equation 6.23, construction cost is estimated by multiplying floor space by construction cost per square foot. Equations 6.24 and 6.25 estimate land-area requirements as a function of net personnel. In equation 6.26, operating cost is computed as a function of net personnel.

Discussion of Major Social Infrastructure Categories

Law Enforcement. This social infrastructure category consists of field services, such as patrolling; staff services, such as collecting information; and supplementary services, such as jail management. These services are provided at the municipal, county, and state levels. The municipal police provide protection for the municipality in which they are located. The County Sheriff's Department provides protection for all rural areas which do not have a local police department. In addition, the county may operate a jail and assist local departments in selected activities. Also, in some states, the county serves warrants and subpoenas, and otherwise services county courts. The State Police are charged with patrolling state highways and assisting local and county police.

Fire Protection. The major purpose of a fire department is to prevent loss of property and life due to fire. Fire departments also try to prevent the occurrence of fires by education and inspection. The fire-protection goal of a small department is usually to offer the capability of handling two large-scale fires simultaneously, for example, a fire in a school and a fire in a business district.

Fire departments are either paid, volunteer, or a combination of the two. Paid-fire departments use salaried personnel who are assigned predefined periods of work and are paid at regular intervals. Volunteer-run fire departments do not have salary outlays. Combination departments are manned by both paid and volunteer personnel. Communities with less than 15,000 residents generally maintain all-volunteer departments, communities with a population between 15,000 and 20,000 could well have combination departments, and large communities are likely to have paid-fire departments.

The unit around which the fire-protection team is organized is the fire company. It operates from a fire station, which is usually situated near the business area or near some other district where there is danger of a serious fire hazard. The type of equipment that the fire station has depends on the size of the unit. A small, all-volunteer fire department is likely to have a pumper, communications equipment, and a staff car. A combination paid/volunteer department may have, in addition, an aerial ladder.

General Government. This category covers the functions of financial administration, general control, public health, and corrections. *Financial administration* includes collecting taxes, managing the budget, and disbursing funds. *General control* consists of municipal planning and conducting elections and various legislative activities. *Public health* involves inspection of water, visiting food establishments, and providing visiting-nurse services. The term *corrections* refers to activities designed to rehabilitate criminals and includes such services as parole administration.

At the municipal level, general government consists primarily of financial administration and general control. Public health functions at the municipal level are usually restricted to protective inspections. At the county level, all four functions—financial administration, general control, public health, and corrections—are performed.

Physical Infrastructure

The physical infrastructure items computed in the Community Planning Model are streets, water supply, sanitary wastewater collection and treatment, storm-water drainage, and solid-waste disposal. Some of these services—for example, water supply—are demanded by business as well as residents. Therefore, the level of physical infrastructure will, in some cases, be a function of both population and secondary employment.

Streets

Equation 6.27: Miles Required. In this equation, the miles of local street required is computed. First, the number of housing units is multiplied by the percentage built in areas without streets. The product of this operation is then multiplied by the street length associated with a single housing unit.

The percentage of homes requiring new streets will be low for townhouses and other multifamily accommodations. However, in the case of single-family homes, this variable could be quite high. Large developers, because of their scale of operations, buy and subdivide tracts of rural land, and the homes they build consequently require new streets.

Equations 6.28 and 6.30: Cost Requirements. In equation 6.28, the construction cost is calculated by multiplying miles of required street by construction cost per mile. In equation 6.30, the operating cost is calculated by multiplying miles of required street by operating cost per mile.

The cost of construction is a function of the type of streets. For example, a 3.5-inch-deep asphalt-surfaced street is more expensive to build than one with a 1.0-inch-deep asphalt surface.

The operating cost per mile is region specific and can be obtained from the financial reports of the municipalities. The operating costs include outlays for snow removal and street lighting.

Equation 6.29: Spatial Requirements., In this equation, the land area is estimated by multiplying miles of street by the input variable, area per mile. This input variable, in square feet, is equal to 5,280 multiplied by the street width in feet (a typical width is 28 feet).

Water Supply and Sanitary Sewage Disposal

The type of infrastructure required to provide water supply is "analytically" analogous to the infrastructure required to dispose of sewage. There is a treatment work in which raw water is made potable, or raw sewage is made dischargeable, as well as a pipe network to convey water from the treatment work to the user, or sewage from the generator to the treatment work. The generic equations used to estimate these requirements are explained, using water as the example.

Equation 6.31: Residential Usage. In this equation, residential water consumption is computed by multiplying population by residential water consumption per capita. The residential-per-capita variable will reflect such uses as drinking, laundry, bathroom, lawn watering, and gardening. The usage is positively correlated to income levels, with wealthy communities having higher per capita ratios. It is negatively related to the rate charged for water.

Equation 6.32: Business Usage. Secondary industrial and commercial water consumption is calculated by multiplying employment by water consumption per employee. The per-employee variable will reflect such industrial applications as process use, cooling, and sanitation. It will also reflect engineering practices; for example, many new plants recycle water and have consequently reduced water consumption while maintaining operating levels. Such recirculation is particularly suited for *indirect-contact cooling water*, which is defined as water that does not come into contact with the product. Even more important than the variation between modern and older plants is the difference between sectors. Service and trade sectors, for example, have much lower water-consumption levels than manufacturing sectors, such as primary metals. Finally, it should be noted that some plants have their own water-supply systems, and their consumption levels from public systems are consequently zero.

Equations 6.33 and 6.34: Total Usage. In equation 6.33, total gross water consumption is calculated by adding residential, business, and primary usage. Primary usage is an exogenous input, the value of which is provided by the primary facility owner.

Before consumption can be used as a basis for calculating capacity, existing surplus capacity must be taken into account. In equation 6.34, the baseline surplus is deducted from gross consumption to give net consumption. The surplus variable reflects the ability of the existing treatment system to handle a higher load than it currently does.

Equation 6.35: Required Treatment Capacity. In equation 6.35, required treatment capacity is calculated by multiplying net water consumption by the ratio of required capacity to consumption. The ratio is greater than 1.0 and reflects the need to have capacity to meet peak requirements. During hot summer days and during large fires, the requirement for water is at a level significantly in excess of average consumption.

Equation 6.36: Treatment Construction Cost. In equation 6.36, construction cost is estimated by multiplying capacity, which is expressed in millions of gallons per day (MGD), by the construction cost per MGD.

The *central water system* is defined here as including withdrawal and storage as well as treatment facilities. The type of *withdrawal equipment* depends on the source of water. For example, if water is being drawn from a lake, equipment which can make withdrawals at a depth sufficient to avoid freezing in the winter is required. This particular equipment would be unnecessary for a ground water source. *Storage facilities* are generally designed to hold untreated water to help in times of peak demand. A common form of storage is in an elevated tank.

Treatment facilities are designed to convert raw water into a form that can be used for residential and industrial applications. A typical treatment system might involve sedimentation, filtration and disinfection, and odor and taste removal. The purpose of sedimentation is to settle out the solids suspended in the water, which is done by retaining the water in tanks. Filtration involves passing the water through sand and gravel filters, and disinfection entails the addition of chlorine. Odor and taste removal can be performed by adding carbon particles and then refiltering the water.

Equation 6.37: Required Main Length. The length of the water mains required to distribute the treated water is estimated in equation 6.37. The number of miles of new street is multiplied by the ratio of main length to street length.

Equation 6.38: Main-Construction Cost. In equation 6.38, the construction cost for the water-distribution system is calculated by multiplying miles of water main by the construction cost per mile. The cost per mile depends on the region. In areas where the terrain is very flat or changes significantly, booster pumps may be required.

Equations 6.39 through 6.41: Cost Aggregates and Spatial Requirements. In equation 6.39, total water system construction cost is computed by summing central system costs, from equation 6.36, and the distribution system costs, predicted by equation 6.38.

In equation 6.40, operating costs for the central and distribution systems are computed. For central systems, the operating cost is a function of capacity in MGD, and for the distribution systems, the cost is a function of the length of the mains.

In equation 6.41, the land area associated with the central system is computed by multiplying capacity in MGD by land area per MGD.

Stormwater Drainage

A stormwater-drainage system is designed to convey the runoff created by rain or snow to a receiving body of water. In the absence of an adequate drainage system, flooding may result. In rural areas, stormwater drainage may take the form of a natural network, such as streams, helped by open ditches alongside the local roads. In areas where there are paved roads, the drainage system will generally be in the form of underground pipes. Appurtenances, such as manholes, are associated with the pipes.

Equation 6.42: Miles Required. In this equation, the length of the storm sewers that will be required is estimated. The basis for estimating the length of new sewers is the number of miles of new street. It is assumed that when such streets are built, a certain percentage of them will be accompanied by sewers.

Equations 6.43 and 6.44: Costs. In these equations, the construction costs and operating costs for storm sewers are determined by multiplying mileage by a cost-per-mile variable. Construction costs depend on the depth of burial of the pipe, the diameter of the pipe, and the topography of the region. Operating costs are related to the inspection and cleaning of the pipes and associated appurtenances.

Solid-Waste Disposal

Increased economic and demographic activity generates waste matter of various kinds. In the Simpact system, the generation of solid wastes and the facilities required to dispose of them are determined. *Solid waste* is defined as excluding hazardous wastes, which consist largely of chemical residues from industrial sources and, under the Resource Conservation and Recovery Act (RCRA) of 1976 (P.L. 94-580), require special disposal.

Equation 6.45: Solid-Waste Generated. This equation computes the total solid waste generated. Residential solid-waste generation is computed by multiplying in-migrant population by a residential solid-waste-per-capita variable. Business solid-waste generation is computed by multiplying employment by a waste-per-employee variable. Primary solid-waste generation is exogenously added in.

Equations 6.46 and 6.47: Collection Costs. In equation 6.46, the capital costs associated with solid-waste collection are computed; and equation 6.47 computes the operating costs associated with solid-waste collection. Both capital and operating costs are a function of the volume of solid waste generated.

The collection and transfer of solid waste to a disposal site represent a significant component of overall solid-waste management costs. Residential wastes typically are collected in a 20-cubic-yard rear-loader. Such loaders take the waste to a transfer station, where the waste from various loaders is transferred to a larger vehicle. The cost of collection on a per-ton-of-solid-waste basis depends on frequency of collection, type of collection vehicles, and the distances involved.

Equations 6.48 through 6.50: Disposal Cost. In equation 6.48, the dimensions of the site required to dispose of the solid waste generated are estimated. The size is calculated by multiplying the amount of solid waste in tons by a variable to convert it into landfill in acre-feet. In equation 6.49, capital costs are estimated by multiplying landfill in acre-feet by the capital cost per acre-foot. In equation 6.50, operating costs are calculated by multiplying solid waste generated by the operating disposal cost per ton.

The solid wastes are disposed in sanitary landfills. Open dumps, a common disposal method, have been prohibited by the RCRA. In a landfill, the wastes are first compacted to reduce their volume, and the compacted wastes are then placed on the land and covered with soil.

Equations 6.51 and 6.52: Total Costs. In equation 6.51, the total capital costs associated with solid-waste services are calculated by summing the capital costs of collection and the capital costs of disposal. In equation 6.52, the total operating costs are determined in an analogous manner. These equations conclude the Community Planning Model.

Appendix 6A: Equations

Listed here are the equations in the Community Planning Model. The format used to present these equations is similar to that used to list the equations of the Economic and Demographic Model. In this model, all output variables are denoted by YC and input variables by XC. The Y indicates input, the X indicates output, and the C stands for Community Planning. All variables are accompanied by a numeric to identify the order of appearance. Thus, the first output variable is YC_1 and the first input variable XC_1.

In obtaining the output variables of the Community Planning Model, there are in fact two types of input variables. The first are those in the XC series. The second class of input variables are the solutions from the Economic and Demographic Model. For example, the output variable from the Economic and Demographic Model—YE_{24} = total in-migrant population—is an input in generating the solutions of the Community Planning Model.

$$YC_{1(c)} = YE_{14(c)} - XC_{1(c)} \tag{6.1}$$

where $YC_{1(c)}$ = Net employees in sector c

$\qquad YE_{14(c)}$ = Secondary employees in sector c

$\qquad XC_{1(c)}$ = Baseline excess capacity in sector c

$$YC_{2(c)} = YC_{1(c)} \times XC_{2(c)} \tag{6.2}$$

where $YC_{2(c)}$ = Floor space required in sector c

$\qquad YC_{1(c)}$ = Net employees in sector c

$\qquad XC_{2(c)}$ = Floor space per employee in sector c

$$YC_{3(c)} = YC_{2(c)} \times XC_{3(c)} \tag{6.3}$$

where $YC_{3(c)}$ = Construction cost in sector c

$\qquad YC_{2(c)}$ = Floor space required in sector c

$\qquad XC_{3(c)}$ = Construction cost per square foot in sector c

$$YC_{4(c)} = YC_{1(c)} \times XC_{4(c)} \tag{6.4}$$

where $YC_{4(c)}$ = Land area required in sector c

$YC_{1(c)}$ = Net employees in sector c

$XC_{4(c)}$ = Land area per employee in sector c

$$YC_{5(c)} = YC_{4(c)} \times XC_{5(c)} \tag{6.5}$$

where $YC_{5(c)}$ = Open and paved land area in sector c

$YC_{4(c)}$ = Land area required in sector c

$XC_{5(c)}$ = Percentage of land area in sector c which is open and paved

$$YC_{6(g)} = \overset{de}{\Sigma\Sigma} (YE_{22(d,e)} \times XC_{6(d,e,g)}) \tag{6.6}$$

where $YC_{6(g)}$ = Housing units of type g demanded by movers

$YE_{22(d,e)}$ = Mover households in income group d and family group e

$XC_{6(d,e,g)}$ = Percentage of mover household in income group d and family group e who demand housing-unit type g

$$YC_{7(g)} = \left(\overset{d}{\Sigma} YE_{18(d)} \right) \times XC_{7(g)} \times XC_{8(g)} \tag{6.7}$$

where $YC_{7(g)}$ = Housing units of type g demanded by weeklies

$YE_{18(d)}$ = Weeklies employees in income group d

$XC_{7(g)}$ = Percentage of weeklies who demand housing-unit type g

$XC_{8(g)}$ = Weeklies' doubling-up factor for housing unit g

$$YC_{8(g)} = YC_{6(g)} + YC_{7(g)} \tag{6.8}$$

where $YC_{8(g)}$ = Required number of housing units of type g

$YC_{6(g)}$ = Housing units of type g demanded by movers

$YC_{7(g)}$ = Housing units of type g demanded by weeklies

$$YC_{9(g)} = YC_{8(g)} \times XC_{7(g)} \tag{6.9}$$

where $YC_{9(g)}$ = Floor space of housing type g required

$YC_{8(g)}$ = Required number of housing units of type g

$XC_{7(g)}$ = Floor space per unit of housing type g

$$YC_{10(g)} = YC_{9(g)} \times XC_{10(g)} \tag{6.10}$$

where $YC_{10(g)}$ = Construction cost for housing type g

$YC_{9(g)}$ = Floor space of housing type g required

$XC_{10(g)}$ = Construction cost per square foot of housing type g

$$YC_{11(g)} = YC_{8(g)} \times XC_{11(g)} \qquad (6.11)$$

where $YC_{11(g)}$ = Land area required for housing type g

$YC_{8(g)}$ = Required number of housing units of type g

$XC_{11(g)}$ = Land area per unit of housing type g

$$YC_{12(g)} = YC_{8(g)} \times XC_{12(g)} \qquad (6.12)$$

where $YC_{12(g)}$ = Open and paved land area required for housing type g

$YC_{8(g)}$ = Required number of housing units of type g

$XC_{12(g)}$ = Land area required per unit of housing type g

$$YC_{13(f)} = YE_{27(f)} \times XC_{13(f)} \qquad (6.13)$$

where $YC_{13(f)}$ = Gross public school enrollment in educational group f

$YE_{27(f)}$ = In-migrating children in educational group f

$XC_{13(f)}$ = Percentage of in-migrating children in group f who attend public schools

$$YC_{14(f)} = YC_{13(f)} - XC_{14(f)} \qquad (6.14)$$

where $YC_{14(f)}$ = Net public school enrollment in educational group f

$YC_{13(f)}$ = Gross public school enrollment in educational group f

$XC_{14(f)}$ = Baseline pupil surplus in educational group f

$$YC_{15(f)} = YC_{14(f)} \times XC_{15(f)} \qquad (6.15)$$

where $YC_{15(f)}$ = Floor space required for educational group f

$YC_{14(f)}$ = Net public school enrollment in educational group f

$XC_{15(f)}$ = Floor space per pupil in educational group f

$$YC_{16(f)} = YC_{15(f)} \times XC_{16(f)} \qquad (6.16)$$

where $YC_{16(f)}$ = Construction cost for schools in educational group f

$YC_{15(f)}$ = Floor space required for educational group f

$XC_{16(f)}$ = Construction cost per square foot of floor space in schools of type f

$$YC_{17(f)} = YC_{14(f)} \times XC_{17(f)} \qquad (6.17)$$

where $YC_{17(f)}$ = Land area required for educational group f

$YC_{14(f)}$ = Net public school enrollment in educational group f

$XC_{17(f)}$ = Land area per pupil in educational group f

$$YC_{18(f)} = YC_{17(f)} \times XC_{18(f)} \qquad (6.18)$$

where $YC_{18(f)}$ = Open and paved land area required for educational group f

$YC_{17(f)}$ = Land area required for educational group f

$XC_{18(f)}$ = Percentage of land area in educational group f which is open and paved

$$YC_{19(f)} = YC_{13(f)} \times XC_{19(f)} \qquad (6.19)$$

where $YC_{19(f)}$ = Operating cost for schools in educational group f

$YC_{13(f)}$ = Gross public school enrollment in educational group f

$XC_{19(f)}$ = Operating cost per pupil in educational group f

$$YC_{20(g)} = YE_{25} \times XC_{20(g)} \qquad (6.20)$$

where $YC_{20(g)}$ = Gross personnel requirements for social infrastructure group g

YE_{25} = Total in-migrant population

$XC_{20(g)}$ = Personnel requirements per capita for social infrastructure group g

$$YC_{21(g)} = YC_{20(g)} - XC_{21(g)} \qquad (6.21)$$

where $YC_{21(g)}$ = Net personnel requirements for social infrastructure group g

$YC_{20(g)}$ = Gross personnel requirements for social infrastructure group g

$XC_{21(g)}$ = Baseline personnel surplus for social infrastructure group g

$$YC_{22(g)} = YC_{21(g)} \times XC_{22(g)} \qquad (6.22)$$

where $YC_{22(g)}$ = Floor space requirements for social infrastructure group g

$YC_{21(g)}$ = Net personnel requirements for social infrastructure group g

$XC_{22(g)}$ = Floor space per personnel for social infrastructure group g

$$YC_{23(g)} = YC_{22(g)} \times XC_{23(g)} \qquad (6.23)$$

where $YC_{23(g)}$ = Construction cost for social infrastructure group g

$YC_{22(g)}$ = Floor space requirements for social infrastructure group g

$XC_{23(g)}$ = Construction cost per square foot of social infrastructure group g floor space

$$YC_{24(g)} = YC_{21(g)} \times XC_{24(g)} \qquad (6.24)$$

where $YC_{24(g)}$ = Land area required for social infrastructure group g

$YC_{21(g)}$ = Net personnel requirements for social infrastructure group g

$XC_{24(g)}$ = Land area per personnel for social infrastructure group g

$$YC_{25(g)} = YC_{24(g)} \times XC_{25(g)} \qquad (6.25)$$

where $YC_{25(g)}$ = Open and paved land area requirded for social infrastructure group g

$YC_{24(g)}$ = Land area required for social infrastructure group g

$XC_{25(g)}$ = Percentage of land area for social infrastructure group g which is open and paved

$$YC_{26(g)} = YC_{21(g)} \times XC_{26(g)} \qquad (6.26)$$

where $YC_{26(g)}$ = Operating cost for social infrastructure group g

$YC_{21(g)}$ = Net personnel requirements for social infrastructure group g

$XC_{26(g)}$ = Operating cost per personnel for social infrastructure group g

$$YC_{27} = \Sigma \, (YC_{8(g)} \times XC_{27(g)} \times XC_{28(g)}) \qquad (6.27)$$

where YC_{27} = Miles of street required

$YC_{8(g)}$ = Required number of housing units of type g

$XC_{27(g)}$ = Percentage of housing units of type g built in areas requiring streets

$XC_{28(g)}$ = Length of street associated with a housing unit of type g

$$YC_{28} = YC_{27} \times XC_{29} \tag{6.28}$$

where YC_{28} = Construction cost for streets

YC_{27} = Miles of street required

XC_{29} = Construction cost per mile of street

$$YC_{29} = YC_{27} \times XC_{30} \tag{6.29}$$

where YC_{29} = Paved land area associated with streets

YC_{27} = Miles of street required

XC_{30} = Paved land area per mile of street

$$YC_{30} = YC_{27} \times XC_{31} \tag{6.30}$$

where YC_{30} = Operating cost for streets

YC_{27} = Miles of street required

XC_{31} = Construction cost per mile of street

$$YC_{31(h)} = YE_{24} \times XC_{32(h)} \tag{6.31}$$

where $YC_{31(h)}$ = Residential water consumption/sewage generation

YE_{24} = Total in-migrant population

$XC_{32(h)}$ = Residential water consumption/sewage generation per capita

$$YC_{32(h)} = \Sigma^{c}(YE_{14(c)} \times XC_{33(c,h)}) \tag{6.32}$$

where $YC_{32(h)}$ = Secondary industrial water consumption/sewage generation

$YE_{14(c)}$ = Secondary employees in sector c

$XC_{33(c,h)}$ = Water consumption/sewage generation per employee in sector c

$$YC_{33(h)} = YC_{31(h)} + YC_{32(h)} + XC_{34(h)} \tag{6.33}$$

where $YC_{33(h)}$ = Total gross water consumption/sewage generation

$YC_{31(h)}$ = Residential water consumption/sewage generation

$YC_{32(h)}$ = Secondary industrial water consumption/sewage generation

$XC_{34(h)}$ = Primary facility's water consumption/sewage generation

$$YC_{34(h)} = YC_{33(h)} - XC_{35(h)} \qquad (6.34)$$

where $YC_{34(h)}$ = Net water consumption/sewage generation

$YC_{33(h)}$ = Total gross water consumption/sewage generation

$XC_{35(h)}$ = Baseline surplus water/sewage

$$YC_{35(h)} = YC_{34(h)} \times XC_{36(h)} \qquad (6.35)$$

where $YC_{35(h)}$ = Required central water/sewer system capacity in million gallons per day (MGD)

$YC_{34(h)}$ = Net water consumption/sewage generation

$XC_{36(h)}$ = Ratio of required capacity to consumption/generation

$$YC_{36(h)} = YC_{35(h)} \times XC_{37(h)} \qquad (6.36)$$

where $YC_{36(h)}$ = Construction cost for central water sewer system

$YC_{35(h)}$ = Required central water/sewer system capacity in MGD

$XC_{37(h)}$ = Construction cost per MGD of central water/sewer capacity

$$YC_{37(h)} = YC_{27} \times XC_{38(h)} \qquad (6.37)$$

where $YC_{37(h)}$ = Miles of water/sewer main required

YC_{27} = Miles of street required

$XC_{38(h)}$ = Ratio of water/sewer main length to street length

$$YC_{38(h)} = YC_{37(h)} \times XC_{39(h)} \qquad (6.38)$$

where $YC_{38(h)}$ = Construction cost for water/sewer distribution system

$YC_{37(h)}$ = Miles of water/sewer main required

$XC_{39(h)}$ = Construction cost associated with a mile of water/sewer main

$$YC_{39(h)} = YC_{36(h)} + YC_{38(h)} \qquad (6.39)$$

where $YC_{39(h)}$ = Total water/sewer system construction cost

$YC_{36(h)}$ = Construction cost for central water/sewer system

$YC_{38(h)}$ = Construction cost for water/sewer distribution system

$$YC_{40(h)} = YC_{34(h)} \times XC_{40(h)} \qquad (6.40)$$

where $YC_{40(h)}$ = Land area associated with central water/sewer system

$YC_{34(h)}$ = Required central water/sewer system capacity in MGD

$XC_{40(h)}$ = Land area associated with one MGD of central water/sewer system capacity

$$YC_{41(h)} = (YC_{35(h)} \times XC_{41(h)}) + (YC_{37(h)} \times XC_{42(h)}) \qquad (6.41)$$

where $YC_{41(h)}$ = Operating cost for the water/sewer system

$YC_{35(h)}$ = Required central water/sewer capacity in MGD

$XC_{41(h)}$ = Operating cost per MGD of water/sewer capacity

$YC_{37(h)}$ = Miles of water/sewer main required

$XC_{42(h)}$ = Operating cost per mile of water/sewer main

$$YC_{42} = YC_{27} \times XC_{43} \qquad (6.42)$$

where YC_{42} = Miles of storm sewer required

YC_{27} = Miles of street required

XC_{43} = Ratio of storm-sewer length to street length

$$YC_{43} = YC_{42} \times XC_{44} \qquad (6.43)$$

where YC_{43} = Construction cost for storm sewers

YC_{42} = Miles of storm sewer required

XC_{44} = Construction cost per mile of storm sewer

$$YC_{44} = YC_{42} \times XC_{45} \qquad (6.44)$$

where YC_{44} = Operating cost for storm sewers

YC_{42} = Miles of storm sewer required

XC_{45} = Operating cost per mile of storm sewer

$$YC_{45} = (YE_{25} \times XC_{46}) + \overset{c}{\Sigma}(YE_{14(c)} \times XC_{47}) + XC_{48} \qquad (6.45)$$

where YC_{45} = Total solid-waste generation

        YE_{25} = Total in-migrant population

        XC_{46} = Residential solid-waste generation per capita

        $YE_{14(c)}$ = Secondary employees in sector c

        XC_{47} = Solid waste per employee in sector c

        XC_{48} = Primary facility's solid-waste generation

$$YC_{46} = YC_{45} \times XC_{49} \qquad (6.46)$$

where YC_{46} = Capital costs associated with solid-waste collection

        YC_{45} = Total solid-waste generation

        XC_{49} = Capital cost associated with collecting 1 ton of solid waste

$$YC_{47} = YC_{45} \times XC_{50} \qquad (6.47)$$

where YC_{47} = Operating costs associated with solid-waste collection

        YC_{45} = Total solid-waste generation

        XC_{50} = Operating cost associated with collecting 1 ton of solid waste

$$YC_{48} = YC_{45} \times XC_{51} \qquad (6.48)$$

where YC_{48} = Acres of landfill required

        YC_{45} = Total solid-waste generation

        XC_{51} = Acres of landfill associated with 1 ton of solid waste

$$YC_{49} = YC_{48} \times XC_{52} \qquad (6.49)$$

where YC_{49} = Capital costs associated with solid-waste disposal

        YC_{48} = Acres of landfill required

        XC_{52} = Capital cost associated with 1 acre of landfill

$$YC_{50} = YC_{45} \times XC_{53} \qquad (6.50)$$

where YC_{50} = Operating costs associated with solid-waste disposal

YC_{45} = Total solid-waste generation

XC_{53} = Operating cost per ton of solid-waste disposal

$$YC_{51} = YC_{46} + YC_{49} \qquad (6.51)$$

where YC_{51} = Capital costs for solid-waste system

YC_{46} = Capital costs associated with solid-waste collection

YC_{49} = Costs associated with solid-waste disposal

$$YC_{52} = YC_{47} + YC_{50} \qquad (6.52)$$

where YC_{52} = Operating costs for solid-waste system

YC_{47} = Operating costs associated with solid-waste collection

YC_{50} = Operating costs associated with solid-waste disposal

7 The Fiscal Model

The fiscal changes associated with the construction and operation of a new facility can be quite significant, especially when the host community happens to be small and rural. Because fiscal issues are of prime concern to the local citizenry, most environmental impact statements (EISs) attempt to address this area seriously. Nonetheless, their analyses are often inadequate, not because the subject matter is complex, but because fiscal changes are analyzed independently, while they are in fact, a corollary of economic, demographic, and infrastructure-requirement developments. In Simpact, a comprehensive Fiscal Model has been built, in which revenues are closely linked to the solutions from the Economic and Demographic Model and expenditures are tied to the output of the Community Planning Model.

It must be pointed out that the Fiscal Model of Simpact is the least generalized of the models. Because of regional variations in tax structure, some components have to be changed for each new application. The model is illustrated in this chapter by assuming that the region of analysis is in Pennsylvania.

The chapter is organized into four sections. The first section describes the form of local government in Pennsylvania, and the second section presents an overview of the model. The third section explains the equations used to project the revenues from taxes and intergovernmental transfers, and the fourth section explains the equations used to compute operating and capital expenditures.

Form of Local Government

The Commonwealth of Pennsylvania is organized into the following major forms of government: counties, municipalities, authorities, and school districts. In the Simpact fiscal analysis, the impact on each fiscal unit is modeled separately.

Counties

The structure, powers, and responsibilities of counties are defined by the Pennsylvania Constitution and County Code, although counties can, if they wish, redefine their respective roles by adopting a Home Rule Charter. As defined by the County Code, the county government consists of a three-member

Board of County Commissioners elected for concurrent 4-year terms. Also elected, and largely independent of the commissioners, are the so-called row officers. The commissioners direct the financial operations in such matters as the setting of tax rates and the assessing of property. The row officers include the treasurer, coroner, and sheriff.

The services provided by the county are largely of an ancillary nature, and they tend to be of the type that cannot be provided by the municipalities because of the scale of operations involved. The county usually performs correction-related functions, for example, maintaining a county jail. It may also run a vocational school, provide health care, and manage welfare distribution.

In Pennsylvania, counties are classified into one of eight classes. Classification is important, since statutory powers with regard to taxing authority vary by class. The classification is based on population. For example, counties with population in excess of 1.8 million are class 1; those with population between 800,000 and 1.8 million are class 2; and those with population between 500,000 and 800,000 are class 3.

Municipalities

Municipalities can take the form of townships, boroughs, or cities, and they have structures, powers, and responsibilities similar to those of the counties. Cities do have a greater range of enumerated powers, but many of these powers may be exercised by boroughs or townships under specific grants.

The municipalities provide a wide range of services to their citizens, including police and fire protection and the maintenance and construction of local roads. Because of these responsibilities, municipalities have the authority to impose a wide range of taxes, chief of which are the property and personal income taxes.

For illustrative purposes, the governmental structure of townships is discussed here. Townships in Pennsylvania are classified as first class if they have more than 300 people per square mile and second class if they do not. Second-class townships are governed by a three-member board of supervisors elected for staggered 6-year terms. The board is both the executive and legislative arm of the township. It appoints the various town officials, who may include a secretary/treasurer, a solicitor, an engineer, police officers, sanitation officers, and park board members.

Authorities

An *authority* is a special corporate unit established by one or more municipalities for the purpose of constructing and operating a specific public facility.

Typical facilities run by authorities include airports, waterworks, sewage-treatment works, transportation facilities, hospitals, and industrial-development projects.

The authority is managed by a board appointed by the board of the parent municipalities. A major management objective is fiscal self-sufficiency: costs, both operating and debt related, are supposed to be met by revenues. In the case of a sewer authority, for example, sewer-use charges are set at a rate high enough to cover both operating costs and amortized capital costs. To raise capital, the authority is empowered to float its own bonds. In fact, the authority concept was initially set up in Pennsylvania to avoid the statutory debt limitations imposed by the Constitution of Pennsylvania.

School Districts

In Pennsylvania, school districts, which can encompass several municipalities, are managed by a board consisting of nine members elected for overlapping 6-year terms. To finance school construction and operation, the board is authorized to levy taxes and issue bonds. It is also entrusted with hiring personnel, buying supplies, and providing other school-related administrative functions. The day to day administration is carried out by a district superintendent, and school teachers and other personnel are recommended by him for appointment to the board.

School districts in Pennsylvania are classified into size classes. The classification is again according to total population. Class 1 school districts, for example, are those with a population in excess of 1.5 million, and class 2 districts are those with a population between 500,000 and 1.5 million.

Overview of the Model

In the Fiscal Model, separate analyses are performed at the state, county, municipal, and school district levels. There is no fiscal analysis for authorities since they are self-supporting entities.

The Fiscal Model draws on solutions from the Economic and Demographic and Community Planning Models. In discussing these earlier models, no mention was made of the regional scheme. In actuality, all analysis is performed at the municipality level. For the purpose of the Fiscal Model, the municipal solutions are aggregated to a school district, county, and multicounty level. Thus the same solution variable—for example, population—is available at different area levels of aggregation.

It should be emphasized that the analysis focuses only on those municipalities likely to be impacted severely. A typical regional scheme would analyze ten municipalities, six school districts, and three counties. In such a setup, the remaining municipalities and school districts would be aggregated into an "other" category. The state, in such an analysis, would equal the sum of the three counties.

A fiscal impact model involves three sequential analytical stages: revenue, cost, and budget. In the first stage, the increased revenue that will be generated by the new economic and demographic activity is computed. In the second stage, the operating and capital costs associated with providing the public infrastructure demands created by such activity are determined; and the capital costs are then annualized and added to operating costs to give total annual costs. In the third stage, the net budgetary change is calculated by comparing revenues to total annualized costs.

Figure 7-1 presents a schematic synopsis of the Simpact Fiscal Model. For the state, only a revenue analysis is performed. For the county, municipality, and school district, revenue, cost, and budget analyses are made.

State and county revenue computations, as the flowchart arrow indicates, are based only on solutions from the Economic and Demographic Model. Municipal and school district revenue projections also depend on solutions from the Community Planning Model. The output of the Community Planning Model, used in the revenue calculations, consists of the business and housing construction cost variables, which form the basis for calculating municipal and school district property tax revenues.

Figure 7-1 depicts the fiscal analyses of the state, county, municipality, and school district as being independent of each other. In fact, this is not the case. The Fiscal Model includes equations for intergovernmental transfers, a source of revenue which is very important for both municipalities and school districts. An example of an intergovernmental transfer is the motor fuel tax. There are procedures built into the model to ensure that state motor fuel tax revenues are distributed to the counties and then from the counties to the municipalities.

Figure 7-2 describes the state revenue analysis. In the figure, solutions from the Economic and Demographic Model are identified by a circle and the solutions of the Fiscal Model are identified by a triangle.

The major sources of revenue to the state of Pennsylvania are the sales, corporate income, personal income, and motor fuel taxes, which together account for more than three-quarters of the state's tax revenue. The remaining tax revenue comes from taxes on cigarettes, alcoholic beverages, realty transfer, intangible property, horse racing, and severance, as well as motor vehicle license fees. In the model, projections are made for the following state revenue categories:

1. Sales tax
2. Corporate income tax
3. Personal income tax

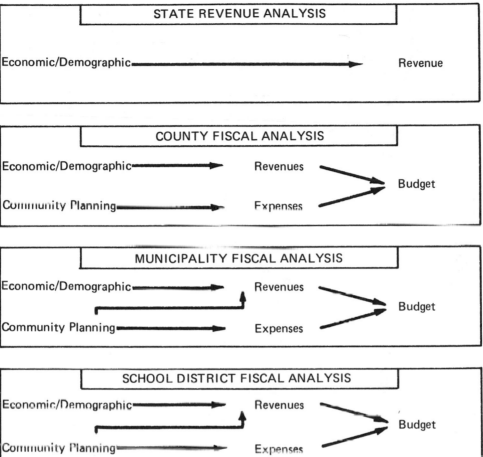

Figure 7-1. Fiscal Model Components

4. State fuel tax
5. Miscellaneous taxes
6. Total revenues

The state tax computations are based on the following Economic and Demographic Model solutions: production, employment, and population. Sales and corporate income taxes are both computed from production. The personal income tax is based on employment, and fuel and miscellaneous taxes are functions of population.

Total state revenue changes are calculated by summing the revenues from

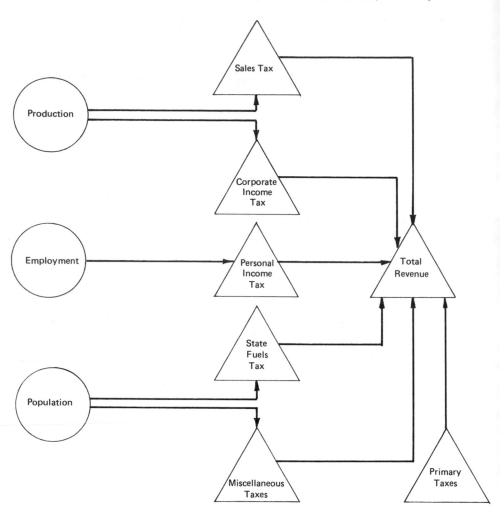

Figure 7-2. State Revenue Analysis

the just enumerated taxes and the corporate taxes paid by the primary facility. The taxes paid by the primary facility are calculated outside the model. While it is certainly possible to treat the taxes on primary production in the same manner as taxes on other production, the relative importance of this source warrants special attention. The appropriate procedure—and the one used in Simpact—is to derive a value for primary taxes in consultation with the company accountants and the government tax officials, and then to enter this offline figure into the model to calculate total revenue.

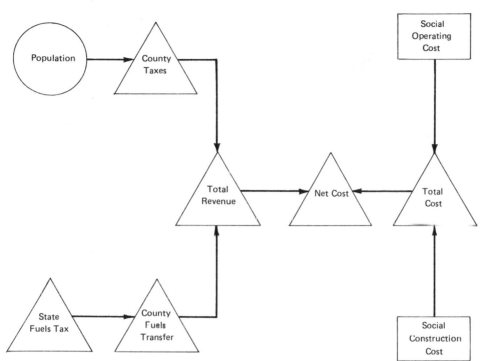

Figure 7-3. County Fiscal Analysis

Figure 7-3 presents a schematic exposition of the county fiscal analysis. The figure contains three types of symbols: triangles for the Fiscal Model, circles for the Economic and Demographic Model, and rectangles for the Community Planning Model.

There are two sources of county revenues calculated in the model: taxes and motor fuel transfers. Taxes are calculated as a function of population; motor fuel transfers to the county are based on the state motor fuel tax receipts.

Operating and capital costs for the county are based on solutions from the Community Planning Model. In that model, the cost of operating and constructing various infrastructure items had been computed. Here the infrastructure items that are the county's responsibilities, such as county parks and general government, are selected and aggregated. Next the annualized capital and operating costs associated with such infrastructure are summed to give total annual costs. These costs are then compared with total revenues to derive the net budgetary impact.

Figure 7-4 describes the logic of municipality fiscal analysis. Because of its small base of operations, the municipality, along with the school district, is

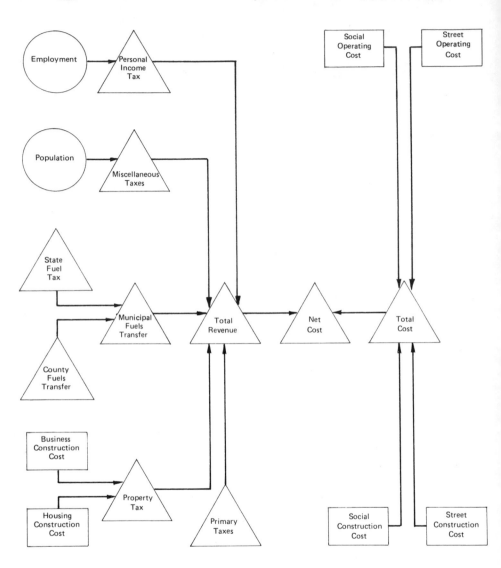

Figure 7-4. Municipality Fiscal Analysis

relatively the most severely impacted fiscal unit. Even in an absolute context, municipal changes can be quite dramatic. This is the case because municipalities have the responsibility for providing, and therefore financing, a wide range of essential services. In the model, municipal revenues are projected for the following categories:

1. Personal income tax
2. Property tax
3. Miscellaneous taxes and fees
4. Fuel tax transfers
5. Total revenues

Personal income tax is calculated as a function of employment, and miscellaneous taxes are based on population, with both employment and population coming from the Economic and Demographic Model. Municipal property tax payments are based on the business and housing construction cost solutions from the Community Planning Model. Fuel tax transfers to the municipality are based on state motor fuel tax revenues and the county motor fuel receipts from the state. Total revenues are calculated by summing the receipts from the various categories and adding the corporate taxes paid by the primary facility. Taxes paid by the primary facility are, as before, an exogenous input to the model.

Operating and capital costs for the municipality are based on solutions from the Community Planning Model. The costs cover social infrastructure items, such as law enforcement and fire protection, and other services, such as local streets and solid-waste collection and disposal. The total annual costs for the municipality are calculated as the sum of operating and annualized capital costs. It should be noted that the capital costs, as calculated in the Community Planning Model, are adjusted to reflect construction subsidies. In the final step of the municipal fiscal analysis, the net budgetary impact is computed as the excess of costs over revenue.

Figure 7-5 visually describes the school district fiscal analysis. A comparison of this figure with figure 7-4 indicates that the tax structure of the school district is almost identical with that of the municipality, with a major difference only in the area of intergovernmental transfers.

School district revenues are projected in the Fiscal Model for the following categories:

1. Personal income tax
2. Property tax
3. Miscellaneous taxes and fees
4. State and federal subsidies
5. Total revenues

The procedures for calculating personal income tax, property tax, miscellaneous taxes, and total revenue are identical with those applied in the municipal analysis. State and federal subsidies, a major source of school district revenue, are calculated as a function of public school enrollment, a variable which is the output of the Community Planning Model.

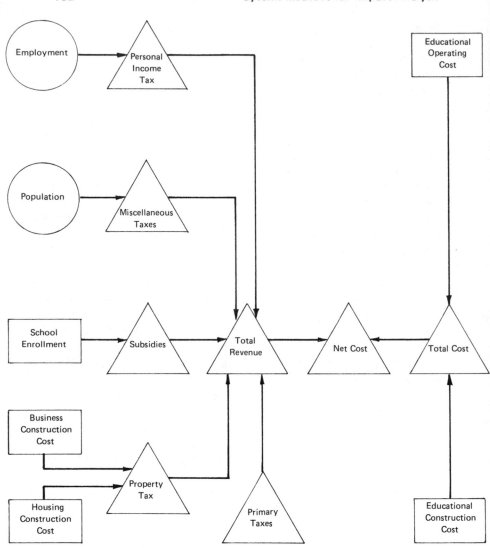

Figure 7-5. School District Fiscal Analysis

In the Community Planning Model, the cost of operating and constructing educational infrastructure had been computed. Here these costs become the basis for calculating annualized school district expenditures. As in the case of municipalities, capital costs are adjusted down to reflect the construction subsidies received from the state.

Revenues

The purpose of this section is to provide an equation-by-equation explanation of the procedures used to forecast impact-related revenues. The equations are grouped in this section under the four fiscal units: state, county, municipality, and school district.

State

Equation 7.1: Sales Tax. The equation for state sales tax involves two steps: first, the percentage of wholesale and retail business activity subject to sales tax is computed; second, the sales tax rate is applied to that portion of sales which is taxable. Wholesale and retail business activity is a variable that has been calculated in the Economic and Demographic Model as part of the secondary production computations.

The percentage of retail business activity which is taxable varies by item. In Pennsylvania, food consumed off premises is exempt from sales tax, as are sales of apparel, cigarettes, and gasoline. Items on which sales taxes are levied include automobiles, furniture, and lumber. Some activities are partially exempt; for example, only the prescription sales of drug stores are not subject to sales tax. In aggregate, it is reasonable to assume that about 60 percent of wholesale and retail trade sales in Pennsylvania are taxed.

The sales tax is 7 cents on the dollar in Pennsylvania. This tax was enacted in 1951 at 1 percent. It has been raised four times since then: 1957, 1960, 1964, and 1968.

Equation 7.2: Corporate Income Tax. The equation for state corporate income tax revenues involves two steps: first, taxable profits are estimated by multiplying business activity by the profit rate; and second, the state income tax rate is applied to taxable profits.

Taxable income in Pennsylvania is that portion of the corporation's income attributable to its facilities in the state. Some corporations are totally exempted, for example, building and loan associates, savings associations, trust companies, agricultural cooperatives, and insurance companies.

The corporate income tax rate in Pennsylvania at 9½ percent is among the highest in the country. Since its enactment in 1935, the tax has varied considerably, particularly in the last decade. The rate was increased from 6 to 7 percent in 1967, and in 1969 it went to 12 percent.

Equations 7.3 and 7.4: Personal Income Tax. Equation 7.3 estimates the number of employees who live in the state, and equation 7.4 computes the personal income tax paid by these employees. State personal income taxes in Pennsylvania are levied on a place-of-residence basis. This means, for example, that an individual working in Ohio but living in Pennsylvania has to pay taxes to Pennsylvania, while someone working in Pennsylvania but living in Ohio has to pay taxes to Ohio.

This place-of-residence rule raises the issue of the type of demographic activity variable that should be used. Since the region of analysis is in Pennsylvania, total employment could be used. This would assume that everybody who works in that region lives in the state. As has been discussed in chapter 5, employees fall into various demographic groups, chief of which are the original residents and the movers who have permanent residence in the region and the weeklies and commuters who have permanent residences outside the region. If the facility is located in central Pennsylvania, a significant percentage of the weeklies and commuters could in fact be residents of Pennsylvania. This clearly need not be the case if the region of analysis is near the state border.

In equation 7.3, total employment is multiplied by a variable, which defines the percentage of employees in each demographic and income group who live in the state. This operation gives the number of employees living in the state classified by income group (the detail on demographic group being removed by summation).

In equation 7.4, the state personal income tax revenue is calculated by multiplying the number of employees in each income group by the tax paid by a single member of an income group.

In Pennsylvania, the personal income tax, which was enacted in 1971, is currently 2 2/10 percent. The income that is subject to tax includes compensation, dividends, interest, royalties, rent income, capital gains from sale of property, gambling and lottery winnings, and trust income. Except for poverty-related provisions, there are no exemptions or deductions allowed in Pennsylvania. Poverty exemptions are restricted to individuals with annual income in the $5,000 range. Specifically, the provisions apply to single individuals earning annually $3,000, taxpayers with one dependent earning $4,200, taxpayers with two dependents earning $4,950, taxpayers with three dependents earning $5,600, and so on. Because the impact-generated employees are not expected to be in the poverty bracket, the Pennsylvania tax can be treated as if it were a flat 2 2/10 percent.

Equation 7.5: Motor Fuel Tax. The revenues from this tax are estimated by multiplying population by gasoline consumption per capita and by the motor fuel tax rate, which is 9 cents on the gallon in Pennsylvania.

Equation 7.6: Miscellaneous State Revenues. The revenue from miscellaneous sources is estimated by multiplying population by a miscellaneous-revenues-per-capita variable. In Pennsylvania, miscellaneous sources of revenue include motor vehicle registration fees and taxes on cigarettes, liquor, realty transfer, and inheritance. The per capita contribution from these sources can be calculated from the historical revenue records of the state. The mean value for the last few years can be used as input to the model, or if a trend is apparent, the value can be extrapolated using regression analysis.

Equation 7.7: Total State Revenues. The aggregate change in state revenues is obtained by summing the revenues from sales tax, corporate income tax, personal income tax, motor fuel tax, miscellaneous sources, and the exogenously derived taxes paid by the primary facility.

County

Equations 7.8 through 7.10: Taxes and Transfers. Equation 7.8 estimates the tax revenue using a per capita approach; that is, population is multiplied by a county-tax-per-capita variable. There are a variety of taxes and fees at the county level—for example, a tax on intangible personal property—but their value does not justify a more detailed treatment.

Equation 7.9 estimates the funds that will be transferred from the state to the county. In Pennsylvania, counties receive 0.5 cent of the 9 cents on the gallon that is collected by the state. The county receipts are calculated by multiplying the state motor fuel tax revenue, solved in equation 7.5, by the county's share. Equation 7.10 calculates total county revenue by summing the solutions from the preceding two equations.

Equations 7.11 and 7.12: Property Assessment. For the purpose of property tax calculations, the value of real property has to be assessed. In Pennsylvania, the assessed values are developed by the county and are made for the benefit of the political subdivisions they contain, namely, the municipalities and the school districts. It is these entities that levy a tax against the assessed valuations.

Property is classified into real, personal tangible, and personal intangible. *Real property* consists of land and the buildings on it. *Tangible personal property* consists of machinery, inventories, automobiles, and so on. *Intangible personal property* consists of paper wealth such as stock, bonds, and cash. Because personal property taxes are hard to administer, they are not widely used, and the preeminent form of property tax is the real property tax.

In Pennsylvania, various properties are exempt from the real property tax. These exemptions are similar to the ones granted in other states and include property owned by churches, educational institutions, hospitals, and public institutions. All nonexempt properties are appraised at periodic intervals, with the property being appraised at full market value. However, the assessment ratio need not be 100 percent. For example, in Erie County the assessment ratio is 40 percent, and in Crawford County it is 30 percent. Therefore, assessed value is some fraction of market value, and market value is, in turn, some multiple of construction cost.

In the Economic and Demographic Model, the construction cost of secondary business infrastructure and housing has been computed. In equation 7.11, business construction cost is multiplied by a market-value-to-construction-cost ratio and an assessment-to-market-value ratio. These operations give the assessed value of secondary business property. Equation 7.12 performs a similar operation to compute the assessed value of housing.

Municipalities

Equations 7.13 and 7.14: Property Tax. The real property tax revenues accruing to the municipality are calculated in these two equations. In equation 7.13, assessed business value is multiplied by a property tax rate to give business property tax; and equation 7.14 performs the same type of operations to compute housing property tax.

The property tax rate is traditionally expressed in mills, where a mill is equal to 0.1 cent. A tax rate of 10 mills would mean a tax payment of $10 for every $1,000 of assessed valuation. In Pennsylvania, there are statutory limits on the property tax rate. In first-class townships, for example, the rate is restricted to 30 mills, although additional levies are allowed for predefined purposes.

The real property tax is a significant revenue raiser for many municipalities, second only to the personal income tax. This popularity is attributable to a number of reasons. First, real property is hard to conceal and its value can be clearly defined, which makes the administration of the tax easy. Second, real property is a major category of community wealth, which means that it constitutes a sizable revenue base. Third, the property base increases steadily over time, and so the revenue from this source can be expected to increase. Despite these advantages, the property tax has been widely attacked, particularly in areas where land values have inflated rapidly, and communities are seeking to diversify their tax base to avoid overreliance on this source.

Equation 7.15: Personal Income Tax. The personal income tax is the most important municipal revenue source. Equation 7.15 calculates personal income tax by multiplying mover employees, classified by income group, by the tax payable by an employee in a particular income group. The choice of demographic variable requires some explanation.

In computing state personal income tax, total employment, which includes weeklies and commuters, was used, the rationale being that even commuters may live in the state. This is not the case for a municipality. A person who is a commuter or weekly does not live in the municipality, and so, assuming tax is levied on a region-of-residence basis, such a person does not pay tax. This is why mover employment, rather than total employment, is used to compute municipal personal income tax revenues.

The tax rate for Pennsylvania municipalities is set in conjunction with the school districts. It is stipulated that the joint personal income tax levy should not exceed 1 percent, with the school district receiving at least half. For example, the municipal rate could be 0.4 of 1 percent and the school district 0.6 of 1 percent.

Equation 7.16: Miscellaneous Tax Revenue. Apart from the property and personal income taxes, municipalities are empowered to use a variety of taxes, including per capita, occupation, mercantile, real estate transfer, and amusement. The contribution from such miscellaneous taxes is estimated in equation 7.16 using a per capita approach.

Equation 7.17: Transfers. For the purpose of street maintenance, municipalities receive funds from the state, and they usually also receive funds from the county. These funds constitute a significant proportion of total revenues. The state distributes approximately 20 percent of its motor fuel tax directly to municipalities. As discussed earlier, the state also gives a portion of the motor fuel tax to counties, which the counties may, if they wish, distribute to the municipalities. In equation 7.17, the funds received by a municipality are calculated by multiplying the state motor fuel revenues by a state-municipality transfer rate and multiplying the county motor fuel revenues by a county-municipality transfer rate.

The transfer rate is based on 50 percent on a municipality's population and 50 percent on its street mileage. Because the impacted municipality is experiencing an induced population and street growth, its transfer rate will increase above its historical value. This suggests that the transfer rate shall be endogenized; that is, it should be solved within the model. Although not shown here, this can, in fact, be done. Population solutions are available from the Economic and Demographic Model and street solutions from the Community Planning Model. Together these variables constitute the input necessary to calculate a new transfer rate.

Equation 7.18: Total Revenues. The total revenues obtained by a municipality are calculated in this equation by summing the solutions generated in the preceding equations. Total revenues include contributions from the property tax, personal income tax, miscellaneous taxes and fees, transfers from the state, transfers from the county, and taxes paid by the primary facility. As noted earlier, taxes paid by the primary facility are derived externally of the model.

School District

Equations 7.19 through 7.21: Taxes. The tax structure of a Pennsylvania school district is very similar to that of a municipality. The major sources of revenue are the property tax and the personal income tax, with the property tax playing a proportionately larger role. The procedures to compute revenues from these sources are identical with those described for the municipality. Equation 7.19 and 7.20 compute property tax revenues from secondary business and housing, and equation 7.21 calculates the revenues generated by the school district's personal income tax.

Equations 7.22 and 7.23: Subsidies. The school district receives subsidies from the state and federal governments. The state subsidies account for a significant portion of the school district's revenue. The most important state program is the basic instructional subsidy. The so-called state categorical aid programs account for the remainder of operating aid received from the state.

The total basic instructional subsidy to a school district (P) is based on weighted school enrollment (W) and an aid ratio (Q). Mathematically, it can be expressed as $P = \$750 \times W \times Q$. Total subsidy can be put on a per pupil basis by the following transformation: $A = (\$750 \times Q) \times (W/E)$, where E is the actual as opposed to weighted enrollment.

The aid ratio is negatively related to the ratio of the assessed value per pupil in the school district and to the assessed value per pupil in the state as a whole. This means that relatively wealthy communities will have a low Q and consequently obtain relatively low subsidies on a per pupil basis.

The categorical programs include transportation, special education, vocational education within high schools, driver education, and medical and dental services. The operating revenue from these categorical programs and other sources can also be put on a per pupil basis.

In equation 7.22, the aid received by school districts from the state is estimated by multiplying school enrollment by state aid per pupil. The input variable, state aid per pupil, includes revenues from the basic instructional subsidy and the categorical programs.

Equation 7.23 estimates the aid received by the school district from the federal government. The approach used is identical with that applied in the preceding equation. Federal aid is calculated by multiplying enrollment by the input variable, federal aid per pupil.

Equations 7.24 and 7.25: Miscellaneous Total Revenues. In equation 7.25, the total operating revenues received by a school district are calculated by summing the receipts from the property tax, the personal income tax, miscellaneous taxes and fees, state subsidies, federal contributions, and the externally determined taxes paid by the primary facility. The revenues from miscellaneous taxes and fees are calculated in equation 7.24 using a per capita approach.

Note on Federal Revenue Sharing

In the Simpact Fiscal Model, revenues obtained through the federal government's revenue-sharing program are not quantified. The revenue-sharing process is essentially a three-stage process. First, revenue is allocated to the states. Second, the amount allocated to the state is distributed to the state and counties. And third, the funds allocated to a county are distributed among the local governments within the county.

The allocations are governed by statutory formulas that use such variables as personal income and population. The impacts created by the new facility and related developments will change the allocation variables. This means that the share of the impacted region of federal revenues will change. However, the extent of the change will also depend on how the allocation variables are changing in other regions of the state. Because it is difficult to obtain projections of the variables for the nonimpacted regions, federal revenue-sharing changes are not computed in Simpact.

Expenditures and Finances

In developing governmental impact budgets, it is also necessary to calculate the operating and debt-service costs associated with providing the required infrastructure. This information, when used along with the revenue projections, can indicate whether or not the budget of a particular fiscal unit will be negatively or positively impacted. The purpose of this section is to describe the procedures used in Simpact to calculate the operating and capital costs by governmental unit.

Equations 7.26 through 7.28: Operating Costs. These three equations correspond to the operating costs of counties, municipalities, and school districts. The operating costs of various infrastructure items, already computed in the Community Planning Model, are grouped in these equations by the fiscal unit assumed to be responsible for operating them.

Equations 7.29 through 7.31: Capital Requirement. These three equations calculate the amount of capital that must be raised by the county, municipality, and school district. The capital costs for a given governmental entity are calculated by multiplying construction cost by the percentage of construction cost that will not be subsidized.

In the Community Planning Model, the construction cost associated with various infrastructure items has been computed. For example, the cost of constructing new schools has been determined in that model. However, total construction costs for schools are an overstatement of the amount of capital that must be raised by the school district. This is so because a significant percentage of the construction costs for schools is subsidized by the state. Therefore, total construction cost must be adjusted to take subsidies into account.

It should be noted that there are statutory limitations on the amount of debt that can be incurred. The existence of these statutory limitations implies that the solutions from equations 7.29 through 7.31 should be checked to ensure that the limits are not exceeded. In Pennsylvania, a municipality cannot incur any new debt if this debt, plus any other nonelectoral debt outstanding, would cause the total debt to exceed 250 percent of its borrowing base. The borrowing base is defined as the 3-year average of total revenues, with total revenues including all monies received, except subsidies, revenues pledged to self-liquidating debt, interest on sinking funds which are pledged for payment of outstanding debt, grants designated for a specific project, and nonrecurring receipts, such as sales of capital assets.

Equations 7.32 through 7.34: Annual Debt Costs. The capital expenditures that are not subsidized are assumed to be financed by debt. The borrowing instrument is the municipal bond, which actually refers to bonds issued not only by municipalities, but also by the state or any of its political subdivisions.

The most striking feature of municipal bonds is that the interest they pay is exempt from federal income tax. Furthermore, while municipal bonds do not have to be exempt from state income taxes, many states with income taxes have granted such exemption. As a result of their tax-exempt status, municipal bonds can find purchasers, while offering relatively low rates of interest. For example, to an individual in the 50 percent tax bracket, a municipal bond paying 6 percent gives the same yield as a corporate bond paying 12 percent.

While municipal bonds, as a class, pay lower rates, there are variations between municipal bonds. The interest rate at which a particular municipality can borrow is influenced by the quality rating assigned to it by the two investors services, Moodys and Standard and Poors. The rating is based on the ability of a municipality to honor its commitment. For example, a municipality with a high ratio of debt per capita to income per capita could be regarded as a high-risk candidate.

Municipal bonds can be categorized in a number of ways. The most important classifications are according to security pledged and method of retirement. In connection with security, there are two chief classes of bonds— general obligation and limited obligation. A *general-obligation bond* is one that is unconditionally backed by the complete taxing authority of the issuing municipality. *Limited-obligation bonds* are supported only from the revenues of the project that they were borrowed to finance.

If method of retirement is used as a basis for classification, there are serial bonds and term bonds. *Serial bonds* mature at intervals determined at the time at which the bonds are issued. For example, a municipality may issue $10 million worth of bonds with $1 million coming to maturity each year. In the *term issue,* all the bonds mature on the same date. For example, $10 million worth of bonds could be issued with all of them coming to maturity at the end of 5 years.

Equations 7.32 through 7.34 compute the annual debt-related cost for the county, municipality, and school district, respectively. Annual debt-service cost is defined here as the sum of the repayment of principal and the payment of interest. A constant annual debt cost is calculated by multiplying required capital, computed in equations 7.29 through 7.31, by an amortization factor.

The procedure described in equations 7.32 through 7.34 assumes a term issue. In practice, serial bonds are the more popular borrowing mechanism. Under a serial bond issue, annual debt-related costs are not constant, but decline each year. This is so because interest payments are based on the unpaid principal, which, because some bonds are falling due each year, is a decreasing amount.

Equations 7.35 through 7.37: Net Annual Costs. These three equations calculate net annual costs for the county, municipality, and school district. *Net annual cost* is defined as the excess of costs over total revenue, with *cost* defined as the sum of operating costs and annual debt-service costs. Of course, net annual costs can be negative, which would imply a revenue surplus.

There are no new input variables involved in the net annual cost equations. These three equations merely bring together solutions generated in the earlier equations. For example, in the case of municipalities, operating costs have been calculated in equation 7.27, annual debt-service costs in equation 7.33, and total revenues in equation 7.18. The net-cost equations conclude the Fiscal Model.

Appendix 7A: Equations

Listed here are the equations in the Fiscal Model. The output variables in the model are denoted by YF and the input variables by XF. The solutions of this model also use as inputs, solutions from the Economic and Demographic and Community Planning Models. The analysis in these earlier models has been on a municipality basis. For the Fiscal Model, these municipal solutions are aggregated to school district, county, and multicounty level. Thus the same solution variable—for example, YE_{24} population—is available at different levels of aggregation. The regional schema is not specifically noted in labeling the variables. For example, population at the county level is not identified by a code that is any different from the one used for population at the municipality level. This omission is not likely to cause any confusion, since the definitions that follow the equation identify the regional unit being modeled.

$$YF_1 = YE_{13(c=4)} \times XF_1 \times XF_2 \qquad (7.1)$$

where YF_1 = State sales tax revenue

$YE_{13(c=4)}$ = Secondary production in sector $c = 4$ (sector 4 is wholesale and retail trade)

XF_1 = Percentage of the activity in sector $c = 4$ subject to sales tax

XF_2 = State sales tax rate

$$YF_2 = \overset{c}{\Sigma} (YE_{13(c)} \times XF_{3(c)}) \times XF_4 \qquad (7.2)$$

where YF_2 = State corporate income tax revenue

$YE_{13(c)}$ = Secondary production in sector c

$XF_{3(c)}$ = Ratio of profit to production in sector c

XF_4 = State corporate income tax rate

$$YF_{3(d)} = \overset{b}{\Sigma} (YE_{17(b,d)} \times XF_{5(b,d)}) \qquad (7.3)$$

where $YF_{3(d)}$ = Employees in income group d living in the state

$YE_{17(b,d)}$ = Total employees in demographic group b who are in income group d

$XF_{5(b,d)}$ = Percentage of employees in demographic group b and income group d who live in the state

113

$$YF_4 = \overset{d}{\Sigma} (YF_{3(d)} \times XF_{6(d)}) \qquad (7.4)$$

where YF_4 = State personal income tax revenue

$YF_{3(d)}$ = Employees in income group d living in the state

$XF_{6(d)}$ = Personal income tax paid by an employee in income group d

$$YF_5 = YE_{25} \times XF_7 \times XF_8 \qquad (7.5)$$

where YF_5 = State motor fuel tax revenue

YE_{25} = Total in-migrant population

XF_7 = Gasoline consumption per capita

XF_8 = Motor fuel tax per gallon

$$YF_6 = YE_{24} \times XF_9 \qquad (7.6)$$

where YF_6 = Miscellaneous state revenues

YE_{24} = Total in-migrant population

XF_9 = Miscellaneous state revenues per capita

$$YF_7 = YF_1 + YF_2 + YF_4 + YF_5 + YF_6 + XF_{10} \qquad (7.7)$$

where YF_7 = Total state tax revenues

YF_1 = State sales tax revenue

YF_2 = State corporate income tax revenue

YF_4 = State personal income tax revenue

YF_5 = State motor fuel tax revenue

YF_6 = Miscellaneous state revenues

XF_{10} = State taxes paid by primary facility

$$YF_8 = YE_{25} \times XF_{11} \qquad (7.8)$$

where YF_8 = County tax revenues

$YE25$ = Total in-migrant population

XF_{11} = County tax revenues per capita

$$YF_9 = YF_5 \times XF_{12} \tag{7.9}$$

where YF_9 = State motor fuel tax transfers to county

YF_5 = State motor fuel tax revenue

XF_{12} = State to county transfer rate

$$YF_{10} = YF_8 + XF_9 \tag{7.10}$$

where YF_{10} = Total county revenues

YF_8 = County tax revenues

XF_9 = State transfers to county

$$YF_{11} = \overset{c}{\Sigma}(YC_{13(c)} \times XF_{13(c)} \times XF_{14(c)}) \tag{7.11}$$

where YF_{11} = Assessed value for secondary business property

$YC_{13(c)}$ = Construction cost in sector c

$XF_{13(c)}$ = Ratio of market value to construction cost in sector c

$XF_{14(c)}$ = Ratio of assessed value to market value for sector c

$$YF_{12} = \overset{g}{\Sigma}(YC_{10(g)} \times XF_{15(g)} \times XF_{16(g)}) \tag{7.12}$$

where YF_{12} = Assessed value of housing

$YC_{10(g)}$ = Construction cost for housing type g

$XF_{15(g)}$ = Ratio of market value to construction cost for housing type g

$XF_{16(g)}$ = Ratio of assessed value to market value for housing type g

$$YF_{13} = YF_{11} \times XF_{17} \tag{7.13}$$

where YF_{13} = Municipal property tax revenues from secondary business

YF_{11} = Assessed value for secondary business property

XF_{17} = Municipal property tax rate

$$YF_{14} = YF_{12} \times XF_{17} \tag{7.14}$$

where YF_{14} = Municipal property tax revenues from housing

YF_{12} = Assessed value of housing

XF_{17} = Municipal property tax rate

$$YF_{15} = \overset{d}{\Sigma}(YE_{18(d)} \times XF_{18(d)}) \tag{7.15}$$

where YF_{15} = Municipal personal income tax revenues

$YE_{18(d)}$ = Mover employees in income group d

$XF_{18(d)}$ = Municipal personal income tax paid by an employee in income group d

$$YF_{16} = YE_{25} \times XF_{19} \tag{7.16}$$

where YF_{16} = Miscellaneous municipal revenues

YE_{25} = Total in-migrant population

XF_{19} = Municipal revenues per capita

$$YF_{17} = (YF_5 \times XF_{20}) + (YF_9 \times XF_{21}) \tag{7.17}$$

where YF_{17} = Motor fuel tax transfers to municipality

YF_5 = State motor fuel tax revenues

XF_{20} = State to municipality transfer rate

YF_9 = State motor fuel tax transfers to county

XF_{21} = County to municipality transfer rate

$$YF_{18} = YF_{12} + YF_{14} + YF_{15} + YF_{16} + YF_{17} + XF_{22} \tag{7.18}$$

where YF_{18} = Total municipal revenues

YF_{12} = Municipal property tax revenues from secondary business

YF_{14} = Municipal property tax revenues from housing

YF_{15} = Municipal personal income tax revenues

YF_{16} = Miscellaneous municipal revenues

YF_{17} = County motor fuel tax transfers to municipality

XF_{22} = Municipal taxes paid by the primary facility

$$YF_{19} = YF_{11} \times XF_{23} \tag{7.19}$$

where YF_{19} = School district property tax revenues from secondary business

YF_{11} = Assessed value for secondary business property

XF_{23} = School district property tax rate

$$YF_{20} = YF_{12} \times XF_{23} \tag{7.20}$$

where YF_{20} = School district property tax revenues from housing

YF_{12} = Assessed value of housing

XF_{23} = School district property tax rate

$$YF_{21} = \overset{d}{\Sigma}(YE_{18(d)} \times XF_{24(d)}) \tag{7.21}$$

where YF_{21} = School district personal income tax revenues

$YE_{18(d)}$ = Mover employees in income group d

$XF_{24(d)}$ = School district personal income tax paid by an employee in income group d

$$YF_{22} = (\overset{f}{\Sigma} YC_{13(f)}) \times XF_{25} \tag{7.22}$$

where YF_{22} = State instructional subsidy and categorical aid received by the school district

$YC_{13(f)}$ = Gross public school enrollment in educational group f

XF_{25} = State instructional subsidy and categorical aid per pupil

$$YF_{23} = \overset{f}{\Sigma}(YC_{13(f)} \times XF_{26(f)}) \tag{7.23}$$

where YF_{23} = Federal aid to school district

$YC_{13(f)}$ = Gross public school enrollment in educational group f

$XF_{26(f)}$ = Federal aid per pupil of group f

$$YF_{24} = YE_{25} \times XF_{27} \tag{7.24}$$

where YF_{24} = Miscellaneous school district revenues

YE_{25} = Total in-migrating population

XF_{27} = Miscellaneous school district revenues per capita

$$YF_{25} = YF_{19} + YF_{20} + YF_{21} + YF_{22} + YF_{23} + YF_{24} + XF_{28} \quad (7.25)$$

where YF_{25} = Total school district revenues

YF_{19} = School district revenues from secondary business

YF_{20} = School district property tax revenues from housing

YF_{21} = School district personal income tax revenues

YF_{22} = State instructional subsidy and categorical aid received by the school district

YF_{23} = Federal aid to school district

YF_{24} = Miscellaneous school district revenues

XF_{28} = School district taxes paid by the primary facility

$$YF_{26} = \overset{g}{\Sigma} YC_{26(g=c)} \quad\quad (7.26)$$

where YF_{26} = Operating costs for county

$YC_{26(g=c)}$ = Operating costs for county social infrastructure group g

$$YF_{27} = \overset{g}{\Sigma} YC_{26(g=m)} + YC_{30} + YC_{52} \quad\quad (7.27)$$

where YF_{27} = Operating costs for municipality

$YC_{26(g=m)}$ = Operating costs for municipality social infrastructure group g

YC_{30} = Operating cost for streets

YC_{52} = Operating costs for solid-waste system

$$YF_{28} = \overset{f}{\Sigma} YC_{19(f)} \quad\quad (7.28)$$

where YF_{28} = Operating costs for school district

$YC_{19(f)}$ = Operating cost for schools in educational group f

$$YF_{29} = (YC_{23(g=c)} \times XF_{29(g)}) \quad\quad (7.29)$$

where YF_{29} = Capital funds to be raised by the county

$YC_{23(g=c)}$ = Construction cost for county social infrastructure item g

$XF_{29(g)}$ = Percentage of construction cost that must be financed by the county

$$YF_{30} = \overset{g}{\Sigma}(YC_{23(g=m)} \times XF_{30(g)}) + (YC_{28} \times XF_{31}) + YC_{51} \quad (7.30)$$

where YF_{30} = Capital funds to be raised by municipality

$YC_{23(g=m)}$ = Construction cost for municipality infrastructure group g

$XF_{30(g)}$ = Percentage of construction cost for group g that must be financed by the municipality

YC_{28} = Construction costs for street

XF_{31} = Percentage of street construction costs that must be financed by the municipality

YC_{51} = Capital costs for solid-waste system

$$YF_{31} = \overset{f}{\Sigma}(YC_{16(f)} \times XF_{32(f)}) \quad (7.31)$$

where YF_{31} = Capital funds to be raised by school district

$YC_{16(f)}$ = Construction cost for schools in educational group f

$XF_{32(f)}$ = Percentage of construction costs for group f that must be financed by the school district

$$YF_{32} = YF_{29} \times XF_{33} \quad (7.32)$$

where YF_{32} = Debt-service costs for county

YF_{29} = Capital funds to be raised by county

XF_{33} = Amortization factor

$$YF_{33} = YF_{30} \times XF_{33} \quad (7.33)$$

where YF_{33} = Debt-service costs for municipality

YF_{30} = Capital funds to be raised by municipality

XF_{33} = Amortization factor

$$YF_{34} = YF_{31} \times XF_{33} \quad (7.34)$$

where YF_{34} = Debt-service costs for school district

YF_{31} = Capital funds to be raised by school district

XF_{33} = Amortization factor

$$YF_{35} = (YF_{26} + YF_{32}) - YF_{10} \qquad (7.35)$$

where YF_{35} = Net annual costs for county

YF_{26} = Operating costs for county

YF_{32} = Debt-service costs for county

YF_{10} = Total county revenues

$$YF_{36} = (YF_{27} + YF_{33}) - YF_{18} \qquad (7.36)$$

where YF_{36} = Net annual costs for municipality

YF_{27} = Operating costs for municipality

YF_{33} = Debt-service costs for municipality

YF_{18} = Total municipality revenues

$$YF_{37} = (YF_{28} + YF_{34}) - YF_{25} \qquad (7.37)$$

where YF_{37} = Net annual costs for school district

YF_{28} = Operating costs for school district

YF_{34} = Debt-service costs for school district

YF_{25} = Total school district revenues

8 Environmental Model

Attention in the EIS process is focused on the physical environmental problems created by the primary facility. Most important are the pollutant-concentration levels at the property line of the plant site. However, the regional air-quality impacts of the secondary economic and demographic activity may also be very significant. For example, increased traffic in the subject region will affect carbon monoxide concentration levels, which is already the major air problem in U.S. urban areas, with the automobile the predominant cause. While the secondary environmental analysis is important, it should be emphasized that, in terms of effort, it nevertheless constitutes only a small fraction of the overall physical environmental analysis. Modeling the site-specific environmental impacts created by the primary facility is a complicated task, a description of which could fill several volumes.

The Environmental Model of Simpact is designed to project the air emissions and water-effluent loadings resulting from secondary developments. The Environmental Model does not constitute the sum total of the Simpact secondary environmental analysis. The water-consumption, solid-waste generation, and land-use projections of the Community Planning Model are also of interest to environmentalists.

The material in this chapter has been organized into four sections. The first section contains a summary of U.S. environmental legislation, and the second section contains an overview of the Simpact Environmental Model. The third section explains the equations used to predict secondary air emissions, and the fourth section explains the equations used to project secondary water discharges. The equations themselves are listed in appendix 8A.

Environmental Legislation

The laws to protect our environment are largely administered by the Environmental Protection Agency (EPA). The EPA is an independent federal agency which sets and enforces regulations for maintaining the quality of the environment. It came into being in December 1970, absorbing environmentally related units that were scattered among existing agencies. These units included the National Air Pollution Control Administration from the Department of Health, Education and Welfare and the Federal Water Quality Program from the Department of Interior.

121

Air-Quality Legislation

In connection with air-quality legislation, it is necessary to understand the distinction between emission levels and ambient levels. *Emission levels* refer to the amount of the pollutant discharged to the airshed, for example, tonnage of sulfur dioxide (SO_2) emitted. *Ambient levels* refer to the concentration of the pollutant in the airshed, for example, micrograms of SO_2 per cubic meter. Note that the ultimate objective is ambient quality, but the way to maintain ambient quality is by restricting emissions.

The Clean Air Act of 1970 (P.L. 91-604) and the 1977 amendments (P.L. 95-95) have set up a comprehensive framework, administered by the EPA, for controlling emission levels and enhancing ambient quality.

Emission standards are set by discharging sources, both stationary and mobile. *Stationary standards* express the allowable emission discharge as a function of the production level, for example, SO_2 emitted from a sulphuric acid plant should be less than 0.2 of 1 percent of the sulphuric acid produced. *Mobile emission standards* are set as a function of vehicle mileage, for example, carbon monoxide (CO) emitted should be less than 3.4 grams per mile traveled.

In setting emission standards, consideration is given to ambient goals and to economic attainability. Prior to setting emission standards, EPA conducts technological and economic studies to identify demonstrated pollution-control technologies, and the promulgated emission standards reflect an assumption about these technologies.

National ambient air quality standards (NAAQS), as defined by EPA, are to be maintained in each of the country's air quality control regions (AQCRS). Standards are set for "criteria pollutants," which are pollutants that are deemed because of their ubiquity and deleterious effects to warrant special attention. There are two types of NAAQS, primary and secondary. Primary standards are set at a level which is judged necessary to protect public health. Secondary standards are more onerous and are set to protect the public welfare from any known or anticipatory effect of the pollutant.

NAAQS have been set for the following six criteria pollutants: sulfur dioxide (SO_2), carbon monoxide (CO), nitrogen dioxide (NO_2), hydrocarbons (HC), total suspended particulates (TSP), and photochemical oxidants.

Air quality control regions (AQCR) are classified according to whether or not they meet the standards. Areas which violate the standards are termed *nonattainment* areas, and areas which meet them are called *attainment* areas or *prevention of significant deterioration* (PSD) areas. It is possible for a single AQCR to have a multiple classification; for example, an AQCR may be nonattainment for CO but attainment for SO_2.

Although they meet standards, PSD regions are still subject to growth controls to prevent a significant degradation in their air quality. In this context, PSDs are classified into three classes, and maximum allowable increments in ambient concentration are promulgated for each class. The classification is based on environmental and economic factors. For example, PSD class 1 areas, which include national parks and wilderness areas, are restricted to the smallest allowable ambient pollutant increments of the three classes.

Water-Quality Legislation

The Federal Water Pollution Control Act Amendments of 1972 (P.L. 92-500), as further amended by the Clean Water Act of 1977 (P.L. 92-217), are the analogue to the Clean Air Act. They set up a comprehensive framework, administered by the EPA, for water-quality management.

In discussing this legislation, a distinction must again be made between ambient and effluent standards. The *ambient standards* specify the permissible level of concentration of a pollutant in the watercourse; for example, the level of total dissolved solids in the stream should not exceed 500 milligrams per liter. The *effluent standards* specify the allowable pollutant discharge; for example, the suspended solids discharge should not exceed 0.04 pounds per ton of production. The ultimate objective of the legislation is improved ambient quality, and this is to be realized by minimizing effluent discharge.

In the setting of effluent standards, EPA plays a preeminent role. Not all facilities, however, are subject to effluent standards. In particular, facilities that are at zero discharge are not regulated. Facilities that discharge to sewers are to comply with EPA set pretreatment standards, which define the quality of the wastestream prior to discharge to the sewer; and the remaining facilities—the direct dischargers—must comply with EPA regulations defining the quality of the wastestream that can be discharged to so-called navigable waters.

In the setting of ambient water standards, EPA has only an advisory role. It periodically publishes ambient criteria based on the latest scientific knowledge on the effects of water-quality conditions on health and welfare. The criteria do not have the force of law, and the actual standards are set by the states, subject to EPA approval. In setting the standards, of course, the states take into consideration the EPA criteria.

Each state must promulgate ambient standards for all intrastate waters. These standards are to be reviewed, and if necessary modified, every 3 years. The standards reflect the uses to which the watercourse is put, since the quality requirements depend on the application. For example, alkalinity is a factor in the protection of aquatic life, but its presence or absence does not affect the use of water for drinking purposes.

Overview of the Model

There are basically three discrete stages involved in a complete air- or water-quality impact analysis. In the first stage, the amount of the pollutant discharged to the receiving airshed or waterbody is predicted. In the second stage, the change in the ambient air and water quality resulting from the increased discharge is quantified. In the third stage, the effect of the changed ambient quality on life, health, and property is estimated.

Procedures for modeling the first and second stages are reasonably well developed. Techniques for modeling the third stage are in a very experimental phase. In Simpact, the environmental modeling is restricted to the first stage. The second stage—the so-called dispersion or diffusion modeling—is highly site-specific and cannot be incorporated within the structure of a system like Simpact.

This section contains a summary of the three modeling stages and an overview of the Simpact Environmental Model's air and water components.

Air-Quality Modeling Concepts

Stage 1. Emissions modeling takes the form of multiplying emission factors by a pollution-causing activity level. The emission factor is in terms of the level of pollutant emitted per unit of activity, for example, grams of CO per automobile traveled. The activity level for the preceding example would be the number of automobile miles traveled.

In connection with emission sources, a distinction is made between point sources and area sources. A *point source* is a single, large, stationary source of pollution, such as a power plant. *Area sources* include homes, automobiles, and other polluting sources too small to be individually identified. The distinction between point sources and area sources has implications for the second modeling stage.

Stage 2. In the second stage of diffusion modeling, the objective is to determine the effect of the emission level of a pollutant on its concentration in the atmosphere. Because point sources are large-volume dischargers and since they typically emit the pollutants through stacks, the characteristics of the model used to translate their emission levels into changes in ambient air quality will differ from those used to quantify the ambient air-quality impacts of area sources. For example, point-source diffusion models will use stack height as an input, but this is not a relevant input for an area diffusion model.

In translating changes in emission levels to changes in ambient quality, the simplest model is the proportional rollback. According to this model, a reduction (or increase) in emission will cause a corresponding reduction (or increase) in ambient concentration levels.

More sophisticated diffusion models take into account the physical and chemical forces that affect a pollutant after it has been discharged into the air. Among these forces are wind, rain, and the dilution of the pollutant in the atmosphere. Inputs to these models describe the characteristics of the generating source as well as various meteorological parameters.

Stage 3. In this stage, the damage resulting from a change in ambient air quality is estimated. Damage will include losses to property and life. Corroding of property and increased incidence of lung disease and heart attack are among the problems caused by air pollution. Carbon monoxide, for example, has a particularly harmful effect on patients with angina pectoris, a form of heart disease.

The development of a damage function relating changes in ambient quality to a societal cost index is a very ill-defined area. There is inadequate empirical evidence on the precise effects on property and life of changed air quality, and the assignment of a monetary value to these effects is highly subjective.

Simpact Air Model Overview. Figure 6-1 contains a schematic overview of the air component of the Simpact Environmental Model. The circles denote Economic and Demographic Model solutions and diamonds indicate Environmental Model Solutions.

Predicted in the model are the emissions from automobiles, trucks, residential energy combustion, and secondary industrial energy combustion. The emissions from specific point sources are exogenously added in to give total emissions.

Automobile and truck emissions are predicted as a function of vehicle miles traveled (VMT). The VMT is determined by the employment and population solutions of the Economic and Demographic Model. Combustion-related emissions are naturally predicted as a function of the energy usage. The energy consumption rates are also determined from solutions of the Economic and Demographic Model.

Water-Quality Modeling Concepts

Stage 1. In this stage, the volume of discharge to the watercourse is predicted and its composition characterized. In characterizing the discharge, the important parameters are biochemical oxygen demand (BOD), suspended solids, total dissolved solids, oil and grease, inorganic nitrogen, and inorganic phosphate.

Effluent modeling takes the form of multiplying an activity variable by a unit wastewater-generation rate to get the wastewater discharged and then multiplying wastewater by effluent rates. In the case of a zinc smelter, the activity variable would be tons of zinc produced, the wastewater rate would be gallons of discharge per ton of production, and the effluent rates would consist of such variables as pounds of BOD per gallon of discharge.

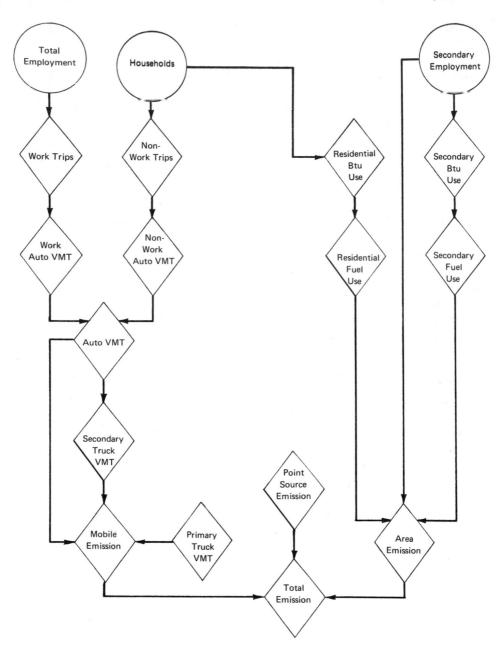

Figure 8-1. Air-Emissions Projections

Stage 2. In the second stage, the effect of the effluent discharge on ambient water quality is computed. It is possible, for example, to predict the effect on the dissolved oxygen (DO) content in the waterbody of a BOD discharge. When organic wastes enter a waterbody, they are decomposed and assimilated, in the process reducing the DO content of the stream. The BOD content of a discharge is a measure of the amount of oxygen required to decompose the organic wastes in the discharge, and the greater the BOD, the worse the effect on DO. The DO content of a stream is important because very low DO levels will kill aquatic life. Therefore, it is of interest to predict the effect of a BOD discharge on DO. The effect of BOD on DO is expressed in the form of a U-shaped oxygen-sag curve. The maximum reduction in DO will occur some distance from the point of discharge. Then it will usually begin to rise again. The shape of the curve can be predicted using models which require as inputs BOD discharge rates and various hydrological parameters.

Stage 3. In this stage, the losses resulting from the decreased ambient water quality are estimated. Doing this will require determining how each waterbody use is impaired by the increased pollutant concentration and assigning a monetary value to this impairment. In some cases there may be straightforward ways to make this assignment. For example, degradation in the water quality will result in higher treatment costs to make it potable, and this incremental expenditure represents the cost of the pollution in this application. For other uses, highly subjective procedures will have to be used to develop a monetary cost. The loss of swimmable water is an example of a use to which it is hard to assign a dollar estimate.

Simpact Water Model Overview. Figure 8-2 is a schematic depiction of the water component of the Simpact Environmental Model. The circles stand for Economic and Demographic Model solutions, the rectangles for Community Planning Model solutions, and the diamonds for the Environmental Model solutions.

The model predicts wastewater discharges by different sources. There are three major categories: runoff, industrial discharges, and sewer, that is, publicly owned treatment works (POTW), discharges.

Runoff is water which travels overland and enters the stream from myriad sources. Rainfall ends up as runoff unless it is infiltrated into the soil, evaporates, or is otherwise intercepted. The degree of interception is lower for unpaved than for paved areas. In the Simpact Environmental Model, incremental runoff flows are predicted as a function of paved land area.

Industrial discharges are predicted as a function of sectoral employment. The function takes into account the possibility that industry might be at zero discharge or discharging to a POTW.

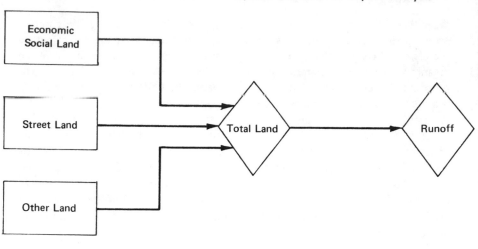

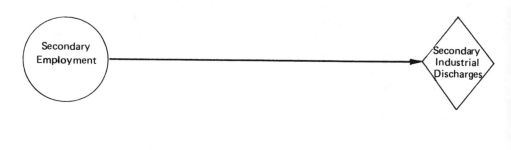

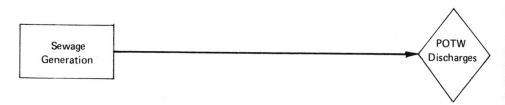

Figure 8-2. Water-Effluent Projections

After treating sewage, the POTW will probably discharge some of residues to a receiving stream. In Simpact, POTW discharges are predicted as a function of their sewage intake.

Air Emissions Modeling

The purpose of the air analysis is to predict the emissions of five of the six criteria pollutants. The model predicts emissions of the four gaseous pollutants—sulfur dioxide, nitrogen dioxide, carbon monoxide, and hydrocarbons—and of total suspended particulates. The model does not attempt to handle the sixth criteria pollutant, photochemical oxidants. This pollutant is produced by the interaction during sunlight between hydrocarbons and nitrogen dioxide and cannot be predicted using emission factors.

Emission Sources

The major source of sulfur dioxide emissions is the burning of fossil fuels, in particular coal and oil. Utilities generate about half the total national sulfur dioxide emissions, as they burn fuel to generate electricity. Coal-fired utilities contribute relatively more, because in obtaining a given heat, coal causes more than twice the sulfur dioxide emissions that would be generated by oil and many thousand times the emissions that would result from natural gas. The application of scrubbers or the use of low-sulfur coal can substantially reduce the utility coal-emission problem.

About 40 percent of the national nitrogen dioxide emissions are caused by fossil-fuel-fired electric utilities and industrial fuel burning. In connection with NO_2 emissions, it should be noted that coal, oil, and natural gas for a given heat production generate approximately the same emissions. Residential burning of oil and gas for space heating and the use of vehicles are the other major sources of NO_2. Among the mobile sources, heavy-duty diesel trucks are on a unit basis large polluters; each mile they travel causes almost ten times as much NO_2 as does a car traveling the same distance.

Vehicles are responsible for most of the carbon monoxide emissions and a significant percentage of hydrocarbon emissions. Important stationary contributors to the hydrocarbon problem are the petroleum and petrochemical industries.

Particulates are the most ubiquitous of the pollutants. They are generated by electric utilities, industrial and residential fuel combustion, industrial processes, and vehicle travel.

To model emissions, it is clearly necessary to have predictions of vehicle miles traveled (VMT); utility, industrial, and residential fossil-fuel consumption; and industrial production. Given these predictions, forecasts of emissions simplify to multiplying the activity level by an appropriate emissions factor. Forecasts of industrial production have already been generated in the Economic and Demographic Model, but the Simpact Environmental Model has to predict VMT and energy consumption to provide the complete activity base for the emission calculations. The emission factors themselves are available in the EPA document, *Compilation of Air Pollutant Emission Factors*. This publication is referred to as "AP-42" and is updated by periodic supplements.

Mobile Source Emissions

The increased economic and demographic activity will augment the flow of traffic in the region. The unit to measure this flow is vehicle miles traveled. The projection of VMT is in itself a discipline around which a wide body of literature has grown. Most VMT projections are performed as part of transportation planning studies and consequently are stand-alone studies without the benefit of economic and demographic inputs. In Simpact, the VMT projections can draw on the variables predicted in the Economic and Demographic Model. Because of this, the VMT analysis of Simpact is much simpler than that used in transportation planning studies. It is useful, nevertheless, to start with a brief review of conventional stand-alone VMT modeling.

VMT Models. Stand-alone VMT modeling involves three steps: trip generation, trip distribution, and trip assignment. Trip generation involves predicting how many trips will be produced from zone i (T_i) and how many trips will be attracted to zone j (T_j). In the trip-distribution stage, trip interchanges (T_{ij}) are calculated, with trip interchanges defined as the number of trips produced from zone i that end up in zone j. Trip assignment consists of simulating the effect that trip interchanges (T_{ij}) will have on road network.

Trip generation is based on regression analysis. The number of trips that will be produced from a zone is estimated by entering the demographic characteristics of the community—such variables as income and population—into a regression equation in which such characteristics are the independent variables and trips produced is the dependent variable. Predicting trip attraction involves analagous procedures. Trips attracted to a zone will be the dependent variable, and variables such as retail floorspace and employment will be the independent variables.

There are various trip-distribution models that can be used in computing the number of trips that start in zone i and end in zone j. In the gravity model, one of the most popular of the trip-distribution models, T_{ij} is a positive function of both T_i and T_j and a negative function of C_{ij}, where C_{ij} is defined as the distance or some other measure of the impedance between the two zones.

In trip assignment, the actual routes that the trip interchanges will involve are approximated. A coded description of the highway network is entered into the program, and the computer uses an algorithm to find the minimum impedance route between zones, in the process determining traffic loads by route.

Simpact VMT Coverage. For the purpose of the Environmental Model, all that is required is a VMT forecast. Disaggregation by highway route is not necessary, so trip assignment can be excluded. Similarly, there is only one zone of analysis, so trip distribution is also not necessary. Therefore, in Simpact, the VMT analysis reduces to predicting the number and length of trips attracted to and produced from a region. In the model, VMT is disaggregated by automobile, light-duty gasoline trucks (less than 6,000 pounds gross vehicle weight), heavy-duty gasoline trucks (more than 6,000 pounds), and heavy-duty diesel trucks. This disaggregation is largely motivated by the different emission characteristics of these vehicle types.

Equation 8.1: Work-Related Automobile Trips. In this equation, the number of automobile work-related trips is computed. First, employees are multiplied by a trip factor to give the annual number of person trips in the region. The trip factor is equal to twice the annual workdays, since there is a daily trip from home to work and from work back to home. Then person trips are converted to vehicle trips by multiplying by a car-occupancy factor. The occupancy factor is the reciprocal of the car-pooling rate: for example, three people per car would translate into an occupancy factor of 0.33. There are separate occupancy factors for each demographic group, because commuting construction workers, for example, tend to have a much greater tendency to car pool.

Equation 8.2: Work-Related VMT. In this equation, work-related automobile VMT is computed by multiplying work-related automobile trips by the average trip length. Since the objective of the analysis is restricted to predicting emissions in the region of analysis, the trip length must include only the distance traveled within the region.

Equations 8.3 through 8.5: Nonwork-Related Automobile VMT. In equation 8.3, the number of nonwork-related person trips is computed as a function of the number of households. Surveys have been made to determine the number of nonwork-related person trips taken by a household; a typical value is around 1,000 with higher values for wealthy households or those in rural communities.

In equation 8.4, person trips are converted to automobile trips by multiplying by a car-occupancy rate; and in equation 8.5, automobile trips are converted to VMT by multiplying by an average nonwork-related trip length.

Equation 8.6: Total Automobile VMT. In this equation, total automobile VMT is computed by summing work-related VMT from equation 8.2 and nonwork-related VMT from equation 8.5.

Equations 8.7 and 8.8: Truck VMT. In equation 8.7, truck VMT is computed as a function of automobile VMT. Typical ratios of truck to automobile VMT are published in the EPA's AP-42 publication. It reports light-duty gasoline truck VMT at 14.7 percent of automobile VMT, heavy-duty gasoline truck VMT at 5.7 percent, and heavy-duty diesel truck VMT at 4.0 percent.

The EPA published ratios do not allow for the especially high heavy-duty diesel truck VMT created by a large-scale project. In equation 8.8, total truck VMT is calculated by adding an exogenous estimate of primary truck VMT to the solution of equation 8.7.

Equations 8.9 and 8.10: Automobile and Truck Emissions. In equation 8.9, automotive emissions of the five criteria pollutants are calculated by multiplying automobile VMT by emission factors, which give the grams of pollutant emitted per VMT. The emission factors depend on a number of forces, most important of which is the fleet composition, since new cars have much lower emission rates. Other determinants of the emission rate are the ambient temperature and the vehicle speed. Procedures to derive "composite emission factors" which incorporate these forces are explained in AP-42. In equation 8.10, truck emissions are calculated in an analagous manner.

Stationary Emissions

Stationary emissions include area sources, such as homes and small businesses which are too small to individually identify, and point sources, such as major industrial facilities which emit pollutants through stacks. Generally most, if not all, of the secondary emissions will be of the area type. Supermarkets, department stores, and other such secondary activities are all area sources. In Simpact, area emissions from residential and industrial energy combustion are predicted. Point-source emissions, if any, are exogenously added in.

Equations 8.11 through 8.13: Residential Energy Consumption. In the last few years, highly sophisticated econometric models of energy demand have been built. Such sophistication is not warranted for an impact analysis, in which energy consumption only constitutes the input to emissions computations. However, such an analysis can make use of predictions generated by such models. A useful source in this context is the Energy Information Administration, which is responsible for modeling and forecasting within the Department of Energy.

In Simpact, residential energy consumption in physical units—that is, in gallons of oil, million cubic feet of gas, and kilowatt hours of electricity—is predicted in a three-step procedure. In equation 8.11, total residential energy consumption in British thermal units (Btus) is computed by multiplying population by a residential-energy-consumption-per-capita variable. In equation 8.12, consumption of oil, gas, and electricity in Btus is computed by multiplying the solution from the preceding equation by the shares accounted for by each of the three energy forms. In equation 8.13, the fuel consumption in physical units is calculated by dividing the Btu solutions of the preceding equations by the appropriate conversion factors.

Equation 8.14: Residential Emissions. In this equation, residential emissions are calculated by multiplying energy-consumption-by-fuel, as predicted by equation 8.13, by emission factors. The emission factor for oil and gas can be directly read from AP-42. Deriving an emission factor for electricity is more complicated and warrants some explanation.

Oil- and gas-burning emissions occur in the home in which the fuel is used, but the use of electricity does not result in any emissions at the place of use, rather the emissions occur at the utility at which the electricity is generated. The emission factor for electricity is a product of two terms: the fossil-fuel units required to generate a kilowatthour and the emission per fossil fuel unit. Since the type of fossil fuels used vary by utility, the emission factor is utility-specific.

Equations 8.15 through 8.17: Industrial Energy Consumption. The procedures to calculate secondary industrial consumption are similar to those used to derive residential consumption. In equation 8.15, energy consumption by sector (in Btus) is calculated by multiplying sectoral employment by an energy-consumption-per-employee variable. In equation 8.16, the industrial consumption by fuel type—oil, gas, coal, and electricity—is estimated by multiplying the prediction of the preceding equation by fuel shares. In equation 8.17, the Btu predictions of equation 8.16 are put on a physical-unit basis by using conversion factors.

Equations 8.18 and 8.19: Industrial Emissions. In equation 8.18, combustion-related emissions are calculated by multiplying industrial fuel consumption by emission factors. In equation 8.19, noncombustion-related industrial emissions are calculated as a function of sectoral employment.

Equation 8.20: Total Emissions. In this equation, total emissions are calculated by summing pollutants generated by automobiles, trucks, residential energy use, industrial energy use, and industrial processes.

Water-Effluent Modeling

The purpose of water modeling is to predict the volume of effluent discharged. The effluents predicted include BOD, suspended solids, and dissolved solids. The sources modeled are POTW discharges, secondary industrial discharges, and runoff.

Equations 8.21 and 8.22: POTW Discharges. In equation 8.21, the volume of treated sewage that is discharged by the publicly owned treatment works is computed. Discharge levels are solved as a function of sewage intake, a variable that has been computed in the Community Planning Model. In equation 8.22, the chemical composition of the POTW discharge, in terms of such parameters as BOD, is determined by multiplying the discharge by effluent parameters.

The effluent composition of the discharge will depend on the treatment technology of the POTW. For a new POTW, treatment will generally involve primary and secondary processing as well as removal of phosphorous and ammonia. Primary treatment involves removal of solid materials, and secondary treatment involves the use of processes to biologically decompose degradable wastes.

Equations 8.23 and 8.24: Industrial Discharges. In equation 8.23, the volume of secondary industrial discharge by sector is predicted as a function of sectoral employment. In equation 8.24, effluent loadings are calculated by multiplying the discharge by effluent factors.

Not all industrial facilities discharge to navigable waters. Some facilities are at zero discharge; that is, they do not have any discharges, but dispose of their water through such techniques as evaporation. Others discharge to POTWs. In developing discharge factors, these considerations must be kept in mind, as must the environmental legislation stipulating the allowable discharges. All point-source dischargers must obtain a national pollutant discharge elimination system (NPDES) permit, which will define the concentration and volume of effluents that can be discharged.

Equations 8.24 through 8.26: Runoff. In equation 8.25, the volume of runoff is predicted by multiplying paved land area by an incremental runoff-per-acre factor. In equation 8.26, the effluent characteristics of the runoff are calculated by multiplying the runoff volume by effluent factors. The open and paved land-area input to equation 8.25 is generated in equation 8.24 as the sum of the land areas associated with industry, housing, educational infrastructure, social infrastructure, and streets. These individual land-area solutions have been computed in the Community Planning Model.

Runoff which enters a waterbody from myriad sources is among the most serious of the water-pollution problems. Considerable progress has been made in controlling discharges by the point sources, such as POTWs and industrial facilities, but the problem of runoff has not yet been addressed. The volume of runoff depends on the precipitation in the region as well as its topography. For example, in areas with heavy rainfall, there is likely to be a high volume of runoff. The effluent characteristics of the flow will also be region-specific. The composition of agricultural runoff, for example, is quite different from that of urban stormwater runoff.

The increased urbanization resulting from a large-scale project increases the volume of runoff in the region, because runoff from paved areas is much greater than from unpaved areas, since the paved areas will not intercept the flow of water toward a receiving waterbody. The incremental runoff coefficient used in equation 8.24 is designed to account for this; it is equal to the excess of runoff per acre of paved area over the runoff per acre of unpaved area.

The runoff equations conclude the Secondary Environmental Model of Simpact. Off-line analysis is required to put the output into a form that is usable. In the case of water-quality analysis, this may take the form of identifying the impacted waterbodies and gauging the change in their ambient quality resulting from the increased effluent discharge.

Appendix 8A:
Equations

This appendix lists the equations in the Simpact Environmental Model. The output variables are denoted by YN, the Y indicating output and the N indicating environmental; the input variables are identified by XN. The variables are numbered by the order of their appearance. Thus YN_1 is the first output variable of this model and XN_1 is the first input variable. This model also makes use of solutions from the Economic Demographic Model (identified by YE) and the Community Planning Model (YC).

$$YN_1 = \Sigma[\overset{b}{\Sigma}(\overset{d}{YE}_{17(b,d)}) \times XN_1 \times XN_{2(b)}] \tag{8.1}$$

where YN_1 = Number of work-related automobile trips

$YE_{17(b,d)}$ = Total employees in demographic group b who are in income group d

XN_1 = Annual number of person trips per employee

$XN_{2(b)}$ = Automobile work-related car occupancy rate for demographic group b

$$YN_2 = YN_1 \times XN_3 \tag{8.2}$$

where YN_2 = Work-related automobile VMT

YN_1 = Number of work-related automobile trips

XN_3 = Average work-related trip length in region

$$YN_3 = \overset{de}{\Sigma\Sigma}(YE_{23(d,e)} \times XN_{4(d,e)}) \tag{8.3}$$

where YN_3 = Number of nonwork-related person trips

$YE_{23(d,e)}$ = Mover households in income group d and family group e

$XN_{4(d,e)}$ = Number of nonwork-related person trips per household of income group d and family group e

$$YN_4 = YN_3 \times XN_5 \tag{8.4}$$

where YN_4 = Number of nonwork-related automobile trips

YN_3 = Number of nonwork-related person trips

XN_5 = Automobile nonwork-related car occupancy rate

$$YN_5 = YN_4 \times XN_6 \qquad (8.5)$$

where YN_5 = Nonwork-related automobile VMT

YN_4 = Number of nonwork-related person trips

XN_6 = Average nonwork-related trip length in the region

$$YN_6 = YN_2 + YN_5 \qquad (8.6)$$

where YN_6 = Total automobile VMT

YN_2 = Work-related automobile VMT

YN_5 = Nonwork-related automobile VMT

$$YN_{7(i)} = YN_6 \times XN_{7(i)} \qquad (8.7)$$

where $YN_{7(i)}$ = Secondary truck VMT in truck category i

YN_6 = Total automobile VMT

$XN_{7(i)}$ = Ratio of truck VMT of category i to automobile VMT

$$YN_{8(i)} = YN_{7(i)} + XN_{8(i)} \qquad (8.8)$$

where $YN_{8(i)}$ = Total truck VMT in truck category i

$YN_{7(i)}$ = Secondary truck VMT in truck category i

$XN_{8(i)}$ = Primary truck VMT in truck category i

$$YN_{9(j)} = YN_6 \times XN_{9(j)} \qquad (8.9)$$

where $YN_{9(j)}$ = Automobile-generated emissions of pollutant j

YN_6 = Total automobile VMT

$XN_{9(j)}$ = Automobile emission factor for pollutant j

$$YN_{10(j)} = \overset{i}{\Sigma}(YN_{8(i)} \times XN_{10(i,j)}) \qquad (8.10)$$

where $YN_{10(j)}$ = Truck-generated emissions of pollutant j

$YN_{8(i)}$ = Total truck VMT in truck category i

$XN_{10(i,j)}$ = Emission factor for truck category i for pollutant j

$$YN_{11} = YE_{25} \times XN_{11(r)} \tag{8.11}$$

where YN_{11} = Total residential energy consumption in Btus

     YE_{25} = Total in migrating population

    $XN_{11(r)}$ = Residential energy consumption in Btus per capita

$$YN_{12(r)} = YN_{11} \times XN_{12(r)} \tag{8.12}$$

where $YN_{12(r)}$ = Residential energy consumption of fuel type r in Btus

     YN_{11} = Total residential energy consumption in Btus

    $XN_{12(r)}$ = Residential share of fuel type r

$$YN_{13(r)} = YN_{12(i)} + XN_{13(i)} \tag{8.13}$$

where $YN_{13(r)}$ = Residential energy consumption in physical units of fuel type r

    $YN_{12(r)}$ = Residential energy consumption of fuel type r in Btus

    $XN_{13(r)}$ = Conversion factor for fuel type r

$$YN_{14(j)} = \overset{r}{\Sigma}(YN_{13(r)} \times XN_{14(r,j)}) \tag{8.14}$$

where $YN_{14(j)}$ = Residential combustion-generated emissions of pollutant j

    $YN_{13(r)}$ = Residential energy consumption in physical units of fuel type r

    $XN_{14(r,j)}$ = Emission of pollutant j for residential consumption of a unit of fuel type r

$$YN_{15(c)} = YE_{14(c)} \times XN_{15(c)} \tag{8.15}$$

where $YN_{15(c)}$ = Total energy consumption in Btus by sector c

    $YE_{14(c)}$ = Secondary employees in sector c

    $XN_{15(c)}$ = Energy requirement in Btus per sector c employee

$$YN_{16(c,r)} = YN_{15(c)} \times XN_{16(c,r)} \tag{8.16}$$

where $YN_{16(c,r)}$ = Consumption by sector c of fuel type r in Btus

    $YN_{15(c)}$ = Total energy consumption in Btus of sector c

$XN_{16(c,r)}$ = Share of fuel type r in sector c

$$YN_{17(r)} = \overset{c}{\Sigma}(YN_{16(c,r)} \div XN_{13(r)}) \tag{8.17}$$

where $YN_{17(r)}$ = Secondary industrial fuel consumption of fuel type r in physical units

$YN_{16(c,r)}$ = Consumption by sector c of fuel type r in Btus

$XN_{13(r)}$ = Conversion factor for fuel type r

$$YN_{18(j)} = \overset{r}{\Sigma}(YN_{17(r)} \times XN_{17(r,j)}) \tag{8.18}$$

where $YN_{18(j)}$ = Secondary industrial combustion-generated emissions of pollutant j

$YN_{17(r)}$ = Secondary industrial fuel consumption of fuel type r in physical units

$XN_{17(r,j)}$ = Emissions of pollutant j for industrial consumption of a unit of fuel type r

$$YN_{19(j)} = \overset{c}{\Sigma}(YE_{14(c)} \times XN_{18(c,j)}) \tag{8.19}$$

where $YN_{19(j)}$ = Secondary industrial noncombustion-related emissions of pollutant j

$YE_{14(c)}$ = Secondary employees in sector c

$XN_{18(c,j)}$ = Noncombustion-related emissions in sector c of pollutant j

$$YN_{20(j)} = YN_{9(j)} + YN_{10(j)} + YN_{14(j)} + YN_{18(j)} + YN_{19(j)} + XN_{19(j)} \tag{8.20}$$

where $YN_{20(j)}$ = Total emissions of pollutant j

$YN_{9(j)}$ = Automobile-generated emissions of pollutant j

$YN_{10(j)}$ = Truck-generated emissions of pollutant j

$YN_{14(j)}$ = Residential-combustion-generated emissions of pollutant j

$YN_{18(j)}$ = Secondary industrial combustion-generated emissions of pollutant j

$YN_{19(j)}$ = Secondary industrial noncombustion-related emissions of pollutant j

$XN_{19(j)}$ = Point-source emissions of pollutant j

$$YN_{21} = YC_{33(h=2)} \times XN_{20} \qquad (8.21)$$

where YN_{21} = POTW discharge

$YC_{33(h=2)}$ = Total gross sewage generation

XN_{20} = Ratio of POTW discharge to sewage intake

$$YN_{22(m)} = YN_{21} \times XN_{21(m)} \qquad (8.22)$$

where $YN_{22(m)}$ = POTW discharges of effluent m

YN_{21} = POTW discharge

$XN_{21(m)}$ = Factor for effluent m for POTWs

$$YN_{23(c)} = YE_{14(c)} \times XN_{22(c)} \qquad (8.23)$$

where $YN_{23(c)}$ = Secondary industrial point-source discharge for sector c

$YE_{14(c)}$ = Secondary employees in sector c

$XN_{22(c)}$ = Point discharge per employee in sector c

$$YN_{24(m)} = \overset{c}{\Sigma}(YN_{23(c)} \times XN_{23(c,m)}) \qquad (8.24)$$

where $YN_{24(m)}$ = Secondary industrial discharges of effluent m

$YN_{23(c)}$ = Secondary industrial point-sources discharges for sector c

$XN_{23(c,m)}$ = Factor for effluent m for sector c

$$YN_{25} = \overset{c}{\Sigma}(YC_{5(c)} + \overset{n}{\Sigma} YC_{12(n)} + \overset{f}{\Sigma} YC_{18(f)} + \overset{g}{\Sigma} YC_{25(g)} + YC_{29} \qquad (8.25)$$

where YN_{25} = Total open and paved land area

$YC_{5(c)}$ = Open and paved land area in sector c

$YC_{12(n)}$ = Open and paved land area for housing type n

$YC_{18(f)}$ = Open and paved land area for educational group f

$YC_{25(g)}$ = Open and paved land area for social infrastructure group g

YC_{29} = Paved land area associated with streets

$$YN_{26} = YN_{22} \times XN_{24} \qquad (8.26)$$

where YN_{26} = Runoff

YN_{22} = Total open and paved land area

XN_{24} = Runoff differential per acre of paved area

$$YN_{27(m)} = YN_{26} \times XN_{25(m)} \qquad (8.27)$$

where $YN_{27(m)}$ = Effluent m runoff

YN_{26} = Runoff

$XN_{25(m)}$ = Effluent m runoff factors

9 Conclusions

The preceding chapters have presented a complete description of a generalized socioeconomic impact system. This concluding chapter discusses some of the political and institutional factors involved in designing a system and disseminating its results. The material is presented from the perspective of a consultant working for a corporation to prepare the socioeconomic component of its environmental impact assessment (EIA).

Preproject Interactions

The legislative and institutional background against which the consulting system designer must work is far from conducive to product development. Reviewing and critiquing his work are a diverse collection of special interest groups, most of whom know little about socioeconomic impact modeling but all of whom nevertheless have very legitimate interests in the analysis. Among the more important groups with whom the consultant must interact are the applicant, the lead agency, other agencies with major reviewing responsibilities, and local public-interest consortiums.

It will be necessary for the consultant to educate these groups about his system and incorporate their recommendations where appropriate. Prior to undertaking this educational role, the consultant will have to define to his own satisfaction the form his system will take on the particular project. This section explores both issues: the customization of a system to a project and the consultants interaction with the groups.

System Customization

Assuming that the consultant has a system such as Simpact, he will still find that plenty of work remains to be done on each new case in order to adapt his system to the specific characteristics of the project. An example is the best way to illustrate this issue. A project built in a truly desolate region, whose only attraction is its energy base, will have unique features. First, the construction workers will probably be housed in a camp site. Second, a complete new town may have to be built for the operation workers. Third, the owner of the proposed project may have to play a large role in providing housing and other supporting infrastructure. The situation described here is clearly somewhat different from that for which Simpact was developed and so will require a restructured system.

Restructuring a system will involve expanding portions of some models and deleting parts of others. If the original system has been programmed in a modular manner, such modifications need not be particularly expensive. By *modularization* is meant a system in which each model can be, if desired, run independently of the rest of the system.

To decide what type of customization is required, the system designer will have to thoroughly familiarize himself with the new project. He will have to interview the owner of the proposed facility, the construction contractor, and local officials. The familiarization thus acquired can allow him to specify the system for the new project.

Task Force Interactions

Once the specification has been completed, the designer must seek to get it approved. Failure to do so can be costly. When the EIA is turned over to the lead agency, the agency might find it unacceptable; or when the lead agency issues the draft environmental impact statement (DEIS), the reviewing agencies and public groups could find it inadequate. The likelihood of these problems can be minimized if the consultant, rather than working alone, confers early with both the lead agency and the reviewing groups.

An interagency task force should be set up prior to the EIA writing. The task force should consist of the applicant, the lead agency, the chief reviewing agencies, and local groups. The task force should meet at regular intervals to review the work being performed by the consultant. These meetings will ensure that there is an understanding of the techniques being used by the consultant and an appreciation of the data limitations and other constraints under which the consultant must work.

As far as the socioeconomic impacts are concerned, the most important issue on which an early consensus should be reached is the system specification. To obtain such agreement, it is necessary to educate the task force about the system. They should be provided with a fairly complete documentation of the conceptual characteristics of the system. The documentation will include flowcharts and a list of equations. Since many members of the task force will have no familiarity with quantitative modeling, it will also be necessary to provide an intuitive description of the system logic.

Postproject System Applications

Once the project's environmental impact statement has been approved, the role played by the socioeconomic system should not end. It can be used as a tool for planning and monitoring. The ideal group to use the system for this purpose is what will be referred to here as the Regional Impact Commission (RIC).

The RIC would have been formed at the start of the EIS process and will have participated in the task force meetings. It will be made up of decision makers and planners from the impacted municipalities, water and sewer authorities, school districts, and counties. It will also include representatives from the applicant, private housing developers, and the state economic agency. The main purpose of the RIC will be to coordinate the building of infrastructure in each of the fiscal units.

At the time the project is approved, the RIC will have in its hands an EIS describing, year by year, the types of infrastructure that will be required as a result of the project. The EIS can be converted into a physical master plan which will identify each required infrastructure type and where and when it should be built. The plan will contain more detail than the EIS and may disagree with it in some respects. For example, the EIS might indicate that a new wing must be added to a school if a pupil-per-classroom ratio of 25 is to be maintained, but the RIC in specifying their plan could decide not to build it, thereby accepting a rise in the pupil-per-classroom ratio.

Once the plan has been finalized, construction bids on the priority infrastructure items can be requested. These are items that are required early and which provide an absolutely essential service.

To the extent possible, the RIC should try to defer requesting construction bids. This will give them an opportunity to assess, in light of early experience with the project, the accuracy of the forecasts on which their master plan is based. For example, it may be that the project's first 2 years indicate that in-migration is at a rate that is far lower than has been predicted in the EIS. Then the system can be rerun to determine how this affects the forecasts of infrastructure requirements and the master plan can be revised in this light. Thus the system can be used as a flexible monitoring device.

In conclusion, it should be noted that system methods are not a panacea. By definition, they contain rigidities that would not be present in a qualitative approach. However, as this book has hopefully demonstrated, system methods can provide comprehensive and consistent socioeconomic forecasts that can help the potential host communities in deciding whether or not they want a project. And if they do want the project, the forecasts can then help them in planning for the project and monitoring it as it progresses.

Bibliography

Books

Baram, Michael S. *Environmental Law and the Siting of Facilities.* Cambridge, Mass.: Ballinger, 1976.

Burchell, Robert W., and David Listokin. *The Environmental Impact Handbook.* New Brunswick, N.J.: Center for Urban Policy Research, Rutgers University, 1975.

Burchell, Robert W., and David Listokin. *The Fiscal Impact Handbook.* New Brunswick, N.J.: Center for Urban Policy Research, Rutgers University, 1978.

Forrester, Jay W. *Urban Dynamics.* Cambridge, Mass.: M.I.T. Press, 1969.

Harris, Curtis C. *Regional Economic Effects of Alternative Highway Systems.* Cambridge, Mass.: Ballinger, 1974.

House, Peter W. *Trading Off Environment, Economics, and Energy: EPA's Strategic Environmental Assessment System.* Lexington, Mass.: Lexington Books, 1977.

House, Peter W., and John McLeod. *Large-Scale Models for Policy Evaluation.* New York: Wiley, 1977.

Isaard, Walter. *Ecologic-Economic Analysis for Regional Development.* New York: Free Press, 1972.

Isaard, Walter, and Thomas W. Langford. *Regional Input-Output Study.* Cambridge, Mass.: M.I.T. Press, 1971.

Mills, Edwin S. *Studies in the Structure of the Urban Economy* Baltimore, Md.: John Hopkins Press, 1972.

Moak, Lennox L., and Albert M. Hillhouse. *Concepts and Practices in Local Government Finance.* Chicago, Ill.:Municipal Finance Officers Association, 1975.

Pugh, Robert E. *Evaluation of Policy Simulation Models.* Washington: Information Resources Press, 1977.

Rodgers, Joseph Lee. *Environmental Impact Assessment, Growth, Management, and the Comprehensive Plan.* Cambridge, Mass.: Ballinger, 1976.

Rogers, Andrei. *Matrix Analysis of Interregional Population Growth and Distribution.* Berkeley, Calif.: Univ. of California Press, 1968.

Articles

Aidala, James V. "Computer-Assisted Social Profiling: Some Uses of Computerized Data Banks on Social Impact Assessment." In Kurt Finsterbusch and C.P. Wolf, eds., *Methodology of Social Impact Assessment.* Stroudsburg, Penn.: Dowden, Hutchinson & Ross, 1977, pp. 167-171.

147

Caprio, Rosalie. "The Role of Secondary Impacts under NEPA." *Environmental Affairs* 6 (1977):127-154.

Cesario, Frank J. "Toward the Estimation of Transportation-Related Pollution." In Walter Isaard and Frank J. Cesario, eds., *Working Papers on the Use of Regional Science Techniques in Environmental Management*. Ithaca, N.Y.: Center for Urban Development Research, Cornell University, 1974, pp. 115-140.

Chern, Wen S., and William W. Lin. "Energy Demand for Space Heating in the United States" In G.S. Maddala, Wen S. Chern, and Gurmukh S. Gill, eds., *Econometric Studies in Energy Demand and Supply*, New York: Praeger, 1978, pp. 60-74.

Deutsch, Stuart L. "The National Environmental Policy Act's First Five Years," *Environmental Affairs* 4 (1975):3-80.

Erickson, Rodney A. "Sub-Regional Impact Multipliers: Income Spread Effects from a Major Defense Installation." *Economic Geography* 53 (1977): 283-294.

Gibson, James A. "A Review of Recent Extensions of Linear Economic Models to Regional Environmental Quality Analysis." *Journal of Environmental Systems* 6 (1976-1977):147-172.

Guldberg, Peter H., Frank H. Benesh, and Thomas McCurdy. "Secondary Impacts of Major Land Use Projects." *Journal of the American Institute of Planners* 43 (1977):260-270.

Isaard, Walter, "Regional Science and Research on Environmental Management." In Walter Isaard and Frank J. Cesario, eds., *Working Papers on the Use of Regional Science Techniques in Environmental Management*. Ithaca, N.Y.: Center for Urban Development Research, Cornell University, 1974, pp. 1-40.

Isaard, Walter, and Robert E. Kuenne. "The Impact of Steel Upon the Greater New York-Philadelphia Industrial Regions." *The Review of Economics and Statistics* 35 (1953):289-301.

Kohn, Robert E. "Input-Output Analysis and Air Pollution Control." in Edwin S. Mills, ed., *Economic Analysis of Environmental Problems*. New York: Columbia University Press, 1975, pp. 239-274.

Kornbluh, Marvin, and Denis Little. "The Nature of a Computer Simulation Model." *Technological Forecasting and Social Change* 9 (1976):3-26.

Lajic, J.E., and W.Y. Svrcek. "Environmental Impact Statement Preparation." *Journal of Environmental Systems* 5 (1975):115-120.

Lapping, Mark B. "Environmental Impact Methodologies: A Critique." *Environmental Affairs* 4 (1975):123-134.

Nelson, Paul E., and John S. Perrin. "A Short Cut for Computing Final Demand Multipliers: Some Empirical Results." *Land Economics* 54 (1978):82-91.

Peterson, George L., and Robert S. Gemmell. "Social Impact Assessment: Comments on the State of the Art." In Kurt Finsterbusch and C.P. Wolf, eds., *Methodology of Social Impact Assessment.* Stroudsbury, Penn.: Dowden, Hutchinson & Ross, 1977, pp. 374-387.

Putman, Stephen H. "Urban Land Use and Transportation Models: A State-of-the-Art Summary." *Transportation Research* 9 (1975):187-202.

Reiche, Johann-Michael. "Investigations into Regional Infrastructure Equipments." *Regional and Urban Economics* 2 (1972):1-24.

Schlager, Kenneth J. "A Land Use Plan Design Model." In David C. Sweet, ed., *Models of Urban Structure.* Lexington, Mass.: Lexington Books, 1972, pp. 53-67.

Sears, David W., Michael F. DiGiano, and Kenneth L. Hoagland. "Simulation of Residential Mobility: The Decision to Move Process and the Search for Selection Process." *Computers and Urban Society* 1 (1975):1-9.

Tipton, William R. "Environmental Considerations in Project Management." *Journal of Metals* (1977):18-21.

Documents

Arthur D. Little. *Report on the Environmental Impacts of U.S. Steel Corporation's Proposed Lakefront Plant.* Cambridge, Mass., 1978.

Battelle-Columbus Laboratories. *A Review of Environmental Impact Assessment Methodologies.* Springfield, Va.: National Technical Information Service, 1974.

Bjornstad, D.J. *Fiscal Impacts Associated with Power Reactor Siting: A Paired Case Study.* Oakridge, Tenn.: Oakridge National Laboratory, 1977.

Cohen, Alan S., and Kenneth W. Costello. *Regional Energy Modeling: An Evaluation of Alternative Approaches.* Springfield, Va.: National Technical Information Service, 1975.

Edelston, Bruce S. *The Development and Use of Employment Multipliers in Socioeconomic Impact Assessment.* Pittsburgh, Penn.: Westinghouse Electric Corporation, 1976.

Ford, Andrew. *Users Guide to the BOOMI Model.* Los Alamos, N.M.: Los Alamos Scientific Laboratory, 1977.

Ingram, Gregory K. *TASSIM: A Transportation and Air Shed Simulation Model.* Washington: Office of the Secretary, Department of Transportation, 1973.

Leistritz, Larry F., Edlon C. Schriner, and Steven H. Murdock. "An Assessment of Social and Economic Research Needs Related to Western Energy Development." Paper presented at Energy Research and Development Administration Public Meeting in Denver, Colorado, May 17-18, 1976.

Marks, David H. "Models in Water Resources." In Saul I. Gass and Roger L. Sisson, eds., *A Guide to Models in Governmental Planning and Operation.* Springfield, Va.: National Technical Information Service, 1974, 103-137.

Minnesota Energy Agency, Research Division. *MINTOM: Minnesota Tradeoff*

Model, Energy/Economy/Environment. St. Paul, Minn.: Research Division, 1975.

Murphy/Williams Urban Planning and Housing Consultants. *Socioeconomic Impact Assessment: A Methodology Applied to Synthetic Fuels.* Washington: U.S. Government Printing Office, 1978.

Pittenger, Donald B. "Practical Perspectives on Regional Demographic-Economic Forecast Models." In *Report of the Conference on Economic and Demographic Methods for Projecting Population.* Washington: American Statistical Association, 1977.

Rose, Adam Z. *A Dynamic Interindustry Model for the Economic Analysis of Air Pollution Abatement.* Ithaca, N.Y.: Center for Urban Development Research, Cornell University, 1976.

Sanderson, Debra, and Michael O'Hare. *Predicting the Local Impacts of Energy Development: A Critical Guide to Forecasting Methods and Models.* Cambridge, Mass.: Laboratory of Architecture and Planning, Massachusetts Institute of Technology, 1977.

Schaffer, William A., Eugene A. Laurent, and Ernest M. Sutter. *Using the Georgia Economic Model.* Atlanta, Ga.: College of Industrial Management, Georgia Institute of Technology, 1972.

Shields, Mark A. *Social Impact Assessment: An Analytic Bibliography.* Springfield, Va.: National Technical Information Service, 1974.

Singpurwalla, Nozer D. "Models in Air Pollution." In Saul I. Gass and Roger L. Sisson, eds., *A Guide to Models in Governmental Planning and Operation.* Springfield, Va.: National Technical Information Service, 1974, pp. 61-102.

Slidell, John B. *A Users Guide to the GE-UNC New Towns Financial Feasibility Model-Long Program.* Chapel Hill, N.C.: Center for Urban and Regional Studies, University of North Carolina at Chapel Hill, 1972.

State of Wyoming, Department of Economic Planning and Development. *Coal and Uranium Development of the Powder River Basin: An Impact Analysis.* Cheyenne, Wy.: Department of Economic Planning and Development, 1974.

Stenehjem, Erik J. *Forecasting the Local Economic Impacts of Energy Resource Development: A Methodological Approach.* Argonne, Ill.: Argonne National Laboratory, 1975.

Stone, Richard. *Demographic Accounting and Model Building.* Paris: Organization for Economic Cooperation and Development, 1971.

Toman, Norman E., Norman L. Dalsted, Arlen G. Leholm, Randall C. Coon, and Larry F. Leistritz. *Economic Impacts of Construction and Operation of the Coal Creek Electrical Generation Complex and Related Mine.* Fargo, N.D.: Department of Agricultural Economics, North Dakota State University, 1976.

Urbanomics Research Associates. *The Economic Impact of Kaiser Steel Corporation-Fontana on the Southern California Economy.* Claremont, California, 1975.

U.S. Department of Commerce, National Bureau of Standards. *Guidelines for Documentation of Computer Programs and Automated Data Systems.* Washington: U.S. Government Printing Office, 1976.

U.S. Department of Transportation, Federal Highway Administration, Urban Planning Division. *Urban Transportation Planning.* Washington: U.S. Government Printing Office, 1972.

U.S. Department of Transportation, Federal Highway Administration, Urban Planning Division. *Trip Generation Analysis.* Washington: U.S. Government Printing Office, 1975.

U.S. Environmental Protection Agency, Office of Air Quality Planning and Standards. *Compilation of Air Pollutant Emission Factors,* 2d ed. Research Triangle Park, North Carolina, Environmental Protection Agency, 1973.

Wakelin, Michael H. "Approaches to Impact Management." Paper presented at Atomic Industrial Forum Conference on Land Use and Nuclear Facility Siting, Denver, Colorado, July 20, 1976.

Watkins, George. *Development of a Social Impact Assessment Methodology (SIAM).* Columbus, Ohio: Battelle-Columbus Laboratories, undated.

Index

Index

Access systems, low and high speed, 14, 16
Accommodations, multifamily, 77
Age classification, 59
Agencies: federal, 2, 12, 23-25, 28, 121; lead, 25-26; local, 25; reviewing, 25-26, 144; state, 25
Aid: federal school, 108, 117-118; programs, 1, 108
Air: emissions, 3, 12, 28, 33, 121, 129-130; pollution, 125, 130; quality, 5, 121-125
Airports, 95; 24
Alkalinity, effects of, 123
Ambient: air quality, 124-125; temperature, 132; water quality, 122-123, 127
Ammonia, removal of, 134
Amortization, factor of, 95, 119
Amusement tax, 107
Apartments, 67
Apl language, 16, 38
Aquatic life, protection of, 24, 123
Arthur D. Little, Inc., 3, 12, 14-16
Assessment and assessed valuations, 94, 105-106, 115-117
Assets, capital, 110
Attainment areas, 122
Authority, definition of, 94-95
Automobile(s), 103, 121, 124; emission problem of, 125, 132, 138, 140; occupancy factor and car pooling, 131, 137-138; registration fees for, 105; speed and traffic factor of, 5, 132; work and nonwork related trips, 33, 131, 137-138

Base and baseline values, 45, 49, 74, 110
Biochemical oxygen demand (BOD), 125, 127, 133-134
Bonds: flotation of, 5, 95; general and limited obligation, 110; issuance of, 95; municipal, 110; serial, 110-111; term, 110-111

Borrowing activities, 110
Boroughs. See Towns and Townships
Budgets and budgetary problems, 31-34, 76, 96-99, 109
Building construction cost data, 71
Business: construction costs, 100, 102, 106; professional developers, ; properties, 115, 117; secondary, 108, 118; water usage, 78; wholesale and retail activities, 103

Canned routines, methods of, 16
Capital: annualized, 99, 101; assets, 110; costs, 80-81, 91-92, 95-96, 101-102; expenditures, 93; funds, 118-119; gains, 104; requirements, 109
Car pools, 131
Carbon monoxide (CO), 35, 121-122, 125, 129
Card storage, 15, 38; and computers, 21
Central water system, 79
Checklists, 27
Chemical residues, 3, 80, 124
Children, 68; age groups of, 59; in-migrating, 59, 66, 73, 85-86
Churches, 105
Clean Air Acts, 122-123
Coal: coking, 50; consumption of, 8-10; emission problems of, 129; exploitation of, 1; low sulfur, 9, 129; metallurgical, 9; steam, 9; and utilities, 129
Cobol written programs, 38, 43
Codes and coding, 4, 12, 9, 21, 24, 93
Collections: data, 11, 13, 20-21; information, 75; of sanitary waste water, 77
Commerce, Department of, 17, 25
Commercial sector, 5, 71, 78
Communications, means of, 11, 14, 40, 76

Community: host, 28, 49, 145; hosti-
tility, 28; rural, , 131; small, 67;
wealthy, 1, 106
Community Planning Model, 3-4, 9-10,
30-35, 57, 59, 67, 69, 81, 96, 101,
121
Commuters, viable factor of, 4, 31-34,
51-57, 104-107
Computer systems and computeri-
zation, 1-17, 20-21, 37, 43, 45
Conceptual Design Paper, 4, 7, 11-14,
18, 20
Constitution, Pennsylvania, 93, 95
Construction: bids, 145; costs, 4,
28-29, 34, 54, 68-71, 74-79, 83-90,
99-102, 106, 109, 115; educational,
102; housing, 1, 34, 67, 69, 96,
100-102; industry, 53, 55; for
schools, 95, 109-110, 118-119;
street, 100, 118; water system, 79;
workers, 2-3, 12, 31, 53-54, 131,
143
Consultants and consulting companies,
2, 25, 143
Consumers, 31, 56
Contaminant, 5. See also Pollution and
Pollutants
Contractor, 144
Control systems, 10, 15, 18, 38, 48
Corps of Engineers, 23
Corporate income taxes, 96-98, 101,
105, 113-114
Costs: annual, 110-111; capital, 80-81,
91-92, 95-96, 101-102; construction, 4, 28-29, 34, 54, 68-71,
74-79, 83-90, 99-102, 106, 109,
115; county, 118, 120; debt-
service, 109-111, 119-120; minimization of, 38; muniicpal, 118,
120; operating, 16, 75, 91-92, 95,
99-100, 109, 111, 118, 120; requirements, 71-72, 75; societal,
99-100, 25
County: Board of Commissioners, 94;
Codes, 93; debt service costs, 118,
120; fiscal analysis, 97, 109; jail,
94; operating costs, 118, 120;
parks, 99; responsibilities, 93; sher-

iff's department, 76; tax revenues,
99, 105, 114-115; transfers, 100,
107, 115

Data: and documentation, 20-21, 29;
files, 47; processing, 17; records, 7,
18, 37; tests, 8
Debts: amount of, 110; service,
109-111, 119-120; statutory limitations on, 95
Debugging, purpose of, 8, 17
Decisions and decision-makers, 14, 17,
145
Demography and demographic: activities, 30-34, 96, 121; characteristics,
130; composition, 2; development,
29; employee mix, 53-54; group-
ings, 56-58, 113; impact, 49, 93,
137; models, 3-4, 8-9; split, 4
Dental services, 08
Department stores, 132
Design objectives, 37-39
Development and developers, 16,
20-21, 29, 53-54, 77, 95, 145
Diesel trucks, heavy-duty, 129-132
Discharges: BOD, 127; effluent, 34-35,
127; industrial, 127-128, 133-134;
POTW, 35, 133-134; wastewater, 2,
34, 127
Disks, storage of, 16-19
Disposal of solid wastes, 77-81, 92
Dissolved oxygen (DO), 127
Documentation types, 11, 20-21
Draft environmental impact statement
(DEIS), 26, 144
Drainage systems, stormwater, 77-80

Economic: activities, 5, 67, 96, 121;
impacts, 2, 49, 93, 128; infrastructure, 67-71; models, 3-4, 8-9,
30-34; studies, 122-123, 128
Education: components of, 59; driver,
108; groups, 85-86, 117; infrastructure, 69, 73-75, 134; institutions for, 05; role of, 33, 141,
143; special, 108; staff requirements, 10; vocational, 108

Effluent: discharges, 34-35, 127; parameters, 134, 141; runoff factors, 142; water, 3, 12, 28, 34, 121, 123, 133-135

Electricity: consumption of, 132-133; generating of, 9, 129

Emissions: air, 3, 12, 28, 33, 121, 129-130; automobile, 125, 132, 138, 140; carbon monoxide, 129; combustion related, 125; control levels of, 122; factor of, 35, 124; gas, 133; hydrocarbon, 129; industrial, 133; nitrogen dioxide, 129; oil, 133; and pollutants, 124, 139-140; residential, 133; sources of, 5, 122, 24, 129-132; standards, 122; stationary, 132-133; sulfur dioxide, 3, 8-10, 129; sulfur dioxide, 3, 8-10; truck, 125, 132, 138, 140

Employee(s), 55, 62; floor-space variables for, 67, 71; income groups, 113-114; indirect, 51, 55-56, 62-64; induced, 63-64; mover, 64-65, 116-117; primary, 51-54, 61, 63; secondary, 51-53, 64, 83, 128; supplier, 51, 55, 64; weeklies, 57-58, 66, 84

Employment: analysis of, 57; functions of, 4, 30-31, 35, 97-98, 101-102; gross, 71; low, 28; net, 69-71; new source of, 1, 57; and production, 51-57; sectoral, 127, 133-134; total, 104-107; variables of, 49-50

Energy: combustion of, 34, 125, 132; consumption of, 35, 125, 129, 132-133, 139; forms of, 1, 9, 33; industrial, 35, 125, 132-133; nuclear development of, 1; residential, 35, 125, 139

Energy, Department of, 132

Energy Information Administration, 132

Enforcement: of laws, 75-76, 101; mechanism of, 2

Engineers and engineering practices, 2, 23, 78, 94

Enrollment, school, 69, 73-74, 101-102, 117

Environment: biotic, 24; changes in, 3, 123; human, 24, 27; legislation on, 134; models of, 5, 31-35; physical, 2, 24, 121; pseudo interactive, 38; variables, 30, 42

Environmental impact assessment (EIA), 2-3, 12-13, 26, 143-144

Environmental impact statement (EIS), 2, 4-5, 12, 23-29, 93, 121, 145

Environmental Protection Agency (EPA), 2, 25-26, 121-123, 130, 132

Error diagnostics, 18-19, 48

Exec programs, 28, 38-43

Executive Order 11514, 23

Exogenous variables, 9-10, 71

Factories, 34, 67

Family-size groups, 58-59, 65, 72, 137

Federal: agencies, 2, 12, 23-25, 28, 121; aid, 108, 117-118; regulations, 23; revenue sharing, 109; subsidies, 101; taxes, 55, 110

Federal Register, cited, 26

Federal Water Pollution Control Act, The, 123

Federal Water Quality Program, 121

Files and filing structure, 43-45, 48

Final environmental impact statement (FEIS), 26

Financing, private and public, 29, 67, 76

Fire protection, 34, 67, 69, 75-76

Fiscal: analysis, 97, 101-102, 109; changes, 2, 30, 93; forecasts, 2; model, 3, 5, 8, 31-34; self-sufficiency, 95

Floor space, availability of, 34, 67-71, 74, 83-86

Flow charts, 49, 144

Forecasting, systems of, 2, 29, 37, 145

Fortran-written programs, 16, 19, 38, 43, 45, 48

Fuel: consumption, 31, 140; boiler, 9; fossil, 129; industrial, 129, 140; residential, 129; tax transfers, 34,

Fuel: continued
    96-101, 104-107, 114-116
Functional specialists, 12-13, 20-21,
    40

Gas and gaseous pollutants, 129, 133
Gasoline, 103; consumption of, 114,
    132; trucks, 131-132
Geopolitics, factor of, 29
Guidelines for Documentation of the
    Computer Programs and Auto-
    mated Data Systems, 17

Hardware selections, 14-17
Hazardous wastes, 80
Health, Education and Welfare, De-
    partment of, 121
Health care, factor of, 76, 94
High school populations, 73, 108
High-speed access systems, 14-15
Highways, patrolling of, 76, 131. See
    also Streets
Hospitals, 95, 105
Households, 28, 52, 55, 68, 131; in-
    comes of, 72; in-migrating, 30, 34,
    51; mover, 58-59, 65-66, 71, 84,
    137; population of, 32, 57-59
Housing, 28, 54, 108, 134, 143; asses-
    sed value of, 115-117; and devel-
    opers, 145; predictions for, 29; and
    property taxes, 106; requirements
    of, subsidization of, 69; types, 4,
    141; units, 42, 67, 70-73, 84-88
Housing and Urban Development,
    Department of, 54
Houston-Galveston area, 54-56, Uni-
    versity of, 54
Human environmental, 24, 27
Hydrocarbons (HC), 122, 129
Hydrological parameters, 127

Identification and identifiers, types of,
    40, 46-47
Income: group, 58, 64-66, 72, 84,
    104, 113-114, 137; gross, 71;
    household, 72; levels of, 57, 72,
    109, 130; rental, 104; tax, 34, 94,
    96, 100-110, 114, 116; trust, 104

Independent variables, 130
Indirect: employees, 51, 55-56, 62-64;
    production, 50-51, 55, 62, 64
Industrial: discharges, 127-128,
    133-134; emissions, 80, 133; energy
    consumption, 35, 125, 132-133;
    fuel burning, 129, 40; processes,
    5, 129; sectors, 9, 71; water con-
    sumption, 78, 89
Industry, factor of, 9, 55, 95, 129,
    134
In-migrants, 3-4, 49, 54, 45
In-migrating: households, 30, 34, 51;
    population, 4, 30, 50, 58-59, 66,
    88, 91, 114-117; workers, 1
Inpt Exec program, 39-40, 43-48
Input variables, 10-14, 20-21, 28,
    37-38, 45-47, 51, 56, 61, 71, 73,
    83, 113
Institutions: public, 105, 143; sub-
    sidies for, 108, 117
Intangible personal property, 105
Interdisciplinary systems, 7
Interest, rates of, 104, 110-111
Intergovernmental transfers, 93, 96,
    101
Interior, Department of, 121
Intermodular relationships, 9

Labor force, availability of, 3, 49, 53,
    61
Land: areas, 28-29, 34, 67-74, 77, 79,
    83-87, 90, 134, 141-142; economic
    social, 128; fills, 67-70, 81, 91;
    rural, 77; street, 128; use of, 12,
    24, 121; values, 106
Large-scale analytical systems, 37-39
Law-enforcement requirements, 75-76,
    101
Lead agencies, 25-26
Legislation and legislative changes, ,
    122-123, 134, 143
Local: agency officials, 25, 144; gov-
    ernment, 93-95; groups, 144;
    streets, 69, 77; taxes, 55; unions,
    53
Lotax file, 41, 44, 47-48

Management and Budget, Office of, 25
Managing and management, impact of,
    75-76, 99
Manpower required, 53
Market values, 106, 115
Married people and households, 58, 65
Master plans, 145
Mathematical techniques, 37, 51
Matrix inversion, 16, 27
Medical services, 108
Meteorological parameters, 9, 27, 125
Modularization, 30-31, 144
Motor fuel tax revenues, 96, 101,
    104-107, 114-116
Movers, 31-34, 51-57, 104; employees,
    64-65, 116-117; households, 58-59,
    65-66, 71, 84, 137; population,
    65-66
Multifamily accommodations, 73, 77
Municipalities, activities of, 2, 34, 76,
    94, 97, 100, 106-107, 110, 113-116

National Air Pollution Control Admin-
    istration, 121
National Ambient Air quality stan-
    dards (NAAQS), 122
National Bureau of Standards, 17
National Environmental Protection
    Act (NEPA), 1-2, 23
National Marketing Institute, 72
National Oceanic and Atmospheric
    Administration, 25
National Pollutant discharge elimina-
    tion system (NPDES), 2, 134
Navigable waters, 2, 123, 134
Nitrogen, inorganic, 125
Nitrogen dioxide emissions (NO^2),
    122, 129
Nonattainment areas, 122
Nonelectoral debt, 110
Nonexmpt properties, 105
Nonurbanized regions, 51

Occupancy rate, car, 131, 137-138
Occupational groups, 53-56, 61-64
Ohio, 3, 104
Oil: burning of, 9; consumption of,
    125, 129, 132; crude, 3; emission

factor for, 133; shale, 1; tankers, 3
Operating costs, county, 118, 120
Operationalization, 4, 8-11
Oprin file, 40-41, 44-47
Oprout file, 44
Organic wastes, 127
Original residents, 4, 31-32, 51-57,
    104
Otpt Exec programs, 39, 42, 45
Output: analysis, 51; clarity, 38-39;
    format, 39; retrieval, 38-39, 42-43;
    terminal, 42-43; variables, 10-14,
    30, 40, 42, 61, 113
Oxygen, dissolved, 127

Parameterization, 4, 8-11, 18, 37, 134
Parking lot areas, 74
Parks and parklands, 94, 99, 123
Particulates, suspended, 22, 129
Pennsylvania, 3, 94-95; local govern-
    ment of, 93; school districts of,
    108; taxes in, 103-104, 107
Performance attributes, 16, 18
Personal income tax revenues, 105,
    117
Personnel: hiring of, 95; requirements,
    69, 75, 86; salaried, 76
Petrochemical complexes, 3, 129
Petroleum, 129; refineries, 3, 54-55
Phosphate, inorganic, 125
Phosphorous, removal of, 134
Photochemical oxidants, 122, 129
Physical: environment, 2, 24, 121;
    infrastructure analysis, 70, 77
Planners and planning, regional, 2, 76,
    145
Plant sites, 121
Play areas, 74
Police protection, 34, 67, 76, 94
Pollution and pollutants: air, 125,
    130; concentration of, 121, 127;
    control technologies, 122; criteria,
    122; gaseous, 129, 133; levels of,
    124, 129, 138-140; water, 134
Population: analysis, 57, 59; factor of,
    8-9, 28, 31, 35, 52, 68-70, 75,
    95-99, 102, 109, 125, 130; house-
    hold, 32, 57-59; in-migrating, 4, 30,

Population: continued
   50, 58-59, 66, 88, 91, 114-117;
   school, 73, 108; variables, 49-50
Prepoc program, 43-48
Prevention of significant deterioration
   (PSD), 122-123
Primary: employees, 51-54, 61, 63;
   facilities, 49-51, 54, 121; production, 31, 55; supplier, 63
Printouts and printing, 15, 42
Private: infrastructure, 34, 67-71; financing, 29, 67, 76; schools, 73
Production: and employment, 51-57;
   factor of, 49-50, 97-98; indirect,
   50-51, 55, 62, 64; primary, 31, 55,
   61-64; secondary, 50, 63-64, 13;
   spinoff, 49; supplier, 31, 50-55,
   61-62; total, 50, 64
Profits, ratio of, 103, 113
Programmers and programs, 11, 14-20
Property: assessment of, 94, 105-106;
   business, 115, 117; nonexempt,
   105; personal, 105; real, 105-106;
   sale of, 104; tax on, 28, 34, 94, 96,
   100, 102, 106-107, 15-117
Pseudo-interactive environment, 38
Public: financing, 29, 67, 76; groups,
   25; infrastructure demands, 34, 67,
   96; institution, 105, 143; interest
   consortiums, 143; school enrollment, 69, 73-74, 85-86, 101-102,
   117; services, 54; welfare, 122
Publicly owned treatment work systems (POTWS), 34, 35, 127,
   133-134, 141
Pupils, federal aid for, 108, 117-118

Quality: air, 122-125; legislation on,
   122-123; water, 25, 23-127, 135,
   145

Rainfall, 5, 35, 124, 127, 134
Raw sewage, 78
Raw water treatment facilities, 78-79
Real estate and realtors, 72, 96, 105,
   107
Recursive systems, 10-11

Refractory materials, 3, 50
Regional Impact Commission (RIC),
   145
Regionalism, framework of, 2, 5,
   29-30, 76, 121, 145
Regression analysis, 10, 37, 130
Regulations, imposing of, 23
Rent, income from, 71, 104
Report generation stage, 20, 43, 45
Rept program, 44-45
Reqst program, 45
Research and researchers, 9-12
Residences: and emissions, 133; en-
   ergy consumption, 35, 125, 139;
   and fuel combustion, 129; per-
   manent, 104, 107; and water con-
   sumption, 21, 78, 88-89; wastes
   from, 80
Residents, original, 4, 31-32, 51-57,
   104
Resource Conservation and Recovery
   Act (RCRA), 80
Retail: floorspace, 130; trade, 51, 103,
   113
Retrieval operations, 38-39, 42-43
Revenue(s), 5, 31; changes in, 3; government, 28; from motor fuels, 96,
   101, 104-107, 114-116; municipal,
   107; from property, 34, 96,
   115-117; school districts, 117-118;
   sharing, 109; state, 96-98, 105,
   113-114; and taxes, 12, 93, 96,
   113-117
Reviewing agencies and groups, 25-26,
   144
Robert Snow Means Company, Inc.,
   71
Rollbacks, proportional, 124
Runoffs, factor of, 5, 31-35, 79,
   127-128, 133-135, 142
Rural areas, 3, 76-77, 80, 93

Sales: of property, 104; taxes on,
   96-98, 103
Sanitary: landfills, 81; sewage disposal,
   31, 77-78
Sanitation facilities, 1, 4, 67, 94
Scenario files, 41, 47

School(s), 28, 34, 67; administration
of, 95; district, 3-5, 95, 99, 108,
113, 145; enrollments, 69, 73-74,
80-86, 101-102, 117; fiscal analysis,
97, 101-102; in Pennsylvania, 108;
population, 73, 108; private, 73;
revenues, 96, 117-118; space for,
74; taxes, 108, 118; teachers, 95;
vocational, 93-94; water use by, 1
Scrubbers, application of, 10, 129
Secondary: business, 108, 118; economic infrastructure, 67-71; employees, 51-53, 64, 83, 128; environmental changes, 3, 123;
production, 50, 63-64, 113; truck
VMT, 138
Sedimentation, factor of, 79
Selection and selectivity, 14-17, 38, 47
Self-sufficiency, fiscal, 95, 110
Serial bonds, 110-111
Service sectors, 1, 15, 34, 54, 56, 75
Sewage, 35, 70; generation, 69, 88-89,
128; raw, 78; sanitary disposal, 31,
77-78; treatment works, 95, 134
Sewer distribution systems, 69-70, 80,
89-91, 123, 127, 145
Shale oil, 1
Simpact system, 3, 7, 13-16, 19-20,
23, 35-39, 45, 49, 96
Single-family homeowners, 71-73;
housing units, 77; mover employ-
ees, 65; people, 58
Sinking funds, interest on, 110
Site-specific environmental impact,
121
Snow, runoff of, 35
Social: disruptions, 1; environment, 2;
infrastructure categories, 67-69, 75,
86-87, 101, 118, 128, 134, 141;
scientists, 7; services, 1, 34
Socioeconomic impact system, 2, 5,
12, 23, 28, 143-145
Sociology and sociologists, 2, 4, 12,
31, 49
Software decisions and selections, 14,
16, 37
Solid waste(s), 12, 70; collection, 101;
disposal, 34, 77-81, 92; dissolved,

125, 133; generation rates, 20,
80-81, 91-92, 121; landfills, 67, 69;
system for, 81, 118-119
Spatial requirements, 71-74, 77, 79
Specialists, functional, 12-13, 20-21,
40
Specification, tasks of, 4, 9, 11
Spinoff productions, 4, 49
Staff requirements, educational, 10,
75
Standard and Poors financial service,
110
Standardization, degrees of, 74,
122-123
State: agencies, 25; highways, 76, 131;
income taxes, 106, 110; instructional aid, 117; motor fuel tax rev-
enues, 97-99, 101, 103, 105,
113-115; police, 76; subsidies, 108,
117; transfers, 107
Stationary emissions, 122, 132-133
Statutory limitations, 110
Steel: industry, 9, 50; mills, 3, 31
Storage facilities: disk, 16, 18-19; files,
15; tape, 16; water, 79
Stores and supermarkets, 67, 132
Storm sewer network, 69-70, 80,
90-91
Storm waters, drainage systems for,
77-80, 134
Streets, construction and maintenance
of, 3-4, 67-70, 74-77, 87-90, 107,
128, 131, 134, 141
Studies, socioeconomic, 5; transportation, 130
Subsidies: federal, 101; housing, 69;
instructional, 108, 117; state,
101-102, 108
Sulfur dioxide (SO^2), 3, 8-10, 35, 122,
129
Sulphuric acid plants, 122
Supplier: employees, 50-55, 64; primary, 63; and production, 31,
50-55, 61-64
Supplies, purchasing systems of, 21,
55, 95
Suspended: particulates, 122, 129;
solids, 125, 133

Swimmable, water, loss of, 127

Tankers, oil, 3
Tapes, use of, 15-16
Task forces, 14
Taxes and tax system: alcoholic beverages, 96, 105; amusement, 107; and assessed valuations, 05; collecting of, 76; county, 99, 105, 114-115; cuts in, 41; exempt status factor, 110; federal, 55, 110; income, 34, 94, 96, 100-110, 114, 116; inheritance, 105; local, 55; motor fuel transfer, 34, 96-101, 104-107, 114-116; and officials, 98; in Pennsylvania, 103-104, 107; and profits, 103; property, 28, 34, 94-96, 100, 102, 106-107, 115-117; revenues from, 12, 93, 96, 113-117; sales, 96-98, 103, 113-114; school district, 108, 118; structure of, 29, 42, 93-95; state, 103, 106, 110, 113-114
Teaching profession, 95
Technicians and technical support techniques, 10-11, 15, 18, 122
Temperature, ambient, 132
Tennessee Valley Authority (TVA), 53
Term bonds, 110-111
Terminal: hookup charges, 15; output, 42-43; portable, 39; printouts, 42; screen, 39
Terrestrial life, 24
Tests and testing procedures, 8, 7, 20
Textual editing and files, 4, 38, 45, 48
Time, turnaround, 15-18
Time-series table, 39
Time-sharing services, 14-16
Topography, factor of, 80
Townhouses, 77
Towns and townships, 1, 12, 29, 67, 94
Trade, retail and wholesale, 51, 103, 113
Tradeoffs, policy of, 24, 27, 38
Traffic models, 1, 5, 12, 28, 31, 121

Transfers: county, 100, 107, 115; fuel revenues, 34, 96-101, 114-116; intergovernmental, 93, 96, 101; municipal, 00; reality, 96, 105, 107; state, 107
Transportation, Department of, 25
Transportation programs, 95, 108, 130
Treasury officials, 94
Treatment facilities, water, 78-79, 95, 134
Trips, work and nonwork related, 130-131, 137-138
Trucks: categories of, 138; diesel, 129-132; emissions from, 125, 132, 138, 140; gasoline, 131-132; traffic from, 5; VMT (vehicle miles traveled), 138
Turnaround time, 15-18

Unions, local, 53
United States Steel Corporation, 3
Urbanization, increase in, 121, 134-135
User orientation, 38-43, 49
User's Manual, 7, 17-19
Utilities, 34; electric, 9, 129

Value: assessment market ratio, 106, 115-117; and income, 72; of land, 106; real property, 105-106
Vehicle miles traveled (VMT), work and nonwork related, 33-35, 122, 125, 129-132, 138
Vendors, time-sharing, 5-16
Vocational education, 73, 94, 108

Wages, 55, 76
Wastes: hazardous, 80; organic, 127; residential, 80; and water discharges, 2, 34-35, 125, 127
Water: components, 4-5; consumption, 21, 69, 78, 88-89, 121; effluents, 3, 12, 28, 33-34, 121, 123, 133-135; industrial, 78, 80, 89; inspection of, 76; intrastate, 123; navigable, 2, 123, 134; mains, 79; pollution,

134; quality, 25, 123-127, 135;
recycling, 78; residential, 21, 78,
88-89; school, 1; and sewers, 145;
standards, 123; storage facilities,
79; storm, 77-80, 134; swimmable,
127; supply systems, 21, 34, 67,
77-78, 89-90, 95; terminals, 3;
treatment facilities, 69, 78-79, 95,
134; and wastes, 2, 34-35, 127
Watercourses, 95, 123-125
Weeklies categories, 31-34, 51-52, 56,
104-107; employees, 57-58, 66, 84;
housing units, 72; income group,

65; pool, 53-54
Welfare distribution, 94, 122
Wholesale trade, 51, 113
Wilderness areas, 123
Wind, factor of, 124
Work and non-work related vehicle
trips, 130-131, 137-138
Workers, in-migrating,   1
Working papers and worksheets, 20-21
Wylbur language program, 38-39, 43,
45, 47

Zinc smelters, 125

About the Author

Glenn R. DeSouza received the B.Com. from the University of Madras, graduating in the top 1 percent of his class, and the M.A. and Ph.D. in Economics from Fordham University, where he held a fellowship. He is a senior member of the Industry Modeling and Policy Econometrics Unit at Arthur D. Little and has been a consultant on large-scale modeling to federal agencies, corporations, and public utilities. His clients include the U.S. Environmental Protection Agency, the U.S. Department of Energy, the U.S. Department of Commerce, the U.S. State Department, the National Science Foundation, the U.S. Chamber of Commerce, American Telephone and Telegraph, General Electric, U.S. Steel, Pacific Gas and Electric, and the Illinois Power Company. In addition to consulting, Dr. DeSouza is engaged in teaching and has taught courses in economic theory and quantitative methods at the undergraduate and graduate levels.

DATE DUE